THE

FOOD

REPORT CARD

12,000 Favorite Foods—Including Brand-Name Products—
Graded A, B, C, or D for Nutritional Value

THOMAS YANNIOS, M.D.

MACMILLAN • USA

MACMILLAN
A Simon & Schuster Macmillan Company
1633 Broadway
New York, NY 10019-6785

Macmillan Publishing books may be purchased for business or sales promotional use.
For information please write:
Special Markets Department, Macmillan Publishing USA, 1633 Broadway, New York, NY 10019.

Library of Congress Cataloging-in-Publication Data

Yannios, Thomas.
    The food report card : 12,000 favorite ... / Thomas Yannios.
        p.   cm.
    Includes index.
    ISBN 0-02-038965-5 : $15.95
      1. Food—Composition—Tables. 2. Nutrition—Tables. 3. Convenience foods—Composition—Tables. 4. Brand name products—Composition—Tables. I. Title.
    TX551.Y36   1996
    641.1—dc20   95-24968
                                                                   CIP

Printed in the United States of America

10 9 8 7 6 5 4 3 2 1

This publication contains the opinions and ideas of its authors. It is intended to provide helpful and informative material on the subject matter covered. It is sold with the understanding that the author and publisher are not engaged in rendering medical or other professional services in this book. If the reader requires personal medical or health assistance or advice, a competent professional should be consulted.

The author and publisher specifically disclaim any responsibility for liability, loss, or risk, personal or otherwise, which is incurred as a consequence, directly or indirectly, of the use and application of any of the contents in this book.

Contents

Acknowledgments

This book was a Herculean task, and I thank all the people who helped with the various aspects of the process: Nick Yannios and Tony Bye who designed and manipulated the software that organized and processed the seemingly endless stream of data; the people at Preferred Data Inc. of Schenectady, New York, for data entry; Scott Brown for his assistance in hardware selection; the editors at Macmillan who tirelessly chiseled the imposing raw manuscript into a finished form; Registered Dietitians Brenda Mayette, Angela Gray, and Mary Yannios for their often needed advice; Amy DeMarco for word processing; my partner Dr. Peter Weinberg for helpful tips and indefatigable encouragements; and my agent, Jane Dystel, for making this entire endeavor possible.

Last, but not least, I thank my wife, Edith, who, when all else failed, roamed the supermarket aisles with calculator in hand to collect the newest data and solve the legion of problems forever being encountered.

Author's Note

The foods you see on the supermarket shelves are the results of a very dynamic process. New products are constantly being introduced, tested, retained, or discarded. Even old foods and classic products are periodically being reformulated. Of course, the composition of raw, unprocessed, natural foods such as bulk grains, fruits and vegetables, and meats, changes very little over time.

The food-composition data of brand-name products used to derive the information in this book was obtained directly from the actual product labels. This book does not rely on any independent testing or laboratory analysis. Some foods appearing in these listings will have been discontinued or renamed by the time this book sees print. Other foods will have been reformulated without any indication of this on the label. This reformulation may effect caloric density and/or the qualitative rating given the food. I have observed that common reformulations of an established product usually varies the calorie per serving value by about 10% in either direction. Where reformulations have effected the grade, it is rarely by more than one step. Many new foods resemble their discontinued predecessors fairly closely.

For brand-name products, we have relied on the product labels, so any errors or omissions in the information on which we relied could affect the validity of our findings. Also, manufacturers modify their product ingredients from time to time, and there may be variations within products. Anyone who knows of data that may alter the evaluation of the products and foods reviewed in this book is encouraged to make this information available to me by writing in care of Macmillan Publishing USA, 1633 Broadway, New York, NY 10019. I will consider all such information so that any revisions, if necessary, can be made in future editions.

Furthermore, I would like readers to let me know what they think about *The Food Report Card*. What did you like? Where could it be improved? I look forward to hearing from you.

Introduction

Foods: What You Really Need to Know

Forty-four percent of the foods on your supermarket shelves contain more fat than is safe for your long-term health. The same can be said about the sodium content of an astounding sixty-two percent of foods! And only fifteen percent can be considered minimally adequate sources of fiber. Would you be able to tell any of that from a *quick* glance at a food label? Probably not. To really know what's in a product, you'd have to calculate percentages, add up nutrients, and decipher ingredients. Fortunately, *The Food Report Card* can help you pick your way through this minefield.

In *The Food Report Card*, I will show you just how easy it is to eat intelligently. Since so many of my patients are in intensive care units, I have spent many a tense night standing at the bedside of a person whose incredibly desperate and complex medical problems were nothing more than the extreme consequences of a lifetime of poor eating habits. This irony has left a compelling impression, and has motivated me to simplify what are literally volumes of nutritional information and advice so that everyone can benefit without having to study, calculate, and worry. I've seen the difficulties people have changing the way they eat even after realizing they've developed serious medical problems, and it has become obvious to me that the problem with public nutrition in this society is not one of negligence or motivation but of confusion.

With the explosion of nutrition-related information over the past decade, most Americans realize that they must adjust their diets. Minimizing your chances for what is the number one risk to your life, atherosclerosis, depends significantly upon what foods you *routinely* eat. I'm sure I don't have to tell you that. I probably also don't have to tell you just how difficult it is to translate the advice you are receiving from the medical community, the Surgeon General, the FDA, the media, product labels, and even all the consumer-oriented diet and health books being published, into concrete food item selections. With the straightforward A, B, C, D ratings presented in this book, you can immediately identify which foods are good for your heart and your blood pressure, will help you lose weight and lower your cholesterol, and may even help increase your physical endurance.

In *The Food Report Card*, I have analyzed virtually every brand name and generic food item you're likely to encounter in your food store, plus the foods found in the nationwide fast-food outlets—most of the foods Americans *really* eat—and given each a simple letter grade: A, B, C, or D. The criteria of analysis are based on the Surgeon General's, The American Heart Association's, and the American Diabetes Association's guidelines for reducing all risk factors for cardiovascular disease. You can make an enormous impact on your long-term health, and even on your appearance, if you do nothing else during your normal food shopping but select the A- and B-rated foods, and leave the C's and D's on the shelves back at the store.

The Food–Health Connection

Winding its way through the rolling farmlands of upstate New York, the New York Thruway is supported by large, inviting food emporiums. During a trip I stopped at one to get a drink. In the Burger King, while leaning against a booth, I could hear the woman sitting behind me announce she wouldn't touch the fruits and vegetables from the roadside farm stands because all New York farms used pesticides. All the time she was munching on some drippy version of a mega burger and the requisite side order of fries!

This is exactly what I mean by "confusion." People can't filter or prioritize the chaos of nutritional information, warnings, and advice barraging them from all sources. Even if you have become adept at analyzing foods, just what is it you are looking for? The answer has been muddled and everyone is being distracted by what are, as important as they might be, secondary issues. We are being told in quite an indiscriminate way that there's an entire world of food factors out there to worry about: fat, cholesterol, unsaturated fat, polyunsaturated fat, pesticides, sugar, additives, colors, preservatives, salt, radiation, heavy metals. . . The list goes on and on, and so do the consequences: strokes, heart attack, kidney stones, anemia, stomach cancer, breast cancer, colon cancer, bladder cancer, thyroid disease, high blood pressure, nervousness, inattentiveness, depression, cavities—just to name a very few.

And the list seems to expand daily. Some problems seem connected to diet, but in many cases that connection is tenuous. What is crystal-clear and incontestable is that the greatest threat to your life and the quality of your life, as well as that of your family, is the insidious, silent process of atherosclerosis, "hardening of the arteries," and the cardiovascular diseases it causes: coronary artery disease, heart attacks, cerebrovascular disease, strokes, kidney failure, high blood pressure, and peripheral vascular disease. Half of all Americans will succumb to one of these problems and almost *all* of us, as we age, will be plagued by some manifestation of them. That can't be said of any other medical problem—nothing even comes close!

You're in Control

What is also fact is that, with the exception of the smoking-related diseases, there is no other significant medical problem that can be so decisively altered by lifestyle changes. Atherosclerosis is a disease process that begins when you're a child. It is fated by your genes but modulated by your lifestyle. Those modulating risk factors are smoking, blood pressure, diabetes, weight, cholesterol and other blood lipid levels, stress, and physical activity. Genetics not only predisposes you to developing the disease, but also can predispose you to developing one or more of the risk factors that can lead to it. However, except in the most extreme cases, you can alter those risks. What and how much you eat can be a major determinant of your weight, your cholesterol levels and lipid ratios, and can even significantly affect your blood pressure.

Thus, food significantly impacts both directly and indirectly upon most of the major risk factors for the number one threat to your life; and this variable is 100% under your control. There is no gene forcing you to eat bacon.

This intimate food-atherosclerosis connection is, then, *the* issue demanding our focused attention; and it is the issue which my A-B-C-D ratings directly address.

Diet advice is a multi-billion dollar industry. Yet despite all of the money, time, and energy that has been devoted to improving how Americans eat, statistics show we are a population becoming more overweight, less fit, and still as likely to suffer from cardiovascular disease as ever. Virtually *half* of all Americans have undesirable cholesterol levels, and in the latest study, the majority of adult Americans were found to be significantly overweight. Even children and adolescents are becoming fatter. The only good things that can be said is that yes, finally, high as they are, our cholesterol levels are beginning to inch downward—but only inch—and, that one is less likely to actually die from a heart attack. But this latter reality has as much to do with the advances in interventional cardiology, cardiovascular surgery, and the elaborate care given to people once *advanced* disease has stricken, as it does with prevention.

How can this be? I refer back to my original statement: People are confused. The fact that you're reading these pages attests to that, and you're not alone. The food figures I quoted in the beginning of the book attest to the necessity of arming yourself with some method for choosing relatively healthful foods. Actually figuring out what to eat, though, is a science.

Why the A-B-C-D System Was Developed

Most people concerned about their diet and their health at some point make an effort to learn about foods and nutrition to help them select what to eat. Unfortunately, like any other scientific discipline, the language of nutrition is very foreign to the layperson. The relation of calories to units of weight, the variability of this relationship as it pertains to different nutrients, the plethora of nutrients themselves as well as the categories and subcategories of each, and the confusing claims attached to each kind of nutrient have successfully frustrated most people's attempts to gain control of their diet. I think I'll be ringing a familiar bell when I tell you how often I see patients purchase a diet or nutrition book and think they're prepared to intelligently food shop, only to become instantly bewildered upon encountering the array of numbers and units on the package labels.

Before writing this book, I did what I advise all patients to do: go food shopping with a calculator. If you know how to use the numbers and, with calculator in hand, analyze every food label you choose, you can become quite adept at picking the right foods. But in this busy society, how many of us realistically can do this? Who has time to even follow the volumes of recipes presented in so many health books. Eating right can literally be a full-time occupation! And there's no getting around it, whether you're in an organized diet plan or following a doctor's guidelines, a nutrition or "food-counter" book, or recipes, you either have to do the math or follow precalculated and very regimented eating plans.

The final factor motivating me to write this book was the FDA food label. This was heralded as the revolution in consumer education finally making a food-package label user friendly. While it represents a gigantic improvement, study after study clearly shows most people are still mystified by these labels.

I presented the label below to a dozen doctors with the simple question: "Is this food good for you?" Most looked at it for a while and embarrassedly shrugged. The most thoughtful evasion was, "Well, in what context?" No context. Given a choice of similar products on the shelf, is this the one you should buy? That's what I want YOU to know, and you want to determine the answer in about ONE second.

Nutrition Facts
Serving Size 1oz. (28g /
Servings Per Container 5

Amount Per Serving	
Calories 130	Calories from Fat 50
	% Daily Value*
Total Fat 6g	**9%**
Saturated Fat 0.5g	**3%**
Polyunsaturated Fat 2g	
Monounsaturated Fat 3.5g	
Cholesterol 0mg	**0%**
Sodium 110mg	**5%**
Total Carbohydrate 18g	**6%**
Dietary Fiber 1g	**4%**
Sugars Less than 1g	
Protein 2g	
Vitamin A 0% • Vitamin C 10%	
Calcium 0% • Iron 2%	

Even if you know how to use the FDA labels, they still transform each day's healthful eating into a math project. Here's what I mean; in order to translate what these numbers mean to your body, you have to do the following:

1. Divide the fat calories by the total calories and make sure the number is less than .3.
2. Divide milligrams sodium into calories and make sure it is more than .8.
3. Multiply grams sugar by 4, then divide that by total calories. It shouldn't be more than .25.
4. Divide grams fiber into calories. The result should be less than 66.

If that's too much computation, the alternative approach is to carry a pad and pen with you at all times and make at least 4 columns: calories, fat, saturated fat, sodium. Then each time you eat something, divide the stated serving size into *your* serving size and multiply that result by the respective percent number listed on the right side of the label of each nutrient. Then list that result in the appropriate column on your record. As the day goes by, you must add each column, planning or adjusting your intake not to exceed 100 in any column. And that's if you're on a 2,000 calorie diet. It works, but it's quite a project!

The depicted food appears in *The Food Report Card* as a C. C tells you not to buy it. More specifically, it tells you the food will deliver 30% to 40% of its calories as fat (which is far too much fat for its caloric value), has little appreciable fiber, and is okay for sodium. There's nothing for you to calculate, and if you're weight conscious, you only need to keep track of your daily calorie total. With only one parameter to track, you can do that in your head.

What You Really Need to Know about Foods

I was sitting in a Mexican restaurant filled with a mix of college students and professionals from a nearby university and hospital. I won't tell you what I was eating, but the woman at the next table was scolding her boyfriend for ordering a chicken chimichanga. Meanwhile, she was using her tortilla chips to steamroll through a heaping plate of oily guacamole dip. When he commented on what she was eating, she smugly replied, "But this is vegetarian."

Just as the last three decades of scientific and epidemiological research incontestably proved that the major food-mediated health threat to you is atherosclerosis in all of its manifestations, it has also pinpointed dietary fat as a specific, major culprit. But translating that single morsel of awareness into consistent and comprehensively safe eating is a major problem not just for the woman in the Mexican restaurant, but for just about everybody.

What you must understand about what constitutes a safe food is quite less elaborate than what an academic physician, a research scientist, or a Ph.D. nutritionist needs to know.

A safe food is a food that will not contribute to *any* of the risk factors for atherosclerosis. All of these risk factors are intimately interrelated and the presence of each one makes all the others worse either in their actual intensity or in their ultimate effects on the body. The converse is also true. Those are key points to understand, because much of the confusion comes from experts who are focused on a specific nutrient or a single risk factor; their focused studies become widely publicized without the proper context.

If you were to integrate the information accumulated over the last ten years, you'd reach an interesting conclusion: whether you are trying to lose weight, lower blood lipids, do aerobic exercise, minimize a diabetic condition, or lower blood pressure, you'll probably turn to the same foods for each problem. And the common denominator is that practically all these foods are low in fat. And that's key. Unless you're one of those people we will discuss later who needs more fat in your diet, your total fat intake should be less than 30% of total calories. Many people tolerate diets with 20% or even 10% fat. For those people, the less fat, the better! Don't focus on milligrams of cholesterol, grams saturated versus unsaturated, animal versus vegetable. Fat is fat. True, saturated fats directly promote atherosclerosis, but *all* fats more efficiently promote fat deposition in your body. Heart disease risk has been correlated with both saturated and total fat ingestion. First, a gram of fat is so much more calorie dense than other foods. Second, calorie for calorie, fats only require a fifth of the energy as your other big calorie source, carbohydrates, need for their metabolism. Thus, 100 calories of carbohydrates may deliver 75 of those calories as energy to be stored in your body while 100 calories of fat deliver 95 of those calories for storage. That more efficient weight gain, regardless of the food source, amplifies all the other atherosclerosis risk factors.

The American Heart Association's dietary guidelines with respect to fats form the minimal core of virtually every medically sound diet plan published. They are the results of decades of study. They state:

Less than 30% of your total calories should come from fat.
Less than 10% of total calories from saturated fat.
Up to 10% of total calories from polyunsaturated fat.
Approximately 10% of total calories from monosaturated fat.
Always consume less than 300 mg per day of cholesterol.

The problem with the 30% fat rule is in how you are traditionally instructed to apply it. Dietary guidelines are almost always derived from the perspective of the *total* daily food mix. The onus falls on you to keep track of what's in everything you're eating and to know how much of anything, like bacon, you can eat in any given meal to keep the proportions of fat within the guidelines.

Aside from planning your entire day of eating in advance, this kind of approach requires you to dissect the contents of individual meals and keep an account of the nutrient accumulations over the course of the day. That's why the new product labels are structured the way they are. This kind of dietary approach is too complicated and unrealistic.

Wouldn't it be better if you could just look at a food and know: "yes," "no," or "sometimes"?

I have taken the 30% fat rule and applied it to *each individual* food. Ultimately, this means I am characterizing the quality of every *calorie* you are eating rather than instructing you on how you can increase the quality of each *meal* you are eating. By knowing that every calorie of food you are eating fulfills certain healthful criteria, you don't have to worry about whether your entire meal is safe because the whole meal can't be different from the sum of its parts. When one does that, an interesting thing happens; it becomes impossible to eat too much fat, and almost as impossible to eat too much saturated fat and cholesterol. It also becomes almost impossible to cheat. You also never have to do a single calculation and usually don't even have to look at a food label! You just have to know how the food is rated: A, B, C, or D.

It's not a perfect solution, but it is an incredibly more effective way to eat a healthful diet. I can say this because most of the foods that are less than 30% fat, and even more certainly the foods that are less than 15% fat, have a higher proportion of mono or unsaturated fats in their fat composition. In my scheme, there are foods that just should *not* appear on your table except as a rare indulgence.

Nutrients to Watch

Fat

With some important exceptions, fatty foods should be avoided, period. You theoretically only need a small amount for metabolic purposes, from 5% to 10% of calories.

All fats are equally calorie-dense, packing too many calories into relatively small amounts of food. So all fats promote easy weight gain, and excess weight itself causes cholesterol levels to rise. But saturated fats will raise cholesterol levels without a weight gain, and even most polyunsaturated fats have the nasty ability to make cholesterol particles more avidly stick to the walls of your arteries. Only monounsaturated fats and the fats called "Omega-3's" found in seafood won't promote atherosclerosis.

Complex Carbohydrates

Complex carbohydrates are generally the perfect foods. They should constitute 50% to 60% of your daily calories. Some people even do very well with 70% or higher complex carbohydrates. You can find complex carbohydrates in grains and grain products such as breads, cereals, and pastas, as well as vegetables like beans and potatoes. Because they are often bulky foods, complex carbohydrates have the added benefit in that they fill you up faster with less calories than will fats or sugars.

Sugar

While the issues of complex carbohydrates and fats are relatively clear cut, the sugar problem is not. Sugars are single- and double-molecule carbohydrates naturally occurring in many fruits, vegetables, and honey. Refined sugars such as table sugar have been separated from their native sources and added in great abundance to a wide variety of foods such as baked goods, confections, candies, snacks, sodas, and to otherwise healthful breakfast cereals and yogurts.

Probably no other major nutrient's effects on your body is so dependent upon the "context" of its ingestion. How sugar will be metabolized is very dependent upon the amount consumed, what form it's in, its temperature, what it's consumed with, and most importantly, what you are doing when you are eating the sugar. If you are regularly exercising, sugar ingested during or any time around the period of exercise gets immediately consumed or stored as energy reserve in your muscles. That is exactly what you want to happen. The more you exercise, the wider this "window" of optimal metabolism becomes and the more sugary treats you can safely enjoy.

However, if you're sedentary, the way your sugar is metabolized may be quite different and highly dependent on the other factors I've mentioned. These factors will determine, among other things, whether the sugar becomes energy or fat. An even bigger problem with sugar-laden foods is that a few hours after eating them you feel hungry again and frequently turn to that same sugary treat to satisfy that hunger. This promotes snacking between meals with low bulk, calorie dense foods. This is one of the most potent eating habits promoting weight gain and can become quite a trap.

Most A and B foods are mainly either protein or complex carbohydrates. The high sugar foods usually also contain large amounts of fat causing them to fall into the C and D categories. There are significant exceptions to this, however, and most of those exceptions have been dealt with by sequestering those categories of foods where this is a systematic problem into the separate "Frivolous Foods" table.

HIGH SUGAR CONTENT FOODS

The following foods are relatively high in sugar:

Canned Fruit
Yogurts
Fresh Fruit
Breakfast Cereals
Commercial Breads
"Frivolous Foods"

As I mentioned just before, be careful about four other categories of foods. One category is canned foods such as fruits and some baked beans which often have large amounts of added sugar. You can detect this in the food lists by watching the calories go up for different versions of the same canned food. The significant calorie difference between "Sliced Pears in Water" and "Sliced Pears in Syrup" is *all* sugar.

Another big group of such foods not sequestered in the "Frivolous Foods" section are yogurts. Most of the calories in most yogurts are sugars.

Third, many breakfast cereals, both cold and hot, have large amounts of sugar added. The flavored hot cereals usually have sugar added whereas the plain hot cereals don't. Cold cereals can be so complicated that I added a special indicator to identify the sugary ones.

The last group I'll warn you about is, surprisingly, fresh fruits. Yes, natural, wholesome fruits! Though the natural fiber content of fruits blunts the effects of their sugars, most of the calories in fruits are simple sugars. For people whose metabolism is sensitive to excess amounts of sugar, even these otherwise wonderful foods may have to be limited to less than 10% of one's calories.

Salt

Salt, or more precisely the sodium half of salt, can be a very significant contributor to one of the more potent risk factors: high blood pressure. I will discuss who has to worry about this in the "−" modifier section to follow.

Protein

The body requires a certain minimal amount of protein, about .8 gram per kg of body weight. That's not very much. Translated, this means that people in the range of 100 to 200 lbs require from $1^1/_3$ oz to $2^1/_2$ oz a day of pure protein. That's far less than is in the average American diet and is the equivalent of 3 to 6 oz of a B-rated meat. Vegetable proteins are of lower effectiveness in meeting this requirement. Therefore, protein should constitute 10% to 15% of total calories or from 3 to 6 oz of an A- or B-rated meat or its vegetable equivalent per day for diets ranging from 1,500 to 3,000 calories a day.

Since animal protein—meat—is the major source of saturated fats and cholesterol, keeping to this rule assures one of never exceeding the saturated fat and cholesterol restrictions we've mentioned. Of course, a diet rich in grain products and legumes like rice and beans—other good protein sources—need never include meats. But since most Americans aren't and never will be vegetarians, modest servings of A and B red meats, fish, and fowl are both safe, adequate, and satisfying. I particularly advise including fish in one's diet at least twice a week.

Again, people who exercise have all the fun. Their protein needs are higher, though it's quite controversial how much higher.

Vitamins and Minerals

A good diet must provide a complete complement of vitamins and minerals. The problem here is the public perception of vitamin and mineral needs and how this has contributed to "food confusion." I think there has been an overemphasis on vitamin and mineral requirements, distracting people from the main problem of what kind of calories they're eating.

There is probably more paper and ink devoted to teaching people how to arrange complicated "balanced" meals to get the daily requirement of vitamins and minerals while not eating too much fat, sugar, and salt, than is devoted to any other aspect of nutrition. Much of the complexity of meal plans stems from people trying to literally mimic the vitamin and mineral content of a multivitamin tablet with *every* meal! So we try the calculations, food exchanges, and unrealistic recipes to create that perfect "balanced" meal as often as possible. Unfortunately, this effort eventually frustrates most people.

It was as a response to this kind of dieting advice that I first thought of rating foods using the calorie as my basic unit of measure. The modern concept of the properly balanced diet involves deriving most of one's calories from cereal and grain products, fruits and vegetables. Concentrating on A and B foods automatically channels you towards these foods without having to "plan" your eating. And by following the protein instructions I've just given you, the healthful balance not just of protein, fat and carbohydrate, but also of vitamins and minerals, is more or less achieved over the course of a day's—or even a few days'—eating.

You shouldn't worry that each meal can't reproduce the vitamin and mineral mix of a pill! Many meals can be mostly composed of only one or two foods. One day may be a pasta day, another dominated by salads and low fat meats. The accumulative variety of A and B foods within the framework of many meals will provide a wide spectrum of vitamins and minerals that should be supplemented with a daily multivitamin with mineral tablet. Between what you're eating and an inexpensive tablet, you'll be assured of the proper kind of calorie intake *and* the proper balance of vitamins and minerals.

This is very iconoclastic advice. It's also very realistic advice, tailored to the way real people really eat. I've saved many lives with the products of pharmaceutical science. I have no problem with people taking vitamin pills to round out the balance of nutrients provided by their diets. There is nothing inferior about manufactured vitamins. The fact that they are pills creates some absorption problems if the pills can't be chewed, but this lack of efficiency in vitamin and mineral absorption is more than made up for by the fact that one receives a concentrated dose—more than you need—of nutrients in the typical high quality vitamin pill. This "bomb" of nutrients presented to your digestive system overcomes the inefficiencies in absorption encountered. Also, remember, such supplements are just that: supplements. They are not to be taken as substitutes. Instead, they give an added margin of nutrient balance to the already adequate diet you are eating.*

When "liberated" from the idea that virtually every "healthful" meal must be a properly proportioned mix of foods from all of the food groups, most people will settle into a certain pattern of eating. They will find the specific A and B foods they particularly enjoy and focus on them, almost to the exclusion of most other foods. I have found the busier the lifestyle, the greater this tendency.

Traditional dietary advice frowns on this, but there is no justification for this attitude. The fact is an average adult would be better off healthwise eating a diet of whole grain bread, salad, and water supplemented with a daily vitamin and an every other day piece of chicken than eating a traditional American mixed diet. I think you'd be terribly bored, but you would probably also never need a cardiologist.

That is an extreme example, but it makes my point. There is nothing wrong with concentrating on a few A and B foods such as pasta, bread, or cereal to provide the overwhelming percentage of your calories. As long as you ensure an adequate vitamin, mineral, and protein intake, you can do quite well with as narrow or broad a range of A or B foods you wish. The choices are yours to make.

What the Food Ratings Mean

"A" Foods

Foods with an "A" rating are very low in fat. This means that not more than 15% of their total caloric content is fat. Depending on the category of food, an A food will be composed mostly of complex carbohydrate, protein, naturally occurring sugar and fiber, or some combination of these elements.

---

*Common exceptions to this are iron and calcium. You may be surprised to know if you are eating a lot of bread or cereal you are getting significant amounts of iron, since these American products are packed with almost as much iron as is in beef. The trick is to eat these foods with a vitamin C source, like fruit juice. The vitamin C maximizes the iron absorption. Otherwise, for an iron source, there's no substitute for red meats and to a less extent other animal proteins. Infants and pregnant women have special needs for iron, which should be discussed with one's doctor. Calcium is discussed at the beginning of the Milk and Dairy section. Alternate sources are dried beans and green leafy vegetables like spinach.

The higher fiber "A" foods, which receive an added "+" designation in the listings, are virtually all fruits, vegetables, or foods with high levels of complex carbohydrates. They are, so to speak, the "perfect" foods.

There are A foods which are meats, and yes, they too are safe foods. Keep in mind though, "A" foods which are meats should still be limited to one serving, or an average of from 3 to 6 ounces per day.

"A" foods which appear in the Frivolous Foods listing of foods contain almost no fat, but are mostly composed of simple sugars. They are foods which should be reserved as occasional treats only and should not constitute more than 5% of your daily calories. If you are actively exercising, you can safely eat more than the recommended allowance for these foods. Overweight people and diabetics should avoid all foods in the Frivolous Foods listings, including A foods.

"B" Foods

Most people will find the majority of their food selections in the B food group. This group contains a wide variety of items which are 16% to 30% fat. Eating B foods will comply with The American Heart Association Step I diet for reducing cholesterol as well as the FDA and Surgeon General's recommendations for a healthy diet. For most people B foods are almost as healthful as A foods. In my opinion, the perfect diet is a mixture of these two groups.

If you have a cholesterol, blood lipid, or weight problem and have tried limiting your fat intake to less than 30% of your total calories to no avail, then you may need to go a step further. Strive to mix A and B foods in roughly equal caloric amounts to achieve a level of less than 25% to 20% dietary fat. This would be equivalent to The American Heart Association Step II diet. The same advice applies to almost all people actively trying to lose weight.

It's important to remember that, as with A foods, B foods which are primarily protein—such as meats, fish, and poultry—should be limited to at most one selection a day.

B foods appearing in the Frivolous Foods listings should be avoided except as a rare treat, as they contain some fat and usually large amounts of simple sugar. Again, if you are actively exercising, you can have more, but even in this case, the "A" selections are superior. Diabetics should avoid these foods entirely.

"C" Foods

C foods are undesirable. They will promote cardiovascular disease and cause you to gain weight. Some are much worse than others but all should be avoided as they contain from 31% to 40% of their calories in fat and very often contain large amounts of sodium. However, occasionally indulging—perhaps once or twice a week—in a C-rated item within the context of a diet consistently composed of A and B foods will not adversely affect you. The C category was constructed to allow this kind of indulgence and add variety to an otherwise healthful diet. However, C foods appearing in the Frivolous Foods listing should always be avoided.

When indulging in a C food, note that the calories per serving are often significantly higher than the corresponding B-rated item. For people for whom weight is a problem, portion sizes should be appropriately reduced or other foods avoided to compensate for this extra calorie load.

"D" Foods

Most D foods are more than 40% fat. There are some D foods whose total fat content is actually low, but the food is particularly high in cholesterol. All are to be avoided except as a *very rare* treat. Even then preference should be given to a corresponding item rated as C.

The only exceptions to this advice pertains to *modest* amounts of high calcium dairy products, soybean products like tofu, the "oily" fish, and the monosaturated—not polyunsaturated—vegetable oils. A few tablespoons of canola oil, the nut oils, high oelic sunflower and safflower oil, and especially olive oil are okay in an otherwise healthful diet. I prefer olive oil because it gives you the most monosaturated fats per calorie of all the oils. These are the *only* D foods I endorse. Yes, they have high fat contents so you must be very careful about calories when eating them, but each conveys such compellingly desirable benefits to various aspects of human metabolism that I cautiously qualify their D rating. Again, a corresponding C-rated item is always preferable when you can find it. Otherwise, my personal advice is that you *rarely* eat a D food; and you should *never* eat a D food appearing in the Frivolous Foods and Fast Foods sections of this book! This Draconian edict is as much for psychological as medical reasons. By consistently avoiding such foods, you might lose the taste for them altogether—and good riddance!

A-B-C-D Modifiers

I have added a "+" or "−", and sometimes both, to the A-B-C-D rating of many foods. These modifiers allow you to identify high sodium and high fiber foods.

"+"

Most nutritionists recommend that you consume from 25 to 35 grams of dietary fiber per day. I have indexed the fiber content of each food against its caloric content (based on an average 2,000 calorie diet). This means that every "+" food has at least 1 gram of fiber for each 66 calories of that food. Thus, if *all* of your food selections contain "+" signs, then you are assured of getting at the very least a 30 gram per day intake of dietary fiber. Be aware that the "+" sign means that the food fulfills this *minimum* requirement; in many cases, a "+" food will have much more fiber than the minimum requirement and may, in fact, fulfill a large part of your daily requirement in one serving. You can check to see exactly how much you are getting by noting the nutritional content label of the product. If there is no "+" then there is no point in checking.

Fiber contents of many foods have yet to be determined, thus some foods were not rated.

"−"

"−" sign refers to sodium content. A food with "−" next to it has a high sodium content relative to its caloric value. Even many "A" foods have "−" signs. The American Heart Association advises that on average, no more than 3 grams of sodium or 7.5 grams of salt be ingested per day. As with fiber, I have indexed the sodium content of a food against its calories so that it is proportional to the amount of calories that food contributes to your overall diet. This is a much more exact evaluation than used by many other guidelines. If none of your selections have a "−" sign, you are absolutely assured that you're not eating more sodium than you should. As with the fiber "+" sign, the "−" sign is more of a signal, or in this case, a warning, than a conveyor of specific information or amounts. When you see it, you should check the exact sodium content of your food; in some cases it will be quite alarming! If there's no "−" sign, you need not check. However, many "−" foods need not be avoided. As I said, the sign is just a warning, signaling you to be aware of how much sodium you are getting. Many "−" foods in moderation can have a place in a healthful diet. And many other "−" foods, such as sauces and condiments, are used in such small amounts that they may not present a problem for you.

Who should worry about this? This sign is particularly important for people with high blood pressure or a history of high blood pressure in their family, as well as people with certain forms of heart and kidney disease. Your doctor is the best advisor about this question. The American Heart Association and the FDA have determined that since it is virtually impossible to predict who of any age is at risk for developing sodium-sensitive high blood pressure and since a substantial minority of the asymptomatic population is at risk, *everyone* should try to keep sodium intake within 3 grams per day.

How This Book Will Help You

If you follow the guidelines set forth in this book and select only the A and B foods from the main food listings, the following transformations in your diet will automatically occur:

1. You will shift your major calorie source from fats and simple sugars to complex carbohydrates.
2. You will consume more bulk and fiber.
3. Your sodium intake will remain at moderate levels.
4. You will find yourself eating less red meats and dairy products and more cereals, grains, and fruits.

You may experience significant health benefits from these changes. Statistically speaking you should experience an average 10% reduction in your total cholesterol level plus a correspondingly favorable reorganization of your blood lipid balance. Remember, for every 1% reduction in your total cholesterol level there is a 2% reduction in your risk for heart disease. That translates into a 20% reduction of your risk just on the basis of the change in fat chemistry of your body! This will lead to a reduced risk for developing the many other medical consequences of atherosclerosis. You will also decrease your risk for developing other non-atherosclerosis related medical problems such as diabetes and certain forms of breast and colon cancers.

The statistics I'm citing are average values obtained when large groups of people are placed on a low-fat diet. Your individual response may be quite different. Because of this, it's everyone's responsibility to keep track of his or her body's response to any major change in one's diet.

In the last few years, research has shown that about 25% to 30% of the population might actually not benefit from adopting a very low-fat diet! This is because some people's metabolism responds to the higher carbohydrate content of the typical low-fat diet by manufacturing the wrong kind of cholesterol particles. It's important to know if this is happening to you when you switch to A and B foods. Fortunately, the body sends up a warning flag when this paradoxical phenomenon occurs: the triglyceride level in your blood rises.

Triglycerides, not cholesterol, are the major lipid form circulating in your blood. It's the form fat assumes after it has been digested and it's the form in which fat is transported in your circulation to provide food to the body. Cholesterol is the more dangerous lipid form but triglyercides are the most common. It is cholesterol that sticks to your arteries.

There's a close linkage between cholesterol metabolism and triglyceride metabolism. When some people shift their major calorie source from fats to carbohydrates, the triglyceride level of their blood ironically rises because all those carbohydrates one is eating can't be burned away quickly enough and get converted to triglycerides. In the wake of all this, bad things happen to the cholesterol particles also circulating with these triglycerides; they become much more prone to forming deposits along one's arteries. The result, one is worse off than when on the higher fat diet.

It's been found that much of this phenomenon is a peculiarity of American culture and the American food industry rather than of the theoretical concept of a low-fat diet. When the typical American resolutely adopts his or her "low-fat diet," the usual result is not a conversion to a healthful rice and beans or whole grain diet, but an increase in Frivolous Food intake as well as the intake of so-called "low fat" commercially prepared foods. Unfortunately, many of these "low fat" foods are also high in added simple sugars. The net effect of all of this sugar ingestion is to raise triglycerides and actually increase the levels of "bad" cholesterol particles in one's system.

This is why I emphasize that sugary foods should remain the exclusive domain of exercisers. Exercise changes one's metabolism to counteract this effect of high sugar intake. But how much exercise does it take?

You will be surprised by the answer: It takes a lot!

The following list of some major sports gives the total amount of exercise needed over one week to achieve what we doctors refer to as "metabolic fitness." Listed along with the *amount* of exercise is the minimal intensity level also required to achieve this effect. "Metabolic fitness" is the ability to use exercise to optimally shift your metabolism to reduce production of triglycerides and the dangerous forms of cholesterol while preferentially increasing production of the beneficial forms of cholesterol called HDL cholesterol.

Burning Calories

A calorie is a unit of energy. You can ingest a calorie or you can "burn" a calorie. Thus, exercise, just as eating, should be conceived of in calories. One mile of running or walking is approximately equal to 100 calories. Studies have shown that the key to achieving "metabolic fitness" is to accumulate about 2,200 calories of exercise each week at an intensity level, or "pace," of about 400 calories an hour. Whether one is trying to lose weight or just stay even, enough exercise is the vital companion to a healthful diet; that way one can be assured that one's metabolism is optimally utilizing the foods one is eating.

Burning 2,200 calories in less than $5^1/_2$ hours:

- Run/walk: 22 miles/wk at 4 mph
- Hiking with 10- to 20-lb pack: 525 cal/hr, 4 hr/wk
- Cycling: 53 miles/wk at 10 mph
- Swimming: 5.5 miles/wk at 1 mph
- Aerobics: 5.2 hr/wk
- Aerobics, high-impact: 4.5 hr/wk
- Handball (good player): 2.5 hr/wk
- Tennis (good player): 4 hr/wk
- Rugby (good player): 3 hr/wk
- Soccer: 4.5 hr/wk
- Canoeing < 4 mph: 10 hr/wk
- Canoeing 4–6 mph: 4.5 hr/wk
- Downhill skiing (expert): 3.9 accumulated continuous hrs/wk
- Cross-country skiing
  < 2 mph: 4.5 hr
  4–5 mph: 3.9 hr
  5–8 mph: 3.5 hr
  uphill fast: 2 hr
  (Sorry, golf doesn't make the list.)

The other side of the low fat, high carbohydrate story is that there are many people who thrive on extremely low-fat diets. For these people, diets consisting of 10% or so of fats—mostly A foods—yield impressive drops in cholesterol values with no adverse effects.

Actual blood tests which reflect the genetic orientation of one's metabolism and which can often predict how that metabolism will respond to a low-fat diet are now available. One test is a determination of the kind of cholesterol particles one has. People with a certain type of particle respond much better than others when placed on a low-fat diet.

Another test characterizes the actual gene contributing to cholesterol metabolism. This test can differentiate not only who is likely to benefit from a low-fat diet, but who may actually *not* tolerate such a diet.

In the Appendix, you can find out more about such important tests.

Regardless of whether you are interested in these new tests, I strongly advise that *any* major change in one's diet be followed in about two months by testing one's blood lipid levels: LDL cholesterol, HDL cholesterol, and triglycerides.

By doing this, you can see how your body metabolism is responding to the A and B food diet. If you see that your triglycerides are rising, you should strive to receive most of your calories from B foods, and you must absolutely stay away from the Frivolous Foods. If you don't see any such rise, and your LDL cholesterol is falling, you should rely more and more on A foods for your major calorie source. Different people have different thresholds. Some do best on a 20% fat diet, some do best on a 15% or 10% fat diet. As with any diet, the only way to tell what's best for you is trial and error.

There are other benefits to consider when changing to A and B foods. Maintaining the A and B diet may also reverse the natural tendency to gain fat weight as you grow older. In fact, total caloric intake being constant, over time you will probably lose a modest amount of weight, about $1/2$ pound per week over the first 6 months. If this happens, you can actually enjoy the luxury of eating more to maintain your baseline weight.

And finally, if you are an exerciser, because of the increase in carbohydrate intake such a diet represents, you will enjoy a noticeable and immediate improvement in sports performance.

These are enormous health benefits for very little effort. Just check the food's grade and pick only the A- and B-rated items.

Losing Weight with A's and B's

People who wish to lose more substantial amounts of weight as well as alter cholesterol levels, must be a touch more technical—but just a touch—in order to properly reduce the amount of total calories they eat. This amount is determined by how much you should weigh. Using the chart in the Appendix, look up the proper weight for your height. Then you must decide how active you are. If you are sedentary, you should multiply the weight in pounds you obtained from the chart by 12. That number represents the daily calories you need. If you're moderately active—that is, walk the equivalent of 2 to 3 miles a day—your daily calorie needs will be 15 times your weight. And if you're very active, running 5 miles a day for instance, you may need from 20 to 25 times your weight in calories. Remember, these are approximate numbers, to be increased or decreased as indicated by your weight loss response.

For effective weight loss, I'm going to reemphasize the point I made earlier about "metabolic fitness." One can't seriously hope to lose weight without engaging in substantial amounts of exercise. The proper diet and physical activity are necessary complements.

In addition to computing your caloric needs, you'll need to keep track of serving sizes and cumulative calorie amounts using the serving size and calorie columns in my listings, but that's all. The A and B ratings take care of all the other calculations—and, oh yes, let me once again emphasize: If you're overweight, keep away from the Frivolous Foods!

One more simple rule, and this applies to almost everyone: Keep meat intake in control. If you eat 1,500 calories a day, your meat intake should be limited to about a 3-oz serving. If you're at the 3,000 calorie level, meat intake shouldn't be more than 6 ozs. For diets in between, the meat portions should likewise be in proportion. The most satisfying way to do this is to "bank" your daily allotment and eat a truly satisfying A- or B-rated portion of meat every few days.

As I said, this rule applies to almost everyone. The exceptions are people engaged in rather extreme levels of physical activity. Competitive athletes, triatheletes, marathoners, century riders, long-distance backpackers, serious bodybuilders and weight lifters are examples of people who may require 25% to 50% additional protein.

Reading the Report Card

The listings are structured to help you easily find a specific food and deliver the exact information you need to know: serving size, its caloric value, and the food's grade.

Food Category
Processing
Brand
Major Description
Minor Description
Serving Size
Calories
Grade

The first column identifies the type of food. The second tells you how it's been processed, for example, frozen, canned, or a mix. The next column gives you the brand name and the next two columns actually name and describe the specific food item. If it's a brand name processed food, the major description might give the title of the food on the label and the minor description will add how it is prepared or what extra items are included. A typical example would be Stouffer's Glazed Ham Steak Frozen Dinner. You would find this as:

Ham Dinner
Frozen
Stouffer's
Steak
Glazed

With more than 15,000 foods lining your supermarket shelves, finding a specific item may seem a daunting task. That's why I've decided to follow this logical format. To make things even easier, I've arranged all varieties of the same food as they would be presented at the market: by listing items alphabetically under brand name. Thus all the Stouffer's frozen ham dinners would be grouped together alphabetically under the "Ham Dinner" heading.

Comparing Calories and Serving Sizes

Another crucial aspect of food is caloric density. Caloric density means how many calories a food contains per unit of measure. We already spoke of this when discussing the nutrients fat, protein, and carbohydrate. Then you learned that a unit of measure such as a gram of fat, was much more densely packed with calories than a gram of carbohydrate or protein. Since foods are mixtures of fat, carbohydrate, and protein, that mix of nutrients will determine how many calories are in a gram of a certain food.

Unfortunately, people don't usually measure the foods they eat by grams. And even if one tried, the serving portion of a food also can contain water and other substances like fiber and non-nutrient "fillers," which add weight but no calories.

Usually switching from a C- or D-rated version of a food to an A- or B-rated selection results in a fall in caloric density; but not always. Because of the variability in the way foods are processed and the serving sizes presented to you by different brands, you have to be careful. Many people actually gain weight when switching to a low-fat diet because they eat too many extra carbohydrate calories hidden in the bigger serving sizes of their low-fat foods!

I've tried to arm you against this phenomenon by making a determined effort to standardize as much as possible, the realistic serving sizes of most of the items listed under a specific food heading. This way you can spot right away if changing to a differently rated food has changed the amount of calories you're getting. That's particularly important for those trying to lose weight. Thus *The Food Report Card* allows you not only to compare grades, but to pick those items sharing the same grade which yield the least calories per serving.

Organization of the Report Card Listings

There are three sections of listings. The first comprises virtually all the nutritionally significant foods you can eat. By nutritionally significant I mean foods that are commonly relied upon as primary sources of calories, protein, vitamins, and minerals. This is the main listing of foods and has been divided alphabetically into major food types in a fashion roughly similar to how foods are organized in the supermarket: Beverages; Condiments, Sauces, Dressings; Cereal and Grain Products; Fruits and Vegetables; Milk and Dairy Products; Soups and Mixes; Frozen and Canned Entrees and Dinners; and Meats, Poultry, and Seafood.

The secondary listing I've titled "Frivolous Foods." These foods are basically snacks, candies, and desserts and are usually very high in simple sugar content. They should never be considered major sources of calories, even when low in fat, so I treat them differently. These foods almost always lack nutritional value; that is, they rarely contain significant amounts of protein, vitamins, or minerals and most are even light on the complex carbohydrates.

Though many people try to, you can't live on these foods. In fact, some nutritionists recommend that you should never eat any of them. I agree, but I am also realistic. If these foods taste good, you are going to eat them, so you might as well get some good advice on them. So I have sequestered them in their own section and ranked them *relative* to each other by applying the same criteria for these foods as I have in the main listing: A's and B's are low in fat and less calorie dense. In these cases though, that means almost without exception they are extremely high in the other problem nutrient, simple sugars.

The third listing, "Fast Foods," I was tempted to subtitle: "Read 'em and weep." The ratings apply the same criteria as in the first section of listings. They speak for themselves. Many of the "D–" foods in this section could effectively be used in biological warfare.

Navigating the Listings: Finding the Food You Want

Just as when you're shopping, it's not always clear where the food you are looking for is located. This is especially true of mixed and prepared foods, so I'll anticipate some of the dilemmas you may have with the following navigational tips.

- The Beverage section mostly involves fat-containing beverages. All sodas, fruit juices, and fruit juice drinks are concentrated solutions of sugar containing from 110 to 130 calories per 8 oz serving. I therefore found no reason for a voluminous listing, and they all should be regarded as would the Frivolous Foods.

- All oils, spreads, spices, herbs, as well as dressings, pasta and tomato sauces, whether they be bottled, canned, dry, or mixes, are found in the Condiments section. The exceptions will be meat and cheese spreads and sauces to be found, respectively, under meat and dairy products.

- The Fruits and Vegetables section will contain all legumes such as beans and all nuts. Additionally, all canned, frozen, and otherwise processed fruits and vegetables will also be found in this section including vegetables with added sauces, spices, etc.

- Vegetarian meats, poultry, and imitation seafood products that are whole foods will be found in the sections they are intended to imitate, not the vegetable section. If they are mixes, they will be in the Soup and Mixes section.

- With the exception of many of the foods in the Condiments section which are packaged as mixes, such as sauce mixes, and those foods which are mixes appearing in the Frivolous Foods section such as cake mixes, all other mixes, regardless of content, will be found under Soups and Mixes.

- The Frozen and Canned Entree and Dinner section was designed to accommodate prepared mixed meals.

- The Meat, Poultry, Seafood, and Meat Products section is divided into four parts: Meat, Poultry, Seafood, and a processed section called "Meat Products." All luncheon meats, "cold cuts," canned, and packaged meats, and composite items such as sausages, franks, and so on are listed alphabetically in this last part.

Though my objective is to provide you with effortlessly accessible food purchasing advice, I do ask you to do some studying.

Take this book and study the lists. Leaf through the pages and peruse the foods. Note the variety of ratings associated with the different foods. Note also how different brands of the same food often have different ratings. Also notice that certain brands consistently carry higher or lower ratings across a wide range of foods. Some companies are more healthful than others. Remember that different kinds of processing or presentation can also drastically alter the ratings of the same food. For example, a normally "A+" artichoke can become a "D–" food once it's canned and marinated.

Despite my experience in nutrition, I learned a lot about the food I eat just from reviewing these charts. I'm now able to see associations and problems I never before appreciated. I hope you'll find these charts helpful not only for the ratings of specific items, but for the general conclusions you can reach about the relative healthfulness of broad categories of foods, processing techniques, and specific companies' product lines.

Beverages

The Beverage section mostly involves fat-containing beverages. All sodas, fruit juices, and fruit juice drinks are concentrated solutions of sugar containing from 110 to 130 calories per 8 oz serving. I therefore found no reason for a voluminous listing, and they all should be regarded as would the "Frivolous Foods."

Food	Processing Category	Brand
Apricot Nectar	Canned or Bottled	
Bloody Mary Mix	Bottled	Holland House Smooth N Spicy
Chocolate Syrup	Canned or in Jars	Generic
Chocolate Syrup	Canned or in Jars	Estee
Chocolate Syrup	Canned or in Jars	Hershey's
Chocolate Syrup	Canned or in Jars	Nestlé Quik
Chocolate-flavored Drink	Canned	Frostee
Chocolate-flavored Drink	Canned	Sego Lite
Chocolate-flavored Drink	Canned	Sego Very Chocolate
Cocoa	Mix	
Cocoa	Mix	Carnation
Cocoa	Mix	Carnation
Cocoa	Mix	Carnation
Cocoa	Mix	Carnation
Cocoa	Mix	Carnation 70 Calorie
Cocoa	Mix	Carnation Sugar Free
Cocoa	Mix	Carnation Sugar Free
Cocoa	Mix	Featherweight
Cocoa	Mix	Featherweight
Cocoa	Mix	Hills Bros.
Cocoa	Mix	Hills Bros. Sugar Free
Cocoa	Mix	Swiss Miss
Cocoa	Mix	Swiss Miss
Cocoa	Mix	Swiss Miss
Cocoa	Mix	Swiss Miss
Cocoa	Mix	Swiss Miss Lite
Cocoa	Mix	Swiss Miss Sugar Free
Cocoa	Mix	Swiss Miss Sugar Free
Cocoa	Mix	Weight Watchers
Coffee	Fluid	
Coffee, Flavored	Mix	General Foods International
Coffee, Flavored	Mix	General Foods International
Coffee, Flavored	Mix	General Foods International
Coffee, Flavored	Mix	General Foods International
Coffee, Flavored	Mix	General Foods International
Coffee, Flavored	Mix	General Foods International
Coffee, Flavored	Mix	General Foods International
Coffee, Flavored	Mix	General Foods International
Coffee, Flavored	Mix	General Foods International
Coffee, Flavored	Mix	General Foods International
Coffee, Flavored	Mix	General Foods International
Coffee, Flavored	Mix	General Foods International
Coffee, Flavored	Mix	Hills Bros. Café Coffee
Coffee, Flavored	Mix	Hills Bros. Café Coffee
Coffee, Flavored	Mix	Hills Bros. Café Coffee
Coffee, Flavored	Mix	Hills Bros. Café Coffee Sugar Free
Coffee, Flavored	Mix	Mjb
Coffee, Flavored	Mix	Mjb
Coffee, Flavored	Mix	Mjb
Coffee, Flavored	Mix	Mjb Sugar Free
Coffee, Flavored	Mix	Mjb Sugar Free
Coffee, Flavored	Mix	Mjb Sugar Free

Major Description	Minor Description	Serving Size	Calories	Grade
		6 fl oz	106	A
		1 fl oz	3	A–
		1 fl oz or 2 Tbsp	82	A
		2 Tbsp	40	D
		2 Tbsp	80	A
		2 Tbsp	100	A
		8 fl oz	200	C
Plain or Dutch		8 fl oz	120	B–
Plain or Malt		8 fl oz	180	A–
Powder		6 fl oz	102	A–
Chocolate Fudge		6 fl oz	110	A
Milk Chocolate		6 fl oz	110	A
Rich Milk Chocolate		6 fl oz	110	A
with Marshmallows, Chocolate	with Marshmallows	6 fl oz	110	A
		6 fl oz	70	A–
Milk Chocolate		6 fl oz	50	A–
Mocha		6 fl oz	50	A–
		6 fl oz	113	B–
Mint		6 fl oz	113	B–
		6 fl oz	220	A
		6 fl oz	80	B–
Amaretto Cream		6 fl oz	120	B–
Chocolate		6 fl oz	110	A
Milk Chocolate		6 fl oz	110	B–
Mint		6 fl oz	110	A–
		6 fl oz	95	A–
Chocolate		6 fl oz	60	A–
Mint		6 fl oz	50	B–
Milk Chocolate	Marshmallow	6 fl oz	60	A–
Brewed		6 fl oz	4	A
Café Amaretto		6 fl oz	50	C
Café Français		6 fl oz	60	D
Café Français	Low Calorie	6 fl oz	35	D
Café Irish Creme		6 fl oz	50	C
Café Vienna		6 fl oz	60	B–
Café Vienna	Low Calorie	6 fl oz	30	D–
Cappuccino		6 fl oz	60	B–
Cappuccino	Low Calorie	6 fl oz	30	D–
Chocolate, Double Dutch		6 fl oz	50	C
Chocolate, Dutch Mint		6 fl oz	50	C–
Mocha		6 fl oz	50	D
Mocha	Low Calorie	6 fl oz	30	D
		6 fl oz	60	B
Orange	Capri	6 fl oz	60	B
Swiss		6 fl oz	60	B
Swiss		6 fl oz	40	D
		6 fl oz	52	B
Cherry		6 fl oz	53	B
Mint		6 fl oz	53	B
Banana Nut		6 fl oz	39	D–
Fudge		6 fl oz	39	D–
Mint		6 fl oz	37	C

"+" indicates the food meets minimum fiber requirements; "–" indicates the food has a high sodium content.

Food	Processing Category	Brand
Coffee, Flavored	Mix	Mjb Sugar Free
Coffee, Substitute	Powder	
Egg Nog	Canned	Borden
Egg Nog	Chilled	
Egg Nog	Chilled	Crowley
Egg Nog	Chilled	Darigold
Egg Nog	Chilled	Darigold Classic
Egg Nog	Chilled	Kemp's
Egg Nog	Chilled	Kemp's
Egg Nog	Mix	
Malted Milk	Mix	Generic
Malted Milk	Mix	Generic
Milkshake	Frozen	Micro Magic
Milkshake	Frozen	Micro Magic
Milkshake	Frozen	Micro Magic
Milkshake	Frozen	Micro Magic
Milkshake	Mix	Weight Watchers
Milkshake	Mix	Weight Watchers
Papaya Nectar	Canned or Bottled	
Peach Juice	Canned or Bottled	Smucker's Naturally 100%
Peach Nectar	Canned or Bottled	
Pear Nectar	Canned	
Piña Colada	Mix	Holland House
Piña Colada	Mix	Holland House
Soy Milk	All Forms	
Soy Milk	All Forms	Ah Soy
Soy Milk	All Forms	Ah Soy
Soy Milk	All Forms	Ah Soy
Soy Milk	All Forms	Soy Moo
Soy Milk	All Forms	Westbrae Natural
Soy Milk	All Forms	Westbrae Natural
Soy Milk	All Forms	Westbrae Natural
Soy Milk	All Forms	Westbrae Natural
Strawberry-flavored Milk	Mix	
Strawberry-flavored Milk	Mix	Carnation Instant Breakfast
Strawberry-flavored Milk	Mix	Carnation Instant Breakfast No Sugar Added
Strawberry-flavored Milk	Mix	Nestlé Quik
Strawberry-flavored Milk	Mix	Pillsbury Instant Breakfast
Tomato Beef Cocktail	Canned or Bottled	
Tomato Beef Cocktail	Canned or Bottled	Beefamato
Tomato Juice	Canned or Bottled	Campbell's
Tomato Juice	Canned or Bottled	Featherweight
Tomato Juice	Canned or Bottled	Hunt's
Tomato Juice	Canned or Bottled	Hunt's No Salt Added
Tomato Juice	Canned or Bottled	Pathmark
Tomato Juice	Canned or Bottled	S & W California
Tomato Juice	Canned or Bottled	S & W/Nutradiet
Tomato Juice	Canned or Bottled	Stokely
Tomato Juice	Canned or Bottled	Welch's
Vanilla Flavor Drink	Canned	Sego Lite
Vanilla Flavor Drink	Canned	Sego Very Vanilla
Vanilla Flavor Drink	Mix	Carnation Instant Breakfast

Major Description	Minor Description	Serving Size	Calories	Grade
Vanilla		6 fl oz	39	C–
		1 tsp	9	A
Nonalcoholic		4 oz	160	D
Nonalcoholic		4 oz	172	D
Nonalcoholic		4 fl oz	180	D
Nonalcoholic		4 fl oz	175	D
Nonalcoholic		4 fl oz	195	C
		4 oz	175	B
	Light	4 oz	120	B
Flavored	Powdered	1 oz	111	A
Chocolate Flavor	Powdered	1 oz	112	A
Natural Flavor	Powdered	1 oz	117	B
Chocolate		7 fl oz	200	B
Chocolate		11.5 fl oz	340	B
Strawberry		11.5 fl oz	340	B
Vanilla		11.5 fl oz	380	C
Chocolate Fudge		1 pkt	70	A–
Orange Sherbert		1 pkt	70	A–
		1 fl oz	18	A
		6 fl oz	90	A
Bottled		6 fl oz	101	A
		1 fl oz	19	A
Bottled		1 fl oz	33	A
Instant		6 fl oz	82	C
Fluid		6 fl oz	54	D
Carob		6 fl oz	160	B
Flavored	Chocolate	6 fl oz	160	B
Flavored	Vanilla	6 fl oz	160	B
		6 fl oz	94	C
Almond, Malted		6 fl oz	250	C
Carob, Malted		6 fl oz	270	C
Java, Malted		6 fl oz	270	C
Vanilla, Malted		6 fl oz	250	C
		6 fl oz	110	A
		6 fl oz	130	A–
		6 fl oz	70	A–
		6 fl oz	80	A
		6 fl oz	130	A–
		6 fl oz	66	A–
		6 fl oz	80	A–
		6 fl oz	40	A–
		6 fl oz	35	A
		6 fl oz	30	A–
		6 fl oz	45	A
		6 fl oz	30	A–
		6 fl oz	35	A–
		6 fl oz	35	A
		6 fl oz	25	A–
		6 fl oz	35	A–
Plain or French		10 fl oz	150	B–
		10 fl oz	225	B–
		1 pouch	130	A

"+" indicates the food meets minimum fiber requirements; "–" indicates the food has a high sodium content.

Food	Processing Category	Brand
Vanilla Flavor Drink	Mix	Carnation Instant Breakfast No Sugar Added
Vanilla Flavor Drink	Mix	Pillsbury Instant Breakfast
Vanilla Flavor Drink	Mix	Pillsbuy Instant Breakfast
Vegetable Juice	Canned or Bottled	Biotta Breuss Juice
Vegetable Juice	Canned or Bottled	Biotta Cocktail
Vegetable Juice	Canned or Bottled	Smucker's
Vegetable Juice	Canned or Bottled	V-8
Vegetable Juice	Canned or Bottled	Veryfine 100%
Wine [1]	Bottled	All wines
Yogurt Drink	Bottled	Danup

[1] *Virtually all wines fall into the 80–100 calorie range per 4 oz. Variability is by brand, not by type of wine, and relates to exact alcohol content.*

Major Description	Minor Description	Serving Size	Calories	Grade
		1 pouch	70	A–
		8 fl oz	300	B
		1 pouch	140	A–
		6 fl oz	67	A–
		6 fl oz	50	A–
All Varieties		8 fl oz	58	A–
All Varieties		6 fl oz	35	A–
		6 fl oz	32	A–
		4 fl oz	91	A
All Flavors		8 oz	190	B

"+" indicates the food meets minimum fiber requirements; "–" indicates the food has a high sodium content.

Cereals and Grains

Fifty to sixty percent of your daily calories should come from the A and B foods in this section. The reduction of total fat and the elimination of cholesterol and saturated fats in one's diet could be achieved if one also relied on products in this section for at least half of one's sources of protein. Good nonmeat protein sources are:

- Beans, prepared as you like: black, great Northern, lima, navy, pinto.
- Soybeans and soybean products such as tofu are another source; but in this case, pay close attention to ratings and calories.

In the chart:

* Indicates simple sugar content of cereal is 25% to 39% of total calories.
** Indicates simple sugar is 40% or greater of total calories.

Food	Processing Category	Brand
Almond Meal	Dry	Generic
Corn Bran	Dry	Generic
Bagel	Fresh	Generic
Bagel	Fresh	Generic
Bagel	Fresh	Generic
Bagel	Fresh	Generic
Bagel	Fresh	Generic
Bagel	Fresh	Generic
Bagel	Fresh	Generic
Bagel	Fresh	Generic
Bagel	Fresh	Generic
Bagel	Fresh	Generic
Bagel	Frozen	International-Baily's
Bagel	Frozen	International-Baily's
Bagel	Frozen	International-Baily's
Bagel	Frozen	Lender's
Bagel	Frozen	Lender's
Bagel	Frozen	Lender's
Bagel	Frozen	Lender's
Bagel	Frozen	Lender's
Bagel	Frozen	Lender's
Bagel	Frozen	Lender's
Bagel	Frozen	Lender's
Bagel	Frozen	Lender's
Bagel	Frozen	Lender's
Bagel	Frozen	Lender's
Bagel	Frozen	Lender's
Bagel	Frozen	Lender's Bagelettes
Bagel	Frozen	Lender's Bagelettes
Bagel	Frozen	Lender's Bagelettes
Bagel	Frozen	Lender's Big N Crusty
Bagel	Frozen	Lender's Big N Crusty
Bagel	Frozen	Lender's Big N Crusty
Bagel	Frozen	Lender's Big N Crusty
Bagel	Frozen	Lender's Big N Crusty
Bagel	Frozen	Sara Lee
Bagel	Frozen	Sara Lee
Bagel	Frozen	Sara Lee
Bagel	Frozen	Sara Lee
Bagel	Frozen	Sara Lee
Bagel	Frozen	Sara Lee
Bagel	Frozen	Sara Lee
Bagel	Frozen	Sara Lee
Bagel	Frozen	Sara Lee
Barley [1]	Cooked	All Brands
Barley Flakes	Dry	Arrowhead Mills
Biscuit	Mix	Arrowhead Mills
Biscuit	Mix	Bisquik
Biscuit	Mix	Healthy Valley
Biscuit	Mix	Martha White Bix Mix
Biscuit	Mix	Robin Hood/Gold Medal Pouch
Biscuit	Packaged	Awrey's

[1] *Serving size equivalent to 2 ozs dry measure.*

Major Description	Minor Description	Serving Size	Calories	Grade
Partially Defatted		1 oz	116	D
Crude		1 oz	64	A+
Buttermilk		1 bagel	127	D–
Cinnamon and Raisin		1 bagel	194	A–
Egg		1 bagel	197	A–
Oat Bran		1 bagel	181	A–
Onion		1 bagel	195	A–
Plain		1 bagel	195	A–
Poppy Seed		1 bagel	195	A–
Pumpernickel		1 bagel	175	A–
Sesame Seed		1 bagel	195	A–
Whole Wheat		1 bagel	175	A–
Garlic		1 bagel	110	A–
Onion		1 bagel	110	A–
Plain		1 bagel	110	A–
Blueberry		1 bagel	190	A–
Egg		1 bagel	150	A–
Garlic		1 bagel	160	A–
Oat Bran		1 bagel	170	A–+
Onion		1 bagel	160	A–
Plain		1 bagel	150	A–
Poppy		1 bagel	160	A–
Pumpernickel		1 bagel	160	A–
Raisin N Honey		1 bagel	200	A–
Rye		1 bagel	150	A–
Sesame		1 bagel	160	A–
Soft		1 bagel	210	A–
Wheat & Raisin		1 bagel	190	A–
Onion		1 bagel	70	A–
Plain		1 bagel	70	A–
Raisin		1 bagel	70	A–
Cinnamon & Raisin		1 bagel	250	A–
Egg		1 bagel	250	A–
Garlic		1 bagel	250	A–
Onion		1 bagel	230	A–
Plain		1 bagel	240	A–
Cinnamon & Raisin		1 bagel	240	A
Cinnamon & Raisin		1 bagel	200	A
Egg		1 bagel	250	A–
Oat Bran		1 bagel	220	A–
Onion		1 bagel	230	A–
Plain		1 bagel	190	A–
Plain		1 bagel	230	A–
Poppy Seed		1 bagel	230	A–
Sesame Seed		1 bagel	240	A–
Pearled		$1/2$ cup	93	A+
		2 oz	200	A+
		1 biscuit	100	A
		1 biscuit	120	B–
Buttermilk		1 biscuit	200	A–+
		1 biscuit	100	B–
		1 biscuit	90	B–
		1 biscuit	160	B–

"+" indicates the food meets minimum fiber requirements; "–" indicates the food has a high sodium content.

Food	Processing Category	Brand
Biscuit	Packaged	Wonder
Biscuit	Refrigerated	1869 Brand
Biscuit	Refrigerated	Ballard Ovenready
Biscuit	Refrigerated	Pillsbury Big Country
Biscuit	Refrigerated	Pillsbury
Biscuit	Refrigerated	Pillsbury
Biscuit	Refrigerated	Pillsbury Big Premium Heat N' Eat
Biscuit	Refrigerated	Pillsbury Country
Biscuit	Refrigerated	Pillsbury Good N' Buttery
Biscuit	Refrigerated	Pillsbury Heat N' Eat
Biscuit	Refrigerated	Pillsbury Hungry Jack
Biscuit	Refrigerated	Pillsbury Hungry Jack
Biscuit	Refrigerated	Pillsbury Hungry Jack
Biscuit	Refrigerated	Pillsbury Hungry Jack
Biscuit	Refrigerated	Pillsbury Hungry Jack
Biscuit	Refrigerated	Pillsbury Hungry Jack
Biscuit	Refrigerated	Pillsbury Tender Layer
Biscuit	Refrigerated	Roman Meal
Biscuit	Refrigerated	Roman Meal
Biscuit	Refrigerated	Roman Meal Premium
Bread [2]	Fresh	Generic
Bread	Fresh	Generic
Bread	Fresh	Generic
Bread	Fresh	Generic
Bread	Fresh	Generic
Bread	Fresh	Generic
Bread	Fresh	Generic
Bread	Fresh	Generic
Bread	Fresh	Generic
Bread	Fresh	Generic
Bread	Fresh	Generic
Bread	Fresh	Generic
Bread	Fresh	Generic
Bread	Fresh	Generic
Bread	Fresh	Generic
Bread	Fresh	Generic
Bread	Fresh	Generic
Bread	Fresh	Generic
Bread	Fresh	Generic
Bread	Fresh	Generic
Bread	Fresh	Generic
Bread	Fresh	Generic
Bread	Fresh	Generic
Bread	Fresh	Generic
Bread	Fresh	Generic
Bread	Fresh	Generic
Bread	Fresh	Generic
Bread	Fresh	Generic
Bread	Fresh	Generic
Bread	Fresh	Generic
Bread	Fresh	Generic

[2] *Serving size based on USDA average recipe, approximately 1 oz per slice.*

Major Description	Minor Description	Serving Size	Calories	Grade
		1 biscuit	80	A–
All Varieties		1 biscuit	100	D–
All Varieties		1 biscuit	50	B–
All Varieties		1 biscuit	100	C–
Butter		1 biscuit	50	B–
Buttermilk		1 biscuit	50	B–
		1 biscuit	140	D–
		1 biscuit	50	B–
	"Fluffy"	1 biscuit	90	D–
Buttermilk		1 biscuit	85	B–
Buttermilk	"Flaky"	1 biscuit	90	C–
Butter Tastin	"Flaky"	1 biscuit	90	D–
Buttermilk	"Fluffy"	1 biscuit	90	C–
Buttermilk	Extra Rich	1 biscuit	50	B–
Honey Tastin	"Flaky"	1 biscuit	90	C–
Southern Style		1 biscuit	80	C–
Buttermilk		1 biscuit	50	B–
		1 biscuit	90	B–
Oat Bran & Honey Nut		1 biscuit	131	C–
White		1 biscuit	127	C–
Banana	Margarine	1 slice	92	B
Banana	Vegetable Shortening	1 slice	96	C
Corn Bread	2% Milk	1 slice	75	B–
Corn Bread	2% Milk & Egg	1 slice	89	B–
Corn Bread	Vegetable Shortening	1 slice	119	B–
Corn Bread	Whole Milk	1 slice	77	B–
Cracked Wheat	Vegetable Shortening	1 slice	65	A–+
Egg	Vegetable Shortening	1 slice	81	B–
French	Vegetable Shortening	1 slice	78	A–
Irish Soda		1 slice	82	B–
Italian Style	Vegetable Shortening	1 slice	77	A–
Mixed or 7 Grain	Vegetable Shortening	1 slice	65	A–+
Oat Bran		1 slice	67	B–+
Oat Bran	Low Calorie	1 slice	57	A–+
Oatmeal		1 slice	73	A–
Oatmeal	Low Calorie	1 slice	60	A–
Pita	White	1 piece	78	A–
Pita	Whole Wheat	1 piece	76	A–
Protein & Gluten		1 slice	70	A–
Pumpernickel		1 slice	71	A–+
Pumpkin		1 slice	94	C
Raisin		1 slice	78	B–
Rice Bran		1 slice	69	B–+
Rye		1 slice	73	A–
Rye	Low Calorie	1 slice	57	A–
Sourdough		1 slice	78	A–
Special, Dark	High Calcium	1 slice	62	A–
Special, Light	High Calcium	1 slice	64	A–
Wheat		1 slice	74	A–+
Wheat	Low Calorie	1 slice	56	A–+
Wheat Bran		1 slice	70	A–
Wheat Germ		1 slice	74	A–
White		1 slice	76	A–

"+" indicates the food meets minimum fiber requirements; "–" indicates the food has a high sodium content.

Food	Processing Category	Brand
Bread	Fresh	Generic
Bread	Fresh	Generic
Bread	Fresh	Generic
Bread	Fresh	Generic
Bread	Packaged	Arnold
Bread	Packaged	Arnold
Bread	Packaged	Arnold
Bread	Packaged	Arnold
Bread	Packaged	Arnold
Bread	Packaged	Arnold Bakery
Bread	Packaged	Arnold Bakery
Bread	Packaged	Arnold Bakery
Bread	Packaged	Arnold Branola
Bread	Packaged	Arnold Branola
Bread	Packaged	Arnold Branola
Bread	Packaged	Arnold Branola Country
Bread	Packaged	Arnold Branola Original
Bread	Packaged	Arnold Brick Oven
Bread	Packaged	Arnold Brick Oven
Bread	Packaged	Arnold Brick Oven
Bread	Packaged	Arnold Country White
Bread	Packaged	Arnold Light Premium
Bread	Packaged	Arnold Stoneground
Bread	Packaged	Awrey's
Bread	Packaged	B & M
Bread	Packaged	B & M
Bread	Packaged	Beefsteak
Bread	Packaged	Beefsteak
Bread	Packaged	Beefsteak
Bread	Packaged	Beefsteak
Bread	Packaged	Beefsteak
Bread	Packaged	Beefsteak Hearty
Bread	Packaged	Beefsteak Hearty
Bread	Packaged	Beefsteak Mild
Bread	Packaged	Beefsteak Robust
Bread	Packaged	Beefsteak Soft
Bread	Packaged	Beefsteak Soft
Bread	Packaged	Boudini
Bread	Packaged	Braun's Old Allegheny
Bread	Packaged	Bread du Jour
Bread	Packaged	Bread du Jour
Bread	Packaged	Brownberry
Bread	Packaged	Brownberry
Bread	Packaged	Brownberry
Bread	Packaged	Brownberry
Bread	Packaged	Brownberry
Bread	Packaged	Brownberry
Bread	Packaged	Brownberry Branola
Bread	Packaged	Brownberry Branola
Bread	Packaged	Brownberry Branola Country
Bread	Packaged	Brownberry Branola Nutty
Bread	Packaged	Brownberry Healthnut
Bread	Packaged	Brownberry Hearth

Major Description	Minor Description	Serving Size	Calories	Grade
White	2% Milk	1 slice	81	B–
White	Low Calorie	1 slice	59	A–+
White	Nonfat Milk	1 slice	78	A
White	Whole Milk	1 slice	82	B
Apple Walnut		1 slice	64	B–+
Cinnamon Raisin		1 slice	67	B–
Pumpernickel		1 slice	70	A–+
Rye & Dill		1 slice	71	A–+
Wheat	Honey Wheatberry	1 slice	77	A–+
Golden Light Wheat		1 slice	44	A–+
Italian Style	Light	1 slice	45	A–+
Oatmeal	Light	1 slice	44	A–+
Dark Wheat		1 slice	83	A–+
Hearty Wheat		1 slice	88	B–+
Nutty Grain		1 slice	85	B–+
Oat		1 slice	90	B–+
		1 slice	85	A–+
Wheat		1 slice	57	B–+
White		1 slice	61	B–
White	Extra Fiber	1 slice	55	A–+
White		1 slice	98	B–
White		1 slice	42	A–+
Whole Wheat		1 slice	48	A–+
Oat Bran		1 slice	50	A–+
Brown	Plain	1 slice	92	A–+
Brown Raisin		1 slice	94	A–+
Hearty Wheat		1 slice	70	A–+
Multigrain Wheat		1 slice	70	A–+
Onion Rye		1 slice	70	A–
Robust White		1 slice	70	A–
Wheatberry Rye		1 slice	70	A–
Rye		1 slice	70	A–
Wheat		1 slice	70	A–+
Rye		1 slice	70	A–
White		1 slice	70	A–
Rye		1 slice	70	A–
Wheat		1 slice	70	A–+
Sourdough	French Style	1 slice	75	A–
Rye		1 slice	70	A–
French Style		1 slice	70	A–
Wheat	Austrian Style	1 slice	70	A–+
Apple Honey Wheat		1 slice	69	B–+
Cinnamon Raisin		1 slice	66	B–
Orange Raisin Oatmeal		1 slice	67	B
Raisin Bran		1 slice	61	B–+
Raisin Walnut		1 slice	68	C–+
Soft Wheat		1 slice	74	B–
Bran		1 slice	85	A–+
Hearty Wheat		1 slice	88	B–+
Oat		1 slice	90	B–+
Nutty Grain		1 slice	85	B–+
Bran		1 slice	71	C–+
Wheat		1 slice	70	B–+

"+" indicates the food meets minimum fiber requirements; "–" indicates the food has a high sodium content.

Food	Processing Category	Brand
Bread	Packaged	Brownberry Light
Bread	Packaged	Brownberry Light Premium
Bread	Packaged	Brownberry Natural
Bread	Packaged	Brownberry Natural
Bread	Packaged	Brownberry Natural
Bread	Packaged	Brownberry Natural
Bread	Packaged	Brownberry Natural Thin
Bread	Packaged	Colombo Brand
Bread	Packaged	Colombo Brand
Bread	Packaged	Colombo Brand BBQ Loaf
Bread	Packaged	Colombo Brand French Stick
Bread	Packaged	Colombo Bread
Bread	Packaged	Country Grain
Bread	Packaged	Daily
Bread	Packaged	DiCarlo
Bread	Packaged	DiCarlo Parisian
Bread	Packaged	Dromedary
Bread	Packaged	Fresh & Natural
Bread	Packaged	Friends
Bread	Packaged	Friends
Bread	Packaged	Hollywood Dark
Bread	Packaged	Hollywood Light
Bread	Packaged	Home Pride
Bread	Packaged	Home Pride
Bread	Packaged	Home Pride
Bread	Packaged	Home Pride 7 Grain
Bread	Packaged	Home Pride Butter Top
Bread	Packaged	Home Pride Butter Top
Bread	Packaged	Home Pride Stoneground
Bread	Packaged	Levy's
Bread	Packaged	Levy's
Bread	Packaged	Monks
Bread	Packaged	Monks
Bread	Packaged	Monks
Bread	Packaged	Monks
Bread	Packaged	Monks 100% Stoneground
Bread	Packaged	Monks Hi Fibre
Bread	Packaged	Oatmeal Goodness
Bread	Packaged	Oatmeal Goodness
Bread	Packaged	Oatmeal Goodness
Bread	Packaged	Oatmeal Goodness
Bread	Packaged	Oatmeal Goodness
Bread	Packaged	Oatmeal Goodness
Bread	Packaged	Oatmeal Goodness
Bread	Packaged	Oatmeal Goodness Light
Bread	Packaged	Pepperidge Farm
Bread	Packaged	Pepperidge Farm
Bread	Packaged	Pepperidge Farm
Bread	Packaged	Pepperidge Farm
Bread	Packaged	Pepperidge Farm
Bread	Packaged	Pepperidge Farm
Bread	Packaged	Pepperidge Farm
Bread	Packaged	Pepperidge Farm

Major Description	Minor Description	Serving Size	Calories	Grade
Italian Style		1 slice	44	A–+
White		1 slice	42	A–+
Caraway Rye		1 slice	73	A–+
Wheat		1 slice	80	A–+
White		1 slice	59	B–
Whole Wheat Bran		1 slice	58	B–+
Rye	Seedless	1 slice	45	A–+
French Style	Extra Sour, Sliced	1 slice	77	A–
French Style	Garlic	1 slice	92	D–
Barbecue		1 slice	69	A–
French Style	Sweet	1 slice	78	A–
French Style	Extra Sour	1 slice	75	A–
Wheat		1 slice	70	A–+
Whole Wheat		1 slice	70	A
Sourdough		1 slice	70	A–
French Style		1 slice	70	A–
Date Nut Roll		1 slice	80	B–
Wheat		1 slice	70	A–+
Brown		1 slice	92	A–+
Brown & Raisins		1 slice	94	A–+
		1 slice	70	A–
		1 slice	70	A–
Buttertop Wheat		1 slice	70	A–+
Wheat	Light	1 slice	40	A–+
White	Light	1 slice	40	A–+
Wheat		1 slice	70	A–
Wheat		1 slice	70	A–
White		1 slice	70	A–
Wheat		1 slice	70	A–+
Rye	Jewish Style, Seeded	1 slice	76	A–+
Rye	Jewish Style, Seedless	1 slice	75	A–+
Cinnamon Raisin		1 slice	70	B
Golden Rice Bran		1 slice	70	A+
Sourdough	Sunflower & Bran	1 slice	70	A+
White		1 slice	60	A–
Whole Wheat		1 slice	70	A–
		1 slice	70	A+
Oatmeal		1 slice	80	A–+
Oatmeal	Light	1 slice	40	A–+
Oatmeal	Sunflower Seed	1 slice	90	B–
Oatmeal	with Bran	1 slice	90	B–
Oatmeal Cinnamon		1 slice	90	B–
Oatmeal Wheat		1 slice	90	B–
Wheat	Light	1 slice	40	A–+
All Varieties		1 slice	40	A–
Cinnamon Raisin Swirl		1 slice	90	B+
Cinnamon Swirl		1 slice	90	B+
Cracked Wheat		1 slice	70	A–
Crunchy Oat		1 slice	95	B–+
Granola, Oat & Honey		1 slice	60	B–+
Oatmeal		1 slice	70	A–
Raisin Cinnamon Swirl		1 slice	90	B
Rye	Dijon Style	1 slice	50	B–+

"+" indicates the food meets minimum fiber requirements; "–" indicates the food has a high sodium content.

Food	Processing Category	Brand
Bread	Packaged	Pepperidge Farm
Bread	Packaged	Pepperidge Farm
Bread	Packaged	Pepperidge Farm
Bread	Packaged	Pepperidge Farm 1 1/2 lb
Bread	Packaged	Pepperidge Farm 1 1/2 lb
Bread	Packaged	Pepperidge Farm 1/2 lb
Bread	Packaged	Pepperidge Farm Family
Bread	Packaged	Pepperidge Farm Family
Bread	Packaged	Pepperidge Farm Family 2 lb
Bread	Packaged	Pepperidge Farm Hearth
Bread	Packaged	Pepperidge Farm Hearth
Bread	Packaged	Pepperidge Farm Hearth
Bread	Packaged	Pepperidge Farm Hearth
Bread	Packaged	Pepperidge Farm Hearty
Bread	Packaged	Pepperidge Farm Hearty
Bread	Packaged	Pepperidge Farm Hearty Country
Bread	Packaged	Pepperidge Farm Large Family 2 lb
Bread	Packaged	Pepperidge Farm Light Style
Bread	Packaged	Pepperidge Farm Party
Bread	Packaged	Pepperidge Farm Party
Bread	Packaged	Pepperidge Farm Party
Bread	Packaged	Pepperidge Farm Thin Sliced 1 lb
Bread	Packaged	Pepperidge Farm Thin Sliced 1 lb
Bread	Packaged	Pepperidge Farm Very Thin
Bread	Packaged	Pepperidge Farm Very Thin
Bread	Packaged	Pepperidge Farm Very Thin
Bread	Packaged	Pepperidge Farms Hearty Slice
Bread	Packaged	Pillsbury
Bread	Packaged	Pillsbury Hearty Grains
Bread	Packaged	Pillsbury Hearty Grains
Bread	Packaged	Pillsbury Hearty Grains
Bread	Packaged	Pillsbury Hearty Grains
Bread	Packaged	Pillsbury Pipin' Hot
Bread	Packaged	Pillsbury Pipin' Hot
Bread	Packaged	Roman Meal
Bread	Packaged	Roman Meal
Bread	Packaged	Roman Meal
Bread	Packaged	Roman Meal
Bread	Packaged	Roman Meal Round Top
Bread	Packaged	Roman Meal Split Top
Bread	Packaged	Roman Meal Sun Grain
Bread	Packaged	Roman Meal Thin Sliced Sandwich
Bread	Packaged	Sahara
Bread	Packaged	Sahara
Bread	Packaged	Sahara
Bread	Packaged	Sahara
Bread	Packaged	Weight Watchers
Bread	Packaged	Weight Watchers
Bread	Packaged	Weight Watchers
Bread	Packaged	Weight Watchers
Bread	Packaged	Weight Watchers
Bread	Packaged	Wonder

Major Description	Minor Description	Serving Size	Calories	Grade
Sprouted Wheat		1 slice	70	B–+
White	Sandwich	1 slice	65	A–
White	Toasting	1 slice	90	A–
Honey Bran		1 slice	90	A–
Oatmeal		1 slice	90	A–
Wheat		1 slice	90	B–+
Pumpernickel		1 slice	80	A–+
Seedless Rye		1 slice	80	A–+
Wheat		1 slice	70	A–+
French Style		1 slice	75	A–
French Style	Twin	1 slice	80	A–
Italian Style		1 slice	80	A–
Sourdough	Vienna Style Thick Sliced	1 slice	70	A–
Rye	Dijon Style	1 slice	70	A–+
Sesame Wheat		1 slice	95	A–+
White		1 slice	95	A–
White		1 slice	70	A–
All Varieties		1 slice	45	A–+
Pumpernickel	Small	1 slice	15	A–+
Rye	Small	1 slice	15	A–+
Seeded Rye		1 slice	80	A–+
White		1 slice	80	B–
Whole Wheat		1 slice	60	A–+
Oatmeal		1 slice	40	B–
White		1 slice	40	A–
Whole Wheat		1 slice	35	A–
7 Grain		1 slice	90	A–
French Style	Crusty	1 slice	60	A–
Cracked Wheat	Honey Twists	1 slice	80	B–
Multigrain		1 slice	80	B–
Oatmeal		1 slice	80	B–
Oatmeal Raisin		1 slice	90	B–
Wheat		1 slice	70	B–
White		1 slice	70	B–
Honey Nut Oat Bran		1 slice	72	B–
Honey Nut Rice Bran		1 slice	71	B–+
Honey Oat Bran		1 slice	71	B–
Rice Bran		1 slice	70	B–+
Mixed Grain		1 slice	67	A–+
Oat Bran		1 slice	68	A–+
Multigrain		1 slice	68	B–+
Mixed Grain		1 slice	55	A–+
Pita	Oat Bran	1 piece	132	A–+
Pita	White	1 piece	158	A–
Pita	White, Mini	1 piece	79	A–
Pita	Whole Wheat	1 piece	150	A–
Multigrain		1 slice	40	A–
Oat Bran		1 slice	40	A–
Rye		1 slice	40	A–
Wheat		1 slice	40	A–
White		1 slice	40	A–
Buttermilk White		1 slice	70	A–

"+" indicates the food meets minimum fiber requirements; "–" indicates the food has a high sodium content.

Food	Processing Category	Brand
Bread	Packaged	Wonder
Bread	Packaged	Wonder
Bread	Packaged	Wonder
Bread	Packaged	Wonder
Bread	Packaged	Wonder
Bread	Packaged	Wonder
Bread	Packaged	Wonder
Bread	Packaged	Wonder 100%
Bread	Packaged	Wonder Country Style
Bread	Packaged	Wonder Family
Bread	Packaged	Wonder Family
Bread	Packaged	Wonder High Fiber
Bread	Packaged	Wonder High Fiber
Bread	Packaged	Wonder Light
Bread	Packaged	Wonder Light
Bread	Packaged	Wonder Soft 100%
Bread	Packaged	Wonder Stoneground
Bread	Packaged	Wonder Thin Sliced
Bread	Refrigerated	Du Jour Austrian
Bread	Refrigerated	Du Jour French
Bread	Refrigerated	Pepperidge Farm
Bread Crumbs	Packaged	Devonsheer
Bread Crumbs	Packaged	Devonsheer
Bread Crumbs	Packaged	Jaclyn's
Bread Crumbs	Packaged	Progresso
Bread Crumbs	Packaged	Progresso
Bread Crumbs	Packaged	Tone's
Bread Dough	Frozen	Bridgford
Bread Dough	Frozen	Bridgford
Bread Dough	Frozen	Rich's
Bread Dough	Refrigerated	Pillsbury
Bread Dough	Refrigerated	Pillsbury
Bread Dough	Refrigerated	Pillsbury Pipin' Hot
Bread Dough	Refrigerated	Pillsbury Pipin' Hot
Bread Dough	Refrigerated	Roman Meal
Bread, Brown	Canned	B & M Friends
Bread, Brown	Canned	B & M Friends
Bread, Brown	Canned	S & W New England
Bread, Sweet	Mix	Aunt Jemima
Bread, Sweet	Mix	Betty Crocker Classics
Bread, Sweet	Mix	Dromedary
Bread, Sweet	Mix	Dromedary
Bread, Sweet	Mix	Martha White Light Crust
Bread, Sweet	Mix	Martha White, Cotton Pickin
Bread, Sweet	Mix	Pillsbury
Bread, Sweet	Mix	Pillsbury
Bread, Sweet	Mix	Pillsbury
Bread, Sweet	Mix	Pillsbury
Bread, Sweet	Mix	Pillsbury
Bread, Sweet	Mix	Pillsbury
Bread, Sweet	Mix	Pillsbury
Bread, Sweet	Mix	Pillsbury Quick
Bread, Sweet	Mix	Pillsbury/Ballard

Major Description	Minor Description	Serving Size	Calories	Grade
Cinnamon Raisin		1 slice	60	A–+
Cracked Wheat		1 slice	70	A–
French Style		1 slice	70	A–
Italian Style	Light	1 slice	40	A–+
Rye		1 slice	70	A–
Sourdough	Light	1 slice	40	A–+
White		1 slice	70	A–
Whole Wheat		1 slice	70	A–+
Wheat		1 slice	70	A–
Italian Style		1 slice	70	A–
Whole Wheat		1 slice	70	A–
White		1 slice	40	A–+
Whole Wheat		1 slice	40	A–+
White		1 slice	40	A–+
Whole Wheat		1 slice	40	A–+
Whole Wheat		1 slice	70	A–+
Whole Wheat		1 slice	80	A–+
White		1 slice	50	B–
Brown & Serve		1 oz slice	70	A–
Brown & Serve		1 oz slice	70	A–
Brown & Serve	Italian Style	1 oz slice	80	A–
Italian Style		1 oz	104	A–
Plain		1 oz	108	A–
Italian Style	Whole Wheat	1 oz	56	C
Italian Style		1 oz	60	A–
Plain		1 oz	60	A–
Plain or Italian Style	Dry Grated	1 oz	48	A–
Honey Walnut		1 oz slice	76	A–
White		1 oz slice	76	A–
White		1 oz slice	60	A–
Cornbread Twists		1 twist	70	D–
Crusty French Style		1 oz slice	65	A–
Wheat		1 oz slice	70	B–
White		1 oz slice	70	B–
		1 oz slice	85	B–
		1 slice	94	A–+
Raisin		1 slice	92	A–+
		1 slice	38	A–
Corn Bread		1 serving	196	B–
Gingerbread		$^{1}/_{12}$ loaf	140	B–
Corn Bread		2" × 2" sq	130	B–
Date Nut		$^{1}/_{12}$ loaf	183	C–
Corn Bread	Yellow	1 oz slice	70	B–
Corn Bread		$^{1}/_{4}$ pan	170	B–
Banana		$^{1}/_{12}$ loaf	170	C
Blueberry Nut		$^{1}/_{12}$ loaf	150	B
Cherry Nut		$^{1}/_{12}$ loaf	180	B
Cranberry		$^{1}/_{12}$ loaf	160	B
Date		$^{1}/_{12}$ loaf	160	B
Gingerbread		3" square	190	B–
Nut		$^{1}/_{12}$ loaf	170	C
Oatmeal Raisin	with 1 Egg	1 oz slice	136	C
Corn Bread		$^{1}/_{6}$ mix	186	B–

"+" indicates the food meets minimum fiber requirements; "–" indicates the food has a high sodium content.

Food	Processing Category	Brand
Bread, Sweet	Mix	Robin Hood/Gold Medal Pouch Mix
Bread, Sweet	Mix	Robin Hood/Gold Medal Pouch Mix
Breadsticks	Packaged	Fattorie & Pandea
Breadsticks	Packaged	Fattorie & Pandea
Breadsticks	Packaged	Fattorie & Pandea
Breadsticks	Packaged	Stella D'oro
Breadsticks	Packaged	Stella D'oro
Breadsticks	Packaged	Stella D'oro
Breadsticks	Packaged	Stella D'oro
Breadsticks	Packaged	Stella D'oro
Breadsticks	Packaged	Stella D'oro
Breadsticks	Packaged	Stella D'oro
Breadsticks	Packaged	Stella D'oro
Breadsticks	Refrigerated	Pillsbury
Breadsticks	Refrigerated	Roman Meal
Breadsticks	Refrigerated	Roman Meal
Buckwheat	Dry	All Brands
Buckwheat Groats [3]	Cooked	Arrowhead Mills
Bulgur	Cooked	All Brands
Bulgur	*See also* Tabbouleh Mix	
Cereal [4]	Hot	3-Minute Brand
Cereal	Hot	3-Minute Brand
Cereal	Hot	3-Minute Brand Quick
Cereal	Hot	3-Minute Brand Regular
Cereal	Hot	Arrowhead Mills
Cereal	Hot	Arrowhead Mills
Cereal	Hot	Arrowhead Mills
Cereal	Hot	Arrowhead Mills
Cereal	Hot	Arrowhead Mills
Cereal	Hot	Arrowhead Mills Bear Mush
Cereal	Hot	Arrowhead Mills Instant
Cereal	Hot	Arrowhead Mills Instant
Cereal	Hot	Arrowhead Mills Instant
Cereal	Hot	Arrowhead Mills Instant
Cereal	Hot	Arrowhead Mills Rise & Shine
Cereal	Hot	Cream of Wheat Instant
Cereal	Hot	Cream of Wheat Quick
Cereal	Hot	H-O Brand
Cereal	Hot	H-O Brand Gourmet
Cereal	Hot	H-O Brand Instant
Cereal	Hot	H-O Brand Instant
Cereal	Hot	H-O Brand Instant
Cereal	Hot	H-O Brand Instant
Cereal	Hot	H-O Brand Instant
Cereal	Hot	H-O Brand Instant
Cereal	Hot	H-O Brand Instant
Cereal	Hot	H-O Brand Instant
Cereal	Hot	H-O Brand Instant
Cereal	Hot	H-O Brand Instant
Cereal	Hot	H-O Brand Instant

[3] *Serving size equivalent to 1 oz dry measure.*
[4] *Hot cereals reported as dry weight or package content where 1 oz equals approximately ¹/₃ cup cooked.*

Major Description	Minor Description	Serving Size	Calories	Grade
Corn Bread	White	$^1/_6$ mix	150	B−
Corn Bread	Yellow	$^1/_6$ mix	150	B−
Pizza		1 piece	20	B−
Sesame		1 piece	22	B−
Whole Wheat		1 piece	19	B−
Garlic		1 piece	35	B−
Onion		1 piece	40	B
Pizza		1 piece	43	B
Plain		1 piece	41	B
Plain	Diet	1 piece	46	B
Sesame		1 piece	51	C
Sesame	Diet	1 piece	49	C
Wheat		1 piece	42	B
	Soft	1 piece	100	B−
		1 piece	117	B−
	Soft	1 piece	117	B−
Whole Grain		$^1/_2$ cup	290	A+
All Varieties		$^1/_2$ cup	90	A+
		1 cup	152	A+
Oatmeal & Oats	Raisins	1 oz	100	B+
Oatmeal & Oats	Raisins & Oat Bran	1 oz	100	B+
Oatmeal & Oats	Oat Bran	1 oz	100	B+
Oat Bran		1 oz	90	B+
Cracked Wheat		1 oz	90	A
Multigrain	4 Grain	1 oz	94	A+
Multigrain	7 Grain	1 oz	100	A+
Oat Bran		1 oz	110	A+
Wheat	Bulger	1 oz	100	A+
Wheat		1 oz	100	A
Oatmeal & Oats		1 oz	100	B+
Oatmeal & Oats	Apples & Spice	1 oz	130	A+
Oatmeal & Oats	Apples, Dates & Almonds	1 oz	130	B+
Oatmeal & Oats	Cinnamon, Raisins & Almonds	1 oz	140	B+
Rice Brown		1 oz	107	A
Wheat		1 oz	100	A
Wheat		1 oz	100	A
Wheat	Farina, Cream	1 oz	80	A+
Oatmeal & Oats		1 oz	100	B+
Oatmeal & Oats		1 pkt	110	B−+
Oatmeal & Oats	Apples & Cinnamon	1 pkt	130	A−+
Oatmeal & Oats	Fiber	1 pkt	110	B−+
Oatmeal & Oats	Fiber, Apples & Bran	1 pkt	130	A+
Oatmeal & Oats	Maple & Brown Sugar	1 pkt	160	A−+
Oatmeal & Oats	Raisin & Bran	1 pkt	150	A+
Oatmeal & Oats	Raisins & Spice	1 pkt	150	A−+
Oatmeal & Oats	Sweet & Mellow	1 pkt	150	A−+
Wheat	Farina	1 pkt	110	A−+
Oatmeal & Oats		1 oz	130	A+
Oatmeal & Oats	Fiber	1 oz	100	B+

"+" indicates the food meets minimum fiber requirements; "−" indicates the food has a high sodium content.

Food	Processing Category	Brand
Cereal	Hot	H-O Brand Quick
Cereal	Hot	H-O Brand Super Bran
Cereal	Hot	Health Valley Natural
Cereal	Hot	Health Valley Natural
Cereal	Hot	Maltex
Cereal	Hot	Maypo 30 Second
Cereal	Hot	Maypo Vermont Style
Cereal	Hot	Mother's
Cereal	Hot	Mother's
Cereal	Hot	Mother's Instant
Cereal	Hot	Mother's Instant
Cereal	Hot	Nabisco
Cereal	Hot	Nabisco
Cereal	Hot	Nabisco Mix N Eat
Cereal	Hot	Nabisco Mix N Eat
Cereal	Hot	Nabisco Mix N Eat
Cereal	Hot	Nabisco Mix N Eat
Cereal	Hot	Oatmeal Swirlers
Cereal	Hot	Oatmeal Swirlers
Cereal	Hot	Oatmeal Swirlers
Cereal	Hot	Oatmeal Swirlers
Cereal	Hot	Oatmeal Swirlers
Cereal	Hot	Oatmeal Swirlers
Cereal	Hot	Pritikin
Cereal	Hot	Pritikin
Cereal	Hot	Quaker
Cereal	Hot	Quaker Extra
Cereal	Hot	Quaker Extra
Cereal	Hot	Quaker Extra
Cereal	Hot	Quaker Instant
Cereal	Hot	Quaker Instant
Cereal	Hot	Quaker Instant
Cereal	Hot	Quaker Instant
Cereal	Hot	Quaker Instant
Cereal	Hot	Quaker Instant
Cereal	Hot	Quaker Instant
Cereal	Hot	Quaker Instant
Cereal	Hot	Quaker Instant
Cereal	Hot	Quaker Instant
Cereal	Hot	Quaker Old Fashioned
Cereal	Hot	Quaker Quick
Cereal	Hot	Quaker Quick/Old Fashioned
Cereal	Hot	Quaker/Mothers
Cereal	Hot	Quaker/Mothers Hot Natural
Cereal	Hot	Ralston High Fiber
Cereal	Hot	Roman Meal
Cereal	Hot	Roman Meal
Cereal	Hot	Roman Meal
Cereal	Hot	Roman Meal
Cereal	Hot	Roman Meal Premium
Cereal	Hot	Roman Meal Premium

Major Description	Minor Description	Serving Size	Calories	Grade
Oatmeal & Oats		1 oz	110	A+
Bran		1 oz	110	B+
Oat Bran	Apples & Cinnamon	1 oz	100	A+
Oat Bran	Raisins & Spice	1 oz	110	A+
Wheat	Wheat & Barley	1 oz	105	A+
Oatmeal & Oats		1 oz	100	A+
Oatmeal & Oats	Maple & Flavor	1 oz	105	A+
Multigrain		1 pkt	130	A+
Whole Wheat		1 pkt	130	A+
Oat Bran		1 pkt	150	B+
Oatmeal		1 pkt	150	B+
Cream of Rice		1 pkt	100	A
Cream of Wheat	All Varieties	1 pkt	100	A
Cream of Wheat	Apples & Cinnamon	1 pkt	100	A–
Cream of Wheat	Brown Sugar & Cinnamon	1 pkt	130	A–
Cream of Wheat	Maple, Brown Sugar	1 pkt	130	A–
Cream of Wheat	Original	1 pkt	100	A–
Oatmeal & Oats	Apples & Cinnamon	1 pkt	160	A
Oatmeal & Oats	Cherry	1 pkt	150	A
Oatmeal & Oats	Chocolate Milk	1 pkt	170	A
Oatmeal & Oats	Cinnamon & Spice	1 pkt	160	A
Oatmeal & Oats	Maple & Brown Sugar	1 pkt	160	A
Oatmeal & Oats	Strawberry	1 pkt	150	A
Apples, Raisins & Spice		1 pkt	170	A+
Multigrain		1 pkt	160	A+
Oat Bran		1 pkt	90	B+
Oatmeal & Oats		1 pkt	95	B–+
Oatmeal & Oats	Apples & Spice	1 pkt	133	A–+
Oatmeal & Oats	Raisins & Cinnamon	1 pkt	129	A+
Oatmeal	Raisin Spice	1 pkt	160	A–+
Oatmeal	Strawberries & Cream	1 pkt	130	A+
Oatmeal	Strawberries & Stuff	1 pkt	150	A
Oatmeal & Oats		1 pkt	94	B–+
Oatmeal & Oats	Cinnamon & Spice	1 pkt	164	A–+
Oatmeal & Oats	Dates & Walnuts	1 pkt	141	B–+
Oatmeal & Oats	Maple & Brown Sugar	1 pkt	152	A–+
Oatmeal & Oats	Peaches & Cream	1 pkt	129	B–+
Oatmeal & Oats	Raisins & Spice	1 pkt	149	A–+
Oatmeal & Oats	Strawberries & Cream	1 pkt	129	A–+
Oats		1 oz	100	B+
Oats		1 oz	100	B+
Oatmeal & Oats		1 oz	99	B+
Oat Bran		1 oz	92	B+
Whole Wheat		1 oz	92	A+
Wheat		1 oz	90	A+
Multigrain	Apples & Cinnamon	1 oz	112	B+
Oatmeal & Oats	Wheat, Rye, Bran & Flax	1 oz	97	A+
Rye, Cream of		1 oz	95	A+
Wheat	Rye, Bran & Flax	1 oz	80	A+
Oatmeal & Oats	Wheat, Dates & Raisins	1 pkt	140	B+
Oatmeal & Oats	Wheat, Honey & Coconut	1 pkt	150	C+

"+" indicates the food meets minimum fiber requirements; "–" indicates the food has a high sodium content.

Food	Processing Category	Brand
Cereal	Hot	Total Instant
Cereal	Hot	Total Instant
Cereal	Hot	Total Instant
Cereal	Hot	Total Instant
Cereal	Hot	Total Quick
Cereal	Hot	Wheat Hearts
Cereal	Hot	Wheatena
Cereal	Hot	Wholesome N Hearty
Cereal	Hot	Wholesome N Hearty Instant
Cereal	Hot	Wholesome N Hearty Instant
Cereal	Ready to Eat Dry	Alpen
Cereal	Ready to Eat Dry	Arrowhead Mills
Cereal	Ready to Eat Dry	Arrowhead Mills
Cereal	Ready to Eat Dry	Arrowhead Mills
Cereal	Ready to Eat Dry	Arrowhead Mills
Cereal	Ready to Eat Dry	Arrowhead Mills
Cereal	Ready to Eat Dry	Arrowhead Mills
Cereal	Ready to Eat Dry	Arrowhead Mills
Cereal	Ready to Eat Dry	Arrowhead Mills
Cereal	Ready to Eat Dry	Arrowhead Mills
Cereal	Ready to Eat Dry	Arrowhead Mills
Cereal	Ready to Eat Dry	Arrowhead Mills
Cereal	Ready to Eat Dry	Arrowhead Mills
Cereal	Ready to Eat Dry	Arrowhead Mills
Cereal	Ready to Eat Dry	Arrowhead Mills
Cereal	Ready to Eat Dry	Arrowhead Mills
Cereal	Ready to Eat Dry	Arrowhead Mills
Cereal	Ready to Eat Dry	Arrowhead Mills
Cereal	Ready to Eat Dry	Arrowhead Mills
Cereal	Ready to Eat Dry	Arrowhead Mills
Cereal	Ready to Eat Dry	Breadshops
Cereal	Ready to Eat Dry	Breadshops
Cereal	Ready to Eat Dry	Breadshops
Cereal	Ready to Eat Dry	Breadshops
Cereal	Ready to Eat Dry	Erewhon Granola
Cereal	Ready to Eat Dry	Erewhon Granola
Cereal	Ready to Eat Dry	Erewhon Granola
Cereal	Ready to Eat Dry	Erewhon Granola
Cereal	Ready to Eat Dry	Erewhon Granola
Cereal	Ready to Eat Dry	Familia
Cereal	Ready to Eat Dry	Familia
Cereal	Ready to Eat Dry	Familia
Cereal	Ready to Eat Dry	Familia
Cereal	Ready to Eat Dry	Familia
Cereal	Ready to Eat Dry	Featherweight
Cereal	Ready to Eat Dry	Featherweight
Cereal	Ready to Eat Dry	General Mills
Cereal	Ready to Eat Dry	General Mills
Cereal	Ready to Eat Dry	General Mills
Cereal	Ready to Eat Dry	General Mills
Cereal	Ready to Eat Dry	General Mills

Major Description	Minor Description	Serving Size	Calories	Grade
Oatmeal & Oats		1 pkt	110	B–+
Oatmeal & Oats	Apples & Cinnamon	1 pkt	150	A+
Oatmeal & Oats	Cinnamon Raisins	1 pkt	170	A+
Oatmeal & Oats	Maple & Brown Sugar	1 pkt	160	A+
Oatmeal & Oats		1 oz	90	B+
Wheat		1 oz	110	A
Wheat		1 oz	100	A+
Oat Bran		1 oz	100	B+
Oat Bran	Apple & Cinnamon	1 pkt	130	A+
Oat Bran	Honey	1 pkt	110	B–+
Mixed Grain	All Varieties	1 cup	330	B+
Amaranth Flakes		1 cup	130	A+
Apple Corns		1 cup	150	A+
Bran Flakes		1 cup	100	A+
Corn Flakes		1 cup	130	A+
Crispy Puffs		1 cup	80	A
Kamut Flakes		1 cup	120	A+
Maple Corns		1 cup	190	A+
Mixed Grain		1 cup	120	B+
Mixed Grain	Granola Maple Nut	1 cup	250	C+
Multigrain Flakes		1 cup	140	A+
Nature O's	Mixed Grain	1 cup	130	A+
Oat Bran Flakes		1 cup	110	B+
Puffed Corn		1 cup	80	A
Puffed Kamut		1 cup	50	A+
Puffed Millet		1 cup	90	A
Puffed Rice		1 cup	90	A
Puffed Wheat		1 cup	90	A+
Spelt Flakes		1 cup	100	A+
Wheat Bran		1 cup	30	A+
Wheat Flakes		1 cup	110	A+
Wheat Germ		1 cup	50	A+
Granola	Blueberries & Cream	1 cup	330	B+
Granola	Oat Bran	1 cup	360	C+
Granola	Raspberries & Cream	1 cup	330	B+
Granola	Strawberries & Cream	1 cup	330	B+
Oat	Bran	1 cup	662	D
Oat	Dates & Nuts	1 cup	660	C+
Oat	Maple	1 cup	660	C+
Oat	Spiced Apples	1 cup	630	C+
Oat	Sunflower Crunch	1 cup	660	C+
Champion		1 cup	200	B
Crunchy		1 cup	460	B
Mixed Grain	No Sugar Added	1 cup	412	B
Muesli	No Sugar Added	1 cup	400	A+
Muesli	Original	1 cup	420	A+*
Corn Flakes		1 cup	90	A
Crisp Rice		1 cup	110	A
Apple & Cinnamon Cheerios	Oat	1 cup	160	B–*
Basic 4		1 cup	170	A–+
Berry Berry Kix		1 cup	110	A–*
Body Buddies	Mixed Grain	1 cup	110	A–**
Booberry	Mixed Grain	1 cup	110	A–**

"+" indicates the food meets minimum fiber requirements; "–" indicates the food has a high sodium content.

Food	Processing Category	Brand
Cereal	Ready to Eat Dry	General Mills
Cereal	Ready to Eat Dry	General Mills
Cereal	Ready to Eat Dry	General Mills
Cereal	Ready to Eat Dry	General Mills
Cereal	Ready to Eat Dry	General Mills
Cereal	Ready to Eat Dry	General Mills
Cereal	Ready to Eat Dry	General Mills
Cereal	Ready to Eat Dry	General Mills
Cereal	Ready to Eat Dry	General Mills
Cereal	Ready to Eat Dry	General Mills
Cereal	Ready to Eat Dry	General Mills
Cereal	Ready to Eat Dry	General Mills
Cereal	Ready to Eat Dry	General Mills
Cereal	Ready to Eat Dry	General Mills
Cereal	Ready to Eat Dry	General Mills
Cereal	Ready to Eat Dry	General Mills
Cereal	Ready to Eat Dry	General Mills
Cereal	Ready to Eat Dry	General Mills
Cereal	Ready to Eat Dry	General Mills
Cereal	Ready to Eat Dry	General Mills
Cereal	Ready to Eat Dry	General Mills
Cereal	Ready to Eat Dry	General Mills
Cereal	Ready to Eat Dry	General Mills
Cereal	Ready to Eat Dry	General Mills
Cereal	Ready to Eat Dry	General Mills
Cereal	Ready to Eat Dry	General Mills
Cereal	Ready to Eat Dry	General Mills
Cereal	Ready to Eat Dry	General Mills
Cereal	Ready to Eat Dry	Health Valley
Cereal	Ready to Eat Dry	Health Valley
Cereal	Ready to Eat Dry	Health Valley
Cereal	Ready to Eat Dry	Health Valley
Cereal	Ready to Eat Dry	Health Valley
Cereal	Ready to Eat Dry	Health Valley
Cereal	Ready to Eat Dry	Health Valley
Cereal	Ready to Eat Dry	Health Valley
Cereal	Ready to Eat Dry	Health Valley
Cereal	Ready to Eat Dry	Health Valley
Cereal	Ready to Eat Dry	Health Valley
Cereal	Ready to Eat Dry	Health Valley
Cereal	Ready to Eat Dry	Health Valley
Cereal	Ready to Eat Dry	Health Valley 100% Natural
Cereal	Ready to Eat Dry	Health Valley 100% Natural
Cereal	Ready to Eat Dry	Health Valley Fiber 7 Flakes
Cereal	Ready to Eat Dry	Health Valley Flakes
Cereal	Ready to Eat Dry	Health Valley Flakes
Cereal	Ready to Eat Dry	Health Valley Flakes
Cereal	Ready to Eat Dry	Health Valley Flakes
Cereal	Ready to Eat Dry	Health Valley Fruit & Fitness
Cereal	Ready to Eat Dry	Health Valley Fruit Lites
Cereal	Ready to Eat Dry	Health Valley Fruit Lites

Major Description	Minor Description	Serving Size	Calories	Grade
Cheerios	Oat	1 cup	90	B–+
Cinnamon Toast	Mixed Grain	1 cup	160	B–*
Clusters	Wheat	1 cup	220	B–+
Cocoa Puffs	Corn	1 cup	110	A–**
Count Chocula	Corn	1 cup	110	A–**
Country Corn	Corn	1 cup	110	A–
Crispy Wheats		1 cup	133	A–+
Fiber One	Mixed Grain	1 cup	120	A–+
Frankenberry	Mixed Grain	1 cup	110	A–**
Golden Grahams	Mixed Grain	1 cup	145	A–
Hidden Treasures	Corn	1 cup	160	A**
Honey Nut Cheerios	Oat	1 cup	145	A–*
Kaboom	Mixed Grain	1 cup	110	A–
Kix	Mixed Grain	1 cup	75	A–
Lucky Charms		1 cup	110	A–
Multi Grain Cheerios	Mixed Grain	1 cup	100	A–+
Oatmeal Crisp		1 cup	220	B–
Oatmeal Crisp	With Apples	1 cup	260	A–*
Raisin Nut Bran	Raisins & Nuts	1 cup	220	B–+
Raisin Oat Bran	Raisins	1 cup	150	A+
Smores Grahams	Corn	1 cup	160	A–
Toasted Oat	Oat	1 cup	130	C
Total	Mixed Grain	1 cup	100	A–+
Total Corn Flakes		1 cup	110	A–
Total Raisin Bran		1 cup	140	A–+
Triples	Mixed Grain	1 cup	145	A–
Trix	Mixed Grain	1 cup	110	A–**
Wheaties		1 cup	100	A–+
Wheaties	Honey Gold	1 cup	130	A–*
10 Bran Os	All Varieties	1 cup	120	A+
Amaranth	Bananas	1 cup	200	B+
Amaranth	Flakes	1 cup	200	B+
Corn Flakes	Corn	1 cup	180	B+
Fat Free Granola	Dates & Almonds	1 cup	270	A+
Fat Free Granola	Raisins & Cinnamon	1 cup	270	A+
Fat Free Granola	Sprouts & Raisins	1 cup	240	A+
Fat Free Granola	Sprouts, Bananas & Fruit	1 cup	270	A+
Fat Free Granola	Tropical Fruit	1 cup	270	A+
Oat Bran Os		1 cup	120	B+
Oat Bran Os	Fruit & Nuts	1 cup	120	B+
Rice Bran Os		1 cup	145	A+
Rice Bran	with Almonds	1 cup	220	B+
Bran	Apples & Cinnamon	1 cup	280	A+
Bran	Raisins	1 cup	280	A+
Mixed Grain		1 cup	200	A+
Bran	Raisins	1 cup	200	A+
Oat Bran		1 cup	200	A+
Oat Bran	Almonds & Dates	1 cup	200	A+
Oat Bran	Raisins	1 cup	200	A+
Mixed Grain	Fruit	1 cup	190	A+
Corn	Fruit	1 cup	90	A
Wheat	Fruit	1 cup	90	A+

"+" indicates the food meets minimum fiber requirements; "–" indicates the food has a high sodium content.

Food	Processing Category	Brand
Cereal	Ready to Eat Dry	Health Valley Healthy Os
Cereal	Ready to Eat Dry	Health Valley Lites
Cereal	Ready to Eat Dry	Health Valley Lites
Cereal	Ready to Eat Dry	Health Valley Lites
Cereal	Ready to Eat Dry	Health Valley Lites
Cereal	Ready to Eat Dry	Health Valley Organic
Cereal	Ready to Eat Dry	Health Valley Organic
Cereal	Ready to Eat Dry	Health Valley
Cereal	Ready to Eat Dry	Health Valley
Cereal	Ready to Eat Dry	Health Valley
Cereal	Ready to Eat Dry	Heartland
Cereal	Ready to Eat Dry	Heartland
Cereal	Ready to Eat Dry	Heartland
Cereal	Ready to Eat Dry	Kashi
Cereal	Ready to Eat Dry	Kashi
Cereal	Ready to Eat Dry	Kellogg's
Cereal	Ready to Eat Dry	Kellogg's
Cereal	Ready to Eat Dry	Kellogg's
Cereal	Ready to Eat Dry	Kellogg's
Cereal	Ready to Eat Dry	Kellogg's
Cereal	Ready to Eat Dry	Kellogg's
Cereal	Ready to Eat Dry	Kellogg's
Cereal	Ready to Eat Dry	Kellogg's
Cereal	Ready to Eat Dry	Kellogg's
Cereal	Ready to Eat Dry	Kellogg's
Cereal	Ready to Eat Dry	Kellogg's
Cereal	Ready to Eat Dry	Kellogg's
Cereal	Ready to Eat Dry	Kellogg's
Cereal	Ready to Eat Dry	Kellogg's
Cereal	Ready to Eat Dry	Kellogg's
Cereal	Ready to Eat Dry	Kellogg's
Cereal	Ready to Eat Dry	Kellogg's
Cereal	Ready to Eat Dry	Kellogg's
Cereal	Ready to Eat Dry	Kellogg's
Cereal	Ready to Eat Dry	Kellogg's
Cereal	Ready to Eat Dry	Kellogg's
Cereal	Ready to Eat Dry	Kellogg's
Cereal	Ready to Eat Dry	Kellogg's
Cereal	Ready to Eat Dry	Kellogg's
Cereal	Ready to Eat Dry	Kellogg's
Cereal	Ready to Eat Dry	Kellogg's
Cereal	Ready to Eat Dry	Kellogg's
Cereal	Ready to Eat Dry	Kellogg's
Cereal	Ready to Eat Dry	Kellogg's
Cereal	Ready to Eat Dry	Kellogg's
Cereal	Ready to Eat Dry	Kellogg's
Cereal	Ready to Eat Dry	Kellogg's Healthy Choice
Cereal	Ready to Eat Dry	Kellogg's Healthy Choice

Major Description	Minor Description	Serving Size	Calories	Grade
Mixed Grain		1 cup	130	A+
Puffed Corn		1 cup	100	A
Puffed Rice		1 cup	100	A
Puffed Wheat		1 cup	100	A+
Rice	Fruit	1 cup	90	A
Bran	Apple & Cinnamon	1 cup	225	A+
Bran	Raisins	1 cup	253	A+
Oat Bran	Almond Crunch	1 cup	375	B+
Oat Bran	Fruit Hawaiian	1 cup	440	B+
Oat Bran	Raisins & Nuts	1 cup	375	B+
Mixed Grain	Coconut	1 cup	500	C+
Mixed Grain	Natural	1 cup	480	B+
Mixed Grain	Raisins	1 cup	480	B+
Mixed Grain	Medley	1 cup	200	A+
Mixed Grain	Puffed	1 cup	70	A+
40% Bran Flakes		1 cup	180	A–+
All-Bran	Extra Fiber	1 cup	100	B–+
All-Bran	Original	1 cup	160	A–+
Apple Cinnamon Squares	Apple & Cinnamon	1 cup	235	A+
Apple Jacks		1 cup	110	A**
Blueberry Squares	Blueberry Filled	1 cup	235	A+
Cocoa Krispies		1 cup	160	A–**
Common Sense	Oat Bran	1 cup	200	A–+
Common Sense	Oat Bran	1 cup	145	A–
Common Sense	Oat Bran & Raisins	1 cup	240	A–+
Complete Bran	Wheat	1 cup	100	A–+
Corn Flakes		1 cup	110	A–
Corn Pops		1 cup	110	A**
Cracklin Oat Bran		1 cup	300	C+*
Crispix	Mixed Grain	1 cup	110	A–
Frosted Flakes	Corn	1 cup	160	A–**
Frosted Krispies	Rice	1 cup	145	A–**
Frosted Mini Wheats	Shredded	1 cup	190	A+*
Fruit & Fibre	Tropical Fruit & Oat Clusters	1 cup	96	B–+
Fruit Loops		1 cup	120	A–**
Fruitful Bran	Fruit	1 cup	165	A–+
Heartwise	Bran	1 cup	90	A–+
Honey Smacks		1 cup	145	A**
Just Right	Fiber Nuggets	1 cup	150	A–+
Just Right	Fruit & Nuts	1 cup	200	A–+
Low Fat Granola	without Raisins	1 cup	420	A*
Low Fat Granola	with Raisins	1 cup	300	A+*
Mueslix	Crispy Blend	1 cup	300	A+*
Product 19		1 cup	110	A–
Raisin Bran		1 cup	170	A–+**
Raisin Squares	Raisin Filled	1 cup	180	A+*
Rice Krispies		1 cup	90	A–
Rice Krispies	Apples & Cinnamon	1 cup	145	A–**
Shredded Wheat	Strawberry Filled	1 cup	180	A+
Special K		1 cup	110	A–
Mixed Grain	Brown Sugar	1 cup	110	A–+
Multigrain Squares	Honey	1 cup	150	A+

"+" indicates the food meets minimum fiber requirements; "–" indicates the food has a high sodium content.

Food	Processing Category	Brand
Cereal	Ready to Eat Dry	Kellogg's Nutri-Grain
Cereal	Ready to Eat Dry	Kellogg's Nutri-Grain
Cereal	Ready to Eat Dry	Kellogg's Nutri-Grain
Cereal	Ready to Eat Dry	Nabisco
Cereal	Ready to Eat Dry	Nabisco
Cereal	Ready to Eat Dry	Nabisco
Cereal	Ready to Eat Dry	Nabisco
Cereal	Ready to Eat Dry	Nature Valley
Cereal	Ready to Eat Dry	Nature Valley
Cereal	Ready to Eat Dry	Nature Valley
Cereal	Ready to Eat Dry	Nature Valley
Cereal	Ready to Eat Dry	Post
Cereal	Ready to Eat Dry	Post
Cereal	Ready to Eat Dry	Post
Cereal	Ready to Eat Dry	Post
Cereal	Ready to Eat Dry	Post
Cereal	Ready to Eat Dry	Post
Cereal	Ready to Eat Dry	Post
Cereal	Ready to Eat Dry	Post
Cereal	Ready to Eat Dry	Post
Cereal	Ready to Eat Dry	Post
Cereal	Ready to Eat Dry	Post
Cereal	Ready to Eat Dry	Post
Cereal	Ready to Eat Dry	Post
Cereal	Ready to Eat Dry	Post
Cereal	Ready to Eat Dry	Post
Cereal	Ready to Eat Dry	Post
Cereal	Ready to Eat Dry	Post
Cereal	Ready to Eat Dry	Post
Cereal	Ready to Eat Dry	Post
Cereal	Ready to Eat Dry	Post
Cereal	Ready to Eat Dry	Post
Cereal	Ready to Eat Dry	Post
Cereal	Ready to Eat Dry	Post
Cereal	Ready to Eat Dry	Post
Cereal	Ready to Eat Dry	Quaker
Cereal	Ready to Eat Dry	Quaker
Cereal	Ready to Eat Dry	Quaker
Cereal	Ready to Eat Dry	Quaker
Cereal	Ready to Eat Dry	Quaker
Cereal	Ready to Eat Dry	Quaker
Cereal	Ready to Eat Dry	Quaker
Cereal	Ready to Eat Dry	Quaker
Cereal	Ready to Eat Dry	Quaker
Cereal	Ready to Eat Dry	Quaker
Cereal	Ready to Eat Dry	Quaker
Cereal	Ready to Eat Dry	Quaker
Cereal	Ready to Eat Dry	Quaker
Cereal	Ready to Eat Dry	Quaker

Major Description	Minor Description	Serving Size	Calories	Grade
Mixed Grain	Almonds & Raisins	1 cup	160	A–+
Mixed Grain	Golden Wheat	1 cup	130	A–+
Wheat	Raisins	1 cup	195	A–+
100% Bran		1 cup	140	B–+
Shredded Wheat		1 cup	170	A+
Shredded Wheat N Bran	Bran	1 cup	135	A+
Spoon Size Mini Wheat		1 cup	90	A+
100% Natural	Cinnamon & Raisins	1 cup	360	B
100% Natural	Mixed Grain	1 cup	390	C
Fruit & Nut	Oat	1 cup	390	C
Toasted Oat		1 cup	390	A
Alpha Bits		1 cup	130	A**
Banana Nut Crunch		1 cup	250	B+
Blueberry Morning		1 cup	184	A
Brannola	Wheat with Raisins	1 cup	400	A+*
Cocoa Pebbles	Rice	1 cup	160	A–**
Fruit & Fibre	Dates, Raisins & Walnuts	1 cup	210	A+*
Fruit & Fibre	Peaches, Raisins & Almonds	1 cup	210	A–+
Fruity Pebbles	Rice	1 cup	125	A–
Golden Crisp	Wheat	1 cup	140	A**
Grape-Nuts		1 cup	110	A–+
Grape-Nuts	Flakes	1 cup	100	A–+
Grape-Nuts	Raisins	1 cup	100	A–+
Grape-Nuts	Wheat & Barley	1 cup	400	A–+
Great Grains	Crunchy Pecans	1 cup	330	B+
Great Grains	Raisin, Dates & Pecans	1 cup	315	B+
Hearty Granola		1 cup	440	C*
Honey Bunches of Oats	Almonds	1 cup	173	B–
Honey Bunches of Oats	Honey Roasted	1 cup	160	A–
Honeycomb	Corn	1 cup	90	A–**
Honeycomb	Mixed Grain	1 cup	83	A–**
Natural Bran Flakes	All Varieties	1 cup	135	A–+
Natural Raisin Bran		1 cup	170	A–+**
Oat Flakes		1 cup	165	A+
Toasties		1 cup	110	A–
Toasties Corn Flakes		1 cup	110	A–
Cap'n Crunch		1 cup	145	A–**
Cap'n Crunch	Peanut Butter	1 cup	145	B–*
Cap'n Crunch	with Crunch Berries	1 cup	130	A–**
Cinnamon Oat Squares		1 cup	230	A+
Crunchy Bran		1 cup	89	A–+
Crunchy Bran		1 cup	120	A–+
Honey Graham Chex		1 cup	110	A–
Honey Graham Ohs		1 cup	122	B–
Kids Favorites	Frosted Flakes	1 cup	145	A–*
Kids Favorites	Marshmallow	1 cup	160	A–**
King Vitamin		1 cup	80	A–
Kretschmer Wheatgerm	Original	2 Tbsp	50	B+
Kretschmer Wheatgerm	Honey	2 Tbsp	60	B+
Life		1 cup	160	A–+

"+" indicates the food meets minimum fiber requirements; "–" indicates the food has a high sodium content.

Food	Processing Category	Brand
Cereal	Ready to Eat Dry	Quaker
Cereal	Ready to Eat Dry	Quaker
Cereal	Ready to Eat Dry	Quaker
Cereal	Ready to Eat Dry	Quaker
Cereal	Ready to Eat Dry	Quaker
Cereal	Ready to Eat Dry	Quaker
Cereal	Ready to Eat Dry	Quaker
Cereal	Ready to Eat Dry	Quaker
Cereal	Ready to Eat Dry	Quaker
Cereal	Ready to Eat Dry	Quaker
Cereal	Ready to Eat Dry	Quaker
Cereal	Ready to Eat Dry	Quaker
Cereal	Ready to Eat Dry	Quaker
Cereal	Ready to Eat Dry	Quaker
Cereal	Ready to Eat Dry	Quaker
Cereal	Ready to Eat Dry	Quaker
Cereal	Ready to Eat Dry	Quaker
Cereal	Ready to Eat Dry	Quaker
Cereal	Ready to Eat Dry	Quaker 100% Natural
Cereal	Ready to Eat Dry	Quaker 100% Natural
Cereal	Ready to Eat Dry	Quaker 100% Natural
Cereal	Ready to Eat Dry	Quaker 100% Natural
Cereal	Ready to Eat Dry	Quaker 100% Natural
Cereal	Ready to Eat Dry	Ralston
Cereal	Ready to Eat Dry	Ralston
Cereal	Ready to Eat Dry	Ralston
Cereal	Ready to Eat Dry	Ralston
Cereal	Ready to Eat Dry	Ralston
Cereal	Ready to Eat Dry	Ralston
Cereal	Ready to Eat Dry	Ralston
Cereal	Ready to Eat Dry	Ralston
Cereal	Ready to Eat Dry	Ralston
Cereal	Ready to Eat Dry	Ralston
Cereal	Ready to Eat Dry	Ralston
Cereal	Ready to Eat Dry	Ralston
Cereal	Ready to Eat Dry	Ralston
Cereal	Ready to Eat Dry	Ralston
Cereal	Ready to Eat Dry	Ralston
Cereal	Ready to Eat Dry	Ralston
Cereal	Ready to Eat Dry	Ralston
Cereal	Ready to Eat Dry	Ralston
Cereal	Ready to Eat Dry	Ralston
Cereal	Ready to Eat Dry	Ralston
Cereal	Ready to Eat Dry	Ralston
Cereal	Ready to Eat Dry	Sun Country
Cereal	Ready to Eat Dry	Sun Country 100% Natural

Major Description	Minor Description	Serving Size	Calories	Grade
Low Fat 100% Natural	Whole Grain with Raisins	1 cup	380	A+*
Oat Bran		1 cup	135	A+
Oat Life	Cinnamon	1 cup	190	A+*
Oat Mms	Toasted	1 cup	110	A–+
Oat Squares		1 cup	220	A+
Ohs	Honey Graham	1 cup	145	B–**
Popeye	Sweet Crunch	1 cup	110	A–**
Popeye	Cocoa Blasts	1 cup	130	A**
Popeye	Fruit Curls	1 cup	120	A–**
Popeye Jeepers	Crispy Corn Puff	1 cup	82	A–**
Popeye Jeepers	Oat	1 cup	82	A–**
Popeye Oat Mms		1 cup	120	A–+
Puffed Rice		1 cup	50	A
Puffed Wheat		1 cup	33	A+
Shredded Wheat	Original Size	2 pieces	145	A+
Sweet Puffs		1 cup	130	A**
Toasted Oatmeal	Honey & Nut	1 cup	200	B+
Toasted Oatmeal	Original	1 cup	160	A–+
Unprocessed Bran		1 cup	90	A+
Mixed Grain		1 cup	500	C+
Mixed Grain	Apple & Cinnamon	1 cup	500	C
Mixed Grain	Raisins & Dates	1 cup	500	C
Oat	Honey	1 cup	440	C
Oat	Honey & Raisins	1 cup	440	C+*
Bran News	Apple Spice or Cinnamon	1 cup	130	A–+
Cookie Crisp	Chocolate Chip	1 cup	110	A–**
Cookie Crisp	Vanilla Wafer	1 cup	110	A–**
Corn Chex		1 cup	88	A–
Crispy Mini Grahams		1 cup	110	A–*
Dinersaurs		1 cup	110	A
Double Chex		1 cup	165	A–*
Frosted Chex Jr.		1 cup	145	A–*
Fruit Muesli	Raisins, Walnuts & Cranberries	1 cup	300	B+
Graham Chex		1 cup	165	A–*
Honey Almond Delight		1 cup	145	B–*
Muesli	Raisin Peaches & Pecans	1 cup	300	B+
Muesli	Raisins, Dates & Almonds	1 cup	280	A+
Muesli	Raspberries & Almonds	1 cup	300	B+
Mueslix	Bananas & Walnuts	1 cup	300	B+
Mueslix	Cranberries & Walnuts	1 cup	300	B+
Mueslix	Dates & Almonds	1 cup	280	A+
Mueslix	Peaches & Pecans	1 cup	300	B+
Multi-Bran Chex	Raspberries & Almonds	1 cup	150	A–+
Rice & Chex		1 cup	100	A–
Sun Flakes		1 cup	100	A–
Tmn Turtles		1 cup	110	A–**
Wheat Chex	Whole Grain	1 cup	150	A–+
Mixed Grain	Granola with Raisins	1 cup	500	C
Mixed Grain	Granola with Almonds	1 cup	520	C

"+" indicates the food meets minimum fiber requirements; "–" indicates the food has a high sodium content.

Food	Processing Category	Brand
Cereal	Ready to Eat Dry	Sun Country 100% Natural
Cereal	Ready to Eat Dry	Sun Country Granola
Cereal	Ready to Eat Dry	Sun Country Granola
Cereal	Ready to Eat Dry	Sunbelt
Cereal	Ready to Eat Dry	Sunbelt
Cereal	Ready to Eat Dry	Sunflakes
Cereal	Ready to Eat Dry	Sunshine
Cereal	Ready to Eat Dry	Sunshine
Cereal Bar	Packaged	Carnation
Cereal Bar	Packaged	Carnation
Cereal Bar	Packaged	Carnation
Cereal Bar	Packaged	Carnation
Cereal Bar	Packaged	Carnation
Cereal Bar	Packaged	Carnation
Cereal Bar	Packaged	Figurines 100 Diet Bar
Cereal Bar	Packaged	Health Valley
Cereal Bar	Packaged	Health Valley
Cereal Bar	Packaged	Health Valley
Cereal Bar	Packaged	Health Valley Apple Bakes
Cereal Bar	Packaged	Health Valley Apple Bakes
Cereal Bar	Packaged	Health Valley Breakfast Bars
Cereal Bar	Packaged	Health Valley Brownie Bars
Cereal Bar	Packaged	Health Valley Fat Free
Cereal Bar	Packaged	Health Valley Fat Free Bakes
Cereal Bar	Packaged	Health Valley Fruit & Fitness
Cereal Bar	Packaged	Health Valley Fruit Bars
Cereal Bar	Packaged	Health Valley Oat Bran Apricot Bakes
Cereal Bar	Packaged	Health Valley Oat Bran Jumbo Fruit
Cereal Bar	Packaged	Health Valley Oat Bran Jumbo Fruit
Cereal Bar	Packaged	Health Valley Oat Bran Jumbo Fruit
Cereal Bar	Packaged	Health Valley Raisin Bakes
Cereal Bar	Packaged	Health Valley Rice Bran Jumbo
Cereal Bar	Packaged	Hershey's
Cereal Bar	Packaged	Hershey's
Cereal Bar	Packaged	Hershey's
Cereal Bar	Packaged	Hershey's
Cereal Bar	Packaged	Kellogg's
Cereal Bar	Packaged	Kellogg's
Cereal Bar	Packaged	Kellogg's Nutri-Grain
Cereal Bar	Packaged	Kellogg's Smart Start
Cereal Bar	Packaged	Kellogg's Smart Start
Cereal Bar	Packaged	Kellogg's Smart Start
Cereal Bar	Packaged	Kellogg's Smart Start
Cereal Bar	Packaged	Kudos
Cereal Bar	Packaged	Kudos
Cereal Bar	Packaged	Kudos
Cereal Bar	Packaged	Kudos
Cereal Bar	Packaged	Kudos
Cereal Bar	Packaged	Kudos
Cereal Bar	Packaged	Kudos

Major Description	Minor Description	Serving Size	Calories	Grade
Mixed Grain	Granola with Raisins & Dates	1 cup	600	C
Mixed Grain	Almonds	1 cup	540	B
Mixed Grain	Raisins & Dates	1 cup	520	B+*
Mixed Grain	Granola, Bananas & Almonds	1 cup	500	B
Mixed Grain	Granola, Fruit & Nuts	1 cup	480	C
Multi-grain		1 cup	100	A–+
Shredded Wheat		2 pieces	180	A
Shredded Wheat	Bite Size	1 cup	165	A
Breakfast	Chocolate Chip	1 bar	150	C
Breakfast	Chocolate Chunk	1 bar	140	A
Breakfast	Chocolate Crunch	1 bar	190	D–
Breakfast	Honey Oat Granola	1 bar	130	B
Breakfast	Peanut Butter	1 bar	140	A
Breakfast	Peanut Butter & Chocolate Chip	1 bar	150	A
All Varieties		1 bar	100	D
Granola	Blueberry Apple	1 bar	140	A+
Granola	Date Almond	1 bar	140	A+
Granola	Raspberry	1 bar	140	A+
Apple		1 bar	100	B+
Date		1 bar	100	B+
Breakfast	All Varieties	1 bar	110	A+
Brownie	All Varieties	1 bar	110	A+
Snack	All Varieties	1 bar	140	A+
Snack	All Varieties	1 bar	90	A+
Fruit		1 bar	100	A+
Fruit	All Varieties	1 bar	100	A+
Oat Bran	Apricot	1 bar	100	B+
Oat Bran	Almond Date	1 bar	170	B+
Oat Bran	Fruit Nut	1 bar	150	B+
Oat Bran	Raisin Cinnamon	1 bar	140	A+
Raisin		1 bar	100	B+
Rice Bran	Almond Date	1 bar	190	B+
Chocolate	Cocoa Cream	1 bar	180	D
Chocolate	Cookies Cream	1 bar	170	D
Chocolate Coated	Chocolate Chip	1 bar	170	D
Chocolate Coated	Peanut Butter	1 bar	180	D
Granola	Low Fat, Apple Spice	1 bar	80	B
Granola	Low Fat, Crunchy Oats	1 bar	80	B
Fruit	All Flavors	1 bar	140	B
Common Sense	Raspberry Filled	1 bar	170	C
Corn Flakes	Mixed Berry	1 bar	170	C
Raisin Bran		1 bar	160	B
Rice Krispies	Almonds	1 bar	130	D
Chocolate Chip		1 bar	120	C
Chocolate Coated	Peanut Butter	1 bar	190	D
Chocolate Nut		1 bar	90	B
Fudge Nutty		1 bar	130	C
Honey Nut		1 bar	90	B
Oatmeal Raisin		1 bar	90	B
Peanut Butter		1 bar	130	C

"+" indicates the food meets minimum fiber requirements; "–" indicates the food has a high sodium content.

Food	Processing Category	Brand
Cereal Bar	Packaged	Nabisco Snack Wells
Cereal Bar	Packaged	Nature Valley
Cereal Bar	Packaged	Nature Valley
Cereal Bar	Packaged	Nature Valley
Cereal Bar	Packaged	Nature Valley
Cereal Bar	Packaged	Quaker Chewy
Cereal Bar	Packaged	Quaker Chewy
Cereal Bar	Packaged	Quaker Chewy
Cereal Bar	Packaged	Quaker Chewy
Cereal Bar	Packaged	Quaker Chewy
Cereal Bar	Packaged	Quaker Chewy
Cereal Bar	Packaged	Quaker Chewy
Cereal Bar	Packaged	Quaker Chewy
Cereal Bar	Packaged	Quaker Chewy Low Fat
Cereal Bar	Packaged	Quaker Chewy Low Fat
Cereal Bar	Packaged	Quaker Granola Dipps
Cereal Bar	Packaged	Quaker Granola Dipps
Cereal Bar	Packaged	Quaker Granola Dipps
Cereal Bar	Packaged	Quaker Granola Dipps
Cereal Bar	Packaged	Quaker Granola Dipps
Cereal Bar	Packaged	Sunbelt
Cereal Bar	Packaged	Sunbelt
Cereal Bar	Packaged	Sunbelt
Cereal Bar	Packaged	Sunbelt
Cereal Bar	Packaged	Sunbelt
Cereal Bar	Packaged	Sunbelt
Cereal Bar	Packaged	Sunbelt
Cereal Bar	Packaged	Sunbelt
Corn Cakes	Packaged	Mother's
Corn Cakes	Packaged	Mother's
Corn Cakes	Packaged	Quaker
Corn Cakes	Packaged	Quaker
Corn Cakes	Packaged	Quaker
Corn Grits	Dry	Generic
Corn Grits	Dry	Albers Hominy Quick Grits
Corn Grits	Dry	Arrowhead Mills
Corn Grits	Dry	Arrowhead Mills
Corn Grits	Dry	Enriched Quaker Quick
Corn Grits	Dry	Enriched Tones
Corn Grits	Dry	Quaker/Aunt Jemima
Corn Grits	Dry	Quaker
Corn Grits	Dry	Quaker
Corn Grits	Dry	Quaker
Corn Grits	Dry	Quaker
Cornmeal	Dry	All Brands
Cornmeal	Dry	All Brands
Cornmeal	Dry	All Brands
Cornmeal	Dry	All Brands
Cornmeal	Dry	All Brands
Cornmeal	Dry	Arrowhead Mills
Cornmeal	Dry	Arrowhead Mills
Cornmeal	Dry	Aunt Jemima

Major Description	Minor Description	Serving Size	Calories	Grade
Fruit	All Flavors	1 bar	120	A
Cinnamon		1 bar	120	C
Oat Bran & Honey Graham		1 bar	110	C
Oats & Honey		1 bar	120	C
Peanut Butter		1 bar	120	D
Chocolate Chip		1 bar	128	C
Chunky	Nuts & Raisin	1 bar	131	C
Granola	Caramel Apple	1 bar	120	B
Oats & Honey		1 bar	125	C
Peanut Butter		1 bar	128	C
Peanut Butter & Chocolate Chip		1 bar	131	C
Raisins & Cinnamon		1 bar	128	C
S'mores		1 bar	126	C
Granola	Apple Berry	1 bar	110	B
Granola	Chocolate Chunk	1 bar	110	B
Chocolate Fudge		1 bar	160	D
Granola	Caramel Nut	1 bar	148	D
Granola	Chocolate Chip	1 bar	139	D
Granola	Chocolate Chip & Peanut Butter	1 bar	174	D
Granola	Peanut Butter	1 bar	170	D
Chewy	Almonds	1 bar	120	D
Chewy	Chocolate Chips	1 bar	150	D
Chewy	Fudge Dipped	1 bar	220	C
Chewy	Raisins	1 bar	150	C
Fudge Dipped, Chewy	Chocolate Chip	1 bar	220	D
Fudge Dipped, Chewy	Oats & Honey	1 bar	190	D
Fudge Dipped, Chewy	Peanuts	1 bar	300	D
Fudge Dipped, Chewy	Raisins	1 bar	200	D
Butter		1 cake	35	A
Popped		1 cake	35	A
Caramel		1 cake	40	A–
Nacho		1 cake	40	A–
White Cheddar		1 cake	40	A–
		1/4 cup	145	A
Instant		1/4 cup	75	A
White		1/4 cup	150	A
Yellow		1/4 cup	150	A
Yellow		1/4 cup	135	A
Yellow		1/4 cup	144	A
White, Enriched		1/4 cup	133	A
Instant	Cheddar Cheese Flavor	1 pkt	104	A–
Instant	Imitation Bacon Bits	1 pkt	101	A–
Instant	Imitation Ham Bits	1 pkt	99	A–+
Instant	White Hominy	1 pkt	79	A–+
Degermed		1/4 cup	138	A
Self-Rising		1/4 cup	109	A–
Self-Rising	Degermed	1/4 cup	120	A–
Self-Rising	Wheat Flour	1/4 cup	157	A–
Whole Grain		1/4 cup	137	A+
Whole Grain	Blue	1/4 cup	138	A+
Whole Grain	Yellow or High Lysine	1/4 cup	138	A+
Self-Rising	White Enriched Bolted	1/4 cup	121	A–

"+" indicates the food meets minimum fiber requirements; "–" indicates the food has a high sodium content.

Food	Processing Category	Brand
Cornmeal	Dry	Aunt Jemima
Cornmeal	Dry	Tones
Cornmeal Mix	Dry	Aunt Jemima
Cornmeal Mix	Dry	Aunt Jemima
Cornmeal Mix	Dry	Aunt Jemima
Cornstarch	Dry	All Brands
Cottonseed Kernels	Dry	All Brands
Cottonseed Meal	Dry	All Brands
Couscous [5]	Cooked	Generic
Couscous	Mix	Casbah
Couscous	Mix	Fantastic Foods
Couscous	Mix	Fantastic Foods
Couscous	Mix	Fantastic Foods
Couscous	Mix	Fantastic Foods
Couscous	Mix	Fantastic Foods
Couscous	Mix	Knorr Pilafs
Couscous	Mix	Near East
Couscous	Mix	Quik Pilaf
Cracker Crumbs & Meal	Packaged	Golden Dipt
Cracker Crumbs & Meal	Packaged	Manischewitz Daily
Cracker Crumbs & Meal	Packaged	Manischewitz Farfel
Crackers	Packaged	Bran Thins
Crackers	Packaged	Carr's
Crackers	Packaged	Carr's
Crackers	Packaged	Carr's Table Water Bite Size
Crackers	Packaged	Cheese Nips
Crackers	Packaged	Cheez-it
Crackers	Packaged	Cheez-it Low Salt
Crackers	Packaged	Chicken in a Biskit
Crackers	Packaged	Combos
Crackers	Packaged	Combos
Crackers	Packaged	Crisp & Light Cracker Bread
Crackers	Packaged	Crown Pilot
Crackers	Packaged	Dandy
Crackers	Packaged	Dar-vida
Crackers	Packaged	Dar-vida
Crackers	Packaged	Devonsheer
Crackers	Packaged	Devonsheer Rounds
Crackers	Packaged	Devonsheer Rounds
Crackers	Packaged	Devonsheer Rounds
Crackers	Packaged	Devonsheer Rounds
Crackers	Packaged	Devonsheer Rounds
Crackers	Packaged	Devonsheer Rounds
Crackers	Packaged	Devonsheer Unsalted
Crackers	Packaged	Devonsheer Unsalted Rounds
Crackers	Packaged	Escort
Crackers	Packaged	Estee
Crackers	Packaged	Estee Snax
Crackers	Packaged	Estee Unsalted
Crackers	Packaged	Featherweight Low Salt
Crackers	Packaged	FFV Crisp
Crackers	Packaged	FFV Crisp
Crackers	Packaged	FFV Crispy Wafer

[5] Serving size where $1/2$ cup cooked equals approximately $1/6$ cup dry.

Major Description	Minor Description	Serving Size	Calories	Grade
White or Yellow, Enriched		$1/4$ cup	136	A
Yellow Bolted		$1/4$ cup	101	A+
Buttermilk, Self-Rising, White		$1/4$ cup	135	A–
White, Bolted		$1/4$ cup	132	A–
Yellow, Self-Rising		$1/4$ cup	133	A–
		$1/2$ cup	244	A
Roasted		$1/2$ cup	372	D
Partially Defatted		$1/2$ cup	170	A
		$1/2$ cup	100	A
Pilaf		$1/2$ cup	100	A
		$1/2$ cup	105	A
Lentils		$1/2$ cup	93	A+
Pilaf	Savory	$1/2$ cup	102	A–+
Whole Wheat		$1/2$ cup	90	A+
Whole Wheat	with Butter	$1/2$ cup	111	B
Spicy		$1/2$ cup	160	A–
		$1/2$ cup	120	A
Pilaf	Savory	$1/2$ cup	94	A–
		.5 oz	50	A
Matzo Meal		1 cup	514	A
Matzo		1 cup	280	A
Bran, Toasted		.5 oz	60	D
Croissant		.5 oz	70	D
Whole Wheat		.5 oz	58	A
Soda or Water		.5 oz	20	C
Cheese Flavor		.5 oz	70	C–
Cheese Flavor		.5 oz	80	D–
Cheese Flavor		.5 oz	80	D
Chicken Flavor		.5 oz	80	D–
Cheese or Cheese Flavor		.5 oz	67	C–
Peanut Butter		.5 oz	67	C–
		1 slice	17	A
Soda or Water		.5 oz	70	B
Soup & Oyster		.5 oz	60	B–
Crisp Bread		1 piece	20	A–
Crisp Bread	Sesame	1 piece	22	D–
Melba Toast	All Varieties	.5 oz	48	B–
Melba Toast	Garlic	.5 oz	56	B–
Melba Toast	Honey Bran	.5 oz	52	B–+
Melba Toast	Onion	.5 oz	51	A–+
Melba Toast	Plain	.5 oz	53	A–+
Melba Toast	Rye	.5 oz	53	A–+
Melba Toast	Sesame	.5 oz	57	B–+
Melba Toast	All Varieties	.5 oz	48	B
Melba Toast	Plain	.5 oz	52	A+
Butter Flavor		.5 oz	70	D–
Melba Toast	Wheat	1 piece	6	A
Melba Toast	Wheat	.5 oz	50	A
		1 piece	15	B
		1 piece	15	B
Sesame		.5 oz	60	B–
Sesame	Wafer	.5 oz	60	B–
Wheat		.5 oz	70	C

"+" indicates the food meets minimum fiber requirements; "–" indicates the food has a high sodium content.

Food	Processing Category	Brand
Crackers	Packaged	FFV Ocean Crisps
Crackers	Packaged	FFV Schooners
Crackers	Packaged	FFV Stoned Wheat Wafer
Crackers	Packaged	Fiberrich
Crackers	Packaged	Finn Crisp
Crackers	Packaged	Finn Crisp Hi-Fiber
Crackers	Packaged	Finn Crisp Hi-Fiber
Crackers	Packaged	Frookies
Crackers	Packaged	Frookies
Crackers	Packaged	Frookies
Crackers	Packaged	Frookies
Crackers	Packaged	Guppies
Crackers	Packaged	Hain
Crackers	Packaged	Hain
Crackers	Packaged	Hain
Crackers	Packaged	Hain
Crackers	Packaged	Hain
Crackers	Packaged	Hain
Crackers	Packaged	Hain
Crackers	Packaged	Hain
Crackers	Packaged	Hain
Crackers	Packaged	Hain
Crackers	Packaged	Hain
Crackers	Packaged	Hain Low Salt
Crackers	Packaged	Hain No Salt Added
Crackers	Packaged	Hain No Salt Added
Crackers	Packaged	Hain No Salt Added
Crackers	Packaged	Hain No Salt Added
Crackers	Packaged	Hain No Salt Added
Crackers	Packaged	Hain Rich
Crackers	Packaged	Hain Rich No Salt Added
Crackers	Packaged	Handi Snacks
Crackers	Packaged	Handi Snacks
Crackers	Packaged	Handi Snacks
Crackers	Packaged	Harvest Crisps
Crackers	Packaged	Harvest Crisps
Crackers	Packaged	Health Valley
Crackers	Packaged	Health Valley Fat Free
Crackers	Packaged	Health Valley Stoned Wheat
Crackers	Packaged	Health Valley Stoned Wheat
Crackers	Packaged	Health Valley Stoned Wheat
Crackers	Packaged	Health Valley Stoned Wheat
Crackers	Packaged	Hickory Farms Old Fashioned
Crackers	Packaged	Hickory Farms Rounds O Rye
Crackers	Packaged	Hickory Farms Rounds O Rye
Crackers	Packaged	Hickory Farms Rounds O Rye
Crackers	Packaged	Hickory Farms Rounds O Rye
Crackers	Packaged	Hickory Farms Salt Free
Crackers	Packaged	Hickory Farms Stoned Wheat
Crackers	Packaged	Hickory Farms Wafers
Crackers	Packaged	Hickory Farms Wafers
Crackers	Packaged	Hickory Farms Wheat Mill Wafers

Major Description	Minor Description	Serving Size	Calories	Grade
Soda or Water		.5 oz	60	B–
		.5 oz	60	B–
Wheat		.5 oz	60	B–
Bran		1 piece	18	A+
Crisp Bread	Dark, Regular or with Caraway Seeds	1 piece	19	A–+
Rye	Light	1 piece	35	B–
Rye	Original	1 piece	40	A–
Garlic & Herb		.5 oz	49	A–
Pepper		.5 oz	49	A
Water		.5 oz	49	A–
Whole Wheat		.5 oz	49	A–
Cheddar Cheese Flavor		.5 oz	40	D–
Cheese Flavor		.5 oz	65	D–
Herb	Fat Free	.5 oz	60	A–
Onion		.5 oz	65	D
Onion	Fat Free	.5 oz	60	A–
Rye		.5 oz	60	B–
Sesame		.5 oz	70	D–
Sour Cream & Chive		.5 oz	65	D
Sourdough		.5 oz	65	D–
Vegetable		.5 oz	65	C–
Vegetable	Fat Free	.5 oz	60	A–
Whole Wheat	Fat Free	.5 oz	50	A–
Sourdough		.5 oz	65	C
Onion		.5 oz	65	D
Rye		.5 oz	60	B
Sesame		.5 oz	70	D
Sour Cream & Chive		.5 oz	65	D
Vegetable		.5 oz	65	C
		.5 oz	65	C
		.5 oz	65	C
Cheese Sandwich		1 pkg	120	D–
Peanut Butter		1 pkg	190	D
with Bacon & Cheese		1 pkg	130	D–
Melba Toast	Oat	.5 oz	60	B–
5 Grain	Mixed	.5 oz	60	B–
Rice Bran		7 pieces	130	B
Whole Wheat	All Varieties	.5 oz	45	A–+
Wheat		.5 oz	55	B+
Wheat	Herb	6 pieces	55	D–+
Wheat	Sesame	6 pieces	60	D+
Wheat	Vegetable, Seven Grain	6 pieces	55	C+
		5 pieces	45	B–
Rye	Barbecue	.5 oz	76	D
Rye	Garlic	.5 oz	73	D
Rye	Natural	.5 oz	78	D
Rye	Sour Cream	.5 oz	78	D
Rye		4 pieces	45	A
Wheat		4 pieces	50	B
Rye		4 pieces	45	B–
Wheat	Cracked	4 pieces	50	B–
Wheat		4 pieces	50	B

"+" indicates the food meets minimum fiber requirements; "–" indicates the food has a high sodium content.

Food	Processing Category	Brand
Crackers	Packaged	Kavli Norwegian
Crackers	Packaged	Keebler
Crackers	Packaged	Keebler
Crackers	Packaged	Keebler
Crackers	Packaged	Keebler Club Low Salt
Crackers	Packaged	Keebler Harvest Wheats
Crackers	Packaged	Keebler Selects
Crackers	Packaged	Keebler Toasteds
Crackers	Packaged	Keebler Toasteds Buttercrisp
Crackers	Packaged	Keebler Town House
Crackers	Packaged	Keebler Town House
Crackers	Packaged	Keebler Town House
Crackers	Packaged	Keebler Town House Jrs.
Crackers	Packaged	Keebler Town House Low Salt
Crackers	Packaged	Keebler Wheatables
Crackers	Packaged	Krispy
Crackers	Packaged	Krispy
Crackers	Packaged	Little Debbie
Crackers	Packaged	Little Debbie
Crackers [6]	Packaged	Manischewitz
Crackers	Packaged	Manischewitz
Crackers	Packaged	Manischewitz
Crackers [7]	Packaged	Manischewitz
Crackers	Packaged	Manischewitz
Crackers	Packaged	Manischewitz
Crackers	Packaged	Manischewitz
Crackers	Packaged	Manischewitz Daily
Crackers	Packaged	Manischewitz Daily Unsalted
Crackers	Packaged	Manischewitz Garlic Tams
Crackers	Packaged	Manischewitz Onion Tams
Crackers	Packaged	Manischewitz Passover Tams
Crackers	Packaged	Manischewitz Passover Tams
Crackers	Packaged	Manischewitz Tam Tams
Crackers	Packaged	Manischewitz Tam Tams
Crackers	Packaged	Manischewitz Wheat Tams
Crackers	Packaged	Meal Mates
Crackers	Packaged	Nabisco
Crackers	Packaged	Nabisco American Classic
Crackers	Packaged	Nabisco American Classic
Crackers	Packaged	Nabisco American Classic
Crackers	Packaged	Nabisco American Classic
Crackers	Packaged	Nabisco American Classic
Crackers	Packaged	Nabisco Bacon Flavor Thins
Crackers	Packaged	Nabisco Better Cheddars
Crackers	Packaged	Nabisco Cheddar Wedges
Crackers	Packaged	Nabisco Cheddar Wedges
Crackers	Packaged	Nabisco Garden Crisp
Crackers	Packaged	Nabisco Premium
Crackers	Packaged	Nabisco Ritz
Crackers	Packaged	Nabisco Ritz Bits
Crackers	Packaged	Nabisco Ritz Bits

[6] *Serving size represents approximately ¹/₂ square.*
[7] *Serving size represents approximately 5 pieces.*

Major Description	Minor Description	Serving Size	Calories	Grade
Crisp Bread		1 piece	35	A+
Cheese Sandwich	Peanut Butter	.5 oz	70	C–
Cheese Sandwich	Wheat & American Cheese	.5 oz	70	D
Peanut Butter	Toast	.5 oz	70	C–
Butter Flavor		.5 oz	60	D–
Wheat	Whole Grain	.5 oz	60	D–
Graham	All Varieties	.5 oz	60	A–
All Varieties		.5 oz	60	D–
Butter Flavor		.5 oz	60	D–
Butter Flavor		.5 oz	70	D–
Cheddar Cheese Sandwich		.5 oz	70	D–
Classic	50% Reduced Fat	.5 oz	70	B–
Cheddar Cheese Flavor		.5 oz	80	D
Butter Flavor		.5 oz	70	D
Whole Wheat		.5 oz	70	C–
Saltine		.5 oz	60	A–
Saltine	Unsalted Tops	.5 oz	60	A–
Peanut Butter	Cheese	.5 oz	65	D–
Peanut Butter	Toasty	.5 oz	70	D–
Matzo	American	.5 oz	57	A
Matzo	Diet, Thin	.5 oz	55	A
Matzo	Egg & Onion	.5 oz	56	A–
Matzo	Miniature	.5 oz	90	A
Matzo	Thin	.5 oz	48	A
Matzo	Whole Wheat	.5 oz	90	A
Matzo	Whole Wheat with Bran	.5 oz	55	A
Matzo	Tea Thin	.5 oz	53	A
Matzo		.5 oz	55	A
Matzo	Garlic	.5 oz	76	D
Matzo	Onion	.5 oz	75	D
Matzo		.5 oz	58	A
Matzo	Egg	.5 oz	55	A
Matzo		.5 oz	73	D
Matzo	No Salt	.5 oz	69	D
Matzo	Wheat	.5 oz	75	D
Sesame	Bread, Wafer	.5 oz	70	C–
Zwieback Toast		.5 oz	60	A
Butter Flavor	Dairy	.5 oz	70	C–
Cracked Wheat		.5 oz	70	D–
Golden Sesame		.5 oz	70	C–
Minced Onion		.5 oz	70	C–
Poppy, Toasted		.5 oz	70	C–
Bacon Flavor		.5 oz	70	D–
Cheese Flavor	Cheddar	.5 oz	70	D–
Cheddar Cheese Flavor		.5 oz	70	C–
Cheddar Cheese Flavor	Low Salt	.5 oz	70	D
Wheat	Crisp	.5 oz	60	B–
Wheat	Multigrain	.5 oz	60	B–
Butter Flavor		.5 oz	70	D–
Butter Flavor		.5 oz	70	D–
Cheese Flavor		.5 oz	70	D–

"+" indicates the food meets minimum fiber requirements; "–" indicates the food has a high sodium content.

Food	Processing Category	Brand
Crackers	Packaged	Nabisco Ritz Bits
Crackers	Packaged	Nabisco Ritz Bits
Crackers	Packaged	Nabisco Ritz Bits
Crackers	Packaged	Nabisco Ritz Bits
Crackers	Packaged	Nabisco Ritz Bits Low Salt
Crackers	Packaged	Nabisco Ritz Low Salt
Crackers	Packaged	Nabisco Snack Wells
Crackers	Packaged	Nabisco Snack Wells
Crackers	Packaged	Nabisco Snorkels
Crackers	Packaged	Nabisco Swiss Cheese
Crackers	Packaged	Nabisco Triscuit
Crackers	Packaged	Nabisco Triscuit Bits
Crackers	Packaged	Nabisco Triscuit Low Salt
Crackers	Packaged	Nabisco Twigs Snack Sticks
Crackers	Packaged	Nabisco Vegetable Thins
Crackers	Packaged	Nabisco Wheat Thins
Crackers	Packaged	Nabisco Wheat Thins
Crackers	Packaged	Nabisco Wheat Thins
Crackers	Packaged	Nabisco Wheat Thins Low Salt
Crackers	Packaged	Nabisco Zings
Crackers	Packaged	Oat Bran Krisp
Crackers	Packaged	Oat Thins
Crackers	Packaged	Old London
Crackers	Packaged	Old London
Crackers	Packaged	Old London
Crackers	Packaged	Old London
Crackers	Packaged	Old London
Crackers	Packaged	Old London
Crackers	Packaged	Old London Rounds
Crackers	Packaged	Old London Rounds
Crackers	Packaged	Old London Rounds
Crackers	Packaged	Old London Rounds
Crackers	Packaged	Old London Rounds
Crackers	Packaged	Old London Rounds
Crackers	Packaged	Old London Rounds
Crackers	Packaged	Old London Unsalted
Crackers	Packaged	Old London Unsalted
Crackers	Packaged	Old London Unsalted
Crackers	Packaged	Oysterettes
Crackers	Packaged	Pepperidge Farm Distinctive
Crackers	Packaged	Pepperidge Farm Distinctive
Crackers	Packaged	Pepperidge Farm Distinctive
Crackers	Packaged	Pepperidge Farm Distinctive
Crackers	Packaged	Pepperidge Farm Distinctive
Crackers	Packaged	Pepperidge Farm Distinctive
Crackers	Packaged	Pepperidge Farm Flutters
Crackers	Packaged	Pepperidge Farm Flutters
Crackers	Packaged	Pepperidge Farm Flutters
Crackers	Packaged	Pepperidge Farm Flutters
Crackers	Packaged	Pepperidge Farm Goldfish
Crackers	Packaged	Pepperidge Farm Goldfish
Crackers	Packaged	Pepperidge Farm Goldfish
Crackers	Packaged	Pepperidge Farm Goldfish

Major Description	Minor Description	Serving Size	Calories	Grade
Cheese Sandwich		.5 oz	80	D–
Cheese Sandwich	Nacho	.5 oz	80	D–
Cheese Sandwich	Pizza	.5 oz	80	D–
Peanut Butter	Sandwich	.5 oz	80	D
Butter Flavor		.5 oz	70	D
Butter Flavor		.5 oz	70	D
Cheese		.5 oz	60	A–
Wheat		.5 oz	50	A–
Cheese	All Flavors	.5 oz	60	B–
Swiss Cheese Flavor		.5 oz	70	C–
All Varieties		.5 oz	60	B–
Wheat		.5 oz	60	B–
Wheat		.5 oz	60	B
Sesame & Cheese		.5 oz	70	D–
Vegetable		.5 oz	70	D–
Wheat		.5 oz	70	C–
Wheat	Multigrain	.5 oz	60	B–
Wheat	Nutty	.5 oz	70	D–
Wheat		.5 oz	70	C
Chips	All Flavors	.5 oz	70	C–
Oat Bran		.5 oz	60	D–+
Oat		.5 oz	70	C–
Melba Toast	Pumpernickel	.5 oz	54	A–
Melba Toast	Rye	.5 oz	52	A–+
Melba Toast	Sesame	.5 oz	55	B–+
Melba Toast	Wheat	.5 oz	51	A–+
Melba Toast	White	.5 oz	51	A–+
Melba Toast	Whole Grain	.5 oz	52	B–+
Melba Toast	Bacon	.5 oz	53	B–+
Melba Toast	Garlic	.5 oz	56	B–
Melba Toast	Onion	.5 oz	52	A–
Melba Toast	Rye	.5 oz	52	A–+
Melba Toast	Sesame	.5 oz	56	B–+
Melba Toast	White	.5 oz	48	A–+
Melba Toast	Whole Grain	.5 oz	54	B–+
Melba Toast	Sesame	.5 oz	55	B+
Melba Toast	White	.5 oz	51	A+
Melba Toast	Whole Grain	.5 oz	53	B+
Soup & Oyster		.5 oz	60	A–
Butter Flavor	Thins	.5 oz	70	C–
Sesame		.5 oz	70	C–+
Soda or Water		.5 oz	70	A–
Wheat	Cracked	.5 oz	100	C–
Wheat	Hearty	.5 oz	100	D–
Wheat	Toasted	.5 oz	80	C–
Butter Flavor		.5 oz	66	C–
Herb Garden		.5 oz	66	C–
Sesame	Golden	.5 oz	73	D–
Wheat	Toasted	.5 oz	73	D–
Cheese Flavor	Parmesan	.5 oz	60	B–
Cheese Flavor	Cheddar	.5 oz	60	B–
Original		.5 oz	65	C–
Pizza		.5 oz	65	C–

"+" indicates the food meets minimum fiber requirements; "–" indicates the food has a high sodium content.

Food	Processing Category	Brand
Crackers	Packaged	Pepperidge Farm Goldfish
Crackers	Packaged	Pepperidge Farm Goldfish Thins
Crackers	Packaged	Pepperidge Farm Snack Sticks
Crackers	Packaged	Pepperidge Farm Snack Sticks
Crackers	Packaged	Pepperidge Farm Snack Sticks
Crackers	Packaged	Pepperidge Farm Snack Sticks
Crackers	Packaged	Premium
Crackers	Packaged	Premium Bits
Crackers	Packaged	Premium
Crackers	Packaged	Premium
Crackers	Packaged	Premium
Crackers	Packaged	Premiumplus
Crackers	Packaged	Rokeach
Crackers	Packaged	Rokeach
Crackers	Packaged	Rokeach
Crackers	Packaged	Royal Lunch
Crackers	Packaged	Rykrisp
Crackers	Packaged	Rykrisp
Crackers	Packaged	Rykrisp
Crackers	Packaged	Rykrisp Twindividuals
Crackers	Packaged	Ryvita Crisp Bread
Crackers	Packaged	Ryvita Crisp Bread
Crackers	Packaged	Ryvita Crisp Bread
Crackers	Packaged	Ryvita Crisp Bread
Crackers	Packaged	Ryvita Original Snackbread
Crackers	Packaged	Sailor Boy Pilot
Crackers	Packaged	Sociables
Crackers	Packaged	Sunshine
Crackers	Packaged	Sunshine Wheats
Crackers	Packaged	Tid Bit
Crackers	Packaged	Uneeda Biscuits Unsalted Tops
Crackers	Packaged	Wasa Crisp Bread
Crackers	Packaged	Wasa Crisp Bread
Crackers	Packaged	Wasa Crisp Bread
Crackers	Packaged	Wasa Crisp Bread
Crackers	Packaged	Wasa Crisp Bread
Crackers	Packaged	Wasa Crisp Bread
Crackers	Packaged	Wasa Crisp Bread
Crackers	Packaged	Wasa Crisp Bread Lite
Crackers	Packaged	Waverly
Crackers	Packaged	Waverly Low Salt
Crackers	Packaged	Weight Watchers
Crackers	Packaged	Weight Watchers
Crackers	Packaged	Wheatsworth Stone Ground
Crackers	Packaged	Zesta
Crackers	Packaged	Zesta
Crackers	Packaged	Zesta
Crackers	Packaged	Zesta
Croissant	Frozen	Pepperidge Farm
Croissant	Frozen	Sara Lee
Croissant	Frozen	Sara Lee
Croissant	Packaged	Awrey's
Croissant	Packaged	Awrey's

Major Description	Minor Description	Serving Size	Calories	Grade
Pretzel		.5 oz	55	B–
Cheese Flavor	Thins	.5 oz	50	C–
Cheese Flavor	Sticks	.5 oz	65	C–
Pretzel		.5 oz	60	B–
Pumpernickel		.5 oz	70	C–
Sesame		.5 oz	70	C–
Saltine		.5 oz	60	B–
Saltine		.5 oz	70	C–
Saltine	Fat Free	.5 oz	50	A–
Saltine	Low Salt	.5 oz	60	B–
Saltine	Unsalted Tops	.5 oz	60	B–
Saltine	Whole Wheat	.5 oz	60	B–
Cheese Flavor		.5 oz	70	D
Saltine		.5 oz	60	B
Snack		.5 oz	65	C
Soda or Water		.5 oz	60	B–
Rye		.5 oz	40	A–+
Rye	Seasoned	.5 oz	45	B–+
Rye	Sesame	.5 oz	60	B–+
Rye	Seasoned	.5 oz	45	B–+
Crisp Bread	High Fiber	.5 oz	40	A+
Rye	Dark	.5 oz	45	A–+
Rye	Light	.5 oz	45	A+
Rye	Sesame, Toasted	.5 oz	55	A+
Wheat		.5 oz	30	A
Soda or Water		1 piece	100	B–
Wheat		.5 oz	70	C–
Soup & Oyster		16 pieces	60	A–
Wheat		.5 oz	50	D–
Cheese Flavor		.5 oz	70	D–
Toast		.5 oz	60	B–
Extra Crisp		.5 oz	58	A–
Fiber Plus		.5 oz	40	B–+
Golden Rye		.5 oz	40	A–+
Hearty Rye		.5 oz	45	A–+
Sesame	Savory	.5 oz	50	B–+
Sesame Wheat		.5 oz	50	C–
Wheat	Whole Grain	.5 oz	50	B–+
Rye	Light	.5 oz	42	A–+
Water		.5 oz	70	C–
Water		.5 oz	70	C
Crisp Bread	Garlic Flavor	2 pieces	30	A–
Crisp Bread	Rice Harvest	2 pieces	30	A–
Wheat		.5 oz	70	C–
Saltine		.5 oz	60	B–
Saltine	Wheat	.5 oz	60	B–
Saltine	Low Salt	.5 oz	60	B–
Saltine	Unsalted Tops	.5 oz	60	B–
Butter	Petite	1 piece	140	D
Butter		1 piece	170	D–
Butter	Petite	1 piece	120	D–
Butter		1 piece	200	D
Margarine		1 piece	250	D–

"+" indicates the food meets minimum fiber requirements; "–" indicates the food has a high sodium content.

Food	Processing Category	Brand
Croissant	Packaged	Awrey's
Croissant	Packaged	Pepperidge Farm Sandwich Quartet
Crouton	Packaged	Brownberry [8]
Crouton	Packaged	Brownberry
Crouton	Packaged	Brownberry
Crouton	Packaged	Brownberry
Crouton	Packaged	Brownberry
Crouton	Packaged	Pepperidge Farm [8]
Crouton	Packaged	Pepperidge Farm
Crouton	Packaged	Pepperidge Farm
Crouton	Packaged	Pepperidge Farm
Crouton	Packaged	Pepperidge Farm
Crouton	Packaged	Weight Watchers
Falafel	Mix	Generic
Falafel	Mix	Casbah
Falafel	Mix	Fantastic Foods Falafil
Falafel	Mix	Near East
Farina	Cooked [9]	All Brands
Farina	Cooked	All Brands
Flour	Dry	All Brands
Flour	Dry	Generic
Flour	Dry	Generic
Flour	Dry	Generic
Flour	Dry	Generic
Flour	Dry	Generic
Flour	Dry	Generic
Flour	Dry	Generic
Flour	Dry	Generic
Flour	Dry	Generic
Flour	Dry	Generic
Flour	Dry	Generic
Flour	Dry	Generic
Flour	Dry	Generic
Flour	Dry	Generic
Flour	Dry	Generic
Flour	Dry	Generic
Flour	Dry	Generic
Flour	Dry	Generic
Flour	Dry	Generic
Flour	Dry	Generic
Flour	Dry	Generic
Flour	Dry	Generic
Flour	Dry	Generic
Flour	Dry	Generic
Flour	Dry	Generic
Flour	Dry	Generic
Flour	Dry	Arrowhead Mills
Flour	Dry	Arrowhead Mills
Flour	Dry	Arrowhead Mills

[8] Serving size of .5 oz of Brownberry and Pepperidge Farm Croutons equivalent to approximately $^1/_3$ cup.
[9] Serving size of $^1/_2$ cup cooked farina equivalent to approximately $1^1/_2$ Tbsp dry.

Major Description	Minor Description	Serving Size	Calories	Grade
Wheat		1 piece	240	D–
		1 piece	170	C–
Caesar Salad		.5 oz	62	C–
Cheddar Cheese		.5 oz	63	C–
Onion & Garlic		.5 oz	60	C–
Seasoned		.5 oz	59	C–
Toasted		.5 oz	56	B–
Cheddar & Romano Cheese		.5 oz	60	B–
Cheese & Garlic		.5 oz	70	C–
Onion & Garlic		.5 oz	70	C–
Seasoned		.5 oz	70	C–
Sour Cream & Chive		.5 oz	70	C–
Seasoned		1 pouch	30	A–
	Fried in Oil	1 oz	94	D
	Pre-Cooked	1 oz	103	B
	Cooked without Oil	1 oz	43	A–
	Cooked in Oil	1.2 oz patty	90	D–
Whole Grain		$^1/_2$ cup	57	A+
Whole Grain	Salted	$^1/_2$ cup	57	A–+
Acorn	Full Fat	$^1/_2$ cup	280	D–
Arrowroot		$^1/_2$ cup	223	A
Buckwheat		$^1/_2$ cup	200	A+
Carob		$^1/_2$ cup	197	A+
Corn	Masa	$^1/_2$ cup	206	A
Corn	Whole Grain	$^1/_2$ cup	204	A+
Cottonseed	Low Fat	$^1/_2$ cup	157	A
Cottonseed	Partially Defatted	$^1/_2$ cup	170	B
Peanut	Defatted	$^1/_2$ cup	196	A
Peanut	Low Fat	$^1/_2$ cup	120	D
Pecan		$^1/_2$ cup	186	A
Potato		$^1/_2$ cup	314	A
Rice	Brown or White	$^1/_2$ cup	290	A
Rye	Dark	$^1/_2$ cup	208	A+
Rye	Light	$^1/_2$ cup	187	A+
Rye	Medium	$^1/_2$ cup	180	A+
Sesame	High Fat	$^1/_2$ cup	149	D
Sesame	Low Fat	$^1/_2$ cup	95	A
Sesame	Partially Defatted	$^1/_2$ cup	109	B+
Soy	Defatted	$^1/_2$ cup	165	A
Soy	Full Fat	$^1/_2$ cup	185	D
Soy	Low Fat	$^1/_2$ cup	144	B
Sunflower Seed	Partially Defatted	$^1/_2$ cup	130	A+
Triticale	Whole Grain	$^1/_2$ cup	220	A+
Wheat, White	All-Purpose	$^1/_2$ cup	200	A
Wheat, White	Bread	$^1/_2$ cup	200	A
Wheat, White	Cake	$^1/_2$ cup	200	A
Wheat, White	Self-Rising	$^1/_2$ cup	220	A–
Wheat, White	Tortilla Mix	$^1/_2$ cup	230	B–
Whole Grain	All Varieties	$^1/_2$ cup	190	A+
Chick Pea		$^1/_2$ cup	200	A+
Corn	Blue	$^1/_2$ cup	210	A+
Corn	Whole Grain Yellow	$^1/_2$ cup	210	A+

"+" indicates the food meets minimum fiber requirements; "–" indicates the food has a high sodium content.

Food	Processing Category	Brand
Flour	Dry	Arrowhead Mills
Flour	Dry	Arrowhead Mills
Flour	Dry	Aunt Jemima
Flour	Dry	Pillsbury Ballard
Flour	Dry	Pillsbury Best
Flour	Dry	Pillsbury Best
Flour	Dry	Pillsbury Best
Flour	Dry	Pillsbury Best
Flour	Dry	Pillsbury Best
Flour	Dry	Pillsbury Best
Flour	Dry	Pillsbury Best
Flour	Dry	Pillsbury's Best Bohemian Style
Grain Cakes	Packaged	Mother's
Grain Cakes	Packaged	Mother's
Millet	Cooked [10]	All Brands
Noodle, Chinese	Dry	Generic
Noodle, Chinese	Dry	Generic
Noodle, Japanese	Dry	Generic
Noodle, Japanese	Dry	Generic
Noodle, Japanese	Dry	Generic
Noodle, Egg	Dry	Generic
Noodle, Egg	Dry	Generic
Noodle, Egg	Dry	Creamette
Noodle, Egg	Dry	Gioia
Noodle, Egg	Dry	Golden Grain
Noodle, Egg	Dry	Goodman's Country Style
Noodle, Egg	Dry	Mrs. Grass
Noodle, Egg	Dry	Mueller's
Noodle, Egg	Dry	P & R
Noodle, Egg	Dry	Prince
Noodle, Egg	Dry	San Giorgio
Oat	Cooked [11]	*See also* Cereal
Oat	Cooked	*See also* Cereal
Oat Bran	Cooked	*See also* Cereal
Oat Bran	Dry	*See also* Cereal
Oat Flakes	Dry	Arrowhead Mills
Oat Groats	Dry	Arrowhead Mills
Pancake	Frozen	Aunt Jemima
Pancake	Frozen	Aunt Jemima
Pancake	Frozen	Aunt Jemima Lite
Pancake	Frozen	Aunt Jemima Original
Pancake	Frozen	Downyflake
Pancake	Frozen	Downyflake
Pancake	Frozen	Downyflake
Pancake	Frozen	Pillsbury Hungry Jack
Pancake	Frozen	Pillsbury Hungry Jack
Pancake	Frozen	Pillsbury Hungry Jack
Pancake	Frozen	Pillsbury Hungry Jack
Pancake	Frozen	Pillsbury Hungry Jack
Pancake	Frozen	Weight Watchers Microwave
See also Waffle		
Pancake & Waffle	Mix	Arrowhead Mills

[10] *Serving size of $1/2$ cup cooked millet equivalent to approximately $1/5$ cup dry.*
[11] *Serving size of $1/2$ cup cooked oat equivalent to $1/4$ cup dry.*

Major Description	Minor Description	Serving Size	Calories	Grade
Millet	Whole Grain	$^1/_2$ cup	185	A+
Oat	Whole Grain	$^1/_2$ cup	200	A+
Wheat, White	Enriched	$^1/_2$ cup	220	A–
All-Purpose		$^1/_2$ cup	200	A
All-Purpose	All Varieties	$^1/_2$ cup	200	A
Bread		$^1/_2$ cup	200	A
Medium Rye		$^1/_2$ cup	200	A+
Rye & Wheat		$^1/_2$ cup	200	A+
Self-Rising		$^1/_2$ cup	190	A–
Shake & Blend		$^1/_2$ cup	200	A
Whole Wheat		$^1/_2$ cup	200	A+
Rye & Wheat		$^1/_2$ cup	200	A+
Rye	No Salt Added	1 cake	35	A+
Wheat	No Salt Added	1 cake	35	A+
		$^1/_2$ cup	144	A
Cellophane or Long Rice		2 oz	257	A
Chow Mein		2 oz	298	D
Soba Buckwheat		2 oz	192	A–
Somen		2 oz	203	A–
Udon Wheat		2 oz	159	A–
Plain		2 oz	217	A
Spinach		2 oz	218	A
Plain		2 oz	221	A
Plain		2 oz	220	A
Plain		2 oz	210	A
Plain		2 oz	220	A
Plain		2 oz	220	A
Plain		2 oz	220	A
Plain		2 oz	220	A
Plain		2 oz	210	A
Plain		2 oz	220	A
Rolled or Oatmeal	Unsalted	$^1/_2$ cup	72	A+
Whole Grain		$^1/_2$ cup	150	B+
Cooked		$^1/_2$ cup	43	B+
Raw		$^1/_2$ cup	115	B+
		$^1/_2$ cup	220	B+
		2 oz	220	B+
Blueberry		3 cakes	220	B–
Low Fat		3 cakes	130	A–+
Buttermilk	Microwave	3.5 oz	140	B–
		3.5 oz	211	B–
		3 cakes	280	B–
Blueberry		3 cakes	290	B–
Buttermilk		3 cakes	280	B–
Blueberry	Microwave	3 cakes	230	A–
Buttermilk	Microwave	3 cakes	260	A–
Harvest Wheat	Microwave	3 cakes	230	A+–
Oat Bran	Microwave	3 cakes	230	A+–
Original	Microwave	3 cakes	240	A–
Buttermilk		$^1/_2$ pkg	140	B–
Blue Corn		Three 4" cakes	330	A

"+" indicates the food meets minimum fiber requirements; "–" indicates the food has a high sodium content.

Food	Processing Category	Brand
Pancake & Waffle	Mix	Arrowhead Mills
Pancake & Waffle	Mix	Arrowhead Mills
Pancake & Waffle	Mix	Arrowhead Mills
Pancake & Waffle	Mix	Arrowhead Mills
Pancake & Waffle	Mix	Aunt Jemima
Pancake & Waffle	Mix	Aunt Jemima
Pancake & Waffle	Mix	Aunt Jemima
Pancake & Waffle	Mix	Aunt Jemima Complete
Pancake & Waffle	Mix	Aunt Jemima Lite Complete
Pancake & Waffle	Mix	Aunt Jemima Original
Pancake & Waffle	Mix	Aunt Jemima Original Complete
Pancake & Waffle	Mix	Betty Crocker
Pancake & Waffle	Mix	Bisquick Shak 'N Pour
Pancake & Waffle	Mix	Bisquick Shak 'N Pour
Pancake & Waffle	Mix	Bisquick Shak 'N Pour
Pancake & Waffle	Mix	Bisquick Shak 'N Pour
Pancake & Waffle	Mix	Bisquick Shak 'N Pour
Pancake & Waffle	Mix	Estee
Pancake & Waffle	Mix	Featherweight
Pancake & Waffle	Mix	Martha White Flapstax
Pancake & Waffle	Mix	Pillsbury Hungry Jack
Pancake & Waffle	Mix	Pillsbury Hungry Jack
Pancake & Waffle	Mix	Pillsbury Hungry Jack
Pancake & Waffle	Mix	Pillsbury Hungry Jack
Pancake & Waffle	Mix	Pillsbury Hungry Jack
Pancake & Waffle	Mix	Pillsbury Hungry Jack
Pancake & Waffle	Mix	Pillsbury Hungry Jack
Pancake & Waffle	Mix	Robin Hood/Gold Medal Pouch Mix
Pancake Batter	Frozen	Aunt Jemima
Pancake Batter	Frozen	Aunt Jemima
Pancake Batter	Frozen	Aunt Jemima
Pasta	Dry [12]	Generic
Pasta	Dry	Generic
Pasta	Dry	Generic
Pasta	Dry	Generic
Pasta	Dry	Generic
Pasta	Dry	Health Valley
Pasta	Dry	Health Valley
Pasta	Dry	Health Valley
Pasta	Dry	Health Valley
Pasta	Dry	Health Valley
Pasta	Dry	Pritikin
Pasta	Dry	Ronzoni
Pasta	Fresh	Homemade
Pasta	Fresh	Homemade
Potato Pancake	Mix	French's Idaho
Potato Starch	Dry	Featherweight
Rice Bran	Dry	Generic
Rice Cake	Packaged	Generic
Rice Cake	Packaged	American Grains Rice Bites
Rice Cake	Packaged	Hain
Rice Cake	Packaged	Hain
Rice Cake	Packaged	Hain

[12] *Serving size of dry pasta calorically equivalent to approximately 1 cup cooked.*

Major Description	Minor Description	Serving Size	Calories	Grade
Buckwheat		Three 4" cakes	270	A
Multigrain		Three 4" cakes	350	A
Oat Bran		Three 4" cakes	200	A
Griddle Lite		Three 4" cakes	260	A
Buckwheat		Three 4" cakes	143	A–+
Buttermilk		Three 4" cakes	122	A–
Whole Wheat		Three 4" cakes	161	A–+
Buttermilk		Three 4" cakes	231	A–
Buttermilk		Three 4" cakes	130	A–
		Three 4" cakes	116	A–
		Three 4" cakes	253	A–
Buttermilk		Three 4" cakes	280	C–
		Three 4" cakes	260	B–
Apple Cinnamon		Three 4" cakes	270	B–
Blueberry		Three 4" cakes	280	B–
Buttermilk		Three 4" cakes	260	B–
Oat Bran		Three 4" cakes	240	A–
		Three 4" cakes	100	A–
		Three 4" cakes	140	A
		Three 4" cakes	300	B–
		Three 4" cakes	250	B–
	Extra Lights	Three 4" cakes	210	B–
	Extra Lights, Complete	Three 4" cakes	190	A–
Blueberry		Three 4" cakes	320	A–
Buttermilk		Three 4" cakes	240	A–
Buttermilk	Complete	Three 4" cakes	180	A–
Buttermilk	Complete Packets	Three 4" cakes	180	A–
		1/8 pouch	100	B–
Blueberry		3.6 oz	204	B–
Buttermilk		3.6 oz	180	A–
Original		3.6 oz	183	A–
Corn	All Varieties & Shapes	2 oz	204	A
Durum Wheat	All Varieties & Shapes	2 oz	210	A
Protein Fortified	All Varieties & Shapes	2 oz	214	A
Spinach	All Varieties & Shapes	2 oz	211	A+
Whole Wheat	All Varieties & Shapes	2 oz	197	A+
Amaranth	Spaghetti	2 oz	170	A+
Oat Bran	Spaghetti	2 oz	120	A+
Whole Wheat	Lasagna/Spaghetti	2 oz	170	A+
Whole Wheat & Spinach	Lasagna	2 oz	170	A+
Whole Wheat & Spinach	Spaghetti	2 oz	170	A+
All Varieties		2 oz	190	A+
All Varieties		2 oz	210	A
Egg		2 oz	180	A
without Egg		2 oz	176	A
Dinner		Three 3" cakes	90	B–
		1/2 cup	310	A
Crude		1 oz	90	D+
Plain		1 cake	40	A
All Varieties		1 cake	3	B–
Apple Cinnamon		1 cake	50	A
Butter		1 cake	45	B–
Caramel		1 cake	50	A

"+" indicates the food meets minimum fiber requirements; "–" indicates the food has a high sodium content.

Food	Processing Category	Brand
Rice Cake	Packaged	Hain
Rice Cake	Packaged	Hain
Rice Cake	Packaged	Hain
Rice Cake	Packaged	Hain
Rice Cake	Packaged	Hain
Rice Cake	Packaged	Hain Mini
Rice Cake	Packaged	Hain Mini
Rice Cake	Packaged	Hain Mini
Rice Cake	Packaged	Hain Mini
Rice Cake	Packaged	Hain Mini
Rice Cake	Packaged	Hain Mini
Rice Cake	Packaged	Hain Mini
Rice Cake	Packaged	Hain Mini
Rice Cake	Packaged	Hain Mini
Rice Cake	Packaged	Hain Mini
Rice Cake	Packaged	Hain Mini
Rice Cake	Packaged	Hain Mini
Rice Cake	Packaged	Hain Mini
Rice Cake	Packaged	Hain Mini
Rice Cake	Packaged	Mother's
Rice Cake	Packaged	Mother's Mini
Rice Cake	Packaged	Mother's Mini
Rice Cake	Packaged	Mother's Mini
Rice Cake	Packaged	Mother's Mini
Rice Cake	Packaged	Pritikin
Rice Cake	Packaged	Quaker
Rice Cake	Packaged	Quaker
Rice Cake	Packaged	Quaker
Rice Cake	Packaged	Quaker
Rice Cake	Packaged	Quaker Mini
Rice Cake	Packaged	Quaker Mini
Rice Cake	Packaged	Quaker Mini
Rice, Basmati	Cooked [13]	Generic
Rice, Basmati	Cooked	Fantastic Foods
Rice, Basmati	Cooked	Fantastic Foods
Rice, Brown	Cooked	Generic
Rice, Glutinous	Cooked	Generic
Rice, White	Cooked	Generic
Rice, White	Cooked	Generic
Rice, White	Cooked	Generic
Roll	Frozen	Bridgford
Roll	Frozen	Pepperidge Farm
Roll	Frozen	Sara Lee
Roll	Frozen	Weight Watchers Microwave
Roll	Frozen	Weight Watchers Microwave
Roll	Frozen	Weight Watchers Microwave
Roll	Packaged	Arnold
Roll	Packaged	Arnold
Roll	Packaged	Arnold 24 Dinner Party
Roll	Packaged	Arnold Dutch
Roll	Packaged	Arnold Francisco
Roll	Packaged	Arnold New England Style
Roll	Packaged	Awrey's

[13] *Serving size $^1/_2$ cup cooked rice equivalent to approximately 1 oz dry.*

Major Description	Minor Description	Serving Size	Calories	Grade
Honey Nut		1 cake	50	A
Nacho Cheese		1 cake	45	B–
Plain		1 cake	35	A–
Sesame		1 cake	40	A
White Cheddar		1 cake	45	B–
Apple Cinnamon		1 cake	9	A
Barbeque		1 cake	10	C
Caramel		1 cake	9	A
Cheese		1 cake	9	B–
Honey Nut		1 cake	9	A
Nacho Cheese		1 cake	10	B–
Plain		1 cake	7	A
Plain	No Salt Added	1 cake	7	A
Popcorn	Butter	1 cake	9	B
Popcorn	Cheddar Mild	1 cake	9	B
Popcorn	Cheddar White	1 cake	9	B
Popcorn	Plain	1 cake	9	A
Ranch		1 cake	10	C–
Teriyaki		1 cake	7	A–
Multigrain		1 cake	35	A
Apple		1 cake	10	A
Caramel		1 cake	10	A
Cinnamon		1 cake	10	A
Plain	Unsalted	1 cake	9	A
All Varieties		1 cake	35	A
Apple Cinnamon		1 cake	50	A
Caramel Corn		1 cake	50	A
Cinnamon Crunch		1 cake	50	A
Multigrain		1 cake	34	A
Buttered Popcorn		1 cake	8	A–
Honey Nut		1 cake	10	A
White Cheddar		1 cake	10	A–
Long Grain	White	1/2 cup	82	A
		1/2 cup	103	A
Brown		1/2 cup	102	A
Long Grain		1/2 cup	100	A
		1/2 cup	117	A
All Grains		1/2 cup	135	A
Parboiled Long Grain		1/2 cup	100	A
Precook or Instant		1/2 cup	80	A
Parker House		1 piece	85	A–
Cinnamon		1 piece	280	D
Cinnamon	All Butter	1 piece	230	D
Apple, Sweet		1/2 pkg	160	B
Cheese		1/2 pkg	180	B
Strawberry		1/2 pkg	170	B
Hamburger		1 piece	115	B–+
Hot Dog		1 piece	100	B–
Dinner		1 piece	51	B–+
Egg Sandwich		1 piece	123	B–+
Kaiser		1 piece	184	A–
Hot Dog		1 piece	108	B–
Dinner	Black Forest	1 piece	50	B–

"+" indicates the food meets minimum fiber requirements; "–" indicates the food has a high sodium content.

Food	Processing Category	Brand
Roll	Packaged	Awrey's
Roll	Packaged	Awrey's
Roll	Packaged	Awrey's
Roll	Packaged	Awrey's
Roll	Packaged	Awrey's
Roll	Packaged	Awrey's
Roll	Packaged	Awrey's
Roll	Packaged	Brownberry Hearth
Roll	Packaged	Colombo Brand
Roll	Packaged	Colombo Brand
Roll	Packaged	Colombo Brand
Roll	Packaged	Colombo Brand
Roll	Packaged	Colombo Brand Twin Pack
Roll	Packaged	Country Grain
Roll	Packaged	Du Jour
Roll	Packaged	Du Jour
Roll	Packaged	Francisco International
Roll	Packaged	Home Pride
Roll	Packaged	Home Pride
Roll	Packaged	Levy's Old Country Deli
Roll	Packaged	Levy's Old Country Deli
Roll	Packaged	Pepperidge Farm
Roll	Packaged	Pepperidge Farm
Roll	Packaged	Pepperidge Farm
Roll	Packaged	Pepperidge Farm
Roll	Packaged	Pepperidge Farm
Roll	Packaged	Pepperidge Farm
Roll	Packaged	Pepperidge Farm
Roll	Packaged	Pepperidge Farm
Roll	Packaged	Pepperidge Farm
Roll	Packaged	Pepperidge Farm
Roll	Packaged	Pepperidge Farm Classic
Roll	Packaged	Pepperidge Farm Deli Classic
Roll	Packaged	Pepperidge Farm Deli Classic
Roll	Packaged	Pepperidge Farm Deli Classic
Roll	Packaged	Pepperidge Farm Deli Classic
Roll	Packaged	Pepperidge Farm Deli Classic
Roll	Packaged	Pepperidge Farm Deli Classic 4/Pkg
Roll	Packaged	Pepperidge Farm Deli Classic 9/Pkg
Roll	Packaged	Pepperidge Farm Family
Roll	Packaged	Pepperidge Farm Hearth
Roll	Packaged	Pepperidge Farm Hearty Classic
Roll	Packaged	Pepperidge Farm Heat N Serve
Roll	Packaged	Pepperidge Farm Old Fashioned
Roll	Packaged	Pepperidge Farm Party
Roll	Packaged	Roman Meal
Roll	Packaged	Roman Meal Original
Roll	Packaged	Roman Meal Original
Roll	Packaged	Wonder
Roll	Packaged	Wonder
Roll	Packaged	Wonder
Roll	Packaged	Wonder
Roll	Packaged	Wonder

Major Description	Minor Description	Serving Size	Calories	Grade
Dinner	Cracked Wheat	1 piece	50	B–
Dinner	Crusty	1 piece	70	A–
Dinner	Plain	1 piece	60	A–
Dinner	Poppy Seed	1 piece	59	B–
Dinner	Sesame Seed	1 piece	60	A–
Hot Dog	Oat Bran	1 piece	110	B–
Sandwich	Oat Bran	1 piece	120	A–
Kaiser		1 piece	152	B–
49er, Sour		1 piece	90	A–
49er, Sweet		1 piece	96	B–
Steak, Sour		1 piece	200	A–
Steak, Sweet		1 piece	206	A–
Luigi		1 piece	146	A–
Hot Dog		1 piece	100	A–
Brown & Serve	French Style Petite	1 piece	230	A–
Brown & Serve	Italian Style Crusty	1 piece	80	A–
French Style		1 piece	108	A–
Dinner	Wheat	1 piece	70	A–
Dinner	White	1 piece	80	B–
Egg		1 piece	146	B–
Onion		1 piece	153	A–
Finger with Poppy Seeds		1 piece	50	C–
French Style	Sourdough	1 piece	100	A–
Hamburger		1 piece	130	A–
Hot Dog		1 piece	140	B–
Hot Dog	Dijon Style	1 piece	160	B–
Parker House		1 piece	60	A–
Party		1 piece	30	B–
Sandwich	Onion with Poppy Seeds	1 piece	150	B–
Sandwich	Potato	1 piece	160	B–
Sandwich	Sesame Seeds	1 piece	140	B–
Dinner	Country Style	1 piece	50	B–
Brown & Serve	Club	1 piece	100	A–
Brown & Serve	French Style	1 piece	240	A–
Crescent Butter		1 piece	110	D–
Hoagie Soft		1 piece	210	B–
Sandwich	Salad	1 piece	110	C–
French Style		1 piece	240	A–
French Style		1 piece	100	A–
Soft		1 piece	100	B–
Brown & Serve		1 piece	50	B–
Potato		1 piece	90	B–
Twist Golden		1 piece	110	D–
Dinner		1 piece	50	C–
Dinner		1 piece	30	B–
Dinner		1 piece	69	B–+
Hamburger		1 piece	113	B–+
Hot Dog		1 piece	104	B–+
Brown & Serve		1 piece	80	B–
Brown & Serve	Buttermilk	1 piece	80	B–
Dinner		1 piece	80	A–
Hamburger		1 piece	120	A–
Hoagie		1 piece	400	B–

"+" indicates the food meets minimum fiber requirements; "–" indicates the food has a high sodium content.

Food	Processing Category	Brand
Roll	Packaged	Wonder
Roll	Packaged	Wonder
Roll	Packaged	Wonder Light
Roll	Packaged	Wonder Light
Roll	Refrigerated	Pillsbury
Roll	Refrigerated	Pillsbury
Roll	Refrigerated	Pillsbury
Roll	Refrigerated	Pillsbury Hungry Jack
Rye Cake	Packaged	Quaker Grain Cakes
Rye Flakes	Dry	Arrowhead Mills
Rye, Whole Grain	Dry	Generic
Semolina, Whole Grain	Dry	Generic
Sesame Meal	Dry	Generic
Sesame Seed	Dry	Generic
Sesame Seed	Dry	Generic
Sorghum Syrup	Dry	Generic
Sorghum, Whole Grain	Dry	Generic
Soy Meal	Dry	Generic
Soybean Flakes	Dry	Arrowhead Mills
Soybean Kernels	Dry	Generic
Stuffing	Frozen	Green Giant Stuffing Originals
Stuffing	Frozen	Green Giant Stuffing Originals
Stuffing	Frozen	Green Giant Stuffing Originals
Stuffing	Frozen	Green Giant Stuffing Originals
Stuffing [14]	Mix	Betty Crocker
Stuffing	Mix	Betty Crocker
Stuffing	Mix	Brownberry
Stuffing	Mix	Brownberry
Stuffing	Mix	Golden Grain
Stuffing	Mix	Homestyle Stove Top Flexible
Stuffing	Mix	Homestyle Stove Top Microwave
Stuffing	Mix	Pepperidge Farm
Stuffing	Mix	Pepperidge Farm
Stuffing	Mix	Pepperidge Farm
Stuffing	Mix	Pepperidge Farm
Stuffing	Mix	Pepperidge Farm Distinctive
Stuffing	Mix	Pepperidge Farm Distinctive
Stuffing	Mix	Pepperidge Farm Distinctive
Stuffing	Mix	Pepperidge Farm Distinctive
Stuffing	Mix	Pepperidge Farm Distinctive
Stuffing	Mix	Savory Stove Top
Stuffing	Mix	Stove Top
Stuffing	Mix	Stove Top
Stuffing	Mix	Stove Top
Stuffing	Mix	Stove Top
Stuffing	Mix	Stove Top
Stuffing	Mix	Stove Top
Stuffing	Mix	Stove Top
Stuffing	Mix	Stove Top
Stuffing	Mix	Stove Top Americana
Stuffing	Mix	Stove Top Flexible Serving

[14] *All brands of stuffing mix prepared with approximately 400 calories margarine per box as per package instructions. If reduced calorie margarine used, rating may rise one level and calories fall by approximately 100 calories per item.*

Major Description	Minor Description	Serving Size	Calories	Grade
Hot Dog		1 piece	80	A–
Pan		1 piece	80	A–
Hamburger		1 piece	80	A–+
Hot Dog		1 piece	80	A–+
Butterflake		1 piece	140	C–
Cinnamon	Iced	1 piece	110	D–
Crescent		1 piece	100	D–
Cinnamon	Iced	1 piece	145	D–
		1 cake	35	A–+
		2 oz	190	A+
		$^1/_2$ cup	280	A+
		$^1/_2$ cup	301	A
Partially Defatted		1 oz	161	D
Kernels Hulled		1 Tbsp	47	D
Whole		1 Tbsp	52	D
		$^1/_2$ cup	424	A
		1 oz	96	A
Defatted		$^1/_2$ cup	207	A+
		2 oz	250	C+
Whole Kernels	Roasted & Toasted	1 cup	490	D
Chicken		$^1/_2$ cup	170	C–
Corn Bread		$^1/_2$ cup	170	C–
Mushroom		$^1/_2$ cup	150	D–
Wild Rice		$^1/_2$ cup	160	C–
Chicken Flavor		$^1/_2$ cup	180	D–
Herb Traditional		$^1/_2$ cup	180	C–
Corn		$^1/_2$ cup	253	D–
Herb		$^1/_2$ cup	250	D–+
All Varieties		$^1/_2$ cup	180	D–
Herb		$^1/_2$ cup	170	D–
Corn Bread		$^1/_2$ cup	160	C–
Corn Bread		$^1/_2$ cup	250	C–
Country Style		$^1/_2$ cup	220	D–
Seasoned Herb		$^1/_2$ cup	250	C–
Seasoned Herb	Cube	$^1/_2$ cup	220	D–
Apples & Raisins		$^1/_2$ cup	229	D–
Chicken, Classic		$^1/_2$ cup	158	D–
Herb	Country Garden Style	$^1/_2$ cup	230	D–
Vegetable Harvest		$^1/_2$ cup	230	D–
Wild Rice & Mushroom		$^1/_2$ cup	260	D–
Herb		$^1/_2$ cup	170	D–
Beef		$^1/_2$ cup	180	D–
Chicken Flavor		$^1/_2$ cup	180	D–
Corn Bread		$^1/_2$ cup	170	D–
Long Grain & Wild Rice		$^1/_2$ cup	180	D–
Mushroom & Onion		$^1/_2$ cup	180	D–
Pork		$^1/_2$ cup	170	D–
Turkey		$^1/_2$ cup	170	D–
with Rice		$^1/_2$ cup	180	D–
San Francisco Style		$^1/_2$ cup	170	D–
Chicken Flavor		$^1/_2$ cup	170	D–

"+" indicates the food meets minimum fiber requirements; "–" indicates the food has a high sodium content.

Food	Processing Category	Brand
Stuffing	Mix	Stove Top Flexible Serving
Stuffing	Mix	Stove Top Flexible Serving
Stuffing	Mix	Stove Top Microwave
Stuffing	Mix	Stove Top Microwave
Stuffing	Mix	Stove Top Microwave
Stuffing	Mix	Traditional Betty Crocker
Taco Salad Shell	Packaged	Azteca
Taco Shell	Packaged	Azteca
Taco Shell	Packaged	Gebhardt
Taco Shell	Packaged	Lawry's
Taco Shell	Packaged	Lawry's Super
Taco Shell	Packaged	Old El Paso
Taco Shell	Packaged	Old El Paso
Taco Shell	Packaged	Old El Paso
Taco Shell	Packaged	Old El Paso
Taco Shell	Packaged	Ortega
Taco Shell	Packaged	Rosarita
Taco Shell	Packaged	Tio Sancho
Taco Shell	Packaged	Tio Sancho Super
Tortilla Shell	Packaged	Azteca
Tortilla Shell	Packaged	Azteca
Tortilla Shell	Packaged	Old El Paso
Tortilla Shell	Packaged	Old El Paso
Tostada Shell	Packaged	Lawry's
Tostada Shell	Packaged	Old El Paso
Tostada Shell	Packaged	Ortega
Tostada Shell	Packaged	Tio Sancho
Waffle	Frozen	Aunt Jemima
Waffle	Frozen	Aunt Jemima
Waffle	Frozen	Aunt Jemima
Waffle	Frozen	Aunt Jemima
Waffle	Frozen	Aunt Jemima
Waffle	Frozen	Aunt Jemima
Waffle	Frozen	Downyflake
Waffle	Frozen	Downyflake
Waffle	Frozen	Downyflake
Waffle	Frozen	Downyflake
Waffle	Frozen	Downyflake
Waffle	Frozen	Downyflake
Waffle	Frozen	Downyflake Crisp & Healthy
Waffle	Frozen	Downyflake Crisp & Healthy
Waffle	Frozen	Downyflake Hot & Buttery
Waffle	Frozen	Downyflake Jumbo
Waffle	Frozen	Eggo
Waffle	Frozen	Eggo
Waffle	Frozen	Eggo
Waffle	Frozen	Eggo
Waffle	Frozen	Eggo Common Sense
Waffle	Frozen	Eggo Common Sense
Waffle	Frozen	Eggo Homestyle
Waffle	Frozen	Eggo Nutri-Grain
Waffle	Frozen	Eggo Nutri-Grain
Waffle	Frozen	Roman Meal

Major Description	Minor Description	Serving Size	Calories	Grade
Corn Bread		¹/₂ cup	180	D–
Pork		¹/₂ cup	170	D–
Broccoli & Cheese		¹/₂ cup	170	D–
Chicken Flavor		¹/₂ cup	160	C–
Mushroom & Onion		¹/₂ cup	170	C–
Herb		¹/₂ cup	190	D–
Flour		1 piece	200	D
Corn		1 piece	60	D
		1 piece	30	D
		1 piece	50	C–
		1 piece	86	C–
		1 piece	55	D
Corn, White		1 piece	60	D
Mini Shell		1 piece	23	D
Super Shell		1 piece	100	D+
		1 piece	70	D
		1 piece	45	C
		1 piece	64	D
		1 piece	94	D
Corn		1 piece	45	A
Flour	9 Inch	1 piece	130	B–
Corn		1 piece	60	A–
Flour		1 piece	150	B–
		1 piece	73	D–
		1 piece	55	D
		1 piece	50	C
		1 piece	67	D
Apple Cinnamon		1 piece	176	B–
Blueberry		1 piece	175	B–
Buttermilk		1 piece	179	B–
Oat Bran		1 piece	154	B–+
Whole Grain Wheat		1 piece	154	B–+
Original		1 piece	173	B–
Blueberry		1 piece	90	B–
Buttermilk		1 piece	95	B–
Multigrain		1 piece	125	A–
Oat Bran		1 piece	130	D+–
Plain		1 piece	60	B–
Rice Bran		1 piece	105	D+
Apple Cinnamon		1 piece	80	A–
Plain		1 piece	80	A–
		1 piece	90	B–
		1 piece	85	B–
Apple Cinnamon		1 piece	110	C–
Blueberry		1 piece	110	C–
Buttermilk		1 piece	120	C–
Strawberry		1 piece	130	C–
Oat Bran		1 piece	110	B–+
Oat Bran	Fruit & Nuts	1 piece	120	B–+
		1 piece	120	C–
Raisins & Bran		1 piece	130	C–+
Whole Grain Wheat		1 piece	100	B–+
		1 piece	140	D–

"+" indicates the food meets minimum fiber requirements; "–" indicates the food has a high sodium content.

Food	Processing Category	Brand
Waffle	Frozen	Roman Meal
Waffle	Frozen	Weight Watchers Microwave
Wheat Bran	Dry	
Wheat Bran	Dry	Kretschmer
Wheat Bran	Dry	Quaker
Wheat Cake	Packaged	Quaker Grain Cakes
Wheat Flakes	Dry	Arrowhead Mills
Wheat Germ	Dry	
Wheat Germ	Dry	
Wheat Germ	Dry	Arrowhead Mills
Wheat Germ	Dry	Kretschmer
Wheat Gluten	Dry	Arrowhead Mills
Wheat Nuts	Dry	
Wheat Pilaf	Mix	Casbah
Wheat Pilaf	Mix	Near East
Wheat Pilaf	Mix	Near East
Wheat, Sprouted	Dry	
Wheat, Whole Grain	Dry	

Major Description	Minor Description	Serving Size	Calories	Grade
Whole Grain		1 piece	140	D–
Belgian Style		1 piece	120	B–
Crude		$1/4$ cup	33	B+
Toasted		$1/4$ cup	42	C+
Unprocessed		$1/4$ cup	16	B+
		1 cake	34	A–+
		$1/2$ cup	210	A+
Crude		$1/4$ cup	102	B+
Toasted		$1/4$ cup	108	B+
Raw		$1/4$ cup	105	B+
Honey Crunch		$1/4$ cup	105	B+
Vital		1 oz	100	A
All Flavors		1 oz	180	D
		$1/2$ cup	100	A
Pilaf		$1/2$ cup	100	B–+
Tabouli		$1/2$ cup	90	B–+
		$1/2$ cup	107	A+
All Varieties		$1/2$ cup	325	A+

"+" indicates the food meets minimum fiber requirements; "–" indicates the food has a high sodium content.

Condiments

All oils, spreads, spices, herbs, as well as dressings, pasta and tomato sauces, whether they be bottled, canned, dry, or mixes, are found in this Condiments section. The exceptions will be meat and cheese spreads and sauces, to be found under the Meat and Dairy sections, respectively.

Food	Processing Category	Brand
Allspice	Packaged	All Brands
Almond Butter	Jars	Generic
Almond Butter	Jars	Generic
Almond Butter	Jars	Hain
Almond Butter	Jars	Hain Natural
Almond Paste	Packaged	All Brands
Anise Seed	Packaged	All Brands
Apple Butter	Jars	Bama
Apple Butter	Jars	Lucky Leaf/Musselmans
Apple Butter	Jars	Smucker's Autumn Harvest
Apple Butter	Jars	Tap N Apple
Apple Butter	Jars	White House
Baking Powder	Packaged	Davis
Baking Powder	Packaged	Featherweight Low Salt
Baking Powder	Packaged	Tones
Baking Soda	Packaged	All Brands
Barbecue Sauce, *see also* Cooking Sauce		
Barbecue Sauce	Bottled	Bulls-Eye
Barbecue Sauce	Bottled	Bulls-Eye
Barbecue Sauce	Bottled	Enrico's
Barbecue Sauce	Bottled	Enrico's Original
Barbecue Sauce	Bottled	Estee
Barbecue Sauce	Bottled	French's Cattleman's
Barbecue Sauce	Bottled	French's Cattleman's
Barbecue Sauce	Bottled	Golden Dipt
Barbecue Sauce	Bottled	Hain
Barbecue Sauce	Bottled	Heinz
Barbecue Sauce	Bottled	Heinz
Barbecue Sauce	Bottled	Heinz
Barbecue Sauce	Bottled	Heinz
Barbecue Sauce	Bottled	Heinz
Barbecue Sauce	Bottled	Heinz
Barbecue Sauce	Bottled	Heinz Old Fashioned
Barbecue Sauce	Bottled	Heinz Select
Barbecue Sauce	Bottled	Heinz Thick and Rich
Barbecue Sauce	Bottled	Hunt Original
Barbecue Sauce	Bottled	K C Masterpiece
Barbecue Sauce	Bottled	K C Masterpiece
Barbecue Sauce	Bottled	K C Masterpiece
Barbecue Sauce	Bottled	Kraft
Barbecue Sauce	Bottled	Kraft
Barbecue Sauce	Bottled	Kraft
Barbecue Sauce	Bottled	Kraft
Barbecue Sauce	Bottled	Kraft
Barbecue Sauce	Bottled	Kraft
Barbecue Sauce	Bottled	Kraft
Barbecue Sauce	Bottled	Kraft
Barbecue Sauce	Bottled	Kraft
Barbecue Sauce	Bottled	Kraft
Barbecue Sauce	Bottled	Kraft

Major Description	Minor Description	Serving Size	Calories	Grade
Ground		1 tsp	5	C+
Honey & Cinnamon		2 Tbsp	188	D
Plain		2 Tbsp	202	D
Plain	Blanched Toasted	2 Tbsp	220	D
Plain	Raw	2 Tbsp	190	D
		1 Tbsp	63	D
		1 tsp	7	C+
		2 Tbsp	25	A
		2 Tbsp	50	A
		2 Tbsp	24	A
		2 Tbsp	45	A
		2 Tbsp	50	A
		1 tsp	8	A–
		1 tsp	8	A
		1 tsp	5	A–
		1 tsp	0	A–
Honey Mustard		2 Tbsp	60	A–
Original		2 Tbsp	60	A–
Mesquite		2 Tbsp	36	C
		2 Tbsp	36	C
		2 Tbsp	36	A
Mild		2 Tbsp	50	A–
Smoky		2 Tbsp	50	A–
Cajun Style		2 Tbsp	90	D–
Honey		2 Tbsp	24	D–
Cajun Style		2 Tbsp	30	A–
Hawaiian Style		2 Tbsp	38	A–
Hickory Smoke		2 Tbsp	38	A–
Mushroom		2 Tbsp	24	A–
Onion		2 Tbsp	30	A–
Texas Style, Hot		2 Tbsp	30	A–
		2 Tbsp	36	A–
		2 Tbsp	36	A–
All Varieties		2 Tbsp	40	A–
		2 Tbsp	40	A–
Honey Dijon		2 Tbsp	50	B–
Honey Teriyaki		2 Tbsp	60	A–
Original		2 Tbsp	60	A–
		2 Tbsp	45	B–
Char-grill		2 Tbsp	60	A–
Garlic		2 Tbsp	40	A–
Hickory Smoke		2 Tbsp	45	B–
Hickory Smoke	Onion Bits	2 Tbsp	50	B–
Honey	Thick & Spicy	2 Tbsp	60	A–
Hot		2 Tbsp	45	B–
Hot	Hickory Smoke	2 Tbsp	45	B–
Italian Style Seasonings		2 Tbsp	50	B–
Kansas City Style		2 Tbsp	50	B–
Mesquite	Smoke	2 Tbsp	45	B–
Onion	Bits	2 Tbsp	50	B–
Original		2 Tbsp	40	A–

"+" indicates the food meets minimum fiber requirements; "–" indicates the food has a high sodium content.

Food	Processing Category	Brand
Barbecue Sauce	Bottled	Kraft
Barbecue Sauce	Bottled	Kraft
Barbecue Sauce	Bottled	Kraft Thick N Spicy
Barbecue Sauce	Bottled	Kraft Thick N Spicy
Barbecue Sauce	Bottled	Kraft Thick N Spicy
Barbecue Sauce	Bottled	Kraft Thick N Spicy
Barbecue Sauce	Bottled	Kraft Thick N Spicy
Barbecue Sauce	Bottled	Kraft Thick N Spicy Original
Barbecue Sauce	Bottled	La Choy
Barbecue Sauce	Bottled	Lawry's
Barbecue Sauce	Bottled	Lawry's California Grill
Barbecue Sauce	Bottled	Lea & Perrins
Barbecue Sauce	Bottled	Libby's
Barbecue Sauce	Bottled	Maull's
Barbecue Sauce	Bottled	Maull's Genuine
Barbecue Sauce	Bottled	Maull's Lite
Barbecue Sauce	Bottled	Maull's Sweet & Mild
Barbecue Sauce	Bottled	Maull's Sweet & Smokey
Barbecue Sauce	Bottled	Ott's
Barbecue Sauce	Bottled	Texas Best
Barbecue Sauce	Bottled	Texas Best
Barbecue Sauce	Bottled	Texas Best
Barbecue Sauce	Bottled	Texas Best
Barbecue Sauce	Bottled	Texas Best
Bay Leaf	Packaged	Generic
Bearnaise Sauce	Mix	Great Impressions
Bearnaise Sauce	Mix	Knorr
Beef Seasoning	Mix	French's
Beef Stew Seasoning	Mix	French's
Beef Stew Seasoning	Mix	Lawry's
Beef Stew Seasoning	Mix	McCormick/Schilling
Beef Stroganoff Seasoning	Mix	McCormick/Schilling
Beer Batter	Mix	Golden Dipt
Cajun Sauce	Jarred	Golden Dipt
Canola Oil	Bottled	All Brands
Cardamom	Packaged	All Brands
Cardamom	Packaged	All Brands
Cashew Butter	Packaged	All Brands
Celery Salt	Packaged	Tones
Celery Seed	Packaged	All Brands
Chicken Sauce	Mix	Knorr
Chicken Sauce	Mix	Knorr
Chicken Sauce	Mix	McCormick/Schilling Sauce Blends
Chicken Sauce	Mix	McCormick/Schilling Sauce Blends
Chicken Sauce	Mix	McCormick/Schilling Sauce Blends
Chicken Sauce	Mix	McCormick/Schilling Sauce Blends
Chicken Sauce	Mix	McCormick/Schilling Sauce Blends
Chicken Sauce	Mix	McCormick/Schilling Sauce Blends
Chicken Seasoning & Coating	Mix	Featherweight
Chicken Seasoning & Coating	Mix	Golden Dipt
Chicken Seasoning & Coating	Mix	McCormick/Schilling
Chicken Seasoning & Coating	Mix	McCormick/Schilling
Chicken Seasoning & Coating	Mix	Shake 'n Bake

Major Description	Minor Description	Serving Size	Calories	Grade
Salsa		2 Tbsp	45	A–
Teriyaki		2 Tbsp	60	A–
Chunky		2 Tbsp	60	A–
Hickory Smoke		2 Tbsp	50	B–
Kansas City Style		2 Tbsp	60	A–
Mesquite	Smoke	2 Tbsp	50	B–
with Honey		2 Tbsp	60	A–
		2 Tbsp	50	B–
Oriental Style		2 Tbsp	36	A–
Dijon & Honey		2 Tbsp	50	A–
Orange Juice		2 Tbsp	17	B–
Original		2 Tbsp	50	A–
Sloppy Joe with Beef		2 Tbsp	44	D–
All Varieties		2 Tbsp	40	A–
		2 Tbsp	40	A–
		2 Tbsp	24	A–
Sweet		2 Tbsp	54	C–+
Sweet		2 Tbsp	50	C–+
All Varieties		2 Tbsp	28	A–
Cajun Style		2 Tbsp	45	D–
Hawaiian Style		2 Tbsp	60	A–
Mesquite		2 Tbsp	45	A–
Original		2 Tbsp	40	D–
Sweet & Sour		2 Tbsp	60	A–
Dry		1 tsp	2	A
		1/2 cup	351	D–
		1/2 cup	350	D–
Ground	with Onions	1/4 pkg	25	A–
		1/4 pkg	38	A–
		1/4 pkg	33	A–
		1/4 pkg	33	A–
		1/4 pkg	32	A–
		1 oz	100	A–
Cajun Style		1 Tbsp	45	D–+
		1 Tbsp	120	D
Ground		1 Tbsp	44	B+
Seed		1 Tbsp	18	A+
		1 oz	167	D
		1 tsp	6	D–+
Dry		1 tsp	8	D+
Coq au Vin		1/4 cup	40	D–
Dijonnaise		1/4 cup	30	B–
Cacciatore		1 pkg	132	C–
Creole Style		1 pkg	140	C–
Curry		1 pkg	152	C–
Dijon Style		1 pkg	156	C–
Mesquite Marinade		1 pkg	132	B–
Teriyaki		1 pkg	172	B–
		1/4 pkg	18	A–
		2 Tbsp	90	A–
		1/4 pkg	22	A–
Fried		2 Tbsp	16	D–
		1/4 pouch	80	B–

"+" indicates the food meets minimum fiber requirements; "–" indicates the food has a high sodium content.

Food	Processing Category	Brand
Chicken Seasoning & Coating	Mix	Shake 'n Bake
Chicken Seasoning & Coating	Mix	Shake 'n Bake Oven Fry
Chicken Seasoning & Coating	Mix	Shake 'n Bake Oven Fry Extra Crispy
Chicken Seasoning & Coating	Mix	Tone's
Chili Mix	Mix	Fantastic Foods
Chili Mix	Mix	Old El Paso
Chili Mix	Mix	Old El Paso Chili Con Carne
Chili Powder	See Chili Seasoning	
Chili Sauce	Bottled	Chef Boyardee
Chili Sauce	Bottled	Del Monte
Chili Sauce	Bottled	El Molino
Chili Sauce	Bottled	Featherweight
Chili Sauce	Bottled	Gebhardt
Chili Sauce	Bottled	Heinz
Chili Sauce	Bottled	S & W Chili Makins
Chili Sauce	Bottled	Wolf Brand
Chili Seasoning	Mix	Hain
Chili Seasoning	Mix	Lawry's Seasoning Blends
Chili Seasoning	Mix	McCormick/Schilling
Chili Seasoning	Mix	Old El Paso
Chili Seasoning	Mix	Tio Sancho
Chili Seasoning	Packaged	Tone's
Clam Sauce	Canned	Buitoni
Clam Sauce	Canned	Ferrara
Clam Sauce	Canned	Ferrara
Clam Sauce	Canned	Progresso
Clam Sauce	Canned	Progresso
Clam Sauce	Canned	Progresso Authentic Pasta
Clam Sauce	Refrigerated	Contadina Fresh
Clam Sauce	Refrigerated	Contadina Fresh
Cocktail Sauce	Bottled	Del Monte
Cocktail Sauce	Bottled	Estee
Cocktail Sauce	Bottled	Golden Dipt
Cocktail Sauce	Bottled	Great Impressions
Cocktail Sauce	Bottled	Great Impressions Brandy Glow
Cocktail Sauce	Bottled	Great Impressions Low Salt
Cocktail Sauce	Bottled	Heinz
Cocktail Sauce	Bottled	Sauceworks
Cocktail Sauce	Bottled	Stokely
Coconut Oil	Bottled	Generic
Cod Liver Oil	Bottled	Hain
Sauce, Cooking	Bottled or in Jars	Escoffier
Cooking Sauce	Bottled or in Jars	Heinz Thick & Rich
Cooking Sauce	Bottled or in Jars	Knorr
Cooking Sauce	Bottled or in Jars	Knorr
Cooking Sauce	Bottled or in Jars	Knorr
Cooking Sauce	Bottled or in Jars	Knorr
Cooking Sauce	Bottled or in Jars	Knorr
Cooking Sauce	Bottled or in Jars	Knorr
Cooking Sauce	Bottled or in Jars	Kraft
Cooking Sauce	Bottled or in Jars	Kraft
Cooking Sauce	Bottled or in Jars	Lea & Perrins
Cooking Sauce	Bottled or in Jars	Marinade

Major Description	Minor Description	Serving Size	Calories	Grade
Barbecue		¹/₄ pouch	90	B–
Homestyle		¹/₄ pouch	80	B–
		¹/₄ pouch	110	B–
Cajun Style Batter		2 Tbsp	72	A–
with Beans, Vegetarian		¹/₂ cup	104	A–
Beans		¹/₂ cup	108	D–+
		¹/₂ cup	131	C–
		1 Tbsp	24	D–+
Hot Dog		1 Tbsp	15	B–
Tomato		1 Tbsp	17	A–
Green, Mild		1 Tbsp	5	A–
		1 Tbsp	8	A–
Hot Dog		1 Tbsp	10	D–
		1 Tbsp	16	A–
		1 Tbsp	13	A–
Hot Dog		1 Tbsp	17	D–
All Flavors		¹/₄ pkg	30	B–
All Flavors		¹/₄ pkg	143	A–
All Flavors		¹/₄ pkg	27	B–
All Flavors		¹/₄ pkg	26	C–+
All Flavors		¹/₄ pkg	27	B–+
Powder		1 tsp	12	B–+
Red		¹/₂ cup	152	B–
Red		¹/₂ cup	70	B–
White		¹/₂ cup	80	D–
Red		¹/₂ cup	70	C–
White		¹/₂ cup	110	D–
White		¹/₂ cup	130	D–
Red		¹/₂ cup	60	B–
White		¹/₂ cup	190	D–
		1 Tbsp	18	A–
		1 Tbsp	10	D–
Regular or Extra Hot		1 Tbsp	20	A–
		1 Tbsp	21	A–
		1 Tbsp	68	D–
		1 Tbsp	21	A
		1 Tbsp	17	A–
		1 Tbsp	14	A–
		1 Tbsp	18	A–
		1 Tbsp	120	D
Regular or Mint		1 Tbsp	120	D
Diablo		2 Tbsp	40	A–
Buffalo Wing		2 Tbsp	15	A–+
Grilling & Broiling	Chardonnay	2 Tbsp	35	D–
Grilling & Broiling	Spicy Plumb	2 Tbsp	54	B–
Grilling & Broiling	Tequila Lime	2 Tbsp	35	C–
Grilling & Broiling	Tucson Herb	2 Tbsp	35	D–
Microwave	Mandarin Ginger	2 Tbsp	40	D–
Microwave	Parmesano	2 Tbsp	30	C–
Char-grill		2 Tbsp	60	A–
Salsa		2 Tbsp	45	A–
Worcesteshire	Original	2 Tbsp	30	A–
Citrus Grill		2 Tbsp	30	A–

"+" indicates the food meets minimum fiber requirements; "–" indicates the food has a high sodium content.

Food	Processing Category	Brand
Cooking Sauce	Bottled or in Jars	Marinade
Cooking Sauce	Bottled or in Jars	Marinade
Cooking Sauce	Bottled or in Jars	Mr. Marinade
Cooking Sauce	Bottled or in Jars	Mr. Marinade
Cooking Sauce	Bottled or in Jars	Mr. Marinade
Cooking Sauce	Bottled or in Jars	Open Pit
Corn Oil	Bottled	All Brands
Corn Oil	Spray	Mazola No Stick
Corn Syrup	Bottled	Karo
Corn Syrup	Bottled	Karo
Cranberry Sauce	Canned	Generic
Cranberry Sauce	Canned	Ocean Spray
Cream Gravy	Canned	Franco-American
Creole Sauce	Bottled	Enrico's Light
Cumin Seed	Packaged	All Brands
Curry Powder	Packaged	All Brands
Curry Sauce	Mix	Generic
Dill Seasoning	Packaged	McCormick/Schilling Parsley Patch
Dill Seed	Packaged	All Brands
Dill Weed	Packaged	All Brands
Dip	Mix	Fantastic Foods
Dip	Mix	Knorr
Dip	Mix	Knorr
Dip	Mix	Knorr
Dip	Mix	Knorr
Dip	Mix	Knorr
Dip	Mix	Knorr
Dip	Mix	Knorr
Dip	Packaged or in Jars	Bison
Dip	Packaged or in Jars	Breakstone's
Dip	Packaged or in Jars	Breakstone's
Dip	Packaged or in Jars	Breakstone's
Dip	Packaged or in Jars	Breakstone's
Dip	Packaged or in Jars	Breakstone's Gourmet
Dip	Packaged or in Jars	Breakstone's Gourmet
Dip	Packaged or in Jars	Breakstone's Gourmet
Dip	Packaged or in Jars	Breakstone's Gourmet
Dip	Packaged or in Jars	Breakstone's Gourmet
Dip	Packaged or in Jars	Guiltless Gourmet
Dip	Packaged or in Jars	Guiltless Gourmet
Dip	Packaged or in Jars	Guiltless Gourmet
Dip	Packaged or in Jars	Guiltless Gourmet
Dip	Packaged or in Jars	Hain
Dip	Packaged or in Jars	Hain
Dip	Packaged or in Jars	Hain
Dip	Packaged or in Jars	Kemp's
Dip	Packaged or in Jars	Kemp's
Dip	Packaged or in Jars	Kraft
Dip	Packaged or in Jars	Kraft
Dip	Packaged or in Jars	Kraft
Dip	Packaged or in Jars	Kraft
Dip	Packaged or in Jars	Kraft
Dip	Packaged or in Jars	Kraft Premium

CONDIMENTS 75

Major Description	Minor Description	Serving Size	Calories	Grade
Herbs & Garlic		2 Tbsp	20	A–
Lemon Pepper		2 Tbsp	20	D–
Honey Mustard		2 Tbsp	40	A–
Italian Style		2 Tbsp	20	A–
White Wine		2 Tbsp	30	B–
Original		2 Tbsp	50	A–
		1 Tbsp	125	D
		2.5 second spray	6	D
Dark		1 Tbsp	60	A
Light		1 Tbsp	60	A
Sweetened		4 oz	171	A
Whole or Jellied		4 oz	180	A
		1/4 cup	35	D–
Cajun Style		1/2 cup	38	C–
Dry		1 Tbsp	22	D+
Dry		1 tsp	6	C+
		1/2 cup	135	D–
Dry		1 tsp	11	C
Dry		1 tsp	6	D+
Dry		1 tsp	3	A+
Hummus		2 Tbsp	60	D+–
Black Bean		1/16 pkg	10	A–
Chili Caliente		2 Tbsp	100	D–
Cracked Pepper, Ranch		2 Tbsp	100	D–
Dill		2 Tbsp	100	D–
Mexican Bean		1/16 pkg	10	A–
Onion & Chive		2 Tbsp	100	D–
Pesto		2 Tbsp	60	D–
French Onion		2 Tbsp	60	D–
Bacon & Horseradish		2 Tbsp	70	D–
Clam		2 Tbsp	50	D–
Cucumber & Onion		2 Tbsp	50	D–
French Onion		2 Tbsp	50	D–
Bacon & Onion		2 Tbsp	70	D–
Clam		2 Tbsp	50	D–
Jalapeño Pepper	Cheddar	2 Tbsp	70	D–
Mushroom & Herb		2 Tbsp	50	D–
Toasted Onion		2 Tbsp	50	D–
Black Bean		2 Tbsp	25	A–+
Black Bean	Barbecue	2 Tbsp	35	A–+
Pinto Bean		2 Tbsp	25	A+
Pinto Bean	Barbecue	2 Tbsp	25	A–+
Jalapeño Bean	Medium	2 Tbsp	35	A–
Onion	Bean	2 Tbsp	35	A–
Taco	& Sauce	4 Tbsp	25	C–
French Onion	Party Dip	1 oz	50	D–
Vegetable		1 oz	30	D–
Bacon & Horseradish		2 Tbsp	60	D–
Clam		2 Tbsp	60	D–
French Onion		2 Tbsp	60	D–
Green Onion		2 Tbsp	60	D–
Jalapeño Pepper		2 Tbsp	50	D–
Bacon & Horseradish		2 Tbsp	50	D–

"+" indicates the food meets minimum fiber requirements; "–" indicates the food has a high sodium content.

Food	Processing Category	Brand
Dip	Packaged or in Jars	Kraft Premium
Dip	Packaged or in Jars	Kraft Premium
Dip	Packaged or in Jars	Kraft Premium
Dip	Packaged or in Jars	Kraft Premium
Dip	Packaged or in Jars	Kraft Premium
Dip	Packaged or in Jars	Kraft Premium
Dip	Packaged or in Jars	La Victoria
Dip	Packaged or in Jars	Life All Natural
Dip	Packaged or in Jars	Nasoya Vegi-Dip
Dip	Packaged or in Jars	Nasoya Vegi-Dip
Dip	Packaged or in Jars	Nasoya Vegi-Dip
Dip	Packaged or in Jars	Old El Paso
Dip	Packaged or in Jars	Old El Paso
Dip	Packaged or in Jars	Price's
Dip	Packaged or in Jars	Sealtest
Dip	Packaged or in Jars	Sealtest
Dip	Packaged or in Jars	Sealtest
Dip	Packaged or in Jars	Smart Temptations
Dip	Packaged or in Jars	Smart Temptations
Dip	Packaged or in Jars	Smart Temptations
Dip	Packaged or in Jars	Wise
Dip	Packaged or in Jars	Wise
Enchilada Sauce	Canned or in Jars	Del Monte
Enchilada Sauce	Canned or in Jars	Del Monte
Enchilada Sauce	Canned or in Jars	El Molino
Enchilada Sauce	Canned or in Jars	La Victoria
Enchilada Sauce	Canned or in Jars	Las Palmas
Enchilada Sauce	Canned or in Jars	Las Palmas
Enchilada Sauce	Canned or in Jars	Las Palmas
Enchilada Sauce	Canned or in Jars	Old El Paso
Enchilada Sauce	Canned or in Jars	Old El Paso
Enchilada Sauce	Canned or in Jars	Old El Paso
Enchilada Sauce	Canned or in Jars	Ortega
Enchilada Sauce	Canned or in Jars	Rosarita
Enchilada Seasoning	Mix	Lawry's
Enchilada Seasoning	Mix	Old El Paso
Fajita Marinade	Bottled	Old El Paso
Fajita Marinade	Bottled	Tone's
Fajita Sauce	Bottled	Tio Sancho Skillet Sauce
Fennel Seed	Packaged	All Brands
Fenugreek Seed	Packaged	All Brands
Fish Seasoning & Coating	Mix	Golden Dipt
Fish Seasoning & Coating	Mix	Golden Dipt
Fish Seasoning & Coating	Mix	Golden Dipt
Fish Seasoning & Coating	Mix	Golden Dipt
Fish Seasoning & Coating	Mix	Golden Dipt
Fish Seasoning & Coating	Mix	Golden Dipt
Fish Seasoning & Coating	Mix	Golden Dipt
Fish Seasoning & Coating	Mix	Golden Dipt
Fish Seasoning & Coating	Mix	Golden Dipt
Fish Seasoning & Coating	Mix	McCormick/Schilling
Fish Seasoning & Coating	Mix	Shake 'n Bake
Fish Seasoning & Coating	Mix	Tone's

Major Description	Minor Description	Serving Size	Calories	Grade
Bacon & Onion		2 Tbsp	60	D–
Clam		2 Tbsp	45	D–
Creamy Onion		2 Tbsp	45	D–
Cucumber	Creamy	2 Tbsp	50	D–
French Onion		2 Tbsp	45	D–
Jalapeño Pepper	Cheese	2 Tbsp	50	D–
Chili		2 Tbsp	12	B–
Garlic Dressing	with Tofu	2 Tbsp	140	D
Creamy Dill		2 Tbsp	60	D–
Frech Onion		2 Tbsp	50	D–
Garlic Dressing		2 Tbsp	50	C–
Jalapeño	Mild	2 Tbsp	28	A–+
Salsa	All Varieties	2 Tbsp	10	A–+
Jalapeño Pepper	Nacho	2 Tbsp	80	D
Bacon & Horseradish		2 Tbsp	70	D–
Clam		2 Tbsp	50	D–
Cucumber & Onion		2 Tbsp	50	D–
Black Bean	Fat Free All Varieties	2 Tbsp	20	A–+
Garbanzo Bean	Fat Free All Varieties	2 Tbsp	20	A–+
Pinto Bean	Fat Free All Varieties	2 Tbsp	20	A–+
Jalapeño Bean		2 Tbsp	25	A–
Taco		2 Tbsp	12	A–
Hot		1/4 cup	22	A–
Mild		1/4 cup	22	A–
Hot		1/4 cup	32	D–
		1/4 cup	20	D–
Green Chile		1/4 cup	25	D–
Hot		1/4 cup	20	B–+
Original		1/4 cup	15	B–+
Green		1/4 cup	22	A–
Hot		1/4 cup	30	B–
Mild		1/4 cup	25	A–
Hot or Mild		1/4 cup	24	A–
		1/4 cup	14	A–
		2 Tbsp	6	A–
		2 Tbsp	4	A–
		1/8 jar	14	A–
		1 tsp	9	A–
		1 oz	14	C–
Dry		1 tsp	7	C+
Dry		1 tsp	12	B+
Batter, Fish & Chips		1 tsp	16	A–
Blackened Redfish		1 tsp	8	A–
Broiled		1 tsp	8	A–
Fish Fry		1 tsp	15	A–
Fish Fry Cajun Style		1 tsp	15	A–
Seafood		1 tsp	15	A–
Seafood	All-Purpose	1 tsp	8	A–
Seafood	Lemon Pepper	1 tsp	32	A–
Shrimp & Crab, Cajun Style		1 tsp	8	A–
Seafood	Chesapeake Bay Style	1 tsp	8	D–
		1/4 pouch	70	A–
Cajun Style		1 tsp	12	A–

"+" indicates the food meets minimum fiber requirements; "–" indicates the food has a high sodium content.

Food	Processing Category	Brand
Fish Seasoning & Coating	Mix	Tone's
Fish Seasoning & Coating	Mix	Tone's
Flavor Enhancer	Packaged	Accent
Forestiera Sauce	Refrigerated	Contadina Fresh
Fructose	Packaged	Estee
Fruit Spread	Jars	Knott's Berry Farm
Fruit Spread	Jars	Kraft
Fruit Spread	Jars	Polaner All Fruit Spreadable Fruit
Fruit Spread	Jars	Polaner Jam
Fruit Spread	Jars	Polaner Jelly
Fruit Spread	Jars	Polaner Preserves
Fruit Spread	Jars	Smucker's
Fruit Spread	Jars	Smucker's Jam
Fruit Spread	Jars	Smucker's Jelly
Fruit Spread	Jars	Smucker's Low Sugar Spread
Fruit Spread	Jars	Smucker's Preserves
Fruit Spread	Jars	Smuckers Simply Fruit
Fruit Spread	Jars	Sorrell Ridge
Fruit Spread	Jars	Weight Watchers
Garlic Bread Seasoning	Packaged	Lawry's
Garlic Bread Seasoning	Packaged	McCormick/Schilling Garlic Bread
Garlic Bread Seasoning	Packaged	Tone's Garlic Bread Sprinkle
Garlic Powder	Packaged	All Brands
Garlic Salt	Packaged	Lawry's
Garlic Salt	Packaged	Morton
Garlic Salt	Packaged	Tone's
Garlic Seasoning	Packaged	McCormick/Schilling Parsley Patch
Garlic Seasoning	Packaged	McCormick/Schilling Season All
Garlic Spread	Concentrate	Lawry's
Ginger	Packaged	All Brands
Ginger Root	Packaged	All Brands
Gravy	Canned or in Jars	Generic
Gravy	Canned or in Jars	Generic
Gravy	Mix	Generic
Gravy	Mix	Generic
Gravy	Mix	Generic
Gravy	Mix	Generic
Gravy	Canned or in Jars	Franco-American
Gravy	Canned or in Jars	Franco-American
Gravy	Canned or in Jars	Heinz Homestyle
Gravy	Canned or in Jars	Heinz Homestyle
Gravy	Canned or in Jars	Heinz Homestyle
Gravy	Canned or in Jars	Heinz Homestyle
Gravy	Canned or in Jars	Hormel Great Beginnings
Gravy	Canned or in Jars	Hormel Great Beginnings
Gravy	Canned or in Jars	Hormel Great Beginnings
Gravy	Canned or in Jars	McCormick/Schilling
Gravy	Mix	French's
Gravy	Mix	French's
Gravy	Mix	French's
Gravy	Mix	French's
Gravy	Mix	French's
Gravy	Mix	Lawry's

Major Description	Minor Description	Serving Size	Calories	Grade
Seafood		1 tsp	10	D+
Seafood	Chesapeake	1 tsp	8	C–+
		1 tsp	10	A–
		7.5 oz	270	B–
		1 tsp	12	A
All Varieties	Light Preserves	1 Tbsp	8	A
All Varieties		1 Tbsp	50	A
All Flavors		1 Tbsp	42	A
All Flavors		1 Tbsp	50	A
All Flavors		1 Tbsp	50	A
All Flavors		1 Tbsp	50	A
All Flavors		1 Tbsp	54	A
All Flavors		1 Tbsp	54	A
All Flavors		1 Tbsp	54	A
All Flavors		1 Tbsp	24	A
All Flavors		1 Tbsp	54	A
All Flavors		1 Tbsp	48	A
All Flavors	100% Fruit	1 Tbsp	54	A
All Flavors		1 Tbsp	24	A
		1 tsp	30	D
		1 tsp	20	D–
		1 tsp	17	D–
		1 tsp	9	A
		1 tsp	4	B–+
		1 tsp	3	B–
		1 tsp	2	A–+
		1 tsp	13	C
		1 tsp	8	A–
		1 Tbsp	15	D–
Ground		1 tsp	6	B+
Sliced or Ground		$^1/_4$ cup	17	A+
Mushroom		$^1/_4$ cup	30	D–
Turkey		$^1/_4$ cup	31	C
Brown	Prepared with Water	$^1/_4$ cup	19	B–
Mushroom		$^1/_4$ cup	18	A–
Onion		$^1/_4$ cup	19	A–
Turkey		$^1/_4$ cup	22	B–
Beef		$^1/_4$ cup	25	C–
Turkey		$^1/_4$ cup	30	D–
Brown		$^1/_4$ cup	25	C–
Brown	Onions	$^1/_4$ cup	25	C–
Pork		$^1/_4$ cup	25	C–
Turkey		$^1/_4$ cup	25	C–
Beef	with Chunky Beef	$^1/_4$ cup	55	D–
Pork	Chunky Pork	$^1/_4$ cup	60	D–
Turkey	with Chunky Turkey	$^1/_4$ cup	55	D–
Brown		$^1/_3$ cup	30	B–
Brown		$^1/_4$ cup	20	D–
Homestyle		$^1/_4$ cup	20	D–
Mushroom		$^1/_4$ cup	20	D–
Onion		$^1/_4$ cup	25	C–
Pork		$^1/_4$ cup	20	D–
Brown		$^1/_4$ cup	24	A–

"+" indicates the food meets minimum fiber requirements; "–" indicates the food has a high sodium content.

Food	Processing Category	Brand
Gravy	Mix	Lawry's
Gravy	Mix	McCormick
Gravy	Mix	McCormick/Schilling
Gravy	Mix	McCormick/Schilling
Gravy	Mix	McCormick/Schilling
Gravy	Mix	McCormick/Schilling
Gravy	Mix	McCormick/Schilling
Gravy	Mix	McCormick/Schilling
Gravy	Mix	McCormick/Schilling
Gravy	Mix	Pillsbury
Gravy	Mix	Pillsbury
Gravy, Chicken	Canned	Franco-American
Gravy, Chicken	Canned	Franco-American
Gravy, Chicken	Canned	Heinz Homestyle
Gravy, Chicken	Canned	Hormel Great Beginnings
Gravy, Chicken	Mix	French's Gravy for Chicken
Gravy, Chicken	Mix	Lawry's
Gravy, Chicken	Mix	McCormick/Schilling
Gravy, Chicken	Mix	Pillsbury
Gravy, Pork	Mix	Generic
Gravy, Pork	Canned	Franco-American
Guacamole Seasoning	Mix	Lawry's
Guacamole Seasoning	Mix	Old El Paso
Guava Sauce	Canned or in Jars	Generic
Herb & Garlic Sauce	Packaged	Lawry's
Herb Seasoning & Coating	Packaged	McCormick/Schilling Bag 'n Season
Herb Seasoning & Coating	Packaged	Shake 'n Bake
Hollandaise Sauce	Mix	Generic
Hollandaise Sauce	Mix	Generic
Hollandaise Sauce	Packaged	Great Impressions
Hollandaise Sauce	Packaged	Knorr
Hollandaise Sauce	Packaged	Tone's
Honey Butter	All Forms	Honey Butter
Horseradish	Prepared	Kraft
Horseradish Sauce	Bottled	Great Impressions
Horseradish Sauce	Bottled	Heinz
Horseradish Sauce	Bottled	Life All Natural
Horseradish Sauce	Bottled	Sauceworks
Hummus	Fresh	Homemade
Hummus	Mix	Casbah
Hummus	Mix	Fantastic Foods
Jams and Jellies	See Fruit Spread	
Ketchup	Bottled	Generic
Ketchup	Bottled	Generic
Ketchup	Bottled	Del Monte
Ketchup	Bottled	Del Monte No Salt Added
Ketchup	Bottled	Estee
Ketchup	Bottled	Featherweight
Ketchup	Bottled	Hain Natural
Ketchup	Bottled	Hain Natural No Salt Added
Ketchup	Bottled	Heinz
Ketchup	Bottled	Heinz
Ketchup	Bottled	Heinz

Major Description	Minor Description	Serving Size	Calories	Grade
Turkey		$^1/_4$ cup	25	C–
au Jus	Natural Style	$^1/_4$ cup	5	A–
Brown		$^1/_4$ cup	23	B–
Herb		$^1/_4$ cup	20	B–
Homestyle		$^1/_4$ cup	24	B–
Mushroom		$^1/_4$ cup	19	A–
Onion		$^1/_4$ cup	22	B–
Pork		$^1/_4$ cup	25	A–
Turkey		$^1/_4$ cup	22	B–
Brown		$^1/_4$ cup	15	A–
Homestyle		$^1/_4$ cup	15	A–
Chicken		$^1/_4$ cup	45	D–
Chicken	Giblet	$^1/_4$ cup	30	D–
Chicken		$^1/_4$ cup	35	D–
Chicken	Chunky Chicken	$^1/_4$ cup	30	D–
Chicken		$^1/_4$ cup	25	C–
Chicken		$^1/_4$ cup	25	B–
Chicken		$^1/_4$ cup	22	A–
Chicken		$^1/_4$ cup	25	C–
		$^1/_4$ cup	19	B–
		$^1/_4$ cup	40	D–
		1 pkg	60	A–
		1 pkg	49	A–
		$^1/_2$ cup	41	A+
with Lemon Juice		$^1/_4$ cup	36	A–
Italian Style		1 pkg	94	A–
Italian Style		$^1/_4$ pouch	80	A–
	Butterfat	2 Tbsp	30	D–
	Milk and Butter	2 Tbsp	88	D–
		2 Tbsp	192	D
Microwave		2 Tbsp	100	D–
		2 Tbsp	90	D–
		1 Tbsp	50	B
		1 Tbsp	10	A–
		1 Tbsp	74	D–
		1 Tbsp	74	D–
Strong		1 Tbsp	14	A
		1 Tbsp	50	D–
		2 Tbsp	50	D–
		2 Tbsp	55	D
		2 Tbsp	60	D–
		1 Tbsp	14	A–+
Low Sodium		1 Tbsp	14	A+
		1 Tbsp	15	A–
		1 Tbsp	15	A
		1 Tbsp	6	A–
		1 Tbsp	6	A
		1 Tbsp	16	A–
		1 Tbsp	16	A
		1 Tbsp	16	A–
Hot		1 Tbsp	16	A–
Onions		1 Tbsp	19	A–

"+" indicates the food meets minimum fiber requirements; "–" indicates the food has a high sodium content.

Food	Processing Category	Brand
Ketchup	Bottled	Heinz Lite
Ketchup	Bottled	Hunt's
Ketchup	Bottled	Hunt's No Salt Added
Ketchup	Bottled	Life All Natural
Ketchup	Bottled	Smucker's
Ketchup	Bottled	Stokely
Ketchup	Bottled	Weight Watchers
Lemon and Dill Seasoning	Packaged	Generic
Lemon Herb Marinade	Bottled	Golden Dipt
Lobster Sauce	Canned	Progresso
Mace	Packaged	All Brands
Maple Syrup	All Forms	Generic
Maple Syrup, Imitation	Bottled	Generic
Maple Syrup, Imitation	Bottled	Generic
Maple Syrup, Imitation	Bottled	Aunt Jemima Butter Rich
Maple Syrup, Imitation	Bottled	Aunt Jemima Butterlite
Maple Sytrup, Imitation	Bottled	Aunt Jemima Lite
Maple Syrup, Imitation	Bottled	Aunt Jemima Original
Maple Syrup, Imitation	Bottled	Aunt Jemima Pancake & Waffle
Maple Syrup, Imitation	Bottled	Estee
Maple Syrup, Imitation	Bottled	Featherweight
Maple Syrup, Imitation	Bottled	Log Cabin Country Kitchen
Maple Syrup, Imitation	Bottled	Log Cabin Lite
Maple Syrup, Imitation	Bottled	Log Cabin Pancake and Waffle
Maple Syrup, Imitation	Bottled	Mrs. Richardson's Lite
Maple Syrup, Imitation	Bottled	Mrs. Richardson's Original
Maple Syrup, Imitation	Bottled	S & W
Maple Syrup, Imitation	Bottled	Vermont Maid
Margarine	All Forms	All Brands Except as Noted
Margarine	All Forms	All Brands Except as Noted
Margarine	All Forms	All Brands Except as Noted
Margarine	All Forms	Country Morning Light Stick
Margarine	All Forms	I Can't Believe It's Not Butter
Margarine	All Forms	Mazola Diet
Margarine	All Forms	Nucoa Heart Beat
Margarine	All Forms	Nucoa Heart Beat Unsalted
Margarine	All Forms	Parkay Diet
Margarine	All Forms	Weight Watchers Stick
Marinade, see also Cooking Sauce		
Marinade	Mix	Lawry's
Marinade	Bottled	Girard's
Marinade	Bottled	Girard's
Marinade	Bottled	Girard's
Marinade	Bottled	Girard's
Marinade	Bottled	Lawry's
Marinade	Bottled	Lawry's
Marinade	Bottled	Lawry's
Marinade	Bottled	Lawry's
Marinade	Bottled	Lawry's
Marinade	Bottled	Lawry's
Marinade	Bottled	Marinade in Minutes

Major Description	Minor Description	Serving Size	Calories	Grade
		1 Tbsp	8	A–+
		1 Tbsp	15	A–
		1 Tbsp	20	A
		1 Tbsp	17	A
		1 Tbsp	8	A–
		1 Tbsp	20	A–
		1 Tbsp	12	A–
		1 pkg	161	D–
		1 fl oz	130	D–
Rock		$^1/_2$ cup	120	D–
Ground		1 tsp	8	D
		$^1/_2$ cup	397	A
Blend	Cane & Maple	1 Tbsp	50	A
Blend	Light & Dark Corn Syrup	1 Tbsp	59	A
		1 Tbsp	52	A
		1 Tbsp	25	A–
		1 Tbsp	27	A–
		1 Tbsp	54	A
		1 Tbsp	52	A
		1 Tbsp	4	A–
		1 Tbsp	16	A–
		1 Tbsp	50	A
		1 Tbsp	50	A–
		1 Tbsp	50	A
		1 Tbsp	25	A–
		1 Tbsp	52	A
Maple Flavor		1 Tbsp	12	A–
		1 Tbsp	50	A
Reduced Calorie	All Varieties	1 Tbsp	50	D–
Reduced Calorie	Unsalted	1 Tbsp	50	D
Regular Calorie	All Varieties	1 Tbsp	100	D–
		1 Tbsp	60	D–
Sweet		1 Tbsp	90	D
		1 Tbsp	50	D–
		1 Tbsp	25	D–
		1 Tbsp	24	D
		1 Tbsp	50	D–
		1 Tbsp	60	D–
Beef Marinade		$^1/_4$ pkt	12	A–
Honey Mustard		1 Tbsp	20	A–
Italian		1 Tbsp	10	A–
Red Wine		1 Tbsp	15	B–
White Wine		1 Tbsp	15	B–
Citrus Grill		1 Tbsp	15	A–
Herb & Garlic		1 Tbsp	10	A–
Lemon Pepper		1 Tbsp	10	D–
Mesquite		1 Tbsp	5	A–
Teriyaki		1 Tbsp	25	A–
Thai Ginger		1 Tbsp	10	D–
Hickory Grill		1 Tbsp	20	B–

"+" indicates the food meets minimum fiber requirements; "–" indicates the food has a high sodium content.

Food	Processing Category	Brand
Marinade	Bottled	Marinade in Minutes
Marinade	Bottled	Marinade in Minutes
Marinade	Bottled	Marinade in Minutes
Mayonnaise	Bottled or in Jars	Generic & Most Brands
Mayonnaise	Bottled or in Jars	Generic & Most Brands
Mayonnaise	Bottled or in Jars	Generic & Most Brands
Mayonnaise	Bottled or in Jars	Generic & Most Brands
Mayonnaise	Bottled or in Jars	Estee
Mayonnaise	Bottled or in Jars	Featherweight
Mayonnaise	Bottled or in Jars	Hain
Mayonnaise	Bottled or in Jars	Hain
Mayonnaise	Bottled or in Jars	Hain
Mayonnaise	Bottled or in Jars	Hain
Mayonnaise	Bottled or in Jars	Hain
Mayonnaise	Bottled or in Jars	Hain
Mayonnaise	Bottled or in Jars	Hellmann's Light
Mayonnaise	Bottled or in Jars	Kraft Free
Mayonnaise	Bottled or in Jars	Kraft Light
Mayonnaise	Bottled or in Jars	Miracle Whip
Mayonnaise	Bottled or in Jars	Miracle Whip
Mayonnaise	Bottled or in Jars	Miracle Whip Free
Mayonnaise	Bottled or in Jars	Miracle Whip Light
Mayonnaise	Bottled or in Jars	Spin Blend
Mayonnaise	Bottled or in Jars	Spin Blend
Mayonnaise	Bottled or in Jars	Weight Watchers
Mayonnaise	Bottled or in Jars	Weight Watchers
Mayonnaise	Bottled or in Jars	Weight Watchers
Mayonnaise	Bottled or in Jars	Weight Watchers Low Sodium
Mayonnaise, Imitation	Bottled or in Jars	Generic
Mayonnaise, Imitation	Bottled or in Jars	Generic
Mayonnaise, Imitation	Bottled or in Jars	Generic
Mayonnaise, Imitation	Bottled or in Jars	Generic
Mayonnaise, Imitation	Bottled or in Jars	Hain
Mayonnaise, Imitation	Bottled or in Jars	Hain
Mayonnaise, Imitation	Bottled or in Jars	Hellmann's Cholesterol Free
Mayonnaise, Imitation	Bottled or in Jars	Life All Natural
Mayonnaise, Imitation	Bottled or in Jars	Nucoa Heart Beat
Mayonnaise, Imitation	Bottled or in Jars	Weight Watchers Chloresterol Free
Mesquite Sauce	Bottled	Lawry's
Mexican Bean	Dip	Hain
Molasses	Canned or in Jars	Most Brands
Mushroom Sauce	Canned	Franco-American
Mustard	Jars	Featherweight
Mustard	Jars	French's
Mustard	Jars	French's
Mustard	Jars	French's
Mustard	Jars	French's
Mustard	Jars	French's
Mustard	Jars	French's Bold 'n Spicy
Mustard	Jars	Great Impressions
Mustard	Jars	Grey Poupon
Mustard	Jars	Gulden's
Mustard	Jars	Gulden's

Major Description	Minor Description	Serving Size	Calories	Grade
Lemon Garlic		1 Tbsp	30	D–
Mesquite		1 Tbsp	45	D–
Teriyaki		1 Tbsp	20	A–
Light		1 Tbsp	25	D–
Regular	All Varieties	1 Tbsp	100	D
Safflower & Soybean		1 Tbsp	99	D
Soybean		1 Tbsp	99	D
Reduced Calorie		1 Tbsp	45	D–
Reduced Calorie		1 Tbsp	30	D–
Canola		1 Tbsp	100	D
Canola	Low Calorie	1 Tbsp	60	D–
Eggless	No Salt Added	1 Tbsp	110	D
Light	Low Sodium	1 Tbsp	60	D
Regular		1 Tbsp	110	D
Safflower		1 Tbsp	110	D
Reduced Calorie		1 Tbsp	50	D–
Reduced Calorie		1 Tbsp	12	A–
Reduced Calorie		1 Tbsp	50	D–
Coleslaw		1 Tbsp	70	D–
Mayonnaise		1 Tbsp	70	D
Mayonnaise		1 Tbsp	20	A–
Mayonnaise		1 Tbsp	45	D–
Mayonnaise		1 Tbsp	60	D–
Mayonnaise	Cholesterol Free	1 Tbsp	40	D–
Fat Free		1 Tbsp	10	A–
Fat Free	Whipped	1 Tbsp	15	A–
Reduced Calorie		1 Tbsp	50	D–
Reduced Calorie		1 Tbsp	50	D
Milk, Cream		1 Tbsp	15	D–
Soybean		1 Tbsp	35	D–
Soybean	No Cholesterol	1 Tbsp	68	D
Tofu		1 Tbsp	40	D–
Canola	Reduced Calorie	1 Tbsp	60	D–
Eggless	No Salt Added	1 Tbsp	110	D
Reduced Calorie		1 Tbsp	50	D–
Sunflower		1 Tbsp	71	D
		1 Tbsp	40	D–
Reduced Calorie		1 Tbsp	50	D–
with Lime Juice		1/4 cup	24	A–
		4 Tbsp	60	A–
Dark or Light		1 Tbsp	60	A
		1/4 cup	25	C–
	Prepared	1 Tbsp	15	A
Dijon Style	Prepared	1 Tbsp	24	D–
Medford Style	Prepared	1 Tbsp	16	D–
Onion	Prepared	1 Tbsp	24	A–
with Horseradish	Prepared	1 Tbsp	16	D–
Yellow	Prepared	1 Tbsp	10	D–
Spicy	Prepared	1 Tbsp	18	A–
Jalapeño	Prepared	1 Tbsp	11	C–
Dijon Style	Prepared	1 Tbsp	18	D–
Brown, Spicy	Prepared	1 Tbsp	16	A–
Mild, Creamy	Prepared	1 Tbsp	12	A–

"+" indicates the food meets minimum fiber requirements; "–" indicates the food has a high sodium content.

Food	Processing Category	Brand
Mustard	Jars	Gulden's Diablo
Mustard	Jars	Hain Stone Ground
Mustard	Jars	Hain Stone Ground No Salt Added
Mustard	Jars	Heinz
Mustard	Jars	Heinz
Mustard	Jars	Kraft
Mustard	Jars	Kraft
Mustard	Jars	Life All Natural
Newberg Sauce	Canned	Generic
Nutmeg	Ground	Generic
Oil	Bottled	Generic
Oil	Bottled	Generic
Oil	Bottled	Generic
Oil	Bottled	Generic
Oil	Bottled	Generic
Oil	Bottled	Generic
Oil	Bottled	Generic
Oil	Bottled	Generic
Oil	Bottled	Generic
Oil	Bottled	Generic
Oil	Bottled	Generic
Oil	Bottled	Generic
Oil	Bottled	Generic
Oil	Bottled	Generic
Oil	Bottled	Generic
Oil	Bottled	Generic
Oil	Bottled	Generic
Oil	Bottled	Generic
Oil	Bottled or in Jars	Generic
Pancake Syrup, see Maple Syrup		
Paprika	Packaged	All Brands
Pasta Sauce	Canned or in Jars	Buitoni
Pasta Sauce	Canned or in Jars	Chef Boyardee
Pasta Sauce	Canned or in Jars	Chef Boyardee
Pasta Sauce	Canned or in Jars	Chef Boyardee
Pasta Sauce	Canned or in Jars	Chef Boyardee
Pasta Sauce	Canned or in Jars	Chef Boyardee
Pasta Sauce	Canned or in Jars	Chef Boyardee
Pasta Sauce	Canned or in Jars	Classico
Pasta Sauce	Canned or in Jars	Classico
Pasta Sauce	Canned or in Jars	Classico
Pasta Sauce	Canned or in Jars	Classico
Pasta Sauce	Canned or in Jars	Classico
Pasta Sauce	Canned or in Jars	Classico
Pasta Sauce	Canned or in Jars	Classico
Pasta Sauce	Canned or in Jars	Classico
Pasta Sauce	Canned or in Jars	Classico
Pasta Sauce	Canned or in Jars	Del Monte
Pasta Sauce	Canned or in Jars	Enrico's
Pasta Sauce	Canned or in Jars	Enrico's All Natural
Pasta Sauce	Canned or in Jars	Enrico's All Natural No Salt

Major Description	Minor Description	Serving Size	Calories	Grade
Hot	Prepared	1 Tbsp	16	A–
	Prepared	1 Tbsp	14	D–
	Prepared	1 Tbsp	14	D
Mild	Prepared	1 Tbsp	15	C–
Yellow	Prepared	1 Tbsp	9	D–
Horseradish	Prepared	1 Tbsp	14	D–
Pure	Prepared	1 Tbsp	11	D–
English Style	Prepared	1 Tbsp	22	D
		$^1/_4$ cup	90	D–
		1 Tbsp	37	D
Almond		1 Tbsp	120	D
Butter		1 Tbsp	112	D
Cottonseed		1 Tbsp	125	D
Grapeseed		1 Tbsp	125	D
Hazelnut		1 Tbsp	120	D
Nutmeg Butter		1 Tbsp	120	D
Olive	All Varieties	1 Tbsp	120	D
Palm		1 Tbsp	125	D
Palm Kernel		1 Tbsp	125	D
Peanut		1 Tbsp	125	D
Poppy Seed		1 Tbsp	120	D
Rice Bran		1 Tbsp	120	D
Safflower	All Varieties	1 Tbsp	120	D
Soybean		1 Tbsp	125	D
Soybean & Cottonseed	Hydrogenated	1 Tbsp	125	D
Soybean Lecithin		1 Tbsp	125	D
Sunflower		1 Tbsp	120	D
Tomato Seed		1 Tbsp	120	D
Coconut		1 Tbsp	120	D
Sesame		1 Tbsp	125	D
Ground		1 oz	82	D+
Marinara		$^1/_2$ cup	70	C–
Ground Beef		$^1/_2$ cup	99	B–
Meat or Meat Flavor		$^1/_2$ cup	130	D–
Meat or Meat Flavor		$^1/_2$ cup	88	C–
Meatless		$^1/_2$ cup	66	A–
Mushroom or Mushroom Flavor		$^1/_2$ cup	66	A–
Mushroom or Mushroom Flavor		$^1/_2$ cup	88	C–
4 Cheese		$^1/_2$ cup	70	D–
Beef & Pork		$^1/_2$ cup	90	D–
Mushroom & Olive		$^1/_2$ cup	50	B–
Onion & Garlic		$^1/_2$ cup	80	D–
Spice Red Pepper		$^1/_2$ cup	60	C–
Sundried Tomato		$^1/_2$ cup	80	D–
Sweet Pepper & Olive		$^1/_2$ cup	70	D–+
Tomato & Basil		$^1/_2$ cup	50	B–
Tomato & Pesto		$^1/_2$ cup	110	D–
Flavored with Meat		$^1/_2$ cup	70	B–
Mushroom or Mushroom Flavor		$^1/_2$ cup	65	A
Mushroom & Green Pepper		$^1/_2$ cup	65	A–
All Varieties		$^1/_2$ cup	65	A

"+" indicates the food meets minimum fiber requirements; "–" indicates the food has a high sodium content.

Food	Processing Category	Brand
Pasta Sauce	Canned or in Jars	Enrico's Pasta Sauce
Pasta Sauce	Canned or in Jars	Estee
Pasta Sauce	Canned or in Jars	Featherweight
Pasta Sauce	Canned or in Jars	Francesco Rinaldi
Pasta Sauce	Canned or in Jars	Francesco Rinaldi
Pasta Sauce	Canned or in Jars	Francesco Rinaldi
Pasta Sauce	Canned or in Jars	Francesco Rinaldi
Pasta Sauce	Canned or in Jars	Francesco Rinaldi
Pasta Sauce	Canned or in Jars	Healthy Choice
Pasta Sauce	Canned or in Jars	Hunt's
Pasta Sauce	Canned or in Jars	Hunt's
Pasta Sauce	Canned or in Jars	Hunt's
Pasta Sauce	Canned or in Jars	Hunt's
Pasta Sauce	Canned or in Jars	Hunt's
Pasta Sauce	Canned or in Jars	Hunt's
Pasta Sauce	Canned or in Jars	Hunt's
Pasta Sauce	Canned or in Jars	Hunt's
Pasta Sauce	Canned or in Jars	Hunt's
Pasta Sauce	Canned or in Jars	Newman's Own
Pasta Sauce	Canned or in Jars	Newman's Own
Pasta Sauce	Canned or in Jars	Newman's Own
Pasta Sauce	Canned or in Jars	Newman's Own
Pasta Sauce	Canned or in Jars	Newman's Own
Pasta Sauce	Canned or in Jars	Prego
Pasta Sauce	Canned or in Jars	Prego
Pasta Sauce	Canned or in Jars	Prego
Pasta Sauce	Canned or in Jars	Prego
Pasta Sauce	Canned or in Jars	Prego
Pasta Sauce	Canned or in Jars	Prego
Pasta Sauce	Canned or in Jars	Prego
Pasta Sauce	Canned or in Jars	Prego
Pasta Sauce	Canned or in Jars	Prego
Pasta Sauce	Canned or in Jars	Prego
Pasta Sauce	Canned or in Jars	Prego
Pasta Sauce	Canned or in Jars	Prego
Pasta Sauce	Canned or in Jars	Prego
Pasta Sauce	Canned or in Jars	Prego Extra Chunky
Pasta Sauce	Canned or in Jars	Prego Extra Chunky
Pasta Sauce	Canned or in Jars	Prego Extra Chunky
Pasta Sauce	Canned or in Jars	Prego Extra Chunky
Pasta Sauce	Canned or in Jars	Prego Extra Chunky
Pasta Sauce	Canned or in Jars	Prego No Salt Added
Pasta Sauce	Canned or in Jars	Pritikin
Pasta Sauce	Canned or in Jars	Pritikin
Pasta Sauce	Canned or in Jars	Pritikin
Pasta Sauce	Canned or in Jars	Progresso
Pasta Sauce	Canned or in Jars	Progresso
Pasta Sauce	Canned or in Jars	Progresso
Pasta Sauce	Canned or in Jars	Progresso
Pasta Sauce	Canned or in Jars	Progresso
Pasta Sauce	Canned or in Jars	Progresso
Pasta Sauce	Canned or in Jars	Progresso

Major Description	Minor Description	Serving Size	Calories	Grade
Fresh Sliced Mushrooms		1/2 cup	65	A–
		1/2 cup	65	A
Mushroom or Mushroom Flavor		1/2 cup	65	A–
Mushroom & Onion	Chunky Garden Style	1/2 cup	80	B–+
Sausage & Pepper	Genovese Style	1/2 cup	70	C–
Sirloin Beef	Bolognese Style	1/2 cup	70	C–
Tomato & Basil	Neopolitan Style	1/2 cup	80	B–+
Traditional		1/2 cup	90	C–+
Italian-style Vegetables	Extra Chunky	1/2 cup	50	A–+
Flavored with Meat	Homestyle	1/2 cup	60	C–+
Garlic & Herb	Original	1/2 cup	60	B–+
Italian-style Vegetable	Chunky	1/2 cup	60	A–+
Meat or Meat Flavor		1/2 cup	75	B–
Mushroom		1/2 cup	75	B–
Tomato, Garlic & Onion	Chunky	1/2 cup	60	A–+
Traditional	Homestyle	1/2 cup	60	C–+
Traditional	Light	1/2 cup	40	B–+
Traditional	Original	1/2 cup	60	C–+
Marinara		1/2 cup	70	A–
Marinara with Mushroom		1/2 cup	70	B–
Mushroom or Mushroom Flavor		1/2 cup	70	A–
Sockarooni		1/2 cup	60	B–+
Venetian	All Natural	1/2 cup	60	B–+
3 Cheese		1/2 cup	100	B–
Garden-style Combination		1/2 cup	80	B–
Marinara		1/2 cup	100	D–
Meat or Meat Flavor		1/2 cup	140	C–
Mushroom & Diced Tomato	Extra Chunky	1/2 cup	100	B–
Mushroom & Green Pepper	Extra Chunky	1/2 cup	100	C–+
Mushroom or Mushroom Flavor		1/2 cup	130	C–
Onion & Garlic		1/2 cup	110	C–
Sausage & Green Pepper	Extra Chunky	1/2 cup	160	D–
Tomato or Tomato Flavor	& Basil	1/2 cup	100	B–
Traditional	100% Natural	1/2 cup	150	C–
Zesty Basil	Extra Chunky	1/2 cup	130	B–+
Zesty Garlic & Cheese	Extra Chunky	1/2 cup	130	B–+
Zesty Oregano	Extra Chunky	1/2 cup	140	B–+
Extra Spice		1/2 cup	100	B–
Mushroom & Onion		1/2 cup	100	C–
Mushroom & Tomato		1/2 cup	110	B–
Sausage & Green Pepper		1/2 cup	160	D–
Tomato or Tomato-based	& Onion	1/2 cup	110	B–
		1/2 cup	110	D
Chunky Garden Style		1/2 cup	50	A+
Marinara		1/2 cup	60	A–+
Original		1/2 cup	60	A+
Alfredo		1/2 cup	340	D–
Creamy Clam		1/2 cup	100	D–
Marinara		1/2 cup	90	D–
Meat or Meat Flavor		1/2 cup	110	D–
Mushroom		1/2 cup	110	D–
Red Clam		1/2 cup	80	C–
Rock Lobster		1/2 cup	110	D+

"+" indicates the food meets minimum fiber requirements; "–" indicates the food has a high sodium content.

Food	Processing Category	Brand
Pasta Sauce	Canned or in Jars	Progresso
Pasta Sauce	Canned or in Jars	Progresso
Pasta Sauce	Canned or in Jars	Progresso
Pasta Sauce	Canned or in Jars	Progresso
Pasta Sauce	Canned or in Jars	Progresso Authentic Pasta
Pasta Sauce	Canned or in Jars	Progresso Authentic Pasta
Pasta Sauce	Canned or in Jars	Progresso Authentic Pasta
Pasta Sauce	Canned or in Jars	Progresso Authentic Pasta
Pasta Sauce	Canned or in Jars	Progresso Authentic Pasta
Pasta Sauce	Canned or in Jars	Ragu
Pasta Sauce	Canned or in Jars	Ragu
Pasta Sauce	Canned or in Jars	Ragu
Pasta Sauce	Canned or in Jars	Ragu
Pasta Sauce	Canned or in Jars	Ragu
Pasta Sauce	Canned or in Jars	Ragu
Pasta Sauce	Canned or in Jars	Ragu
Pasta Sauce	Canned or in Jars	Ragu
Pasta Sauce	Canned or in Jars	Ragu
Pasta Sauce	Canned or in Jars	Ragu
Pasta Sauce	Canned or in Jars	Ragu
Pasta Sauce	Canned or in Jars	Ragu
Pasta Sauce	Canned or in Jars	Ragu
Pasta Sauce	Canned or in Jars	Ragu
Pasta Sauce	Canned or in Jars	Ragu
Pasta Sauce	Canned or in Jars	Ragu
Pasta Sauce	Canned or in Jars	Ragu
Pasta Sauce	Canned or in Jars	Ragu
Pasta Sauce	Canned or in Jars	Weight Watchers
Pasta Sauce	Canned or in Jars	Weight Watchers
Pasta Sauce	Refrigerated	Contadina Fresh
Pasta Sauce	Refrigerated	Contadina Fresh
Pasta Sauce	Refrigerated	Contadina Fresh
Pasta Sauce	Refrigerated	Contadina Fresh
Pasta Sauce	Refrigerated	Contadina Fresh
Pasta Sauce	Mix	French's
Pasta Sauce	Mix	French's
Pasta Sauce	Mix	French's Pasta Toss
Pasta Sauce	Mix	French's Pasta Toss
Pasta Sauce	Mix	French's Pasta Toss
Pasta Sauce	Mix	Lawry's
Pasta Sauce	Mix	Lawry's Rich & Thick
Pasta Sauce	Mix	McCormick/Schilling
Peanut Butter	Jarred	Generic
Pepper	Packaged	Generic
Pepper	Packaged	Generic
Pepper	Packaged	Generic
Pepper Sauce Hot	Bottled	Generic
Pepper Sauce Hot	Bottled	Tabasco
Pickling Spice	Packaged	Tone's
Pimiento	Spread	Price's
Pizza Sauce	Canned or in Jars	Chef Boyardee
Pizza Sauce	Canned or in Jars	Chef Boyardee Jars
Pizza Sauce	Canned or in Jars	Contadina

Major Description	Minor Description	Serving Size	Calories	Grade
Spaghetti		¹/₂ cup	110	D–
Spaghetti	Meat Flavor	¹/₂ cup	110	D–
Spaghetti	Mushroom	¹/₂ cup	110	D–
White Clam		¹/₂ cup	120	D–
Bolognese Sauce		¹/₂ cup	150	D–+
Marinara		¹/₂ cup	110	D–+
Primavera, Creamy		¹/₂ cup	190	D–
Sicilian Style		¹/₂ cup	30	D–+
White Clam		¹/₂ cup	90	D–
Chunky Mushroom	Light	¹/₂ cup	50	A–
Chunky Mushroom & Onion	Chunky Garden Style	¹/₂ cup	120	B–+
Chunky Tomato, Garlic & Onion	Chunky Garden Style	¹/₂ cup	120	B–+
Garden Harvest	Light	¹/₂ cup	50	A–+
Marinara	Old World Style	¹/₂ cup	90	D–+
Meat	Old World Style	¹/₂ cup	90	C–
Meat Flavor	Thick & Hearty	¹/₂ cup	130	C–+
Mushroom	Thick & Hearty	¹/₂ cup	120	B–+
Mushroom & Green Pepper	Chunky Garden Style	¹/₂ cup	120	C–
Parmesan	Italian Style	¹/₂ cup	100	B–+
Regular		¹/₂ cup	80	D–
Spaghetti Sauce	Thick & Hearty	¹/₂ cup	100	B–
Super Mushroom	Chunky Garden Style	¹/₂ cup	120	B–+
Super Vegetable Primavera	Chunky Garden Style	¹/₂ cup	110	C–+
Tomato & Herb	Fresh Italian	¹/₂ cup	90	B–
Tomato & Herb	Light	¹/₂ cup	60	B–+
Tomato & Herb	Thick & Hearty	¹/₂ cup	120	B–+
Traditional	Old World Style	¹/₂ cup	80	C–+
Meat or Meat Flavor		¹/₂ cup	59	B–
Mushroom		¹/₂ cup	46	A–
Alfredo		¹/₂ cup	356	D
Bolognese Style Sauce		¹/₂ cup	123	D–
Marinara		¹/₂ cup	80	D–
Pesto with Basil		¹/₂ cup	620	D–
Tomato	Chunky	¹/₂ cup	45	A–
Italian Style		¹/₂ cup	80	C–
Mushrooms		¹/₂ cup	80	C–
Cheese & Garlic		¹/₂ cup	80	C–
Italian Style		¹/₂ cup	80	C–
Romanoff		¹/₂ cup	100	C–
Mushrooms	Imported	1 pkg	143	A–
		1 pkg	147	A–
		¹/₂ cup	124	A–
All Varieties		1 Tbsp	c. 100	D
Black		1 tsp	5	A+
Red or Cayenne		1 tsp	6	B+
White		1 tsp	7	A+
		¹/₂ tsp	0	A–
		¹/₂ tsp	2	A–
		1 tsp	10	D+
		1 oz	80	D
	Cheese	¹/₄ cup	50	D–
	Cheese	¹/₄ cup	45	D–
	Italian-style Cheese	¹/₄ cup	30	B–

"+" indicates the food meets minimum fiber requirements; "–" indicates the food has a high sodium content.

Food	Processing Category	Brand
Pizza Sauce	Canned or in Jars	Contadina Pizza Squeeze
Pizza Sauce	Canned or in Jars	Contadina Quick & Easy Original
Pizza Sauce	Canned or in Jars	Enrico's Homemade Style All Natural
Pizza Sauce	Canned or in Jars	Pastorelli Italian Chef
Pizza Sauce	Canned or in Jars	Progresso
Pizza Sauce	Canned or in Jars	Ragu Pizza Quick
Pork Seasoning & Coating	Mix	McCormick/Schilling Bag 'n Season
Pork Seasoning & Coating	Mix	Shake 'n Bake Original Recipe
Pork Seasoning & Coating	Mix	Shake 'n Bake Oven Fry
Potato Salad	Canned	Generic
Potato Salad	Canned	Joan of Arc/Read
Potato Salad	Canned	Joan of Arc/Read
Relish	Canned or in Jars	Claussen
Relish	Canned or in Jars	Heinz
Relish	Canned or in Jars	Heinz
Relish	Canned or in Jars	Heinz
Relish	Canned or in Jars	Heinz
Relish	Canned or in Jars	Heinz
Relish	Canned or in Jars	Old El Paso
Relish	Canned or in Jars	Vlasic
Relish	Canned or in Jars	Vlasic
Relish	Canned or in Jars	Vlasic
Relish	Canned or in Jars	Vlasic
Relish	Canned or in Jars	Vlasic
Rice Seasoning	Mix	Lawry's Seasoning Blends
Rosemary	Packaged	Generic
Safflower Seed Kernel	Packaged	Generic
Safflower Seed Meal	Packaged	Generic
Saffron	Packaged	Generic
Sage	Packaged	Generic
Salad Dressing	Bottled	Generic
Salad Dressing	Bottled	Generic
Salad Dressing	Bottled	Generic
Salad Dressing	Bottled	Generic
Salad Dressing	Bottled	Generic
Salad Dressing	Bottled	Generic
Salad Dressing	Bottled	Generic
Salad Dressing	Bottled	Generic
Salad Dressing	Bottled	Generic
Salad Dressing	Bottled	Generic
Salad Dressing	Bottled	Generic
Salad Dressing	Bottled	Generic
Salad Dressing	Bottled	Generic
Salad Dressing	Bottled	Generic
Salad Dressing	Bottled	Anne's Original 1850 Farmhouse
Salad Dressing	Bottled	Anne's Original 1850 Farmhouse
Salad Dressing	Bottled	Anne's Original 1850 Farmhouse
Salad Dressing	Bottled	Bama
Salad Dressing	Bottled	Bernstein's
Salad Dressing	Bottled	Bernstein's
Salad Dressing	Bottled	Bernstein's
Salad Dressing	Bottled	Bernstein's
Salad Dressing	Bottled	Bernstein's

Major Description	Minor Description	Serving Size	Calories	Grade
		¹/₄ cup	30	B–
		¹/₄ cup	30	B–
		¹/₄ cup	30	A
		¹/₄ cup	45	B–
		¹/₄ cup	35	B–
		¹/₄ cup	46	D–
Chop		1 pkg	103	A–
Barbecue		¹/₈ pouch	40	B–
Extra Crispy		¹/₈ pouch	60	B–
		¹/₂ cup	162	D–
German Style		¹/₂ cup	120	B–
Homestyle		¹/₂ cup	340	D–
Pickle		1 tsp	13	A–
Hamburger		1 tsp	20	A–
Hot Dog		1 tsp	17	A–
Indian Style		1 tsp	17	A–
Piccalilli		1 tsp	15	A–
Sweet		1 tsp	17	A–
Jalapeño		1 tsp	8	A–
Dill		1 tsp	1	A–
Hot Dog		1 tsp	20	B–
Indian Style		1 tsp	15	A–
Piccalilli	Hot	1 tsp	17	A–
Sweet		1 tsp	15	A–
Mexican Style		1 pkg	94	B–+
Dried		1 tsp	4	D+
Dry		1 oz	147	D
Dry	Partially Defatted	1 oz	97	A+
Dry		1 Tbsp	7	B
Ground		1 Tbsp	6	C+
Blue Cheese		1 Tbsp	77	D
Champagne		1 Tbsp	70	D–
French		1 Tbsp	67	D–
French	Low Calorie	1 Tbsp	22	C–
Italian		1 Tbsp	69	D–
Italian	Low Calorie	1 Tbsp	16	D–
Mayonnaise		1 Tbsp	57	D–
Russian		1 Tbsp	76	D–
Russian	Low Calorie	1 Tbsp	23	B–
Sesame & Garlic		1 Tbsp	68	D–
Spinach Salad		1 Tbsp	70	D–
Super Creamy Ranch		1 Tbsp	70	D–
Thousand Island		1 Tbsp	59	D–
Thousand Island	Low Calorie	1 Tbsp	24	D–
Lemon & Pepper Viniagrette	Fat Free	1 Tbsp	10	A–
Vermont Honey Mustard		1 Tbsp	45	D
Vermont Honey Mustard	Fat Free	1 Tbsp	10	A–
Mayonnaise		1 Tbsp	50	D–
Cheese & Garlic Italian		1 Tbsp	55	D–
Cheese Fantastica	Light	1 Tbsp	14	A–
Parmesan Garlic Ranch		1 Tbsp	30	D–
Restaurant Bleu Cheese	Creamy	1 Tbsp	60	D–
Restaurant Recipe Italian		1 Tbsp	70	D–

"+" indicates the food meets minimum fiber requirements; "–" indicates the food has a high sodium content.

Food	Processing Category	Brand
Salad Dressing	Bottled	Cain's
Salad Dressing	Bottled	Cain's
Salad Dressing	Bottled	Cain's
Salad Dressing	Bottled	Cain's
Salad Dressing	Bottled	Cain's
Salad Dressing	Bottled	Cain's
Salad Dressing	Bottled	Cain's
Salad Dressing	Bottled	Catalina
Salad Dressing	Bottled	Catalina Reduced Calorie
Salad Dressing	Bottled	Dorothy Lynch
Salad Dressing	Bottled	Dorothy Lynch Reduced Calorie
Salad Dressing	Bottled	Estee
Salad Dressing	Bottled	Estee
Salad Dressing	Bottled	Estee
Salad Dressing	Bottled	Estee
Salad Dressing	Bottled	Estee
Salad Dressing	Bottled	Estee
Salad Dressing	Bottled	Estee
Salad Dressing	Bottled	Estee
Salad Dressing	Bottled	Featherweight
Salad Dressing	Bottled	Featherweight
Salad Dressing	Bottled	Featherweight
Salad Dressing	Bottled	Featherweight
Salad Dressing	Bottled	Featherweight
Salad Dressing	Bottled	Featherweight
Salad Dressing	Bottled	Featherweight
Salad Dressing	Bottled	Featherweight
Salad Dressing	Bottled	Featherweight
Salad Dressing	Bottled	Featherweight
Salad Dressing	Bottled	Featherweight
Salad Dressing	Bottled	Featherweight
Salad Dressing	Bottled	Featherweight Neu Bleu
Salad Dressing	Bottled	Finast
Salad Dressing	Bottled	Friendship Sour Treat
Salad Dressing	Bottled	Girard's
Salad Dressing	Bottled	Great Impressions
Salad Dressing	Bottled	Great Impressions
Salad Dressing	Bottled	Great Impressions
Salad Dressing	Bottled	Great Impressions
Salad Dressing	Bottled	Great Impressions
Salad Dressing	Bottled	Great Impressions
Salad Dressing	Bottled	Great Impressions
Salad Dressing	Bottled	Hain
Salad Dressing	Bottled	Hain
Salad Dressing	Bottled	Hain
Salad Dressing	Bottled	Hain
Salad Dressing	Bottled	Hain
Salad Dressing	Bottled	Hain
Salad Dressing	Bottled	Hain
Salad Dressing	Bottled	Hain
Salad Dressing	Bottled	Hain
Salad Dressing	Bottled	Hain
Salad Dressing	Bottled	Hain Canola

Major Description	Minor Description	Serving Size	Calories	Grade
Blue Cheese	Country	1 Tbsp	70	D
Caesar	Fat Free	1 Tbsp	15	A–
Honey Mustard	Country	1 Tbsp	45	D–
Italian	Country	1 Tbsp	50	D–
Peppercorn with Parmesan	Country	1 Tbsp	80	D–
Ranch	Country	1 Tbsp	70	D–
Raspberry Viniagrette	Fat Free	1 Tbsp	17	A–
French		1 Tbsp	60	D–
French		1 Tbsp	18	D–
Homestyle		1 Tbsp	55	D–
Homestyle		1 Tbsp	30	A–
Bacon & Tomato		1 Tbsp	8	A–
Blue Cheese		1 Tbsp	8	A–
Dijon	Creamy	1 Tbsp	8	A–
French		1 Tbsp	4	A–
Garlic	Creamy	1 Tbsp	2	A–
Italian	Creamy or Regular	1 Tbsp	4	A–
Red Wine	Vinegar	1 Tbsp	2	A–
Thousand Island		1 Tbsp	8	A–
Cucumber	Creamy	1 Tbsp	4	A–
Dijon	Creamy	1 Tbsp	20	D–
French		1 Tbsp	14	A
Herb		1 Tbsp	6	A
Herb	Garden	1 Tbsp	25	D–
Italian		1 Tbsp	4	A–
Italian	Cheese	1 Tbsp	20	D–
Oriental		1 Tbsp	20	D–
Red Wine	Vinegar	1 Tbsp	6	A–
Russian		1 Tbsp	6	A–
Thousand Island		1 Tbsp	18	A–
Tomato Zesty		1 Tbsp	2	A–
Blue Cheese		1 Tbsp	4	A–
Mayonnaise		1 Tbsp	70	D–
Sour		1 Tbsp	18	D
Old Venice Italian		1 Tbsp	65	D–
Dijon	Mustard	1 Tbsp	57	D–
French	Green Pepper	1 Tbsp	64	D–
Orange Marmalade Fruit		1 Tbsp	87	D
Poppy Seed		1 Tbsp	65	D
Vinegar & Oil	Balsamic Vinegar	1 Tbsp	67	D–
Vinegar & Oil	Red Wine Vinegar	1 Tbsp	64	D–
Vinegar & Oil	White Wine Vinegar	1 Tbsp	63	D–
Caesar	Creamy	1 Tbsp	60	D–
Cucumber	Dill	1 Tbsp	80	D–
Dijon	Vinaigrette	1 Tbsp	50	D–
French	Creamy	1 Tbsp	60	D–
Garlic	& Sour Cream	1 Tbsp	70	D–
Honey & Sesame		1 Tbsp	60	D–
Italian	Cheese Vinaigrette	1 Tbsp	55	D–
Italian	Creamy	1 Tbsp	80	D–
Swiss Cheese Vinaigrette		1 Tbsp	60	D–
Thousand Island		1 Tbsp	50	D–
Citrus Tangy		1 Tbsp	50	D–

"+" indicates the food meets minimum fiber requirements; "–" indicates the food has a high sodium content.

Food	Processing Category	Brand
Salad Dressing	Bottled	Hain Canola
Salad Dressing	Bottled	Hain Canola
Salad Dressing	Bottled	Hain Canola
Salad Dressing	Bottled	Hain Low Salt
Salad Dressing	Bottled	Hain No Oil
Salad Dressing	Bottled	Hain No Oil
Salad Dressing	Bottled	Hain No Oil
Salad Dressing	Bottled	Hain No Oil
Salad Dressing	Bottled	Hain No Salt Added
Salad Dressing	Bottled	Hain No Salt Added
Salad Dressing	Bottled	Hain Old Fashioned
Salad Dressing	Bottled	Hain Rancher's
Salad Dressing	Bottled	Hain Traditional
Salad Dressing	Bottled	Hain Traditional No Salt Added
Salad Dressing	Bottled	Hidden Valley Ranch
Salad Dressing	Bottled	Hidden Valley Ranch
Salad Dressing	Bottled	Hidden Valley Ranch
Salad Dressing	Bottled	Hidden Valley Ranch
Salad Dressing	Bottled	Hidden Valley Ranch
Salad Dressing	Bottled	Hidden Valley Ranch
Salad Dressing	Bottled	Hidden Valley Ranch
Salad Dressing	Bottled	Hidden Valley Ranch
Salad Dressing	Bottled	Hidden Valley Ranch
Salad Dressing	Bottled	Hidden Valley Ranch
Salad Dressing	Bottled	Hollywood
Salad Dressing	Bottled	Hollywood
Salad Dressing	Bottled	Hollywood
Salad Dressing	Bottled	Hollywood
Salad Dressing	Bottled	Hollywood
Salad Dressing	Bottled	Hollywood
Salad Dressing	Bottled	Hollywood
Salad Dressing	Bottled	Hollywood Old Fashion
Salad Dressing	Bottled	Ken's Steak House
Salad Dressing	Bottled	Ken's Steak House
Salad Dressing	Bottled	Ken's Steak House
Salad Dressing	Bottled	Ken's Steak House
Salad Dressing	Bottled	Ken's Steak House
Salad Dressing	Bottled	Ken's Steak House
Salad Dressing	Bottled	Ken's Steak House
Salad Dressing	Bottled	Ken's Steak House
Salad Dressing	Bottled	Ken's Steak House
Salad Dressing	Bottled	Ken's Steak House
Salad Dressing	Bottled	Ken's Steak House
Salad Dressing	Bottled	Ken's Steak House
Salad Dressing	Bottled	Ken's Steak House
Salad Dressing	Bottled	Ken's Steak House
Salad Dressing	Bottled	Ken's Steak House
Salad Dressing	Bottled	Ken's Steak House
Salad Dressing	Bottled	Ken's Steak House
Salad Dressing	Bottled	Ken's Steak House

Major Description	Minor Description	Serving Size	Calories	Grade
Italian		1 Tbsp	50	D–
Mustard Spicy French		1 Tbsp	50	D–
Tomato Vinaigrette		1 Tbsp	60	D–
Caesar	Creamy	1 Tbsp	60	D
Blue Cheese		1 Tbsp	14	D–
French		1 Tbsp	12	A–
Herb		1 Tbsp	2	A–
Italian		1 Tbsp	2	A–
Herb	Savory	1 Tbsp	90	D
Italian	Creamy	1 Tbsp	80	D
Buttermilk		1 Tbsp	70	D–
Poppy Seed		1 Tbsp	60	D–
Italian		1 Tbsp	80	D–
Italian		1 Tbsp	60	D
Coleslaw		1 Tbsp	75	D
Coleslaw	Low Fat	1 Tbsp	17	A–
Creamy Parmesan	Fat Free	1 Tbsp	15	A–
Honey Dijon Ranch	Low Fat	1 Tbsp	17	A–
Nacho Cheese Ranch		1 Tbsp	65	D–
Original Ranch	Creamy Dressing	1 Tbsp	70	D–
Original Ranch	Light	1 Tbsp	40	D–
Original Ranch	Low Fat	1 Tbsp	20	D–
Pizza Ranch		1 Tbsp	70	D–
Taco Ranch		1 Tbsp	65	D–
Caesar		1 Tbsp	70	D
Dijon	Vinaigrette	1 Tbsp	60	D
French	Creamy	1 Tbsp	70	D
Italian		1 Tbsp	90	D–
Italian	Cheese	1 Tbsp	80	D
Italian	Creamy	1 Tbsp	90	D–
Thousand Island		1 Tbsp	60	D
Buttermilk		1 Tbsp	75	D
Balsamic & Basil Vinaigrette		1 Tbsp	55	D–
Blue Cheese		1 Tbsp	65	D–
Caesar		1 Tbsp	85	D–
Caesar	Light	1 Tbsp	35	D–
Country French with Vermont Honey		1 Tbsp	65	D–
Country French with Vermont Honey	Light	1 Tbsp	45	D–
Creamy Cucumber	Light	1 Tbsp	25	D–
Creamy Italian		1 Tbsp	60	D–
Creamy Italian	Light	1 Tbsp	40	D–
Creamy Parmesan		1 Tbsp	85	D–
Creamy Parmesan with Cracked Pepper		1 Tbsp	45	D–
Cucumber & Chive	Fat Free	1 Tbsp	15	A–
French		1 Tbsp	65	D
French	Light	1 Tbsp	35	D–
Greek		1 Tbsp	70	D–
Honey Dijon	Fat Free	1 Tbsp	20	A–
Honey Mustard Vinaigrette	Light	1 Tbsp	45	D–
Honey Mustard Vinaigrette		1 Tbsp	85	D

"+" indicates the food meets minimum fiber requirements; "–" indicates the food has a high sodium content.

Food	Processing Category	Brand
Salad Dressing	Bottled	Ken's Steak House
Salad Dressing	Bottled	Ken's Steak House
Salad Dressing	Bottled	Ken's Steak House
Salad Dressing	Bottled	Ken's Steak House
Salad Dressing	Bottled	Ken's Steak House
Salad Dressing	Bottled	Ken's Steak House
Salad Dressing	Bottled	Ken's Steak House
Salad Dressing	Bottled	Ken's Steak House
Salad Dressing	Bottled	Ken's Steak House
Salad Dressing	Bottled	Ken's Steak House
Salad Dressing	Bottled	Ken's Steak House
Salad Dressing	Bottled	Ken's Steak House
Salad Dressing	Bottled	Ken's Steak House
Salad Dressing	Bottled	Ken's Steak House
Salad Dressing	Bottled	Ken's Steak House
Salad Dressing	Bottled	Ken's Steak House
Salad Dressing	Bottled	Ken's Steak House
Salad Dressing	Bottled	Ken's Steak House
Salad Dressing	Bottled	Ken's Steak House
Salad Dressing	Bottled	Kraft
Salad Dressing	Bottled	Kraft
Salad Dressing	Bottled	Kraft
Salad Dressing	Bottled	Kraft
Salad Dressing	Bottled	Kraft
Salad Dressing	Bottled	Kraft
Salad Dressing	Bottled	Kraft
Salad Dressing	Bottled	Kraft
Salad Dressing	Bottled	Kraft
Salad Dressing	Bottled	Kraft
Salad Dressing	Bottled	Kraft
Salad Dressing	Bottled	Kraft
Salad Dressing	Bottled	Kraft
Salad Dressing	Bottled	Kraft
Salad Dressing	Bottled	Kraft
Salad Dressing	Bottled	Kraft
Salad Dressing	Bottled	Kraft
Salad Dressing	Bottled	Kraft
Salad Dressing	Bottled	Kraft
Salad Dressing	Bottled	Kraft
Salad Dressing	Bottled	Kraft
Salad Dressing	Bottled	Kraft
Salad Dressing	Bottled	Kraft
Salad Dressing	Bottled	Kraft
Salad Dressing	Bottled	Kraft
Salad Dressing	Bottled	Kraft Miracle
Salad Dressing	Bottled	Kraft Presto
Salad Dressing	Bottled	Kraft Reduced Calorie
Salad Dressing	Bottled	Kraft Reduced Calorie
Salad Dressing	Bottled	Kraft Reduced Calorie
Salad Dressing	Bottled	Kraft Reduced Calorie

Major Description	Minor Description	Serving Size	Calories	Grade
Italian		1 Tbsp	75	D–
Italian	Fat Free	1 Tbsp	8	A–
Italian	Light	1 Tbsp	25	D–
Italian with Aged Romano		1 Tbsp	80	D
Olive Oil Vinaigrette	Light	1 Tbsp	30	D–
Peppercorn Ranch	Fat Free	1 Tbsp	13	A–
Ranch		1 Tbsp	90	D–
Ranch	Fat Free	1 Tbsp	15	A–
Ranch	Light	1 Tbsp	50	D–
Raspberry Walnut		1 Tbsp	60	D
Raspberry Walnut	Light	1 Tbsp	40	D–
Red Wine Vinegar & Olive Oil		1 Tbsp	60	D–
Red Wine Vinegar & Olive Oil	Light	1 Tbsp	25	D–
Russian		1 Tbsp	70	D–
Russian	Light	1 Tbsp	30	D–
Spicy Italian		1 Tbsp	80	D–
Sundried Tomato	Fat Free	1 Tbsp	30	A–
Thousand Island		1 Tbsp	70	D–
Thousand Island	Light	1 Tbsp	30	D–
Bacon & Tomato		1 Tbsp	70	D–
Blue Cheese	Chunky	1 Tbsp	60	D–
Blue Cheese	Fat Free	1 Tbsp	23	A–
Buttermilk	Creamy	1 Tbsp	80	D–
Caesar	Golden	1 Tbsp	70	D–
Catalina	Fat Free	1 Tbsp	23	A–
Coleslaw		1 Tbsp	70	D–
Cucumber	Creamy	1 Tbsp	70	D–
French		1 Tbsp	60	D–
French	Fat Free	1 Tbsp	25	A–
Garlic	Creamy	1 Tbsp	50	D–
Honey Dijon	Fat Free	1 Tbsp	25	A–
Italian		1 Tbsp	60	D–
Italian	Creamy with Real Sour Cream	1 Tbsp	50	D–
Italian	Fat Free	1 Tbsp	5	A–
Italian	Zesty	1 Tbsp	50	D–
Oil & Vinegar		1 Tbsp	70	D–
Onion & Chives, Creamy		1 Tbsp	70	D–
Peppercorn	Fat Free	1 Tbsp	13	A–
Ranch	Fat Free	1 Tbsp	25	A–
Russian		1 Tbsp	60	D–
Russian	Creamy	1 Tbsp	60	D–
Russian	Honey	1 Tbsp	23	B–
Thousand Island		1 Tbsp	60	D–
Thousand Island	& Bacon	1 Tbsp	60	D–
Thousand Island	Fat Free	1 Tbsp	23	A–
Vinegar & Oil	Red Wine Vinegar	1 Tbsp	60	D–
French		1 Tbsp	70	D–
Italian		1 Tbsp	70	D–
Bacon & Tomato		1 Tbsp	30	D–
Bacon, Creamy		1 Tbsp	30	D–
Blue Cheese	Chunky	1 Tbsp	30	D–
Buttermilk	Creamy	1 Tbsp	30	D–

"+" indicates the food meets minimum fiber requirements; "–" indicates the food has a high sodium content.

Food	Processing Category	Brand
Salad Dressing	Bottled	Kraft Reduced Calorie
Salad Dressing	Bottled	Kraft Reduced Calorie
Salad Dressing	Bottled	Kraft Reduced Calorie
Salad Dressing	Bottled	Kraft Reduced Calorie
Salad Dressing	Bottled	Kraft Reduced Calorie
Salad Dressing	Bottled	Kraft Reduced Calorie
Salad Dressing	Bottled	Kraft Reduced Calorie
Salad Dressing	Bottled	Kraft Reduced Calorie
Salad Dressing	Bottled	Lawry's Classic
Salad Dressing	Bottled	Lawry's Classic
Salad Dressing	Bottled	Lawry's Classic
Salad Dressing	Bottled	Lawry's Classic
Salad Dressing	Bottled	Lawry's Classic
Salad Dressing	Bottled	Lawry's Classic
Salad Dressing	Bottled	Lawry's Classic
Salad Dressing	Bottled	Life All Natural
Salad Dressing	Bottled	Maple Grove Farms Lite
Salad Dressing	Bottled	Maple Grove Farms Lite
Salad Dressing	Bottled	Maple Grove Farms Lite
Salad Dressing	Bottled	Maple Grove Farms Lite
Salad Dressing	Bottled	Maple Grove Farms of Vermont
Salad Dressing	Bottled	Nasoya Vegi-dressing
Salad Dressing	Bottled	Newman's Own
Salad Dressing	Bottled	Ott's
Salad Dressing	Bottled	Ott's Famous
Salad Dressing	Bottled	Ott's Reduced Calorie Famous
Salad Dressing	Bottled	Pritikin
Salad Dressing	Bottled	Pritikin
Salad Dressing	Bottled	Pritikin
Salad Dressing	Bottled	Pritikin
Salad Dressing	Bottled	Pritikin
Salad Dressing	Bottled	Pritikin
Salad Dressing	Bottled	Pritikin
Salad Dressing	Bottled	Pritikin
Salad Dressing	Bottled	Pritikin
Salad Dressing	Bottled	Pritikin
Salad Dressing	Bottled	Pritikin
Salad Dressing	Bottled	Rancher's Choice
Salad Dressing	Bottled	Rancher's Choice
Salad Dressing	Bottled	Roka
Salad Dressing	Bottled	Roka Brand Reduced Calorie
Salad Dressing	Bottled	S & W/Nutradiet
Salad Dressing	Bottled	S & W/Nutradiet
Salad Dressing	Bottled	S & W/Nutradiet
Salad Dressing	Bottled	S & W/Nutradiet
Salad Dressing	Bottled	S & W/Nutradiet
Salad Dressing	Bottled	S & W/Nutradiet
Salad Dressing	Bottled	Seven Seas
Salad Dressing	Bottled	Seven Seas
Salad Dressing	Bottled	Seven Seas
Salad Dressing	Bottled	Seven Seas
Salad Dressing	Bottled	Seven Seas
Salad Dressing	Bottled	Seven Seas

Major Description	Minor Description	Serving Size	Calories	Grade
Cucumber	Creamy	1 Tbsp	25	D–
French		1 Tbsp	20	D–
Italian	Creamy	1 Tbsp	25	D–
Italian	House	1 Tbsp	30	D–
Italian	No Oil	1 Tbsp	4	A–
Italian	Zesty	1 Tbsp	20	D–
Russian		1 Tbsp	30	B–
Thousand Island		1 Tbsp	20	D–
Caesar		1 Tbsp	130	D–
Chinese Vinegar	Sesame	1 Tbsp	75	D–
Italian	Parmesan Cheese	1 Tbsp	70	D
Red Wine	Cabernet Sauvignon	1 Tbsp	90	D–
San Francisco Style	with Romano Cheese	1 Tbsp	70	D–
Vintage	Sherry Wine	1 Tbsp	55	D–
White Wine	Chardonnay	1 Tbsp	70	D
Creamy	Egg Free	1 Tbsp	39	D
Caesar	Light	1 Tbsp	35	D–
Honey Ranch	Light	1 Tbsp	29	D–
Lemon & Dill	Light	1 Tbsp	40	D–
Pesto Parmesan	Light	1 Tbsp	35	D–
Honey & Lemon Poppy Seed		1 Tbsp	50	D
All Varieties		1 Tbsp	40	D–
Olive Oil & Vinegar		1 Tbsp	75	D
Italian		1 Tbsp	80	D
		1 Tbsp	40	D–
		1 Tbsp	26	D–
Balsamic Vinaigrette		1 Tbsp	15	A–
Dijon	Honey	1 Tbsp	22	A–
Dijon Balsamic	Fat Free	1 Tbsp	15	A–
French		1 Tbsp	18	A–
French	Honey	1 Tbsp	20	A–
Honey Dijon	Fat Free	1 Tbsp	22	A–
Honey French	Fat Free	1 Tbsp	20	A–
Italian		1 Tbsp	10	A–
Raspberry		1 Tbsp	22	A–
Vinaigrette		1 Tbsp	22	A–
Zesty Italian	Fat Free	1 Tbsp	10	A–
Creamy		1 Tbsp	90	D–
Creamy	Reduced Calorie	1 Tbsp	30	D–
Blue Cheese		1 Tbsp	60	D–
Blue Cheese		1 Tbsp	16	D–
Blue Cheese		1 Tbsp	25	D–
French		1 Tbsp	18	A–
Italian	Creamy	1 Tbsp	10	D–
Italian	No Oil	1 Tbsp	2	A–
Russian		1 Tbsp	25	C–
Thousand Island		1 Tbsp	25	D–
Buttermilk		1 Tbsp	80	D–
Buttermilk Ranch		1 Tbsp	50	D–
French	Creamy	1 Tbsp	60	D–
French	Light	1 Tbsp	35	D–
Italian	Creamy	1 Tbsp	70	D–
Italian	Fat Free	1 Tbsp	10	A–

"+" indicates the food meets minimum fiber requirements; "–" indicates the food has a high sodium content.

Food	Processing Category	Brand
Salad Dressing	Bottled	Seven Seas
Salad Dressing	Bottled	Seven Seas
Salad Dressing	Bottled	Seven Seas
Salad Dressing	Bottled	Seven Seas
Salad Dressing	Bottled	Seven Seas Free
Salad Dressing	Bottled	Seven Seas Free
Salad Dressing	Bottled	Seven Seas Free
Salad Dressing	Bottled	Seven Seas Viva
Salad Dressing	Bottled	Seven Seas Viva
Salad Dressing	Bottled	Seven Seas Viva
Salad Dressing	Bottled	Seven Seas Viva
Salad Dressing	Bottled	Seven Seas Viva
Salad Dressing	Bottled	Seven Seas Viva
Salad Dressing	Bottled	Seven Seas Viva
Salad Dressing	Bottled	Seven Seas Viva
Salad Dressing	Bottled	Seven Seas Viva
Salad Dressing	Bottled	Smart Temptations
Salad Dressing	Bottled	Weight Watchers
Salad Dressing	Bottled	Weight Watchers
Salad Dressing	Bottled	Weight Watchers
Salad Dressing	Bottled	Weight Watchers
Salad Dressing	Bottled	Weight Watchers
Salad Dressing	Bottled	Weight Watchers
Salad Dressing	Bottled	Weight Watchers
Salad Dressing	Bottled	Weight Watchers
Salad Dressing	Bottled	Weight Watchers
Salad Dressing	Bottled	Weight Watchers
Salad Dressing	Bottled	Wish-Bone
Salad Dressing	Bottled	Wish-Bone
Salad Dressing	Bottled	Wish-Bone
Salad Dressing	Bottled	Wish-Bone
Salad Dressing	Bottled	Wish-Bone
Salad Dressing	Bottled	Wish-Bone
Salad Dressing	Bottled	Wish-Bone
Salad Dressing	Bottled	Wish-Bone
Salad Dressing	Bottled	Wish-Bone
Salad Dressing	Bottled	Wish-Bone
Salad Dressing	Bottled	Wish-Bone
Salad Dressing	Bottled	Wish-Bone
Salad Dressing	Bottled	Wish-Bone
Salad Dressing	Bottled	Wish-Bone Classic
Salad Dressing	Bottled	Wish-Bone Classic
Salad Dressing	Bottled	Wish-Bone Classic
Salad Dressing	Bottled	Wish-Bone Deluxe
Salad Dressing	Bottled	Wish-Bone Healthy Sensation
Salad Dressing	Bottled	Wish-Bone Healthy Sensation
Salad Dressing	Bottled	Wish-Bone Healthy Sensation
Salad Dressing	Bottled	Wish-Bone Healthy Sensation
Salad Dressing	Bottled	Wish-Bone Healthy Sensation
Salad Dressing	Bottled	Wish-Bone Lite
Salad Dressing	Bottled	Wish-Bone Lite
Salad Dressing	Bottled	Wish-Bone Lite
Salad Dressing	Bottled	Wish-Bone Lite

Major Description	Minor Description	Serving Size	Calories	Grade
Ranch	Fat Free	1 Tbsp	25	A–+
Red Wine Vinegar	Fat Free	1 Tbsp	15	A–
Thousand Island		1 Tbsp	30	D–
Thousand Island	Creamy	1 Tbsp	50	D–
Italian		1 Tbsp	4	A–
Ranch		1 Tbsp	16	A–
Red Wine Vinegar		1 Tbsp	6	A–
Herbs & Spices		1 Tbsp	30	D–
Herbs & Spices		1 Tbsp	60	D–
Italian		1 Tbsp	50	D–
Italian	Creamy	1 Tbsp	45	D–
Italian	Light	1 Tbsp	30	D–
Ranch		1 Tbsp	80	D–
Ranch	Light	1 Tbsp	50	D–
Vinegar & Oil		1 Tbsp	45	D–
Vinegar & Oil	Red Wine Vinegar	1 Tbsp	70	D–
All Varieties	Fat Free	1 Tbsp	10	A–
Caesar		1 Tbsp	4	A–
Cucumber	Creamy	1 Tbsp	18	A–
French		1 Tbsp	10	A–
Italian		1 Tbsp	6	A–
Italian	Creamy	1 Tbsp	50	D–
Peppercorn Creamy		1 Tbsp	8	A–
Ranch	Creamy	1 Tbsp	25	A–
Russian		1 Tbsp	50	D–
Thousand Island		1 Tbsp	50	D–
Tomato Vinaigrette		1 Tbsp	8	A–
Blue Cheese	Chunky	1 Tbsp	75	D–
Caesar		1 Tbsp	77	D–
French	Garlic	1 Tbsp	55	D–
Garlic	Creamy	1 Tbsp	74	D–
Italian		1 Tbsp	46	D–
Italian	Blended	1 Tbsp	37	D–
Italian	Creamy	1 Tbsp	56	D–
Italian	with Cheese	1 Tbsp	89	D–
Olive Oil	Vinaigrette	1 Tbsp	28	D–
Ranch		1 Tbsp	78	D–
Red Wine Vinegar	Vinaigrette	1 Tbsp	51	D–
Russian		1 Tbsp	46	D–
Thousand Island		1 Tbsp	63	D–
Dijon	Vinaigrette	1 Tbsp	60	D–
Italian	Herbal	1 Tbsp	70	D–
Italian Olive Oil		1 Tbsp	34	D–
French		1 Tbsp	60	D–
Chunky Blue Cheese	Fat Free	1 Tbsp	18	A–+
Honey Dijon	Fat Free	1 Tbsp	23	A–
Italian	Fat Free	1 Tbsp	8	A–
Ranch	Fat Free	1 Tbsp	20	A–
Thousand Island	Fat Free	1 Tbsp	20	A–
Blue Cheese	Chunky	1 Tbsp	40	D–
French		1 Tbsp	31	D–
French	Red	1 Tbsp	17	B–
Italian		1 Tbsp	7	B–

"+" indicates the food meets minimum fiber requirements; "–" indicates the food has a high sodium content.

Food	Processing Category	Brand
Salad Dressing	Bottled	Wish-Bone Lite
Salad Dressing	Bottled	Wish-Bone Lite
Salad Dressing	Bottled	Wish-Bone Lite
Salad Dressing	Bottled	Wish-Bone Lite
Salad Dressing	Bottled	Wish-Bone Lite
Salad Dressing	Bottled	Wish-Bone Lite
Salad Dressing	Bottled	Wish-Bone Lite Classic
Salad Dressing	Bottled	Wish-Bone Lite Sweet N Spicy
Salad Dressing	Bottled	Wish-Bone Robusto
Salad Dressing	Bottled	Wish-Bone Sweet N Spicy
Salad Dressing	Mix	Good Seasons
Salad Dressing	Mix	Good Seasons Classic
Salad Dressing	Mix	Good Seasons Farm Style
Salad Dressing	Mix	Good Seasons Lite
Salad Dressing	Mix	Good Seasons Lite
Salad Dressing	Mix	Good Seasons Lite
Salad Dressing	Mix	Good Seasons Lite
Salad Dressing	Mix	Good Seasons No Oil
Salad Dressing	Mix	Hain Fat Free
Salad Dressing	Mix	Hain Fat Free
Salad Dressing	Mix	Hain Fat Free
Salad Dressing	Mix	Hain Fat Free
Salad Dressing	Mix	Hain No Oil
Salad Dressing	Mix	Hain No Oil
Salad Dressing	Mix	Hain No Oil
Salad Dressing	Mix	Hain No Oil
Salad Dressing	Mix	Hain No Oil
Salad Dressing	Mix	Hain No Oil
Salad Dressing	Mix	Hain No Oil
Salsa	Canned or in Jars	Del Monte
Salsa	Canned or in Jars	Del Monte
Salsa	Canned or in Jars	Del Monte
Salsa	Canned or in Jars	Del Monte
Salsa	Canned or in Jars	Del Monte
Salsa	Canned or in Jars	Enrico's Chunky Style
Salsa	Canned or in Jars	Enrico's Chunky Style No Salt
Salsa	Canned or in Jars	Guiltless Gourmet
Salsa	Canned or in Jars	Hain
Salsa	Canned or in Jars	Hain
Salsa	Canned or in Jars	Hot Cha Cha
Salsa	Canned or in Jars	La Victoria
Salsa	Canned or in Jars	La Victoria
Salsa	Canned or in Jars	La Victoria
Salsa	Canned or in Jars	La Victoria
Salsa	Canned or in Jars	La Victoria
Salsa	Canned or in Jars	La Victoria
Salsa	Canned or in Jars	La Victoria
Salsa	Canned or in Jars	La Victoria
Salsa	Canned or in Jars	La Victoria
Salsa	Canned or in Jars	La Victoria
Salsa	Canned or in Jars	Las Palmas Salsa Mexicana
Salsa	Canned or in Jars	Old El Paso
Salsa	Canned or in Jars	Old El Paso

Major Description	Minor Description	Serving Size	Calories	Grade
Italian	Creamy	1 Tbsp	26	D–
Olive Oil	Vinaigrette	1 Tbsp	16	D–
Onion & Chive		1 Tbsp	37	D–
Ranch		1 Tbsp	42	D–
Russian		1 Tbsp	22	B–
Thousand Island		1 Tbsp	36	D–
Dijon	Vinaigrette	1 Tbsp	30	D–
French		1 Tbsp	18	B–
Italian		1 Tbsp	47	D–
French		1 Tbsp	63	D–
All Varieties		1 Tbsp	70	D–
Herb		1 Tbsp	70	D–
Buttermilk		1 Tbsp	60	D–
Italian		1 Tbsp	25	D–
Italian Cheese		1 Tbsp	25	D–
Italian Zesty		1 Tbsp	25	D–
Ranch		1 Tbsp	30	D–
Italian		1 Tbsp	6	A–
Caesar		1 Tbsp	30	A–
Garlic & Cheese		1 Tbsp	30	A–
Herb		1 Tbsp	30	A–
Italian		1 Tbsp	15	A–
Blue Cheese		1 Tbsp	14	D–
Buttermilk		1 Tbsp	11	A–
French		1 Tbsp	12	A–
Garlic & Cheese		1 Tbsp	6	A–
Herb		1 Tbsp	2	A–
Italian		1 Tbsp	2	A–
Thousand Island		1 Tbsp	12	A–
Burrito		2 Tbsp	20	A–
Green Chili	Mild	2 Tbsp	20	A–
Picante	Hot	2 Tbsp	20	A–
Picante	Hot & Chunky	2 Tbsp	15	A–
Roja Mild		2 Tbsp	20	A–
All Varieties		2 Tbsp	8	A–
All Varieties		2 Tbsp	8	A–
All Varieties		2 Tbsp	6	A–
Hot		2 Tbsp	22	A–
Mild		2 Tbsp	20	A–
Texas Style		2 Tbsp	6	A+
Brava		2 Tbsp	12	A–
Casera		2 Tbsp	8	A–
Green Chili		2 Tbsp	6	A–
Green Jalapeño		2 Tbsp	8	A–
Omelette		2 Tbsp	12	A–
Picante		2 Tbsp	8	A–
Ranchera		2 Tbsp	12	A–
Red Jalapeño		2 Tbsp	12	A–
Suprema		2 Tbsp	8	A–
Victoria		2 Tbsp	8	A–
All Varieties		2 Tbsp	10	A–
All Varieties	Picante	2 Tbsp	10	A–
Homestyle	All Varieties	2 Tbsp	5	A–

"+" indicates the food meets minimum fiber requirements; "–" indicates the food has a high sodium content.

Food	Processing Category	Brand
Salsa	Canned or in Jars	Old El Paso
Salsa	Canned or in Jars	Old El Paso
Salsa	Canned or in Jars	Old El Paso
Salsa	Canned or in Jars	Ortega
Salsa	Canned or in Jars	Ortega
Salsa	Canned or in Jars	Ortega
Salsa	Canned or in Jars	Ortega
Salsa	Canned or in Jars	Ortega
Salsa	Canned or in Jars	Rosarita
Sauerkraut	Canned	Generic
Sauerkraut	Canned	A & P
Sauerkraut	Canned	Allen's
Sauerkraut	Canned	Claussen
Sauerkraut	Canned	Del Monte
Sauerkraut	Canned	Finast
Sauerkraut	Canned	Pathmark
Sauerkraut	Canned	Snow Floss
Sauerkraut	Canned	Stokely
Sauerkraut	Canned	Stokely Bavarian
Sauerkraut	Canned	Vlasic Old Fashioned
Seafood Sauce	Bottled or in Jars	Golden Dipt
Seafood Sauce	Bottled or in Jars	Great Impressions
Seafood Sauce	Bottled or in Jars	Great Impressions
Seafood Sauce	Bottled or in Jars	Great Impressions
Seasoning	Mix	Lawry's
Sesame Butter	Bottled or in Jars	All Brands
Sesame Butter	Bottled or in Jars	All Brands
Sesame Butter	Bottled or in Jars	All Brands
Shortening	Canned	All Brands
Shortening	Canned	All Brands
Shortening	Canned	All Brands
Shortening	Canned	All Brands
Shortening	Canned	All Brands
Shrimp Sauce	Bottled or in Jars	Tone's
Sour Cream Sauce Mix	Mix	Generic
Sour Cream Sauce Mix	Mix	McCormick/Schilling
Soy Sauce	Bottled or in Jars	Generic
Soy Sauce	Bottled or in Jars	Generic
Soy Sauce	Bottled or in Jars	Generic
Soy Sauce	Bottled or in Jars	Generic
Soy Sauce	Bottled or in Jars	Kikkoman
Soy Sauce	Bottled or in Jars	Kikkoman Lite
Soy Sauce	Bottled or in Jars	La Choy
Soy Sauce	Bottled or in Jars	La Choy Lite
Steak Sauce	Bottled	A-1
Steak Sauce	Bottled	Estee
Steak Sauce	Bottled	French's
Steak Sauce	Bottled	Heinz
Steak Sauce	Bottled	Heinz 57
Steak Sauce	Bottled	Lea & Perrins
Steak Sauce	Bottled	Life All Natural
Steak Sauce	Bottled	Steak Supreme

Major Description	Minor Description	Serving Size	Calories	Grade
Thick N Chunky	Verde	2 Tbsp	10	A–
Thick N Chunky	Chili	2 Tbsp	3	A–
Thick N Chunky	Mild, Hot or Medium	2 Tbsp	10	A–
Green Chili	Hot	2 Tbsp	10	A–
Green Chili	Mild or Medium	2 Tbsp	8	A–
Picante		2 Tbsp	10	A–
Ranchera		2 Tbsp	12	A–
Taco	Hot or Mild	2 Tbsp	10	A–
Taco	Mild	2 Tbsp	13	A–
in Liquid		$^1/_2$ cup	22	A–+
in Liquid		$^1/_2$ cup	20	A–
Shredded		$^1/_2$ cup	21	A–
in Liquid		$^1/_2$ cup	17	A–
in Liquid		$^1/_2$ cup	25	A–
in Liquid		$^1/_2$ cup	30	A–
in Liquid		$^1/_2$ cup	20	A–
in Liquid		$^1/_2$ cup	28	A–+
Shredded & Chopped		$^1/_2$ cup	20	A–
in Liquid		$^1/_2$ cup	30	A–
in Liquid		1 oz	4	A–
Cocktail		1 Tbsp	20	A–
Creole Style		1 Tbsp	21	A–
Dipping		1 Tbsp	17	C–
Dipping, Polynesian		1 Tbsp	38	A–
Beef Marinade		$^1/_4$ pkg	12	A–
Paste from Whole Sesame		1 Tbsp	95	D+
Tahini	from Raw Kernels	1 Tbsp	89	D+
Tahini	from Roasted Kernels	1 Tbsp	89	D+
Bread	All Varieties	1 Tbsp	113	D
Cake Mix	All Varieties	1 Tbsp	125	D
Confectionery	Coconut and/or Palm Kernel	1 Tbsp	113	D
Confectionery	Fractionated Palm	1 Tbsp	120	D
Frying	Soybean & Cottonseed	1 Tbsp	113	D
		1 Tbsp	30	D+
		1.24 oz pkt	180	A–
		$^1/_4$ pkg	44	D–
from Soy & Wheat Shoyu		1 Tbsp	9	A–
from Soy & Wheat Shoyu	Low Sodium	1 Tbsp	15	A–
from Soy Tamari		1 Tbsp	11	A–
from Vegetable Protein		1 Tbsp	12	A–
from Vegetable Protein		1 Tbsp	10	A–
from Vegetable Protein		1 Tbsp	11	A–
from Vegetable Protein		1 Tbsp	3	A–
from Vegetable Protein		1 Tbsp	3	A–
		1 Tbsp	12	A–
		1 Tbsp	15	D
		1 Tbsp	25	A–
	Traditional	1 Tbsp	12	A–
		1 Tbsp	17	A–
		1 Tbsp	20	B–
		1 Tbsp	11	A
		1 Tbsp	20	A–

"+" indicates the food meets minimum fiber requirements; "–" indicates the food has a high sodium content.

Food	Processing Category	Brand
Steak Seasoning	Bottled	McCormick/Schilling Spice Blends
Steak Seasoning	Bottled	Tone's
Stir-fry Sauce	Bottled	Kikkoman
Stir-fry Sauce	Bottled	Lawry's
Stroganoff Sauce	Mix	Lawry's
Stroganoff Sauce	Mix	McCormick
Stroganoff Sauce	Mix	Natural Touch
Sugar Substitute	Bottled	Featherweight
Sugar Substitute	Packaged	Equal
Sugar Substitute	Packaged	Sweet'n Low
Sugar Substitute	Packaged	Weight Watchers Sweetner
Sugar Substitute	Powder	S & W/Nutradiet
Sugar Substitute	Powder	Sprinkle Sweet
Sugar Substitute	Powder	Sweet 10
Sugar, Beet or Cane	Bulk	Generic
Sugar, Beet or Cane	Bulk	Generic
Sugar, Beet or Cane	Bulk	All Brands
Sugar, Beet or Cane	Bulk	Domino 10-X
Sugar, Dextrose	Powder	All Brands
Sugar, Dextrose	Powder	All Brands
Sugar, Maple	Packaged	All Brands
Sunflower Seed Butter	Packaged	All Brands
Sweet & Sour Sauce	Bottled	Great Impressions
Sweet & Sour Sauce	Bottled	Great Impressions
Sweet & Sour Sauce	Bottled	Hickory Farms
Sweet & Sour Sauce	Bottled	Hickory Farms
Sweet & Sour Sauce	Bottled	Kikkoman
Sweet & Sour Sauce	Bottled	La Choy
Sweet & Sour Sauce	Bottled	La Choy
Sweet & Sour Sauce	Bottled	Lawry's
Sweet & Sour Sauce	Bottled	Sauceworks
Szechwan Sauce	Bottled	La Choy
Taco Salad Seasoning	Packaged	Lawry's Seasoning Blends
Taco Sauce	Bottled or in Jars	Del Monte
Taco Sauce	Bottled or in Jars	El Molino
Taco Sauce	Bottled or in Jars	Enrico's No Salt Added
Taco Sauce	Bottled or in Jars	Estee
Taco Sauce	Bottled or in Jars	Heinz
Taco Sauce	Bottled or in Jars	La Victoria
Taco Sauce	Bottled or in Jars	La Victoria
Taco Sauce	Bottled or in Jars	Lawry's
Taco Sauce	Bottled or in Jars	Lawry's Sauce N Seasoner
Taco Sauce	Bottled or in Jars	Old El Paso
Taco Sauce	Bottled or in Jars	Ortega
Taco Sauce	Bottled or in Jars	Ortega
Taco Sauce	See also Salsa	
Taco Seasoning	Mix	Hain
Taco Seasoning	Mix	Lawry's Seasoning Blends
Taco Seasoning	Mix	McCormick/Schilling
Taco Seasoning	Mix	Old El Paso
Taco Seasoning	Mix	Ortega
Taco Seasoning	Mix	Tio Sancho
Tarragon	Packaged	All Brands

Major Description	Minor Description	Serving Size	Calories	Grade
Broiled		1 tsp	4	A–
Blackened		1 tsp	9	B–
		1 tsp	6	A–
		1 tsp	12	B–
		1 pkg	123	A–
		$^{1}/_{2}$ cup	170	D–
		$^{1}/_{2}$ cup	90	B
Liquid		3 drops		A
		1 pkg	4	A
		1 pkt	4	A
		1 pkt	4	A–
Liquid		$^{1}/_{8}$ tsp		A
		1 tsp	2	A
		$^{1}/_{8}$ tsp		A–
Confectioner's	Sifted	$^{1}/_{2}$ cup	190	A
Granulated	All Varieties	1 tsp	16	A
Brown	All Varieties	1 tsp	c. 15	A
Confectioner's	Sifted	$^{1}/_{2}$ cup	240	A
Anhydrous		2 Tbsp	104	A
Crystallized		2 Tbsp	95	A
		1 oz piece	99	A
		1 Tbsp	93	D
Hawaiian Style		2 Tbsp	102	A
Regular or Hot		2 Tbsp	102	A
Hawaiian Style		2 Tbsp	102	A
Regular		2 Tbsp	102	A
		2 Tbsp	36	A–
		2 Tbsp	60	A–
Duck Sauce		2 Tbsp	52	A–
		2 Tbsp	135	A–
		2 Tbsp	50	A–
Hot & Spicy		2 Tbsp	48	A–
		1 pkg	124	A–
All Varieties		1 Tbsp	4	A–
Red Mild		1 Tbsp	5	A–
Mild		1 Tbsp	7	A–
		1 Tbsp	7	A–
Mild	or Medium	1 Tbsp	6	A
Green		1 Tbsp	4	A–
Red		1 Tbsp	5	A–
Chunky		1 Tbsp	6	B–+
		1 Tbsp	10	A–
All Varieties		1 Tbsp	5	A–
Hot or Mild		1 Tbsp	6	A–
Western Style		1 Tbsp	4	A–
		$^{1}/_{4}$ pkg	25	A–
		$^{1}/_{4}$ pkg	29	A–
		$^{1}/_{4}$ pkg	31	A–
		$^{1}/_{4}$ pkg	24	A–
		$^{1}/_{4}$ pkg	22	A–
		$^{1}/_{4}$ pkg	33	A–+
Ground		1 tsp	5	B+

"+" indicates the food meets minimum fiber requirements; "–" indicates the food has a high sodium content.

Food	Processing Category	Brand
Tartar Sauce	Bottled or in Jars	Golden Dipt
Tartar Sauce	Bottled or in Jars	Golden Dipt Lite
Tartar Sauce	Bottled or in Jars	Great Impressions
Tartar Sauce	Bottled or in Jars	Heinz
Tartar Sauce	Bottled or in Jars	Hellmann's/Best Foods
Tartar Sauce	Bottled or in Jars	Life All Natural
Tartar Sauce	Bottled or in Jars	Sauceworks
Tartar Sauce	Bottled or in Jars	Sauceworks
Tartar Sauce	Bottled or in Jars	Weight Watchers
Teriyaki Sauce	Bottled or in Jars	Generic
Teriyaki Sauce	Mix	Generic
Teriyaki Sauce	Bottled or in Jars	Golden Dipt
Teriyaki Sauce	Bottled or in Jars	Kikkoman
Teriyaki Sauce	Bottled or in Jars	Kikkoman Baste & Glaze
Teriyaki Sauce	Bottled or in Jars	La Choy
Teriyaki Sauce	Bottled or in Jars	La Choy Sauce & Marinade
Teriyaki Sauce	Bottled or in Jars	Lawry's
Teriyaki Sauce	Bottled or in Jars	Lawry's
Thyme	Packaged	All Brands
Tofu Spread	Canned	Natural Touch Tofu Topper
Tofu Spread	Canned	Natural Touch Tofu Topper
Tofu Spread	Canned	Natural Touch Tofu Topper
Tomato Paste	Canned	Contadina
Tomato Paste	Canned	Contadina
Tomato Paste	Canned	Del Monte
Tomato Paste	Canned	Del Monte No Salt Added
Tomato Paste	Canned	Finast No Salt Added
Tomato Paste	Canned	Hunt's
Tomato Paste	Canned	Hunt's
Tomato Paste	Canned	Hunt's No Salt Added
Tomato Paste	Canned	Progresso
Tomato Paste	Canned	S & W
Tomato Puree	Canned	Contadina
Tomato Puree	Canned	Hunt's
Tomato Puree	Canned	Pathmark
Tomato Puree	Canned	Progresso
Tomato Puree	Canned	Progresso
Tomato Puree	Canned	S & W
Tomato Sauce	Canned	Buitoni
Tomato Sauce	Canned	Contadina
Tomato Sauce	Canned	Contadina Thick & Zesty
Tomato Sauce	Canned	Del Monte
Tomato Sauce	Canned	Del Monte
Tomato Sauce	Canned	Del Monte No Salt Added
Tomato Sauce	Canned	Finast
Tomato Sauce	Canned	Health Valley
Tomato Sauce	Canned	Health Valley No Salt Added
Tomato Sauce	Canned	Hunt's
Tomato Sauce	Canned	Hunt's
Tomato Sauce	Canned	Hunt's No Salt Added
Tomato Sauce	Canned	Hunt's Special
Tomato Sauce	Canned	Old El Paso
Tomato Sauce	Canned	Old El Paso

Major Description	Minor Description	Serving Size	Calories	Grade
		1 Tbsp	70	D–
		1 Tbsp	50	D
		1 Tbsp	86	D
		1 Tbsp	71	D–
		1 Tbsp	70	D–
Egg Free		1 Tbsp	38	D
		1 Tbsp	50	D–
Lemon & Herb		1 Tbsp	70	D
		1 Tbsp	35	D–
		1 Tbsp	15	A–
		1 Tbsp	8	A–
Ginger Marinade		1 Tbsp	60	D–
		1 Tbsp	15	A–
		1 Tbsp	27	A–
Thick & Rich		1 Tbsp	20	A–
		1 Tbsp	15	A–
	Pineapple Juice	1 Tbsp	18	A–
Barbecue Marinade		1 Tbsp	41	A–
Ground		1 tsp	4	B+
Green Chili		2 Tbsp	50	D
Herbs & Spices		2 Tbsp	50	D
Mexican Style		2 Tbsp	60	D
		$1/4$ cup	50	B
Italian Style		$1/4$ cup	65	A–
		$1/4$ cup	50	A
		$1/4$ cup	50	A
		$1/4$ cup	50	A
		$1/4$ cup	45	A–
Italian Style		$1/4$ cup	50	A–
		$1/4$ cup	45	A
		$1/4$ cup	50	A
		$1/4$ cup	50	A
		$1/2$ cup	40	A–
		$1/2$ cup	45	A–
		$1/2$ cup	45	A
		$1/2$ cup	45	A
Concentrate		$1/2$ cup	50	A
		$1/2$ cup	60	A
Marinara		$1/2$ cup	70	C–
All Varieties		$1/2$ cup	40	A–
		$1/2$ cup	40	A–
		$1/2$ cup	35	A–
Onions		$1/2$ cup	50	A–
		$1/2$ cup	35	A
		$1/2$ cup	45	A–
		$1/2$ cup	35	A–
		$1/2$ cup	35	A
		$1/2$ cup	30	A–
Italian Style		$1/2$ cup	60	B–
		$1/2$ cup	35	A
		$1/2$ cup	35	A–
Green Chilies		$1/2$ cup	28	A–
Jalapeños		$1/2$ cup	22	B–

"+" indicates the food meets minimum fiber requirements; "–" indicates the food has a high sodium content.

Food	Processing Category	Brand
Tomato Sauce	Canned	Pathmark
Tomato Sauce	Canned	Progresso
Tomato Sauce	Canned	Rokeach
Tomato Sauce	Canned	Rokeach
Tomato Sauce	Canned	Rokeach Low Sodium
Tomato Sauce	Canned	S & W
Tomato Sauce	Canned	Stokely
Tomato Sauce	Refrigerated	Contadina Fresh
Tomato Sauce	Refrigerated	Contadina Fresh
Tomato Sauce	*See also* Pasta Sauce	
Tomato Sauce	*See* Tomato Paste	
Tumeric	Packaged	All Brands
Vegetable Oil	Bottled	All Brands
Vegetable Oil Spray	Bottled	Pam
Vegetable Oil Spray	Bottled	Weight Watchers Spray
Vinegar	Bottled	All Brands
Worcestershire Sauce	*See also* Steak Sauce	
Worcestershire Sauce	Bottled	French's
Worcestershire Sauce	Bottled	Lea & Perrins
Worcestershire Sauce	Bottled	Lea & Perrins
Worcestershire Sauce	Bottled	Life All Natural

Major Description	Minor Description	Serving Size	Calories	Grade
		$^1/_2$ cup	40	A–
		$^1/_2$ cup	27	A–
Italian Style		$^1/_2$ cup	80	B–
Marinara		$^1/_2$ cup	80	B–
		$^1/_2$ cup	75	C–
		$^1/_2$ cup	40	A–
		$^1/_2$ cup	30	A–
Marinara		$^1/_2$ cup	50	C–
Plum with Basil		$^1/_2$ cup	50	C–
Ground		1 tsp	200	B+
All Varieties		1 Tbsp	120	D
All Varieties		1 second spray	2	A
All Varieties		1 second spray	2	A
All Varieties		1 oz	5	B+
Regular or Smoky		1 Tbsp	10	A–
		1 Tbsp	15	A–
White Wine		1 Tbsp	9	A–
		1 Tbsp	10	A

"+" indicates the food meets minimum fiber requirements; "–" indicates the food has a high sodium content.

Frozen and Canned Entrees and Dinners

The frozen and canned entrees and dinners section contains pre-prepared meals. The meals are identified by their major component—for example, beef, chicken, pasta—and are either frozen or canned. Foods are referred to as "entrees" if the item is a single component such as a Salisbury steak in sauce. "Dinner" refers to a mixed meal consisting of a major component such as the same Salisbury steak, and side dishes. This avoids confusion since in most cases, the food package label itself will state "dinner" or "entree." Whenever possible, serving sizes for entrees and dinners are given as the number of ounces for the entire item except where indicated. This allows you to tell if an item has more or less calories because of a size difference or a quality difference.

Note: Serving size value in ounces refers to one whole frozen package or one whole can except where indicated.

Food	Processing Category	Brand
Amaranth Dinner	Canned	Health Valley Fast Menu
Apple Crisp	Frozen	Pepperidge Farm Berkshire
Apple Crisp	Frozen	Weight Watchers
Apple Dumpling	Frozen	Pepperidge Farm
Apple Escalloped	Frozen	Stouffer's
Apple Fritter	Frozen	Mrs. Paul's
Apple Fruit Square	Frozen	Pepperidge Farm
Apple Sticks	Frozen	Farm Rich
Apple, Glazed	Frozen	Budget Gourmet Side Dish
Bean & Frankfurter Dinner	Frozen	Banquet
Bean & Frankfurter Dinner	Frozen	Morton
Bean & Frankfurter Dinner	Frozen	Swanson
Beef Dinner	Frozen	Armour Classics
Beef Dinner	Frozen	Armour Classics
Beef Dinner	Frozen	Armour Classics
Beef Dinner	Frozen	Armour Classics
Beef Dinner	Frozen	Armour Classics
Beef Dinner	Frozen	Armour Classics
Beef Dinner	Frozen	Armour Classics Lite
Beef Dinner	Frozen	Armour Classics Lite
Beef Dinner	Frozen	Armour Classics Lite
Beef Dinner	Frozen	Armour Classics Lite
Beef Dinner	Frozen	Banquet
Beef Dinner	Frozen	Banquet
Beef Dinner	Frozen	Banquet Extra Helping
Beef Dinner	Frozen	Banquet Extra Helping
Beef Dinner	Frozen	Banquet Healthy Balance
Beef Dinner	Frozen	Banquet Healthy Balance
Beef Dinner	Frozen	Budget Gourmet
Beef Dinner	Frozen	Budget Gourmet
Beef Dinner	Frozen	Budget Gourmet
Beef Dinner	Frozen	Budget Gourmet
Beef Dinner	Frozen	Budget Gourmet
Beef Dinner	Frozen	Budget Gourmet Light & Healthy
Beef Dinner	Frozen	Budget Gourmet Light & Healthy
Beef Dinner	Frozen	Budget Gourmet Light & Healthy
Beef Dinner	Frozen	Budget Gourmet Light & Healthy
Beef Dinner	Frozen	Budget Gourmet Light & Healthy
Beef Dinner	Frozen	Freezer Queen
Beef Dinner	Frozen	Freezer Queen
Beef Dinner	Frozen	Freezer Queen
Beef Dinner	Frozen	Healthy Choice
Beef Dinner	Frozen	Healthy Choice
Beef Dinner	Frozen	Healthy Choice
Beef Dinner	Frozen	Healthy Choice
Beef Dinner	Frozen	Healthy Choice
Beef Dinner	Frozen	Healthy Choice
Beef Dinner	Frozen	Kid Cuisine
Beef Dinner	Frozen	Kid Cuisine
Beef Dinner	Frozen	Kid Cuisine Mega Meal
Beef Dinner	Frozen	Kid Cuisine Megameal
Beef Dinner	Frozen	Le Menu
Beef Dinner	Frozen	Le Menu

Major Description	Minor Description	Serving Size	Calories	Grade
with Garden Vegetables		7¹/₂ oz	120	B+
		1 piece	250	B
		3.5 oz	190	B
		3 oz	260	D
		4 oz	130	A
		1 piece	120	C–
		1 piece	220	D
Breaded Fried		4 oz pkg	260	B–
in Raspberry Sauce		5 oz pkg	110	B–
		10 oz	520	D–
		10 oz	350	C–
		10¹/₂ oz	440	C–
Pot Roast, Yankee		10 oz	310	C–
Salisbury Steak		11.25 oz	350	D–
Salisbury Steak	Parmigiana	11.5 oz	410	D–
Short Ribs, Boneless		9.75 oz	380	C–
Sirloin, Roast		10.45 oz	190	B–
Sirloin Tips		10.25 oz	230	B–
Pepper Steak		11.25 oz	220	B–
Salisbury Steak		11.5 oz	300	A–
Steak Diane		10 oz	290	B–
Stroganoff		11.25 oz	250	B–
Chopped Sirloin		11 oz	420	D–
Salisbury Steak		11 oz	500	D
Salisbury Steak		18 oz	910	D
Salisbury Steak	Mushroom Gravy	18 oz	890	D
Meatloaf		11 oz	270	B–
Salisbury Steak		10.5 oz	260	B–
Mexicana		12.8 oz	560	C–
Pot Roast, Yankee		11 oz	380	D–
Salisbury Steak	Sirloin	11.5 oz	410	D–
Sirloin Tips	in Burgundy Sauce	11 oz	310	C–
Swiss Steak		11.2 oz	450	D–
Pot Roast		10.5 oz	230	B–
Salisbury Steak		11 oz	280	B–
Sirloin	in Wine Sauce	11 oz	280	B–
Sirloin	Special Recipe	11 oz	250	B–
Teriyaki		10.75 oz	260	B–
Patty, Charbroiled		10 oz	300	D–
Salisbury Steak		10 oz	380	D–
Sliced Beef	Gravy	10 oz	210	B–
		11 oz	290	B–
Meatloaf		12 oz	340	B–
Pot Roast, Yankee		11 oz	260	A
Salisbury Steak		11.5 oz	300	B–
Sirloin	Barbeque	11 oz	280	A
Sirloin Tips		11.75 oz	290	B
Hot Dog	Bun	6.7 oz	450	C–
Patty & Cheese Sandwich		6.25 oz	400	D–
Hot Dog	Bun	8.25 oz	500	D–
Double Beef Patty	Cheese	9.1 oz	480	C–
		11.5 oz	370	C–
Chopped Sirloin		12.25 oz	430	D–

"+" indicates the food meets minimum fiber requirements; "–" indicates the food has a high sodium content.

Food	Processing Category	Brand
Beef Dinner	Frozen	Le Menu
Beef Dinner	Frozen	Le Menu
Beef Dinner	Frozen	Le Menu
Beef Dinner	Frozen	Le Menu
Beef Dinner	Frozen	Le Menu Lightstyle
Beef Dinner	Frozen	Marie Callender's
Beef Dinner	Frozen	Morton
Beef Dinner	Frozen	Morton
Beef Dinner	Frozen	Morton
Beef Dinner	Frozen	Morton
Beef Dinner	Frozen	Stouffer's Dinner Supreme
Beef Dinner	Frozen	Swanson
Beef Dinner	Frozen	Swanson
Beef Dinner	Frozen	Swanson
Beef Dinner	Frozen	Swanson
Beef Dinner	Frozen	Swanson
Beef Dinner	Frozen	Swanson Hungry-Man
Beef Dinner	Frozen	Swanson Hungry-Man
Beef Dinner	Frozen	Swanson Hungry-Man
Beef Dinner	Frozen	Ultra Slim-Fast
Beef Dinner	Frozen	Ultra Slim-Fast
Beef Dinner	Frozen	Ultra Slim-Fast
Beef Dinner	Frozen	Ultra Slim-Fast
Beef Entree	Canned	Dinty Moore
Beef Entree	Canned	Estee
Beef Entree	Canned	Featherweight
Beef Entree	Canned	Hormel/Dinty Moore Micro-Cup
Beef Entree	Canned	La Choy Bi-Pack
Beef Entree	Canned	La Choy Bi-Pack
Beef Entree	Canned	Libby
Beef Entree	Canned	Nalley's Big Chunk
Beef Entree	Canned	Nalley's Homestyle
Beef Entree	Canned	Wolf Brand
Beef Entree	Freeze-dried	Mountain House
Beef Entree	Freeze-dried	Mountain House
Beef Entree	Freeze-dried	Mountain House
Beef Entree	Frozen	Banquet
Beef Entree	Frozen	Banquet Cookin' Bags
Beef Entree	Frozen	Banquet Cookin' Bags
Beef Entree	Frozen	Banquet Cookin' Bags
Beef Entree	Frozen	Banquet Cookin' Bags
Beef Entree	Frozen	Banquet Cookin' Bags
Beef Entree	Frozen	Banquet Family Entrees
Beef Entree	Frozen	Banquet Family Entrees
Beef Entree	Frozen	Banquet Family Entrees
Beef Entree	Frozen	Banquet Family Entrees
Beef Entree	Frozen	Banquet Family Entrees
Beef Entree	Frozen	Banquet Family Entrees
Beef Entree	Frozen	Banquet Platters
Beef Entree	Frozen	Banquet Supreme Microwave
Beef Entree	Frozen	Budget Gourmet
Beef Entree	Frozen	Budget Gourmet

Major Description	Minor Description	Serving Size	Calories	Grade
Pot Roast, Yankee		10 oz	330	C–
Salisbury Steak		10.5 oz	370	D–
Sirloin Tips		11.5 oz	400	D–
Stroganoff		10 oz	430	D–
Salisbury Steak		10 oz	280	B–
Meatloaf	Mashed Potatoes & Vegetables	14 oz	540	D–
Enchilada & Tamale	Chili	10 oz	300	B–
Patty, Charbroiled	Gravy	9 oz	270	C–
Salisbury Steak		10 oz	300	D–
Sliced Sirloin		10 oz	220	B–
Salisbury Steak	Gravy & Mushrooms	11.63 oz	400	D–
		11.25 oz	310	B–
Beef	in Barbecue Sauce	11 oz	460	C–
Chopped Sirloin		10.75 oz	340	D–
Salisbury Steak		10.75 oz	400	C–
Swiss Steak		10 oz	350	B–
Chopped Steak		16.75 oz	640	D–
Salisbury Steak		16.5 oz	680	D–
Sliced Beef		15.25 oz	450	B–
Beef Tips	Country-style Vegetables	12 oz	230	B–
Meatloaf	in Tomato Sauce	10.5 oz	340	B–
Pepper Steak	Parsley Rice	12 oz	270	A–
Salisbury Steak	Mushrooms	10.5 oz	290	B–
Stew		8 oz	220	D–
Stew		7.5 oz	210	D
Stew		7.5 oz	160	B–
Stew		7.5 oz	190	D–
Chow Mein		4 oz	70	A–
Pepper	Oriental Style	4 oz	80	B–
Stew		7.5 oz	160	B–
Stew		7.5 oz	200	C–
Stew		8 oz	180	B–
Stew		7.75 oz	179	C–
Rice with Onions		1 cup	330	C
Stew		1 cup	260	C
Stroganoff		1 cup	270	D
Pie		7 oz	510	D–
Creamed, Chipped		4 oz	100	C
Patty, Charbroiled	Mushroom Gravy	5 oz	210	D
Salisbury Steak	Gravy	5 oz	190	D
Sliced	Gravy	4 oz	100	D
Sliced	in Barbecue Sauce	4 oz	100	B
Patty	Onion Gravy	8 oz	300	D
Patty, Charbroiled	Mushroom Gravy	8 oz	290	D
Salisbury Steak	Gravy	8 oz	300	D
Sliced	Gravy	8 oz	160	B
Stew		7 oz	140	C
Stroganoff	Noodles	7 oz	190	B
		10 oz	460	D–
Pie		7 oz	440	D–
Oriental Beef		10 oz	290	B–
Pepper Steak	Rice	10 oz	300	B–

"+" indicates the food meets minimum fiber requirements; "–" indicates the food has a high sodium content.

Food	Processing Category	Brand
Beef Entree	Frozen	Budget Gourmet
Beef Entree	Frozen	Budget Gourmet
Beef Entree	Frozen	Budget Gourmet
Beef Entree	Frozen	Budget Gourmet
Beef Entree	Frozen	Budget Gourmet
Beef Entree	Frozen	Budget Gourmet Light & Healthy
Beef Entree	Frozen	Budget Gourmet Light & Healthy
Beef Entree	Frozen	Budget Gourmet Light & Healthy
Beef Entree	Frozen	Budget Gourmet Light & Healthy
Beef Entree	Frozen	Chun King
Beef Entree	Frozen	Chun King
Beef Entree	Frozen	Chun King
Beef Entree	Frozen	Dining Lite
Beef Entree	Frozen	Dining Lite
Beef Entree	Frozen	Dining Lite
Beef Entree	Frozen	Freezer Queen Cook in Pouch
Beef Entree	Frozen	Freezer Queen Cook in Pouch
Beef Entree	Frozen	Freezer Queen Cook in Pouch
Beef Entree	Frozen	Freezer Queen Deluxe Family
Beef Entree	Frozen	Freezer Queen Family Suppers
Beef Entree	Frozen	Freezer Queen Family Suppers
Beef Entree	Frozen	Freezer Queen Family Suppers
Beef Entree	Frozen	Freezer Queen Family Suppers
Beef Entree	Frozen	Freezer Queen in Pouch
Beef Entree	Frozen	Freezer Queen Single Serve
Beef Entree	Frozen	Freezer Queen Single Serve
Beef Entree	Frozen	Healthy Choice
Beef Entree	Frozen	Healthy Choice
Beef Entree	Frozen	Healthy Choice
Beef Entree	Frozen	Hormel
Beef Entree	Frozen	La Choy Fresh & Lite
Beef Entree	Frozen	La Choy Fresh & Lite
Beef Entree	Frozen	La Choy Fresh & Lite
Beef Entree	Frozen	Marie Callender's
Beef Entree	Frozen	Marie Callender's
Beef Entree	Frozen	Micro Magic
Beef Entree	Frozen	Micro Magic
Beef Entree	Frozen	Morton
Beef Entree	Frozen	Myer's
Beef Entree	Frozen	Myer's
Beef Entree	Frozen	Myer's
Beef Entree	Frozen	On-Cor [1]
Beef Entree	Frozen	On-Cor
Beef Entree	Frozen	On-Cor
Beef Entree	Frozen	On-Cor
Beef Entree	Frozen	On-Cor
Beef Entree	Frozen	On-Cor
Beef Entree	Frozen	On-Cor
Beef Entree	Frozen	On-Cor
Beef Entree	Frozen	Pilgrims Pride
Beef Entree	Frozen	Right Course
Beef Entree	Frozen	Right Course

[1] All On-Cor products listed in this section are multiple-meal packages.

Major Description	Minor Description	Serving Size	Calories	Grade
Salisbury Steak	Sirloin	9 oz	280	B–
Sirloin	in Herb Sauce	10 oz	290	C–
Sirloin, Roast		9.5 oz	330	C–
Sirloin, Tips	Country-style Vegetable	10 oz	310	D–
Stroganoff		8.75 oz	280	C–
Oriental Style		10 oz	290	B–
Salisbury Steak		9 oz	220	C–
Sirloin	in Herb Sauce	9.5 oz	250	C–
Stroganoff		8.75 oz	260	C–
Pepper	Oriental Style	13 oz	310	A–
Szechuan		13 oz	340	A–
Teriyaki		13 oz	380	A–
Pepper Steak		9 oz	260	B–
Salisbury Steak		9 oz	200	C–
Teriyaki		9 oz	270	B–
Creamed, Chipped		5 oz	80	B–
Salisbury Steak	Gravy	5 oz	160	D–
Sliced	Gravy	4 oz	60	A–
Sliced	Gravy	7 oz	130	B–
Patty	Onion Gravy	7 oz	200	D–
Patty, Charbroiled	Mushroom Gravy	7 oz	180	D–
Salisbury Steak	Gravy	7 oz	200	D–
Stew		7 oz	150	C–
Patty, Charbroiled	Mushroom Gravy	5 oz	90	B–
& Peppers in Sauce	Rice	9 oz	260	A–
Salisbury Steak, Charbroiled	Vegetable	9 oz	330	D–
Pepper Steak		9.5 oz	250	A–
Ribs	Barbeque	11 oz	330	B–
Salisbury Steak	Extra Portion	11 oz	280	B–
Steak, Breaded		4 oz	370	D
Pepper Steak	Rice & Vegetables	10 oz	280	B–
Steak & Broccoli	Rice	11 oz	260	B–+
Teriyaki	Rice & Vegetables	10 oz	240	B–
Beef Stroganoff	Noodles	13 oz	440	D–
Pot Roast	Old Fashioned Style	13 oz	180	B
Cheeseburger		4.75 oz	450	D–
Hamburger		4 oz	350	D–
Pie		7 oz	430	D–
Creamed, Chipped		3.5 oz	136	D–
Pie		3.5 oz	123	D–
Stroganoff		3.5 oz	112	D–
Chop Suey		8 oz serving	30	B–
Meatballs	Swedish Style	8 oz serving	295	D–
Meatloaf		8 oz serving	518	D–
Patties	Charbroiled	8 oz serving	277	D–
Patties	in Tomato Sauce Italian-style	8 oz serving	316	D–
Salisbury Steak		1 patty	281	D–
Sliced		8 oz serving	90	B–
Stew		8 oz serving	134	A–
Steak	Chicken Fried	3 oz	183	D–
Dijon	Pasta & Vegetables	9.5 oz	290	B–
Fiesta	Corn & Pasta	8.87 oz	270	B–

"+" indicates the food meets minimum fiber requirements; "–" indicates the food has a high sodium content.

Food	Processing Category	Brand
Beef Entree	Frozen	Right Course
Beef Entree	Frozen	Right Course
Beef Entree	Frozen	Stouffer's
Beef Entree	Frozen	Stouffer's
Beef Entree	Frozen	Stouffer's
Beef Entree	Frozen	Stouffer's
Beef Entree	Frozen	Stouffer's
Beef Entree	Frozen	Stouffer's
Beef Entree	Frozen	Stouffer's
Beef Entree	Frozen	Stouffer's
Beef Entree	Frozen	Stouffer's Lean Cuisine
Beef Entree	Frozen	Stouffer's Lean Cuisine
Beef Entree	Frozen	Stouffer's Lean Cuisine
Beef Entree	Frozen	Stouffer's Lean Cuisine
Beef Entree	Frozen	Stouffer's Lean Cuisine
Beef Entree	Frozen	Stouffer's Lean Cuisine
Beef Entree	Frozen	Stouffer's Lean Cuisine
Beef Entree	Frozen	Stouffer's Lean Cuisine
Beef Entree	Frozen	Stouffer's Lean Cuisine
Beef Entree	Frozen	Swanson Homestyle Recipe
Beef Entree	Frozen	Swanson Hungry-Man Pot Pie
Beef Entree	Frozen	Swanson Pot Pie
Beef Entree	Frozen	Tyson Gourmet Selection
Beef Entree	Frozen	Tyson Gourmet Selection
Beef Entree	Frozen	Tyson Gourmet Selection
Beef Entree	Frozen	Tyson Gourmet Selection
Beef Entree	Frozen	Weight Watchers
Beef Entree	Frozen	Weight Watchers
Beef Entree	Frozen	Weight Watchers
Beef Entree	Frozen	Weight Watchers
Beef Entree	Packaged	Hormel Top Shelf [2]
Beef Entree	Packaged	Hormel Top Shelf
Beef Entree	Packaged	Hormel Top Shelf
Beef Entree	Packaged	Hormel Top Shelf
Beef Entree	Packaged	Hormel Top Shelf
Beef Entree	Packaged	Hormel Top Shelf
Beef Pocket Sandwich	Frozen	Hot Pockets
Burrito	Frozen	Hormel
Burrito	Frozen	Hormel
Burrito	Frozen	Hormel
Burrito	Frozen	Hormel
Burrito	Frozen	Hormel Burrito Grande
Burrito	Frozen	Patio
Burrito	Frozen	Patio
Burrito	Frozen	Patio
Burrito	Frozen	Patio Britos
Burrito	Frozen	Patio Britos
Burrito	Frozen	Patio Britos
Burrito	Frozen	Patio Britos
Burrito	Frozen	Patio Britos

[2] *One serving as per package directions, for all Hormel Top Shelf products listed in this section.*

Major Description	Minor Description	Serving Size	Calories	Grade
Pot Roast	Homestyle	9.25 oz	220	B–
Ragout	Rice Pilaf	10 oz	300	B–
Chop Suey	Rice	12 oz	300	B–
Creamed, Chipped		5.5 oz	230	D–
Pepper Steak	Rice	10.5 oz	330	B–
Pie		10 oz	500	D–
Salisbury Steak	Gravy	9.87 oz	250	D–
Short Ribs in Gravy		9 oz	350	D–
Stroganoff	Parsley Noodles	9.75 oz	390	D–
Teriyaki	in Sauce with Rice & Vegetables	9.75 oz	290	B–
Meatballs	Swedish	9.13 oz	290	B–
Meatloaf		9.4 oz	270	C–
Oriental Beef		9 oz	250	B–+
Oriental Beef	in Vegetables-style	8.63 oz	250	B–
Pot Roast		9 oz	210	B–
Salisbury Steak	Italian Sauce with Vegetables	9.5 oz	280	D–
Salisbury Steak	Macaroni & Cheese	9.5 oz	290	C–
Steak Ranchero		9.25 oz	270	B–
Szechwan	with Noodles	9.25 oz	260	C–
Salisbury Steak		10 oz	320	D–
Pie		16 oz	610	D–
Pie		7 oz	370	D–
Champignon		10.5 oz	370	C–
Pepper Steak		11.25 oz	330	B–
Salisbury Steak	Supreme	10 oz	430	D–
Short Ribs		11 oz	470	D–
London Broil	in Mushroom Sauce	7.37 oz	140	B–
Salisbury Steak	Romana	8.75 oz	190	C–
Sirloin Tips	Mushrooms in Wine Sauce	7.5 oz	220	B–
Stroganoff		8.5 oz	290	B–
Pepper Steak	Oriental	1 serving	290	C–
Ribs, Boneless		1 serving	440	D–
Roast	Tender	1 serving	240	B–
Salisbury Steak	Potatoes	1 serving	254	B–
Stroganoff		1 serving	320	C–
Sukiyaki		1 serving	330	B–
& Cheddar Cheese		1 piece	370	D–
Beef		1 piece	205	C–
Cheese		1 piece	210	B–
Chicken & Rice		1 piece	200	B–
Chili	Hot	1 piece	240	B–
		5.5 oz piece	380	C–
Beef & Bean		1 piece	370	C–
Beef & Bean	Green Chili	1 piece	330	C–
Beef & Bean	Red Chili	1 piece	340	C–
Beef & Bean		1 piece	250	C–
Beef & Bean	Nacho	1 piece	270	D–
Cheese Nacho		1 piece	250	C–
Chicken, Spicy		1 piece	250	C–
Chili	Red	1 piece	240	C–

"+" indicates the food meets minimum fiber requirements; "–" indicates the food has a high sodium content.

Food	Processing Category	Brand
Burrito Dinner [3]	Frozen	Old El Paso Festive Dinners
Burrito Dinner [3]	Frozen	Patio
Burrito Entree	Frozen	Healthy Choice Quick Meals
Burrito Entree	Frozen	Healthy Choice Quick Meals
Burrito Entree	Frozen	Healthy Choice Quick Meals
Burrito Entree	Frozen	Old El Paso
Burrito Entree	Frozen	Old El Paso
Burrito Entree	Frozen	Old El Paso
Burrito Entree	Frozen	Old El Paso
Burrito Entree	Frozen	Old El Paso
Burrito Entree	Frozen	Old El Paso
Burrito Entree	Frozen	Old El Paso
Burrito Entree	Frozen	Weight Watchers
Cannelloni Entree	Frozen	Celentano
Cannelloni Entree	Frozen	Dining Lite
Cannelloni Entree	Frozen	Lean Cuisine
Cannelloni Entree	Frozen	Lean Cuisine
Cannelloni Entree	Frozen	Stouffer's Lean Cuisine
Cheese Blintz	Frozen	King Kold
Chicken Dinner	Frozen	Armour Classics
Chicken Dinner	Frozen	Armour Classics
Chicken Dinner	Frozen	Armour Classics
Chicken Dinner	Frozen	Armour Classics
Chicken Dinner	Frozen	Armour Classics
Chicken Dinner	Frozen	Armour Classics
Chicken Dinner	Frozen	Armour Classics
Chicken Dinner	Frozen	Armour Classics Lite
Chicken Dinner	Frozen	Armour Classics Lite
Chicken Dinner	Frozen	Armour Classics Lite
Chicken Dinner	Frozen	Armour Classics Lite
Chicken Dinner	Frozen	Armour Classics Lite
Chicken Dinner	Frozen	Banquet
Chicken Dinner	Frozen	Banquet
Chicken Dinner	Frozen	Banquet Extra Helping
Chicken Dinner	Frozen	Banquet Extra Helping
Chicken Dinner	Frozen	Banquet Extra Helping
Chicken Dinner	Frozen	Banquet Extra Helping
Chicken Dinner	Frozen	Banquet Healthy Balance
Chicken Dinner	Frozen	Banquet Healthy Balance
Chicken Dinner	Frozen	Banquet Healthy Balance
Chicken Dinner	Frozen	Banquet Healthy Balance
Chicken Dinner	Frozen	Budget Gourmet
Chicken Dinner	Frozen	Budget Gourmet
Chicken Dinner	Frozen	Budget Gourmet
Chicken Dinner	Frozen	Budget Gourmet
Chicken Dinner	Frozen	Budget Gourmet Light & Healthy
Chicken Dinner	Frozen	Budget Gourmet Light & Healthy
Chicken Dinner	Frozen	Budget Gourmet Light & Healthy
Chicken Dinner	Frozen	Budget Gourmet Light & Healthy
Chicken Dinner	Frozen	Budget Gourmet Light & Healthy
Chicken Dinner	Frozen	Budget Gourmet Light & Healthy
Chicken Dinner	Frozen	Freezer Queen

[3] Values are for entire dinner.

Major Description	Minor Description	Serving Size	Calories	Grade
Beef & Bean		11 oz	470	B–
		12 oz	517	B–
Beef & Bean	Medium	5.2 oz	270	B–
Beef & Bean	Mild	1 piece	250	B–
Chicken Con Queso		1 piece	280	B–
Bean & Cheese		1 piece	340	C–
Beef & Bean	Hot	1 piece	320	B–
Beef & Bean	Medium	1 piece	330	B–
Beef & Bean	Mild	1 piece	330	B–
Pizza	Cheese	1 piece	320	B–
Pizza	Pepperoni	1 piece	260	C–
Pizza	Sausage	1 piece	260	C–
Chicken		1 piece	310	C–
Florentine		12 oz	350	B–
Cheese		9 oz	310	B–
Beef & Pork	in Mornay Sauce	9.63 oz	260	C–
Cheese	in Tomato Sauce	9.13 oz	260	C–
Cheese		9.13 oz	270	B–
		2.5 oz	113	A–
& Noodles		11 oz	230	B–
Fettuccine		11 oz	260	C–
Glazed		10.75 oz	300	D–
in Wine & Mushroom Sauce		10.75 oz	280	C–
Mesquite		9.5 oz	370	C–
Parmigiana		11.5 oz	370	D–
Sweet & Sour		11 oz	240	A–
à la King		11.25 oz	290	B–
Burgundy		10 oz	210	A–
Marsala		10.5 oz	250	B–
Oriental Style		10 oz	180	A–
Sweet & Sour		11 oz	240	A–
& Dumplings		10 oz	430	D–
Fried		10 oz	400	D–
Fried		16 oz	570	D–
Fried	White Meat	16 oz	570	D–
Nuggets	Barbecue Sauce	10 oz	640	D–
Nuggets	Sweet & Sour Sauce	10 oz	650	D
Enchilada		11 oz	300	A–
Mesquite		10.5 oz	310	B–
Parmesan		10.8 oz	300	B–
Sweet & Sour		10.25 oz	270	A–
Cacciatore		11 oz	300	C–
Mexicana		12.8 oz	510	B–
Roast		11.2 oz	280	B–
Teriyaki		12 oz	360	B–
Breast	Herbed, with Fettuccine	11 oz	240	B–
Breast	Mesquite	11 oz	250	B–
Breast	Parmigiana	11 oz	270	B–
Breast	Stuffed	11 oz	250	B–
Breast	Teriyaki	11 oz	300	A–
Roast	Homestyle Gravy	11 oz	280	B–
Nuggets	Platter	6 oz	410	D–

"+" indicates the food meets minimum fiber requirements; "–" indicates the food has a high sodium content.

Food	Processing Category	Brand
Chicken Dinner	Frozen	Freezer Queen
Chicken Dinner	Frozen	Healthy Choice
Chicken Dinner	Frozen	Healthy Choice
Chicken Dinner	Frozen	Healthy Choice
Chicken Dinner	Frozen	Healthy Choice
Chicken Dinner	Frozen	Healthy Choice
Chicken Dinner	Frozen	Healthy Choice
Chicken Dinner	Frozen	Healthy Choice
Chicken Dinner	Frozen	Healthy Choice
Chicken Dinner	Frozen	Healthy Choice
Chicken Dinner	Frozen	Healthy Choice
Chicken Dinner	Frozen	Healthy Choice
Chicken Dinner	Frozen	Healthy Choice
Chicken Dinner	Frozen	Kid Cuisine
Chicken Dinner	Frozen	Kid Cuisine
Chicken Dinner	Frozen	Kid Cuisine
Chicken Dinner	Frozen	Kid Cuisine
Chicken Dinner	Frozen	Kid Cuisine Mega Meal
Chicken Dinner	Frozen	Kid Cuisine Mega Meal
Chicken Dinner	Frozen	Le Menu
Chicken Dinner	Frozen	Le Menu
Chicken Dinner	Frozen	Le Menu
Chicken Dinner	Frozen	Le Menu
Chicken Dinner	Frozen	Le Menu
Chicken Dinner	Frozen	Le Menu Lightstyle
Chicken Dinner	Frozen	Le Menu Lightstyle
Chicken Dinner	Frozen	Le Menu Lightstyle
Chicken Dinner	Frozen	Marie Callender's
Chicken Dinner	Frozen	Marie Callender's
Chicken Dinner	Frozen	Pillsbury Microwave Classic
Chicken Dinner	Frozen	Pillsbury Microwave Classic
Chicken Dinner	Frozen	Stouffer's Dinner Supreme
Chicken Dinner	Frozen	Stouffer's Dinner Supreme
Chicken Dinner	Frozen	Stouffer's Dinner Supreme
Chicken Dinner	Frozen	Stouffer's Dinner Supreme
Chicken Dinner	Frozen	Stouffer's Dinner Supreme
Chicken Dinner	Frozen	Stouffer's Dinner Supreme
Chicken Dinner	Frozen	Swanson
Chicken Dinner	Frozen	Swanson
Chicken Dinner	Frozen	Swanson
Chicken Dinner	Frozen	Swanson
Chicken Dinner	Frozen	Swanson Hungry-Man
Chicken Dinner	Frozen	Swanson Hungry-Man
Chicken Dinner	Frozen	Swanson Hungry-Man
Chicken Dinner	Frozen	Ultra Slim-Fast
Chicken Dinner	Frozen	Ultra Slim-Fast
Chicken Dinner	Frozen	Ultra Slim-Fast
Chicken Dinner	Frozen	Ultra Slim-Fast
Chicken Dinner	Frozen	Ultra Slim-Fast
Chicken Dinner	Frozen	Ultra Slim-Fast
Chicken Entree	Canned	Featherweight
Chicken Entree	Canned	Featherweight
Chicken Entree	Canned	Heinz
Chicken Entree	Canned	La Choy Bi-Pack

Major Description	Minor Description	Serving Size	Calories	Grade
Pattie Platter		7.5 oz	360	D–
& Pasta Divan		11.5 oz	310	A–
Barbeque		12.75 oz	410	A–
Dijon		11 oz	250	A–
Herb Roasted		11 oz	260	A
Mesquite		10.5 oz	310	A
Oriental Style		11.25 oz	220	A–
Parmigiana		11.5 oz	280	A
Salsa		11.25 oz	240	A–
Southwestern Style		12.5 oz	340	A–
Sweet & Sour		11.5 oz	280	A
Teriyaki		12.25 oz	290	A–
Chicken Nuggets		6.8 oz	360	C–
Fried		7.5 oz	430	C–
Nuggets		6.25 oz	400	C–
Sandwiches		8.2 oz	470	C–
Chicken Nuggets		8.4 oz	470	C–
Fried		10.8 oz	720	C–
à La King		10.25 oz	330	C–
Cordon Bleu		11 oz	460	C–
in Wine Sauce		10 oz	280	B–
Parmigiana		11.75 oz	410	D–
Sweet and Sour		11.25 oz	400	D–
Breast	Glazed	10 oz	230	A–
Herb Roasted		10 oz	240	B–
Sweet & Sour		10 oz	250	B–
Breast	Parmigiana	16 oz	620	C
Country Fried		14 oz	610	C–
& Cheese Casserole		1 pkg	480	D–
Casserole		1 pkg	400	D–
Barbecue		10.5 oz	390	D–
Breast	Baked with Gravy	10 oz	300	C–
Florentine		11 oz	430	C–
Fried		10⅝ oz	450	D–
in Supreme Sauce		11⅜ oz	360	B–
Parmigiana		11.5 oz	360	C–
Fried	Barbecue Flavor	10 oz	540	C–
Fried	Dark Meat	9.75 oz	560	D–
Fried	White Meat	10.25 oz	550	D–
Nuggets		8.75 oz	470	C–
Boneless		17.75 oz	700	C–
Fried	Dark Meat	14.25 oz	860	D–
Fried	White Meat	14.25 oz	870	D–
Chow Mein		12 oz	320	B–
Mesquite		12 oz	350	A
Roasted	in Mushroom Sauce	12 oz	280	B–
Sweet & Sour		12 oz	330	A
Vegetables		12 oz	290	A–
with Fettuccine		12 oz	390	B–
& Dumplings		7.5 oz	160	B
Stew	Wild Rice	7.5 oz	140	A–
Stew	Dumplings	7.5 oz	210	C–
Chow Mein		.75 cup	80	C–

"+" indicates the food meets minimum fiber requirements; "–" indicates the food has a high sodium content.

Food	Processing Category	Brand
Chicken Entree	Canned	La Choy Bi-Pack
Chicken Entree	Canned	Lucks
Chicken Entree	Canned	Swanson
Chicken Entree	Canned	Swanson
Chicken Entree	Canned	Swanson
Chicken Entree	Freeze-dried	Mountain House
Chicken Entree	Frozen	Banquet
Chicken Entree	Frozen	Banquet
Chicken Entree	Frozen	Banquet
Chicken Entree	Frozen	Banquet Chicken Hot Bites
Chicken Entree	Frozen	Banquet Chicken Hot Bites
Chicken Entree	Frozen	Banquet Chicken Hot Bites
Chicken Entree	Frozen	Banquet Chicken Hot Bites
Chicken Entree	Frozen	Banquet Chicken Hot Bites
Chicken Entree	Frozen	Banquet Chicken Hot Bites
Chicken Entree	Frozen	Banquet Chicken Hot Bites
Chicken Entree	Frozen	Banquet Chicken Hot Bites
Chicken Entree	Frozen	Banquet Chicken Hot Bites
Chicken Entree	Frozen	Banquet Chicken Hot Bites
Chicken Entree	Frozen	Banquet Chicken Hot Bites
Chicken Entree	Frozen	Banquet Chicken Hot Bites
Chicken Entree	Frozen	Banquet Cookin' Bags
Chicken Entree	Frozen	Banquet Cookin' Bags
Chicken Entree	Frozen	Banquet Cookin' Bags
Chicken Entree	Frozen	Banquet Family Entree
Chicken Entree	Frozen	Banquet Family Entree
Chicken Entree	Frozen	Banquet Healthy Balance
Chicken Entree	Frozen	Banquet Healthy Balance
Chicken Entree	Frozen	Banquet Healthy Balance
Chicken Entree	Frozen	Banquet Microwave
Chicken Entree	Frozen	Banquet Microwave
Chicken Entree	Frozen	Banquet Microwave
Chicken Entree	Frozen	Banquet Microwave
Chicken Entree	Frozen	Banquet Microwave
Chicken Entree	Frozen	Banquet Platters
Chicken Entree	Frozen	Banquet Platters
Chicken Entree	Frozen	Banquet Platters
Chicken Entree	Frozen	Banquet Platters
Chicken Entree	Frozen	Banquet Platters
Chicken Entree	Frozen	Banquet Snack'n
Chicken Entree	Frozen	Banquet Supreme Microwave
Chicken Entree	Frozen	Banquet/Banquet Hot & Spicy
Chicken Entree	Frozen	Budget Gourmet
Chicken Entree	Frozen	Budget Gourmet
Chicken Entree	Frozen	Budget Gourmet
Chicken Entree	Frozen	Budget Gourmet
Chicken Entree	Frozen	Budget Gourmet Light & Healthy
Chicken Entree	Frozen	Budget Gourmet Light & Healthy
Chicken Entree	Frozen	Budget Gourmet Light & Healthy

Major Description	Minor Description	Serving Size	Calories	Grade
Oriental Style		³/₄ cup	240	A–
& Dumplings		³/₄ cup	240	D–
& Dumplings		7.5 oz	220	D–
à la King		5.25 oz	190	D–
Stew		7.63	160	C–
Stew	Prepared as per Directions	1 cup	230	C
Fried	Breast Portions	5.75 oz	220	D–
Fried	Thighs & Drumsticks	6.25 oz	250	D–
Pie		7 oz	550	D–
Breast, Boneless	Tenders	2.25 oz	150	C–
Breast, Boneless	Tenders	4 oz	260	C–
Breast, Boneless	Tenders, Southern Fried	2.25 oz	160	C–
Drumsnackers		2.63 oz	220	D–
Nuggets		2.63 oz	210	D–
Nuggets	Cheddar Cheese	2.63 oz	250	D–
Nuggets	Hot & Spicy	2.63 oz	250	D–
Nuggets	Southern Fried	2.63 oz	220	D–
Patties	Breast	2.63 oz	210	D–
Patties	Breast, Southern Fried	2.63 oz	210	D–
Sticks		2.63 oz	220	D–
à la King		4 oz	110	D
Primavera	and Vegetable	4 oz	100	B
Sweet & Sour		4 oz	130	A
& Dumplings		7 oz	280	D
Primavera	Vegetable	7 oz	140	B
Breast	Nuggets	2.25 oz	120	B–
Breast	Patties	2.25 oz	120	B–
Breast	Tenders	2.25 oz	120	B–
Nuggets	Hot & Spicy with Barbecue Sauce	4.5 oz	360	D–
Nuggets	Southern Fried with Barbecue Sauce	4.5 oz	370	D–
Nuggets	Sweet & Sour Sauce	4.5 oz	360	D–
Patties	Breast & Bun	4 oz	310	D–
Patties	Southern Fried with Biscuit	4 oz	320	C–
Drumsnackers		7 oz	430	C–
Fried	White Meat	9 oz	430	D
Fried	White Meat, Hot & Spicy	9 oz	430	D
Nuggets		6.4 oz	430	D–
Patties		7.5 oz	380	D–
Hot & Spicy		3.75 oz	140	D–
Pie		7 oz	430	D–
Fried		6.4 oz	330	D–
Egg Noodle with Broccoli		10 oz	450	D–
Marsala		10 oz	250	B–
Sweet & Sour	Rice	10 oz	350	B–
with Fettuccine		10 oz	400	D–
au Gratin		9.1 oz	230	B–
Chinese-style Vegetables		10 oz	280	B–
French Recipe		10 oz	220	C–

"+" *indicates the food meets minimum fiber requirements; "–" indicates the food has a high sodium content.*

Food	Processing Category	Brand
Chicken Entree	Frozen	Budget Gourmet Light & Healthy
Chicken Entree	Frozen	Budget Gourmet Light & Healthy
Chicken Entree	Frozen	Budget Gourmet Light & Healthy
Chicken Entree	Frozen	Budget Gourmet Light & Healthy
Chicken Entree	Frozen	Celentano
Chicken Entree	Frozen	Celentano
Chicken Entree	Frozen	Chun King
Chicken Entree	Frozen	Chun King
Chicken Entree	Frozen	Chun King
Chicken Entree	Frozen	Country Pride
Chicken Entree	Frozen	Country Pride
Chicken Entree	Frozen	Country Pride
Chicken Entree	Frozen	Country Pride
Chicken Entree	Frozen	Country Pride
Chicken Entree	Frozen	Country Pride
Chicken Entree	Frozen	Dining Lite
Chicken Entree	Frozen	Dining Lite
Chicken Entree	Frozen	Dining Lite
Chicken Entree	Frozen	Dining Lite
Chicken Entree	Frozen	Freezer Queen Cook in Pouch
Chicken Entree	Frozen	Freezer Queen Cook in Pouch
Chicken Entree	Frozen	Freezer Queen Deluxe Family
Chicken Entree	Frozen	Freezer Queen Family Suppers
Chicken Entree	Frozen	Freezer Queen Single Serve
Chicken Entree	Frozen	Freezer Queen Single Serve
Chicken Entree	Frozen	Freezer Queen Single Serve
Chicken Entree	Frozen	Green Giant Entrees
Chicken Entree	Frozen	Healthy Choice
Chicken Entree	Frozen	Healthy Choice
Chicken Entree	Frozen	Healthy Choice
Chicken Entree	Frozen	Healthy Choice
Chicken Entree	Frozen	Healthy Choice
Chicken Entree	Frozen	Healthy Choice
Chicken Entree	Frozen	Healthy Choice
Chicken Entree	Frozen	Healthy Choice
Chicken Entree	Frozen	Healthy Choice
Chicken Entree	Frozen	Healthy Choice
Chicken Entree	Frozen	La Choy Fresh & Lite
Chicken Entree	Frozen	La Choy Fresh & Lite
Chicken Entree	Frozen	La Choy Fresh & Lite
Chicken Entree	Frozen	La Choy Fresh & Lite
Chicken Entree	Frozen	Le Menu
Chicken Entree	Frozen	Le Menu Lightstyle
Chicken Entree	Frozen	Le Menu Lightstyle
Chicken Entree	Frozen	Le Menu Lightstyle
Chicken Entree	Frozen	Le Menu Lightstyle
Chicken Entree	Frozen	Marie Callender's
Chicken Entree	Frozen	Morton
Chicken Entree	Frozen	Myer's
Chicken Entree	Frozen	Myer's
Chicken Entree	Frozen	Myer's
Chicken Entree	Frozen	Myer's
Chicken Entree	Frozen	Myer's

Major Description	Minor Description	Serving Size	Calories	Grade
Italian-style Vegetables		10.25 oz	310	B–
Mandarin		10 oz	240	B–
Orange Glazed		9 oz	270	A–
Oriental Style	Vegetables	9 oz	280	B–
Parmigiana		9 oz	330	D–
Primavera		11.5 oz	270	C–
Chow Mein		13 oz	370	A–
Imperial		13 oz	300	A–
Walnut Crunchy		13 oz	310	A–
Chunks		3 oz	240	D–
Chunks	Southern Fried	3 oz	280	D–
Nuggets		3 oz	250	D–
Patties		3 oz	250	D–
Patties	Breast, Southern Fried	3 oz	240	D–
Sticks	Fried	3 oz	240	D–
à la King		9 oz	240	B–
Chow Mein		9 oz	180	A–
Glazed		9 oz	220	B–
with Noodles		9 oz	240	B–
à la King		4 oz	70	A–
Sliced with Gravy		5 oz	80	C–
Nuggets		3 oz	270	D–
Croquettes with Breaded Gravy		7 oz	240	D–
à la King	Rice	9 oz	270	B–
Cacciatore		9 oz	270	B–
Sweet & Sour	Rice	9 oz	300	A–
with Broccoli		9.5 oz	340	C–
à l'Orange		9 oz	260	A
Chow Mein		8.5 oz	220	A–
Fajitas		7 oz	200	A–
Fettuccine		8.5 oz	240	A–
Fiesta		8.5 oz	250	B–
Glazed		8.5 oz	220	A–
Honey Mustard		9.5 oz	310	A–
Mandarin		11 oz	260	A–
Oriental Style	in Peanut Sauce	9.5 oz	340	A–
Stir Fry	Pasta	12 oz	300	A–
Almond	Rice & Vegetables	9.75 oz	270	B–
Imperial	Rice	11 oz	260	B–
Oriental Style	Spicy	9.75 oz	270	A–
Sweet & Sour	Rice & Vegetables	10 oz	260	A–
Kiev		8 oz	530	D–
à la King	Seasoned Rice	8.25 oz	240	B–
Breast, Boneless, Herb Roasted	Rice	7.75 oz	260	B–
Dijon	with Pasta & Vegetables	8.5 oz	240	B–
Empress	with Seasoned Rice	8.25 oz	210	B–
Escalloped Noodles		1 cup	270	B–
Pie		7 oz	420	D–
& Noodles		3.5 oz	136	D–
à la Gratin		3.5 oz	129	D–
à la King		3.5 oz	137	D–
Creamed		3.5 oz	151	D–
Croquettes		3.5 oz	168	C–

"+" indicates the food meets minimum fiber requirements; "–" indicates the food has a high sodium content.

Food	Processing Category	Brand
Chicken Entree	Frozen	Myer's
Chicken Entree	Frozen	On-Cor
Chicken Entree	Frozen	On-Cor
Chicken Entree	Frozen	Pilgrims Pride
Chicken Entree	Frozen	Pilgrims Pride
Chicken Entree	Frozen	Pilgrims Pride
Chicken Entree	Frozen	Pilgrims Pride
Chicken Entree	Frozen	Pilgrims Pride
Chicken Entree	Frozen	Pilgrims Pride
Chicken Entree	Frozen	Pilgrims Pride
Chicken Entree	Frozen	Pilgrims Pride
Chicken Entree	Frozen	Pilgrims Pride Wing Zappers
Chicken Entree	Frozen	Right Course
Chicken Entree	Frozen	Right Course
Chicken Entree	Frozen	Right Course
Chicken Entree	Frozen	Right Course
Chicken Entree	Frozen	Stouffer's
Chicken Entree	Frozen	Stouffer's
Chicken Entree	Frozen	Stouffer's
Chicken Entree	Frozen	Stouffer's
Chicken Entree	Frozen	Stouffer's
Chicken Entree	Frozen	Stouffer's
Chicken Entree	Frozen	Stouffer's
Chicken Entree	Frozen	Stouffer's
Chicken Entree	Frozen	Stouffer's Lean Cuisine
Chicken Entree	Frozen	Stouffer's Lean Cuisine
Chicken Entree	Frozen	Stouffer's Lean Cuisine
Chicken Entree	Frozen	Stouffer's Lean Cuisine
Chicken Entree	Frozen	Stouffer's Lean Cuisine
Chicken Entree	Frozen	Stouffer's Lean Cuisine
Chicken Entree	Frozen	Stouffer's Lean Cuisine
Chicken Entree	Frozen	Stouffer's Lean Cuisine
Chicken Entree	Frozen	Stouffer's Lean Cuisine
Chicken Entree	Frozen	Stouffer's Lean Cuisine
Chicken Entree	Frozen	Stouffer's Lean Cuisine
Chicken Entree	Frozen	Stouffer's Lean Cuisine
Chicken Entree	Frozen	Stouffer's Lean Cuisine
Chicken Entree	Frozen	Stouffer's Lean Cuisine
Chicken Entree	Frozen	Stouffer's Lean Cuisine
Chicken Entree	Frozen	Stouffer's Lean Cuisine
Chicken Entree	Frozen	Stouffer's Lean Cuisine
Chicken Entree	Frozen	Stouffer's Lean Cuisine
Chicken Entree	Frozen	Swanson 1 lb Take-out Pre-fried
Chicken Entree	Frozen	Swanson Homestyle Recipe
Chicken Entree	Frozen	Swanson Homestyle Recipe
Chicken Entree	Frozen	Swanson Homestyle Recipe
Chicken Entree	Frozen	Swanson Homestyle Recipe
Chicken Entree	Frozen	Swanson Hungry-Man
Chicken Entree	Frozen	Swanson Plump and Juicy
Chicken Entree	Frozen	Swanson Plump and Juicy
Chicken Entree	Frozen	Swanson Plump and Juicy
Chicken Entree	Frozen	Swanson Plump and Juicy
Chicken Entree	Frozen	Swanson Pot Pie

Major Description	Minor Description	Serving Size	Calories	Grade
Pie		3.5 oz	129	D–
Breast Tenders	Spaghetti	8 oz	209	B–
Parmigiana		1 piece	260	C–
Breast, Boneless	Fillets	3 oz	195	D–
Breast, Boneless	Tenders	3 oz	181	D–
Cajun Style		3 oz	241	D–
Drumsters		3 oz	200	D–
Fried		3 oz	255	D–
Nuggets		3 oz	202	D–
Patties		3 oz	205	D–
Wings	Southern Fried	3 oz	228	D–
Wings		3 oz	187	D–
Italiano	Fettuccine	9.63 oz	280	B–
Sesame		10 oz	320	B–
Tenderloins	in Barbecue Sauce	8.75 oz	270	B–
Tenderloins	in Peanut Sauce	9.25 oz	330	B–
& Noodles	Homestyle	10 oz	310	D–
à la King	Rice	9.5 oz	290	B–
Cashew	Rice	9.5 oz	380	C–
Chow Mein	Noodles	8 oz	130	B–
Creamed		6.5 oz	300	D–
Divan		8.5 oz	320	D–
Escalloped	Noodles	10 oz	420	D–
Pie		10 oz	530	D–
Baked		8 oz	240	B–
Honey Mustard		7.5 oz	140	A–+
Sweet & Sour		10.4 oz	260	A–
à l'Orange		9 oz	260	A
Chow Mein	Rice	9 oz	210	B–
Enchanadas		9.87 oz	220	B–+
Enchilada Suiza		9 oz	290	B–+
Fettuccine		9 oz	270	B–
Fiesta		8.5 oz	240	B–
Glazed		8.5 oz	240	B–
in Honey Barbecue Sauce		8.75 oz	250	B–+
in Peanut Sauce		9 oz	280	B–
Italiano		9 oz	270	B–
Marsala		8.13 oz	180	B–+
Oriental Style		9 oz	260	B–
Parmesan		10.87 oz	220	B–+
Pie		9.5 oz	320	B–
Vegetables		10.5 oz	240	B–+
Fried		3.25 oz	270	D–
Cacciatore		10.95 oz	260	B–
Fried		7 oz	390	D–
Nibbles		4.25 oz	340	D–
Pie		8 oz	410	D–
Pie		16 oz	630	D–
Fried	Breast Portions	4.5 oz	360	D–
Nibbles		3.25 oz	300	D–
Nuggets		3 oz	230	D–
Thighs & Drumsticks		3.25 oz	290	D–
Pie		7 oz	380	D–

"+" indicates the food meets minimum fiber requirements; "–" indicates the food has a high sodium content.

Food	Processing Category	Brand
Chicken Entree	Frozen	Swift International
Chicken Entree	Frozen	Swift International
Chicken Entree	Frozen	The Budget Gourmet Slim
Chicken Entree	Frozen	The Budget Gourmet Slim
Chicken Entree	Frozen	The Budget Gourmet Slim
Chicken Entree	Frozen	Tyson
Chicken Entree	Frozen	Tyson
Chicken Entree	Frozen	Tyson
Chicken Entree	Frozen	Tyson
Chicken Entree	Frozen	Tyson
Chicken Entree	Frozen	Tyson
Chicken Entree	Frozen	Tyson
Chicken Entree	Frozen	Tyson
Chicken Entree	Frozen	Tyson
Chicken Entree	Frozen	Tyson
Chicken Entree	Frozen	Tyson
Chicken Entree	Frozen	Tyson Chick N Cheddar
Chicken Entree	Frozen	Tyson Chick N Chunks
Chicken Entree	Frozen	Tyson Chick N Chunks
Chicken Entree	Frozen	Tyson Flyers
Chicken Entree	Frozen	Tyson Gourmet Selection
Chicken Entree	Frozen	Tyson Gourmet Selection
Chicken Entree	Frozen	Tyson Gourmet Selection
Chicken Entree	Frozen	Tyson Gourmet Selection
Chicken Entree	Frozen	Tyson Gourmet Selection
Chicken Entree	Frozen	Tyson Gourmet Selection
Chicken Entree	Frozen	Tyson Gourmet Selection
Chicken Entree	Frozen	Tyson Gourmet Selection
Chicken Entree	Frozen	Tyson Gourmet Selection
Chicken Entree	Frozen	Tyson Gourmet Selection
Chicken Entree	Frozen	Tyson Gourmet Selection
Chicken Entree	Frozen	Tyson Microwave
Chicken Entree	Frozen	Tyson Microwave
Chicken Entree	Frozen	Tyson Thick & Crispy
Chicken Entree	Frozen	Weight Watchers
Chicken Entree	Frozen	Weight Watchers
Chicken Entree	Frozen	Weight Watchers
Chicken Entree	Frozen	Weight Watchers
Chicken Entree	Frozen	Weight Watchers
Chicken Entree	Frozen	Weight Watchers
Chicken Entree	Frozen	Weight Watchers
Chicken Entree	Frozen	Weight Watchers
Chicken Entree	Frozen	Weight Watchers
Chicken Entree	Frozen	Weight Watchers
Chicken Entree	Packaged	Hormel Top Shelf
Chicken Entree	Packaged	Hormel Top Shelf
Chicken Entree	Packaged	Hormel Top Shelf
Chicken Entree	Refrigerated	Chicken by George
Chicken Entree	Refrigerated	Chicken by George
Chicken Entree	Refrigerated	Chicken by George
Chicken Entree	Refrigerated	Chicken by George

Major Description	Minor Description	Serving Size	Calories	Grade
Cordon Bleu		6 oz	360	D–
Kiev		6 oz	420	D–
au Gratin		9.1 oz	260	C–
French Style		10 oz	260	C–
Mandarin		10 oz	290	B–
Breast, Boneless	Barbecue, Marinated	3.75 oz	120	B–
Breast, Boneless	Butter-Garlic, Marinated	3.75 oz	160	C–
Breast, Boneless	Chunks	3 oz	240	D–
Breast, Boneless	Fillets	3 oz	190	D–
Breast, Boneless	Italian Style, Marinated	3.75 oz	130	A–
Breast, Boneless	Lemon-Pepper, Marinated	3.75 oz	120	A–
Breast, Boneless	Tenders, Southern Fried	3 oz	220	D–
Breast, Boneless	Teriyaki, Marinated	3.75 oz	130	A–
Diced		3 oz	150	B
Patties		2.6 oz	220	D–
Patties	Breast, Southern Fried	2.6 oz	220	D–
Cheddar, Boneless		2.6 oz	220	D–
Chunks		2.6 oz	220	D–
Chunks	Southern Fried	2.6 oz	220	D–
Wings	All Varieties	3.5 oz or six wings	220	D–
& Beef Luau		10.5 oz	330	B–
à l'Orange		9.5 oz	300	B–
Dijon		8.5 oz	310	D–
Français		9.5 oz	280	D–
Kiev		9.25 oz	520	D–
Marsala		10.5 oz	300	C–
Mesquite		9.5 oz	320	B–
Oriental Style		10.25 oz	270	B–
Parmigiana		11.25 oz	380	D–
Picatta		9 oz	240	C–
Sweet & Sour		11 oz	420	C–
Nuggets		3.5 oz	220	D
Tenders		3.5 oz	230	D
Patties		2.6 oz	220	D–
à l'Orange		8.0 oz	200	A–
à la King		9 oz	240	B–
and Noodles	Homestyle	9 oz	240	B–
Cordon Bleu, Breaded		8 oz	220	C–
Fettuccine		8.25 oz	280	B–
Imperial		9.25 oz	240	A–
Kiev		7 oz	230	C–
Nuggets		5.9 oz	270	C–
Southern Fried		6.5 oz	320	D–
Sweet & Sour	Tenders	10.19 oz	240	A–
Acapulco		1 serving	390	B–
Breast, Glazed		1 serving	210	A–
Sweet & Sour		1 serving	270	A
Blue Cheese, Italian		5 oz	190	C–
Cajun		5 oz	200	D–
Lemon Herb		5 oz	150	B–
Mesquite Barbecue		5 oz	170	B–

"+" indicates the food meets minimum fiber requirements; "–" indicates the food has a high sodium content.

Food	Processing Category	Brand
Chicken Entree	Refrigerated	Chicken by George
Chicken Entree	Refrigerated	Chicken by George
Chicken Entree	Refrigerated	Chicken by George
Chicken Sandwiches	Frozen	Hot Pockets
Chicken Sandwiches	Frozen	Lean Pockets
Chicken Sandwiches	Frozen	Lean Pockets
Chicken Sandwiches	Frozen	Lean Pockets Supreme
Chicken Sandwiches	Frozen	Micro Magic
Chicken Sandwiches	Frozen	Tyson Microwave
Chicken Sandwiches	Frozen	Tyson Microwave
Chicken Sandwiches	Frozen	Tyson Microwave
Chili Entree	Frozen	Marie Callender's
Chili Entree	Frozen	Right Course
Chili Entree	Frozen	Stouffer's
Chili Entree	Frozen	Stouffer's Lean Cuisine
Chili Entree	Frozen	Swanson Homestyle Recipe
Chili Entree	Packaged	Hormel Top Shelf
Chimichanga	Frozen	Old El Paso
Chimichanga	Frozen	Old El Paso
Chimichanga Dinner	Frozen	Old El Paso Festive Dinners
Chimichanga Dinner	Frozen	Old El Paso Festive Dinners
Chimichanga Entree	Frozen	Old El Paso
Chimichanga Entree	Frozen	Old El Paso
Chimichanga Entree	Frozen	Old El Paso
Chimichanga Entree	Frozen	Old El Paso
Clam Entree	Frozen	Gorton's Microwave
Clam Entree	Frozen	Mrs. Paul's
Cod Entree	Frozen	Booth
Cod Entree	Frozen	Booth
Cod Entree	Frozen	Booth
Cod Entree	Frozen	Booth
Cod Entree	Frozen	Frionor Bunch O Crunch
Cod Entree	Frozen	Mrs. Paul's Light
Cod Entree	Frozen	Van de Kamp's Light
Egg Breakfast	Frozen	Aunt Jemima Homestyle
Egg Breakfast	Frozen	Aunt Jemima Homestyle
Egg Breakfast	Frozen	Aunt Jemima Homestyle
Egg Breakfast	Frozen	Downyflake
Egg Breakfast	Frozen	Downyflake
Egg Breakfast	Frozen	Downyflake
Egg Breakfast	Frozen	Downyflake
Egg Breakfast	Frozen	Kid Cuisine
Egg Breakfast	Frozen	Kid Cuisine
Egg Breakfast	Frozen	Swanson Great Starts
Egg Breakfast	Frozen	Swanson Great Starts
Egg Breakfast	Frozen	Swanson Great Starts
Egg Breakfast	Frozen	Swanson Great Starts
Egg Breakfast	Frozen	Swanson Great Starts

Major Description	Minor Description	Serving Size	Calories	Grade
Mustard Country & Dill		5 oz	180	C–
Teriyaki		5 oz	180	B–
Tomato, Herb & Basil		5 oz	190	C–
Pocket	Cheddar Cheese	5 oz	310	C–
Pocket	Oriental Style	4.5 oz	250	B–
Pocket	Parmesan Cheese	4.5 oz	270	B–
Pocket		4.5 oz	280	B–
		4.5 oz	390	C–
Barbecue		4 oz	230	B–
Breast		3.5 oz	275	C
Mini		3.5 oz	230	B
3 Bean	Corn Bread	1 cup	350	C–
Vegetarian		9.75 oz	280	B–
Con Carne with Beans		8.75 oz	260	C–
3 Bean	Corn Bread	9 oz	210	B–+
Con Carne		8.25 oz	270	C–
Con Carne Suprema		1 serving	320	C–
Beef		1 piece	370	D–
Chicken		1 piece	360	D–
Beef		11 oz	540	C–
Beef & Cheese		11 oz	510	D–
Bean & Cheese		1 pkg	380	D–
Beef		1 pkg	380	D
Beef & Pork		1 pkg	340	D–
Chicken		1 pkg	370	D
Strips, Crunchy		3.5 oz	330	D–
Battered, Fried		2.5 oz	200	D–
Fillet	au Gratin	9.5 oz	280	C–
Fillet	Florentine	9.5 oz	244	B–
Fillet	in Lemon Butter Sauce	9.5 oz	567	D–
Fillet	in Mushroom Sauce with Rice	9.5 oz	280	C–
Minced Nuggets Crunchy		4 oz	320	D–
Fillet	Breaded	1 piece	240	D–
Fillet	Breaded	1 piece	250	C–
Scrambled	Cheddar Cheese	5.9 oz	250	D–
Scrambled	Pancakes	5.2 oz	270	D–
Scrambled	Sausages & Hash Browns	5.7 oz	290	D–
Scrambled	Ham & Pecan Twirl	6.25 oz	470	D–
Scrambled	Hash Browns & Sausage	6.25 oz	420	D–
Scrambled	Pecan Twirl	6.25 oz	510	D–
Scrambled	with Ham & Hash Browns	6.25 oz	360	D–
Egg Patties	Cheese	4.8 oz	190	D–
Scrambled		4 oz	280	D–
Omelet	in Cheese & Ham Sauce	7 oz	390	D–
Scrambled	Bacon with Home Fries	5.6 oz	340	D–
Scrambled	Cheese & Cinnamon	3.4 oz	290	D–
Scrambled	Hash Browns	6.5 oz	430	D–
Scrambled	Home Fries	4.6 oz	260	D–

"+" indicates the food meets minimum fiber requirements; "–" indicates the food has a high sodium content.

Food	Processing Category	Brand
Egg Breakfast	Frozen	Swanson Great Starts
Egg Breakfast Sandwich	Frozen	Swanson Great Starts Breakfast
Egg Breakfast Sandwich	Frozen	Swanson Great Starts Breakfast
Egg Breakfast Sandwich	Frozen	Swanson Great Starts Breakfast
Egg Breakfast Sandwich	Frozen	Weight Watchers Microwave
Egg Breakfast Vegetarian	Frozen	Morningstar Farms Country
Egg Breakfast Vegetarian	Frozen	Morningstar Farms Country
Egg Roll	Frozen	Chun King
Egg Roll	Frozen	Chun King
Egg Roll	Frozen	Chun King
Egg Roll	Frozen	Chun King Restaurant Style
Egg Roll	Frozen	Jeno's Snacks
Egg Roll	Frozen	Jeno's Snacks
Egg Roll	Frozen	Jeno's Snacks
Egg Roll	Frozen	La Choy
Egg Roll	Frozen	La Choy
Egg Roll	Frozen	La Choy
Egg Roll	Frozen	La Choy
Egg Roll	Frozen	La Choy
Egg Roll	Frozen	La Choy
Egg Roll	Frozen	La Choy
Egg Roll	Frozen	Worthington
Egg Roll	Restaurant	
Eggplant Entree	Frozen	Celentano
Eggplant Entree	Frozen	Celentano
Eggplant Entree	Frozen	Celentano
Eggplant Entree	Frozen	Celentano
Eggplant Entree	Frozen	Mrs. Paul's
Enchilada Dinner	Frozen	Banquet
Enchilada Dinner	Frozen	Banquet
Enchilada Dinner	Frozen	Healthy Choice
Enchilada Dinner	Frozen	Healthy Choice
Enchilada Dinner	Frozen	Old El Paso Festive Dinners
Enchilada Dinner	Frozen	Old El Paso Festive Dinners
Enchilada Dinner	Frozen	Old El Paso Festive Dinners
Enchilada Dinner	Frozen	Patio
Enchilada Dinner	Frozen	Patio
Enchilada Dinner	Frozen	Swanson
Enchilada Dinner	Frozen	Van de Kamp's Mexican Dinner
Enchilada Dinner	Frozen	Van de Kamp's Mexican Dinner
Enchilada Entree	Frozen	Banquet Family Entrees
Enchilada Entree	Frozen	Budget Gourmet Slim
Enchilada Entree	Frozen	Budget Gourmet Slim
Enchilada Entree	Frozen	Healthy Choice
Enchilada Entree	Frozen	Hormel
Enchilada Entree	Frozen	Hormel
Enchilada Entree	Frozen	Le Menu Lightstyle
Enchilada Entree	Frozen	Legume Mexican
Enchilada Entree	Frozen	Old El Paso
Enchilada Entree	Frozen	Old El Paso
Enchilada Entree	Frozen	Old El Paso
Enchilada Entree	Frozen	Old El Paso

Major Description	Minor Description	Serving Size	Calories	Grade
with Mini Oat Bran		4.75 oz	250	D–
Beefsteak & Cheese		4.9 oz	360	D–
Canadian Bacon & Cheese		5.2 oz	420	D–
Sausage & Cheese		5.5 oz	460	D–
English Muffin		4 oz	230	B–
Scramblers, Hash Browns & Links		7 oz	360	D–
Scramblers, Pancakes & Links		6.8 oz	380	D–
Chicken		1 piece	220	C–
Meat & Shrimp		1 piece	220	C–
Shrimp		1 piece	200	B–
Pork		1 piece	180	B–
Chicken		1 piece	190	D–
Meat & Shrimp		1 piece	200	D–
Shrimp & Cheese		1 piece	190	C–
Almond Chicken	Restaurant Style	1 piece	120	B–
Chicken	Snack Style	1 piece	90	B–
Chicken, Sweet & Sour	Restaurant Style	1 piece	150	B–
Lobster	Snack Style	1 piece	75	B–
Meat & Shrimp	Snack Style	1 piece	80	C–
Pork	Restaurant Style	1 piece	150	B–
Shrimp	Snack Style	1 piece	75	B–
Vegetarian		1 piece	160	C–
Shrimp		1 piece	130	B–
Parmigiana		10 oz	350	D–
Parmigiana		6.25 oz	260	C
Parmigiana		8 oz	280	D–
Rollettes		11 oz	320	C
Parmigiana		5 oz	240	D–
Beef		12 oz	500	B–
Cheese		12 oz	550	C–
Beef		13.4 oz	370	A
Chicken		13.4 oz	320	B–
Beef		11 oz	390	B–
Cheese		11 oz	590	D–
Chicken		11 oz	460	C–
Beef		13.25 oz	520	B–
Cheese		12.25 oz	380	B–
Beef		13.75 oz	480	C–
Beef		12 oz	400	C–
Cheese		12 oz	450	C–
Beef	Chili Gravy	7 oz	270	D
Beef	Sirloin, Ranchero Style	9 oz	290	D–
Chicken	Suiza	9 oz	270	B–
Chicken	Suiza	9.5 oz	270	A–
Beef		1 piece	140	C–
Cheese		1 piece	151	C–
Chicken		8 oz	280	B–
Vegetable	with Tofu & Sauce	11 oz	270	B–+
Beef		11 oz	390	B–
Cheese		11 oz	590	D–
Chicken		11 oz	460	C–
Chicken	in Sour Cream Sauce	1 piece	280	D–

"+" indicates the food meets minimum fiber requirements; "–" indicates the food has a high sodium content.

Food	Processing Category	Brand
Enchilada Entree	Frozen	Stouffer's
Enchilada Entree	Frozen	Stouffer's
Enchilada Entree	Frozen	Stouffer's Lean Cuisine Enchanadas
Enchilada Entree	Frozen	Stouffer's Lean Cuisine Enchanadas
Enchilada Entree	Frozen	Van de Kamp's Mexican Entrees
Enchilada Entree	Frozen	Van de Kamp's Mexican Entrees
Enchilada Entree	Frozen	Van de Kamp's Mexican Entrees
Enchilada Entree	Frozen	Van de Kamp's Mexican Entrees
Enchilada Entree	Frozen	Van de Kamp's Mexican Entrees
Enchilada Entree	Frozen	Van de Kamp's Mexican Entrees
Enchilada Entree	Frozen	Van de Kamp's Mexican Entrees
Enchilada Entree	Frozen	Van de Kamp's Mexican Entrees
Enchilada Entree	Frozen	Weight Watchers
Enchilada Entree	Frozen	Weight Watchers
Enchilada Entree	Frozen	Weight Watchers
Fajita Entree	Frozen	Weight Watchers
Fajita Entree	Frozen	Weight Watchers
Fajita Entree	Refrigerated	Chicken by George
Fettuccine Entree	Frozen	Budget Gourmet
Fettuccine Entree	Frozen	Dining Lite
Fettuccine Entree	Frozen	Green Giant
Fettuccine Entree	Frozen	Green Giant Microwave
Fettuccine Entree	Frozen	Healthy Choice
Fettuccine Entree	Frozen	Healthy Choice
Fettuccine Entree	Frozen	Healthy Choice
Fettuccine Entree	Frozen	Healthy Choice Quick Meals
Fettuccine Entree	Frozen	Marie Callender's
Fettuccine Entree	Frozen	Marie Callender's
Fettuccine Entree	Frozen	Marie Callender's
Fettuccine Entree	Frozen	Stouffer's
Fettuccine Entree	Frozen	Stouffer's Lean Cuisine
Fettuccine Entree	Frozen	Stouffer's Lean Cuisine
Fettuccine Entree	Frozen	Weight Watchers
Fish	Frozen	*See also* Specific Fish Entries
Fish Dinner	Frozen	Kid Cuisine
Fish Dinner	Frozen	Morton
Fish Dinner	Frozen	Swanson
Fish Entree	Frozen	Banquet Platters
Fish Entree	Frozen	Booth Microwave
Fish Entree	Frozen	Frionor Bunch O Crunch
Fish Entree	Frozen	Gorton's
Fish Entree	Frozen	Gorton's Crispy Batter
Fish Entree	Frozen	Gorton's Crispy Batter
Fish Entree	Frozen	Gorton's Crispy Batter
Fish Entree	Frozen	Gorton's Crispy Batter
Fish Entree	Frozen	Gorton's Crispy Batter
Fish Entree	Frozen	Gorton's Crunchy
Fish Entree	Frozen	Gorton's Crunchy
Fish Entree	Frozen	Gorton's Crunchy Microwave
Fish Entree	Frozen	Gorton's Crunchy Microwave
Fish Entree	Frozen	Gorton's Crunchy Microwave Large
Fish Entree	Frozen	Gorton's Light Recipe
Fish Entree	Frozen	Gorton's Light Recipe

Major Description	Minor Description	Serving Size	Calories	Grade
Cheese		10.13 oz	590	D–
Chicken		10 oz	490	D–
Beef	and Bean	9.25 oz	280	C–
Chicken		9.87 oz	270	B–
Beef		1 pkg	270	C–
Beef		$^1/_4$ pkg	150	B–
Beef	Shredded	1 pkg	360	C–
Cheese		1 pkg	300	D–
Cheese		$^1/_4$ pkg	200	D–
Cheese	Ranchero Style	$^1/_2$ pkg	260	D–
Chicken		1 pkg	260	C–
Chicken	Suiza	1 pkg	230	C–
Beef	Ranchero Style	9.12 oz	230	C–
Cheese	Ranchero Style	8.87 oz	360	D–
Chicken	Suiza	9 oz	280	B–
Beef		6.75 oz	250	B–
Chicken		6.75 oz	230	B–
Chicken		5 oz	170	C–
in Meat Sauce		10 oz	290	C–
with Broccoli		9 oz	290	C–
Primavera		1 pkg	230	D–+
Primavera		1 pkg	260	D–+
Alfredo		8 oz	240	B–
Beef & Broccoli		12 oz	290	A–
Turkey & Vegetables		12.5 oz	350	B–
Alfredo		8 oz	240	B–
Alfredo		13 oz	350	D
Broccoli & Chicken		13 oz	230	D–
Primavera	Tortellini	14 oz	310	D
Alfredo		5 oz	480	D–
Alfredo		9 oz	270	B–
Primavera		10 oz	260	B–+
Alfredo		9 oz	210	C–
Nuggets		7 oz	320	D–
		9.75 oz	370	C–
Chips		10 oz	500	C–
		8.75 oz	450	D
Sticks, Breaded	Whole Wheat	2 oz	150	D–
Sticks, Breaded		2.7 oz	210	D–
Florentine Style	in Herb Sauce	1 piece	190	C–
Fillets, Battered		1 piece	145	D–
Fillets, Battered		1 piece	320	D–
Fillets, Battered	Haddock	1 piece	150	D–
Fillets, Battered	Perch	1 piece	150	D–
Sticks, Battered		1 piece	65	D–
Fillets, Battered		1 piece	115	D–
Sticks, Battered		1 piece	53	D
Fillets, Battered		1 piece	170	D
Sticks, Battered		1 piece	57	D
Fillets, Battered		1 piece	320	D–
Fillets, Battered		1 piece	180	C–
Fillets, Battered	Tempura	1 piece	200	D–

"+" indicates the food meets minimum fiber requirements; "–" indicates the food has a high sodium content.

Food	Processing Category	Brand
Fish Entree	Frozen	Gorton's Potato Crisp
Fish Entree	Frozen	Gorton's Potato Crisp
Fish Entree	Frozen	Gorton's Specialty Microwave Large
Fish Entree	Frozen	Gorton's Value Pack
Fish Entree	Frozen	Gorton's Value Pack Portions
Fish Entree	Frozen	Healthy Choice
Fish Entree	Frozen	Healthy Choice
Fish Entree	Frozen	Healthy Choice
Fish Entree	Frozen	Mrs. Paul's
Fish Entree	Frozen	Mrs. Paul's
Fish Entree	Frozen	Mrs. Paul's
Fish Entree	Frozen	Mrs. Paul's Crispy Crunchy
Fish Entree	Frozen	Mrs. Paul's Crispy Crunchy
Fish Entree	Frozen	Mrs. Paul's Crunchy
Fish Entree	Frozen	Mrs. Paul's Light
Fish Entree	Frozen	Mrs. Paul's Light
Fish Entree	Frozen	Mrs. Paul's Light
Fish Entree	Frozen	Mrs. Paul's Light
Fish Entree	Frozen	Mrs. Paul's Portions
Fish Entree	Frozen	Stouffer's Lean Cuisine
Fish Entree	Frozen	Stouffer's Lean Cuisine
Fish Entree	Frozen	Stouffer's Lean Cuisine
Fish Entree	Frozen	Stouffer's Lean Cuisine
Fish Entree	Frozen	Swanson Homestyle Recipe
Fish Entree	Frozen	Van de Kamp's
Fish Entree	Frozen	Van de Kamp's
Fish Entree	Frozen	Van de Kamp's
Fish Entree	Frozen	Van de Kamp's
Fish Entree	Frozen	Van de Kamp's
Fish Entree	Frozen	Van de Kamp's
Fish Entree	Frozen	Van de Kamp's
Fish Entree	Frozen	Van de Kamp's
Fish Entree	Frozen	Van de Kamp's
Fish Entree	Frozen	Van de Kamp's Crisp & Healthy
Fish Entree	Frozen	Van de Kamp's Crisp & Healthy
Fish Entree	Frozen	Van de Kamp's Microwave
Fish Entree	Frozen	Van de Kamp's Microwave
Fish Entree	Frozen	Van de Kamp's Microwave
Fish Entree	Frozen	Van de Kamp's Microwave
Fish Entree	Frozen	Van de Kamp's Value Pack
Fish Entree	Frozen	Weight Watchers
Fish Entree	Frozen	Weight Watchers
Fish Entree	Frozen	Weight Watchers
Flounder Entree	Frozen	Gorton's Crispy Batter
Flounder Entree	Frozen	Gorton's Microwave
Flounder Entree	Frozen	Mrs. Paul's Crunchy
Flounder Entree	Frozen	Mrs. Paul's Light
Flounder Entree	Frozen	Van de Kamp's Light
French Toast	Frozen	Aunt Jemima
French Toast	Frozen	Aunt Jemima
French Toast	Frozen	Downyflake
French Toast	Frozen	Downyflake
French Toast	Frozen	Downyflake Extra Thick

Major Description	Minor Description	Serving Size	Calories	Grade
Fillets, Battered		1 piece	150	D
Sticks, Battered		1 piece	65	D–
Coated Fillets, Ranch		1 piece	330	D–
Sticks, Battered		1 piece	48	D–
Fillets, Battered		1 piece	180	D–
Fillets, Battered		3.5 oz	160	B–
Lemon Pepper		10.7 oz	300	A
Sticks, Breaded		2.4 oz	120	B–
Cakes		1 piece	95	C–
Fillets, Battered		1 piece	165	D–
Sticks Battered		1 piece	52	D–
Fillets, Breaded		1 piece	110	C–
Fillets, Breaded	Minced	1 piece	115	D–
Fillets, Battered		1 piece	140	D–
Dijon		$8^3/_4$ oz	200	B–
Fillets in Butter Sauce		1 piece	140	C–
Florentine		8 oz	220	C–
Mornay		9 oz	230	C–
Fillets, Battered	Minced	1 piece	150	D–
Fillet	Divan	$12^3/_8$ oz	260	B–
Fillet	Florentine	9 oz	230	C–
Florentine	Jardiniere	$11^1/_4$ oz	290	C–
Divan		$10^3/_8$ oz	210	B–
Fries		$6^1/_2$ oz	340	D–
Fillet, Battered	Perch	1 piece	310	D–
Fillet, Breaded	Haddock	1 piece	135	D
Fillets, Battered		1 piece	170	D–
Fillets, Breaded		1 piece	140	D
Fish Nuggets, Battered		1 piece	33	D–
Fish Portions, Battered		1 piece	180	D–
Mini Sticks, Breaded		1 piece	18	D–
Sticks, Battered		1 piece	40	D–
Sticks, Battered		1 piece	50	D–
Fillets, Breaded		1 piece	75	B–
Sticks, Breaded		1 piece	30	A–
Fillet, Breaded	Crispy	1 piece	140	D–
Fish Fillet	Crispy	1 piece	140	D–
Fish Fillet, Large	Crispy	1 piece	290	D–
Fish Sticks	Crispy	1 piece	43	D–
Sticks, Breaded		1 piece	43	D–
au Gratin		9.25 oz	200	B–
Fillet	Fried	7.7 oz	230	C–
Oven Fried		7.08 oz	240	B–
Fillets, Battered		1 piece	150	D–
Stuffed		1 pkg	350	D–
Fillets, Battered		1 piece	110	C–
Fillets, Breaded		1 piece	240	C–
Fillets, Breaded		1 piece	260	D–
Cinnamon Swirl		1 piece	171	B–
Original		3 oz	166	B–
Cinnamon Swirl		1 slice	135	B–
Regular		1 slice	130	B–
		1 slice	150	D–

"+" indicates the food meets minimum fiber requirements; "–" indicates the food has a high sodium content.

Food	Processing Category	Brand
French Toast	Frozen	Farm Rich
French Toast	Frozen	Farm Rich
French Toast	Frozen	Farm Rich
French Toast	Frozen	Weight Watchers Microwave
French Toast Breakfast	Frozen	Aunt Jemima Homestyle
French Toast Breakfast	Frozen	Aunt Jemima Homestyle
French Toast Breakfast	Frozen	Kid Cuisine
French Toast Breakfast	Frozen	Morningstar Farms Country
French Toast Breakfast	Frozen	Swanson Great Starts
French Toast Breakfast	Frozen	Swanson Great Starts
French Toast Breakfast	Frozen	Swanson Great Starts
French Toast Breakfast	Frozen	Swanson Great Starts
French Toast Breakfast	Frozen	Weight Watchers Microwave
Ham & Cheese Breakfast	Frozen	Owens Border Breakfasts
Ham & Cheese Breakfast	Frozen	Swanson Great Starts
Ham & Cheese Loaf	Frozen	Light & Lean
Ham & Cheese Patty	Canned	Hormel
Ham & Cheese Pocket Sandwich	Frozen	Hot Pockets
Ham Dinner	Frozen	Armour Classics
Ham Dinner	Frozen	Le Menu
Ham Dinner	Frozen	Morton
Ham Dinner	Frozen	Stouffer's Dinner Supreme
Ham Entree	Frozen	Banquet Platters
Ham Entree	Frozen	Budget Gourmet Light & Healthy
Ham Entree	Frozen	Budget Gourmet Slim
Ham Entree	Frozen	Budget Gourmet Slim
Ham Entree	Frozen	Stouffer's
Ham Entree	Frozen	Swanson Homestyle Recipe
Lasagna	Canned	Chef Boyardee Microwave
Lasagna	Canned	Chef Boyardee Microwave
Lasagna	Canned	Chef Boyardee Microwave
Lasagna	Canned	Chef Boyardee Microwave
Lasagna	Canned	Nalley's
Lasagna	Canned	Nalley's
Lasagna Dinner	Frozen	Banquet Extra Helping
Lasagna Entree	Frozen	Banquet Family Entrees
Lasagna Entree	Frozen	Budget Gourmet
Lasagna Entree	Frozen	Budget Gourmet
Lasagna Entree	Frozen	Budget Gourmet Light & Healthy
Lasagna Entree	Frozen	Budget Gourmet Light & Healthy
Lasagna Entree	Frozen	Budget Gourmet Slim
Lasagna Entree	Frozen	Buitoni Family Size
Lasagna Entree	Frozen	Buitoni Single Serving
Lasagna Entree	Frozen	Celentano
Lasagna Entree	Frozen	Celentano
Lasagna Entree	Frozen	Dining Lite
Lasagna Entree	Frozen	Dining Lite
Lasagna Entree	Frozen	Freezer Queen Deluxe Family
Lasagna Entree	Frozen	Green Giant Entrees
Lasagna Entree	Frozen	Healthy Choice
Lasagna Entree	Frozen	Healthy Choice Quick Meals
Lasagna Entree	Frozen	Le Menu Light Style

Major Description	Minor Description	Serving Size	Calories	Grade
Sticks	Apple Cinnamon	3 oz	310	D
Sticks	Blueberry	3 oz	310	D
Sticks	Original	3 oz	300	D
	Cinnamon	½ pkg	160	B–
Sticks & Syrup		5.2 oz	400	D–
Wedges & Sausage		5.3 oz	360	D–
		4.11 oz	260	D
Cinnamon Swirl, Vegetarian		6.5 oz	380	C–
	Sausages	5.5 oz	380	D–
Cinnamon Swirl	Sausages	5.5 oz	390	D–
Mini	Sausages	2.5 oz	190	D–
Oatmeal	Light Links	4.65 oz	310	C–
Links		4.5 oz	270	C–
		2 oz	150	C–
Bagel		3 oz	240	B–
		2 slices	90	D
		1 patty	190	D–
		1 piece	360	C–
Steak		10.75 oz	270	B–
Steak		10 oz	300	C–
		10 oz	290	A–
Steak	Glazed	10.5 oz	380	C–
		10 oz	400	C–
Asparagus	au Gratin	8.7 oz	300	D–
Asparagus au Gratin		9 oz	280	C–
with Asparagus	au Gratin	9 oz	280	C–
Asparagus Bake		9.5 oz	510	D–
Scalloped Potatoes		9 oz	300	C–
		7.5 oz	230	C–
		7.5 oz	230	C–
in Garden Vegetable Sauce		7.5 oz	170	A–
in Garden Vegetable Sauce		7.5 oz	170	A–
		7.5 oz	180	B–
		7.5 oz	180	B–
		16.5 oz	645	C–
in Meat Sauce		7 oz	270	C
Cheese	3 Cheese	10 oz	400	C–
Sausage Italian		10 oz	420	D–
in Meat Sauce		9.4 oz	290	C–
Vegetable		10.5 oz	290	C–
in Meat Sauce		10 oz	290	C–
in Sauce		7.3 oz	370	C–
Meat		9 oz	580	B–
		8 oz	370	D–
Primavera		11 oz	330	C–
Cheese		9 oz	260	B–
in Meat Sauce		9 oz	240	B–
in Meat Sauce		7 oz	200	B–
		12 oz	490	C–
in Meat Sauce		9 oz	260	B–
Zucchini		11.5 oz	250	A–
in Meat Sauce		10 oz	290	B–

"+" indicates the food meets minimum fiber requirements; "–" indicates the food has a high sodium content.

Food	Processing Category	Brand
Lasagna Entree	Frozen	Le Menu Light Style
Lasagna Entree	Frozen	Legume
Lasagna Entree	Frozen	Legume Classic
Lasagna Entree	Frozen	Marie Callender's
Lasagna Entree	Frozen	Marie Callender's
Lasagna Entree	Frozen	Mrs. Paul's Light
Lasagna Entree	Frozen	On-Cor
Lasagna Entree	Frozen	On-Cor
Lasagna Entree	Frozen	Stouffer's
Lasagna Entree	Frozen	Stouffer's
Lasagna Entree	Frozen	Stouffer's
Lasagna Entree	Frozen	Stouffer's 21 Oz
Lasagna Entree	Frozen	Stouffer's Lean Cuisine
Lasagna Entree	Frozen	Stouffer's Lean Cuisine
Lasagna Entree	Frozen	Stouffer's Lean Cuisine
Lasagna Entree	Frozen	Stouffer's Lean Cuisine
Lasagna Entree	Frozen	Swanson Homestyle Recipe
Lasagna Entree	Frozen	Tyson Gourmet Selection
Lasagna Entree	Frozen	Ultra Slim-Fast
Lasagna Entree	Frozen	Ultra Slim-Fast
Lasagna Entree	Frozen	Weight Watchers
Lasagna Entree	Frozen	Weight Watchers
Lasagna Entree	Frozen	Weight Watchers
Lasagna Entree	Frozen	Weight Watchers
Linguine Entree	Frozen	Budget Gourmet
Linguine Entree	Frozen	Budget Gourmet Slim
Linguine Entree	Frozen	Healthy Choice
Linguine Entree	Frozen	Lean Cuisine
Macaroni Dinner	Frozen	Banquet
Macaroni Dinner	Frozen	Kid Cuisine
Macaroni Dinner	Frozen	Kid Cuisine
Macaroni Dinner	Frozen	Kid Cuisine Mega Meal
Macaroni Dinner	Frozen	Morton Casserole
Macaroni Dinner	Frozen	Swanson
Macaroni Entree	Canned	Chef Boyardee Beefaroni
Macaroni Entree	Canned	Chef Boyardee Microwave
Macaroni Entree	Canned	Franco-American
Macaroni Entree	Canned	Heinz
Macaroni Entree	Canned	Heinz
Macaroni Entree	Canned	Hormel Micro-Cup
Macaroni Entree	Canned	Lipton Hearty Ones
Macaroni Entree	Canned	Nalley's
Macaroni Entree	Frozen	Banquet Casserole
Macaroni Entree	Frozen	Banquet Family Entrees
Macaroni Entree	Frozen	Budget Gourmet Light & Healthy
Macaroni Entree	Frozen	Budget Gourmet Side Dish
Macaroni Entree	Frozen	Freezer Queen Family Side Dish
Macaroni Entree	Frozen	Green Giant
Macaroni Entree	Frozen	Healthy Choice Quick Meals
Macaroni Entree	Frozen	Healthy Choice Quick Meals
Macaroni Entree	Frozen	Healthy Choice Quick Meals
Macaroni Entree	Frozen	Marie Callender's
Macaroni Entree	Frozen	Marie Callender's

Major Description	Minor Description	Serving Size	Calories	Grade
Vegetable	Garden	10.5 oz	260	B–
Vegetable	with Tofu & Sauce	12 oz	240	B–+
Tofu & Sauce		8 oz	210	C–+
Cheese, Extra		14 oz	330	D–
in Meat Sauce		14 oz	370	D–
Seafood		9.5 oz	290	B–
		1 serving	232	B–
Vegetable		1 serving	229	B–
		10.5 oz	360	C–
Fiesta		10.25 oz	430	D–
Vegetable		10.5 oz	420	D–
		10.5 oz	360	C–
Classic Cheese		$11^1/_2$ oz	290	B–+
Meat Sauce		$10^1/_4$	270	B–+
Tuna		$9^3/_4$ oz	230	B–
Zucchini		11 oz	240	A–+
in Meat Sauce		10.5 oz	400	C–
		11.5 oz	380	C–
Meat Sauce		12 oz	330	B–
Vegetable		12 oz	240	A–
Cheese	Italian Style	11 oz	350	C–
Florentine		10 oz	190	A–+
Garden Style		11 oz	290	B–
in Meat Sauce		11 oz	320	B–
Shrimp	Light	10 oz	280	B–
Scallops & Clams		9.5 oz	280	C–
Shrimp		9.5 oz	230	A–
Clam Sauce		9.63 oz	270	B–
Cheese		10 oz	420	D
Cheese	Mini Franks	9 oz	360	C–
Cheese	Mini Franks Ravioli	9 oz	290	B–
Cheese		12.5 oz	470	B–
Cheese	Pie	6.5 oz	290	D–
Cheese		$12^1/_4$ oz	370	C–
Beef		7.5 oz	220	B–
Beef	Elbows in Beef Sauce	7.5 oz	210	B–
Cheese		$7^3/_8$ oz	170	C–
Beef	in Tomato Sauce	7.5 oz	200	C–
Cheese		7.5 oz	190	C–
Cheese		7.5 oz	189	B–
Shells with Cheddar Cheese		11 oz	367	B–
Beef		7.5 oz	180	A–
Cheese		8 oz	350	D–
Cheese		8 oz	210	B–
Cheese		10.5 oz	330	B–
Cheese		5.3 oz	210	C–
Cheese		4 oz	110	B–
Cheese		1 5.7 oz	230	C–
Beef		8.5 oz	200	A–
Cheese		9 oz	280	B–
Nacho	Cheese	9 oz	280	B–
Beef		14 oz	310	C–+
Cheese	Special	14 oz	420	C–

"+" indicates the food meets minimum fiber requirements; "–" indicates the food has a high sodium content.

Food	Processing Category	Brand
Macaroni Entree	Frozen	Myers
Macaroni Entree	Frozen	On-Cor
Macaroni Entree	Frozen	Stouffer's
Macaroni Entree	Frozen	Stouffer's
Macaroni Entree	Frozen	Stouffer's Lean Cuisine
Macaroni Entree	Frozen	Stouffer's Lean Cuisine
Macaroni Entree	Frozen	Swanson Homestyle Recipe
Macaroni Entree	Frozen	Swanson Pot Pie
Macaroni Entree	Frozen	Weight Watchers
Macaroni Entree	Frozen	Weight Watchers
Manicotti Entree	Frozen	Buitoni Single Serving
Manicotti Entree	Frozen	Celentano
Manicotti Entree	Frozen	Legume Classic
Manicotti Entree	Frozen	Legume Florentine
Manicotti Entree	Frozen	On-Cor
Manicotti Entree	Frozen	The Budget Gourmet
Manicotti Entree	Frozen	Weight Watchers
Meat Loaf Dinner	Frozen	Armour Classics
Meat Loaf Dinner	Frozen	Banquet
Meat Loaf Dinner	Frozen	Freezer Queen
Meat Loaf Dinner	Frozen	Morton
Meat Loaf Dinner	Frozen	Stouffer's Dinner Supreme
Meat Loaf Dinner	Frozen	Swanson
Meat Loaf Entree	Frozen	Banquet Cookin' Bags
Meat Loaf Entree	Frozen	Freezer Queen Family Suppers
Meatball Entree	Frozen	Budget Gourmet
Meatball Entree	Frozen	Budget Gourmet
Meatball Entree	Frozen	Le Menu Lightstyle
Meatball Entree	Frozen	Stouffer's
Meatball Entree	Frozen	Stouffer's Lean Cuisine
Meatball Entree	Frozen	Swanson Homestyle Recipe
Meatball Entree	Frozen	Weight Watchers
Meatball Stew	Canned	Chef Boyardee
Meatball Stew	Canned	Dinty Moore
Menudo	Canned	Old El Paso
Mexican Dinner	Frozen	Banquet
Mexican Dinner	Frozen	Banquet
Mexican Dinner	Frozen	Morton
Mexican Dinner	Frozen	Patio
Mexican Dinner	Frozen	Patio
Mexican Dinner	Frozen	Swanson
Mexican Dinner	Frozen	Swanson Hungry-Man
Noodle Entree	Canned	Heinz
Noodle Entree	Canned	Heinz
Noodle Entree	Canned	Heinz
Noodle Entree	Canned	Hormel/Dinty Moore Micro Cup
Noodle Entree	Canned	Nalleys
Noodle Entree	Canned	Nalleys
Noodle Entree	Canned	Van Camp's Noodle Weenee
Pancake Breakfast	Frozen	Aunt Jemima Homestyle
Pancake Breakfast	Frozen	Aunt Jemima Homestyle
Pancake Breakfast	Frozen	Aunt Jemima Homestyle

Major Description	Minor Description	Serving Size	Calories	Grade
Cheese		3.5 oz	168	D–
Cheese		8 oz	161	B–
Beef		6 oz	170	C–
Cheese		6 oz	250	D–
Beef		10 oz	280	B–
Cheese		9 oz	270	B–
Cheese		10 oz	390	D–
Cheese		7 oz	200	C–
Beef		9.5 oz	230	B–
Cheese		9.0 oz	260	B–+
		9 oz	470	B–
		8 oz	300	C–
Tofu & Sauce		8 oz	220	D–+
Spinach Tofu & Sauce		11 oz	260	B–+
Vegetable		8 oz	200	B–
	with Meat Sauce	10 oz	450	D–
Cheese		9.25 oz	280	B–
		11.25 oz	360	D–
		11 oz	440	D–
		10 oz	350	D–
		10 oz	310	D–
Homestyle		12$^{1}/_{8}$ oz	410	D–
		10.75 oz	360	C–
		4 oz	200	D
in Tomato Sauce		7 oz	230	D–
Italian Style	Noodles	10 oz	310	C–
Swedish Style	Noodles	10 oz	600	D–
Swedish Style	in Sauce with Pasta & Vegetables	8.5 oz	260	B–
Swedish Style	Gravy with Parsley	11 oz	480	D–
Stew		10 oz	250	C–
Swedish Style		8.5 oz	360	D–
Swedish Style		9 oz	280	B–
		8 oz	350	D–
		8 oz	240	D
		$^{1}/_{2}$ can	476	D–
		12 oz	490	C–
Combination		12 oz	520	B–
		10 oz	300	B–
Fiesta		12.25 oz	430	B–
Mexican		13.25 oz	430	C–
Combination		14.25 oz	490	C–
		20.25 oz	820	D–
Beef in Sauce		7.5 oz	170	D–
Chicken		7.5 oz	160	C–
Tuna		7.5 oz	170	B–
Chicken		7.5 oz	180	C–
Chicken		7.4 oz	150	B–
Chicken	Vegetables	7.4 oz	160	B–
Franks		1 cup	245	C–
	Light Syrup	6 oz	260	A–
Light	Light Links	6 oz	310	B–
Sausages		6 oz	420	C–

"+" indicates the food meets minimum fiber requirements; "–" indicates the food has a high sodium content.

Food	Processing Category	Brand
Pancake Breakfast	Frozen	Downyflake
Pancake Breakfast	Frozen	Kid Cuisine
Pancake Breakfast	Frozen	Swanson Great Starts
Pancake Breakfast	Frozen	Swanson Great Starts
Pancake Breakfast	Frozen	Swanson Great Starts
Pancake Breakfast	Frozen	Swanson Great Starts
Pancake Breakfast	Frozen	Weight Watchers Microwave
Pancake Breakfast	Frozen	Weight Watchers Microwave
Pancake Breakfast	Frozen	Weight Watchers Microwave
Pasta Dishes	Canned	Buitoni
Pasta Dishes	Canned	Buitoni
Pasta Dishes	Canned	Chef Boyardee
Pasta Dishes	Canned	Chef Boyardee
Pasta Dishes	Canned	Chef Boyardee
Pasta Dishes	Canned	Chef Boyardee
Pasta Dishes	Canned	Chef Boyardee
Pasta Dishes	Canned	Chef Boyardee Microwave
Pasta Dishes	Canned	Chef Boyardee Microwave
Pasta Dishes	Canned	Dinosaurs
Pasta Dishes	Canned	Dinosaurs
Pasta Dishes	Canned	Franco-American
Pasta Dishes	Canned	Franco-American
Pasta Dishes	Canned	Franco-American
Pasta Dishes	Canned	Franco-American
Pasta Dishes	Canned	Lipton Hearty Ones
Pasta Dishes	Canned	Lipton Hearty Ones
Pasta Dishes	Frozen	Birds Eye Custom Cuisine
Pasta Dishes	Frozen	Birds Eye Custom Cuisine
Pasta Dishes	Frozen	Budget Gourmet Side Dish
Pasta Dishes	Frozen	Green Giant Garden Gourmet
Pasta Dishes	Frozen	Green Giant Garden Gourmet
Pasta Dishes	Frozen	Green Giant One Serving
Pasta Dishes	Frozen	Green Giant One Serving
Pasta Dishes	Frozen	Green Giant Pasta Accents [4]
Pasta Dishes	Frozen	Green Giant Pasta Accents
Pasta Dishes	Frozen	Green Giant Pasta Accents
Pasta Dishes	Frozen	Green Giant Pasta Accents
Pasta Entree	Frozen	Budget Gourmet
Pasta Entree	Frozen	Budget Gourmet Light & Healthy
Pasta Entree	Frozen	Budget Gourmet Light & Healthy
Pasta Entree	Frozen	Buitoni Single Serving
Pasta Entree	Frozen	Celentano
Pasta Entree	Frozen	Celentano
Pasta Entree	Frozen	Celentano
Pasta Entree	Frozen	Healthy Choice
Pasta Entree	Frozen	Healthy Choice

[4] *Serving size for Green Giant Pasta Accents products equals approximately 2 cups.*

Major Description	Minor Description	Serving Size	Calories	Grade
	Sausages	5.5 oz	430	D–
Blueberry		3.5 oz	210	C–
	Bacon	4.5 oz	400	D–
	Sausages	6 oz	460	D–
Silver Dollar	Sausages	3.75 oz	310	D–
Whole Wheat	Light Links	5.5 oz	350	D–
	Light Links	4 oz	220	D–
Blueberry Topping		4.75 oz	200	A–
Strawberry Topping		4.75 oz	200	A–
Rings or Twists	in Sauce	7.5 oz	150	B–
Rings or Twists	Meatballs	7.5 oz	210	B–
ABC's/123's	in Spaghetti Sauce with Cheese Flavor	7.5 oz	180	A–
ABC's/123's	Mini Meatballs	7.5 oz	260	C–
Pac Man	in Chicken Sauce	7.5 oz	170	C–
Tic Tac Toes	in Spaghetti Sauce with Cheese Flavor	7.5 oz	170	A–+
Tic Tac Toes	Meatballs	7.5 oz	250	C–
Shells	in Meat Sauce	7.5 oz	210	B–
Shells	in Mushroom Sauce	7.5 oz	170	A–
	Meatballs	7.5 oz	240	C–+
Dinosaurs	in Spaghetti Sauce with Cheese Flavor	7.5 oz	180	A–+
Circuso's Sporty O's	in Tomato & Cheese Sauce	7.4 oz	170	A–
Circuso's Sporty O's	Meatballs in Tomato Sauce	7.4 oz	210	C–
TeddyO's		7.4 oz	170	A–
TeddyO's	Meatballs	7.4 oz	210	C–
Garden Medley		11 oz	323	A–
Italiano		11 oz	328	A–
Vegetables	in Creamy Sauce	4.6 oz	120	C–
Vegetables	with White Cheese Sauce	4.6 oz	150	C–
Alfredo	Broccoli	5.5 oz	200	C–
Dijon		8 oz	260	D–+
Florentine		8 oz	155	B–+
Marinara		5.5 oz	180	B–
Parmesan	Sweet Peas	5.5 oz	170	B–
Creamy Cheddar		6.8 oz serving	130	B–
Garden-style Herb		6.8 oz serving	116	B–
Garlic Seasoning		6.8 oz serving	135	C–
Primavera		6.8 oz serving	156	C–
Shells	Beef	10 oz	340	C–
Linguini	Scallops & Clams	9.5 oz	280	C–
Penne Pasta	in Tomato Sauce with Italian Sausage	10 oz	320	B–
Shells	Stuffed	9 oz	460	B–
Baked & Cheese		6 oz	290	D
Cavatelli		3.2 oz	250	A
Shells	Stuffed	8 oz	330	B–
Chicken Cacciatore		12.5 oz	310	A–
Italiano		12 oz	350	A–

"+" indicates the food meets minimum fiber requirements; "–" indicates the food has a high sodium content.

Food	Processing Category	Brand
Pasta Entree	Frozen	Healthy Choice
Pasta Entree	Frozen	Healthy Choice
Pasta Entree	Frozen	Healthy Choice
Pasta Entree	Frozen	Healthy Choice Quick Meals
Pasta Entree	Frozen	Legume Provencale
Pasta Entree	Frozen	Marie Callender's
Pasta Entree	Frozen	Marie Callender's
Pasta Entree	Frozen	On-Cor
Pasta Entree	Frozen	Stouffer's
Pasta Entree	Frozen	Stouffer's
Pasta Entree	Frozen	Stouffer's
Pasta Entree	Frozen	Stouffer's
Pasta Entree	Frozen	Stouffer's
Pasta Entree	Frozen	Stouffer's
Pasta Entree	Frozen	Stouffer's Lean Cuisine
Pasta Entree	Frozen	The Budget Gourmet
Pasta Entree	Frozen	Tyson Gourmet Selection
Pasta Entree	Frozen	with Sauce Celentano
Pasta Entree	Frozen	Weight Watchers
Pasta Entree	Frozen	Weight Watchers
Pasta Entree	Frozen	Weight Watchers
Peppers, Stuffed Entree	Frozen	Celentano
Peppers, Stuffed Entree	Frozen	On-Cor
Peppers, Stuffed Entree	Frozen	Stouffer's
Pizza	Frozen	Celentano
Pizza	Frozen	Celentano Thick Crust
Pizza	Frozen	Celeste
Pizza	Frozen	Celeste
Pizza	Frozen	Celeste
Pizza	Frozen	Celeste
Pizza	Frozen	Celeste
Pizza	Frozen	Celeste Pizza for One
Pizza	Frozen	Celeste Pizza for One
Pizza	Frozen	Celeste Pizza for One
Pizza	Frozen	Celeste Pizza for One
Pizza	Frozen	Celeste Pizza for One
Pizza	Frozen	Celeste Suprema
Pizza	Frozen	Fox Deluxe
Pizza	Frozen	Fox Deluxe
Pizza	Frozen	Fox Deluxe
Pizza	Frozen	Fox Deluxe
Pizza	Frozen	Jeno's 4 Pack
Pizza	Frozen	Jeno's 4 Pack
Pizza	Frozen	Jeno's 4 Pack
Pizza	Frozen	Jeno's 4 Pack
Pizza	Frozen	Jeno's 4 Pack
Pizza	Frozen	Jeno's Crisp N Tasty
Pizza	Frozen	Jeno's Crisp N Tasty
Pizza	Frozen	Jeno's Crisp N Tasty
Pizza	Frozen	Jeno's Crisp N Tasty
Pizza	Frozen	Jeno's Crisp N Tasty

Major Description	Minor Description	Serving Size	Calories	Grade
Shells	in Tomato Sauce	12 oz	330	A–
Shrimp & Vegetables		12.5 oz	270	A–
Teriyaki Chicken		12.6 oz	350	A
Italiano	Vegetables	10 oz	220	A–
Shells, Stuffed	Vegetables	11 oz	240	D–+
Delux		1 cup	350	D–
Primavera	Chicken	1 cup	310	D–
Mostaccioli	Meatballs	8 oz	220	C–
Carbonara		9.75 oz	620	D–
Casino		9.25 oz	300	B–
Mexicali		10 oz	490	D–
Oriental Style		9.87 oz	300	D–
Primavera		10.75 oz	540	D–
Shells	Cheese in Tomato Sauce	9.25 oz	330	D–
Angel Hair		10 oz	210	B–+
Shells	Beef	10 oz	340	C–
Trio		11 oz	450	C–
Shells	Stuffed	10 oz	410	C–
Angel Hair		10 oz	210	B–
Primavera		8.5 oz	260	C–
Rigati		10.63 oz	300	B–
Sweet Red		13 oz	350	D–
		8 oz	168	D–
	with Beef in Tomato Sauce	7.75 oz	200	B–
Cheese		2.7 oz	150	B–
Cheese		4.3 oz	290	C–
Cheese		1/4 pie	317	D–
Deluxe		1/4 pie	378	D–
Pepperoni		1/4 pie	368	D–
Sausage		1/4 pie	376	D–
Vegetable		1/4 pie	310	D–
Cheese		1 pie	497	D–
Deluxe		1 pie	582	D–
Pepperoni		1 pie	546	D–
Sausage		1 pie	571	D–
Vegetable		1 pie	490	D–
		1/4 pie	381	D–
Golden Topping		1/4 pie	120	D–
Hamburger		1/4 pie	130	D–
Pepperoni		1/4 pie	125	D–
Sausage		1/4 pie	130	D–
Cheese		1 pie	160	D–
Combination		1 pie	180	D–
Hamburger		1 pie	180	D–
Pepperoni		1 pie	170	D–
Sausage		1 pie	180	D–
Canadian Bacon		1/4 pie	125	C–
Cheese		1/4 pie	135	D–
Hamburger		1/4 pie	145	D–
Pepperoni		1/4 pie	140	D–
Sausage		1/4 pie	150	D–

"+" indicates the food meets minimum fiber requirements; "–" indicates the food has a high sodium content.

Food	Processing Category	Brand
Pizza	Frozen	Jeno's Microwave for One
Pizza	Frozen	Jeno's Microwave for One
Pizza	Frozen	Jeno's Microwave for One
Pizza	Frozen	Jeno's Microwave for One
Pizza	Frozen	Jeno's Snacks
Pizza	Frozen	John's
Pizza	Frozen	John's
Pizza	Frozen	John's 3 Pack
Pizza	Frozen	John's 3 Pack
Pizza	Frozen	John's Deluxe
Pizza	Frozen	Mr. P's
Pizza	Frozen	Mr. P's
Pizza	Frozen	Mr. P's
Pizza	Frozen	Mr. P's
Pizza	Frozen	Mr. P's
Pizza	Frozen	Pappalo's Pan Pizza
Pizza	Frozen	Pappalo's Pan Pizza
Pizza	Frozen	Pappalo's Pan Pizza
Pizza	Frozen	Pappalo's Pan Pizza
Pizza	Frozen	Pappalo's Thin Crust
Pizza	Frozen	Pappalo's Thin Crust
Pizza	Frozen	Pappalo's Thin Crust
Pizza	Frozen	Pappalo's Thin Crust
Pizza	Frozen	Stouffer's
Pizza	Frozen	Stouffer's
Pizza	Frozen	Stouffer's
Pizza	Frozen	Stouffer's
Pizza	Frozen	Stouffer's Extra Cheese
Pizza	Frozen	Tombstone
Pizza	Frozen	Tombstone
Pizza	Frozen	Tombstone
Pizza	Frozen	Tombstone
Pizza	Frozen	Tombstone Deluxe
Pizza	Frozen	Tombstone Deluxe
Pizza	Frozen	Tombstone Double Top
Pizza	Frozen	Tombstone Double Top
Pizza	Frozen	Tombstone Double Top
Pizza	Frozen	Tombstone Italian Thin Crust
Pizza	Frozen	Tombstone Microwave
Pizza	Frozen	Tombstone Microwave
Pizza	Frozen	Tombstone Thin Crust
Pizza	Frozen	Tombstone Thin Crust
Pizza	Frozen	Totino's Microwave
Pizza	Frozen	Totino's Microwave
Pizza	Frozen	Totino's Microwave
Pizza	Frozen	Totino's Microwave
Pizza	Frozen	Totino's Party
Pizza	Frozen	Totino's Party
Pizza	Frozen	Totino's Party
Pizza	Frozen	Totino's Party
Pizza	Frozen	Totino's Party
Pizza	Frozen	Totino's Party

Major Description	Minor Description	Serving Size	Calories	Grade
Cheese		1 pie	226	C–
Combination		1 pie	257	D–
Pepperoni		1 pie	250	D–
Sausage		1 pie	250	D–
Cheese	Snack Tray	4 pieces	130	D–
Golden Topping		1/4 pie	120	D–
Sausage		1/4 pie	130	D–
Cheese		1 pie	300	C–
Sausage		1 pie	300	C–
Sausage		1/4 pie	130	D–
Combination		1/4 pie	130	D–
Golden Topping		1/4 pie	120	D–
Hamburger		1/4 pie	130	D–
Pepperoni		1/4 pie	125	D–
Sausage		1/4 pie	130	D–
Combination		1/4 pie	340	C–
Hamburger		1/4 pie	310	C–
Pepperoni		1/4 pie	330	C–
Sausage		1/4 pie	540	D–
Combination		1/4 pie	390	C–
Hamburger		1/4 pie	360	B–
Pepperoni		1/4 pie	405	C–
Sausage		1/4 pie	375	C–
Cheese		1/4 pie	160	D–
Deluxe		1/4 pie	185	D–
Pepperoni		1/4 pie	175	D–
Sausage		1/4 pie	180	D–
Cheese		1/4 pie	185	D–
Canadian Bacon		1/4 pie	340	C–
Cheese		1/4 pie	330	C–
Cheese & Hamburger		1/4 pie	360	C–
Cheese & Pepperoni		1/4 pie	380	D–
Pepperoni		1/4 pie	380	D–
Sausage		1/4 pie	350	C–
Cheese	3 Cheese	1/4 pie	490	D–
Hamburger & Cheese	Double Cheese	1/4 pie	530	D–
Sausage & Cheese	Double Cheese	1/4 pie	510	D–
Cheese & Hamburger		1/4 pie	320	D–
Cheese & Pepperoni		1 pie	530	D–
Sausage	Deluxe	1 pie	520	D–
Cheese	2 Cheese	1/4 pie	330	D–
Pepperoni & Cheese		1/4 pie	330	D–
Cheese		1 pie	250	C–
Combination		1 pie	290	D–
Pepperoni		1 pie	270	D–
Sausage		1 pie	280	D–
Canadian Bacon		1/4 pie	145	C–
Cheese		1/4 pie	140	C–
Combination		1/4 pie	170	C–
Hamburger		1/4 pie	160	C–
Pepperoni		1/4 pie	165	C–
Sausage		1/4 pie	170	C–

"+" indicates the food meets minimum fiber requirements; "–" indicates the food has a high sodium content.

Food	Processing Category	Brand
Pizza	Frozen	Totino's Party Family Size
Pizza	Frozen	Totino's Party Family Size
Pizza	Frozen	Totino's Party Family Size
Pizza	Frozen	Totino's Party Family Size
Pizza	Frozen	Totino's Party Pizza
Pizza	Frozen	Weight Watchers
Pizza	Frozen	Weight Watchers
Pizza	Frozen	Weight Watchers
Pizza	Frozen	Weight Watchers
Pizza	Frozen	Weight Watchers
Pizza	Frozen	Weight Watchers
Pizza Dinner	Frozen	Kid Cuisine
Pizza Dinner	Frozen	Kid Cuisine
Pizza Dinner	Frozen	Kid Cuisine Megameal
Pizza Roll	Frozen	Jeno's
Pizza Roll	Frozen	Jeno's
Pizza Roll	Frozen	Jeno's
Pizza Roll	Frozen	Jeno's
Pizza Roll	Frozen	Jeno's Microwave
Pizza Roll	Frozen	Jeno's Microwave
Pizza, Croissant Pastry	Frozen	Pepperidge Farm
Pizza, Croissant Pastry	Frozen	Pepperidge Farm
Pizza, Croissant Pastry	Frozen	Pepperidge Farm
Pizza, French Bread	Frozen	Banquet Zap
Pizza, French Bread	Frozen	Banquet Zap
Pizza, French Bread	Frozen	Banquet Zap
Pizza, French Bread	Frozen	Healthy Choice Quick Meals
Pizza, French Bread	Frozen	Healthy Choice Quick Meals
Pizza, French Bread	Frozen	Healthy Choice Quick Meals
Pizza, French Bread	Frozen	Healthy Choice Quick Meals
Pizza, French Bread	Frozen	Pappalo's
Pizza, French Bread	Frozen	Pappalo's
Pizza, French Bread	Frozen	Pappalo's
Pizza, French Bread	Frozen	Pappalo's
Pizza, French Bread	Frozen	Pillsbury Microwave
Pizza, French Bread	Frozen	Pillsbury Microwave
Pizza, French Bread	Frozen	Pillsbury Microwave
Pizza, French Bread	Frozen	Pillsbury Microwave
Pizza, French Bread	Frozen	Stouffer's [5]
Pizza, French Bread	Frozen	Stouffer's
Pizza, French Bread	Frozen	Stouffer's
Pizza, French Bread	Frozen	Stouffer's
Pizza, French Bread	Frozen	Stouffer's
Pizza, French Bread	Frozen	Stouffer's
Pizza, French Bread	Frozen	Stouffer's
Pizza, French Bread	Frozen	Stouffer's
Pizza, French Bread	Frozen	Stouffer's
Pizza, French Bread	Frozen	Stouffer's
Pizza, French Bread	Frozen	Stouffer's Double Cheese
Pizza, French Bread	Frozen	Stouffer's Lean Cuisine
Pizza, French Bread	Frozen	Stouffer's Lean Cuisine
Pizza, French Bread	Frozen	Stouffer's Lean Cuisine
Pizza, French Bread	Frozen	Stouffer's Lean Cuisine

[5] *Serving size of 1 piece for Stouffer's regular French Bread Pizza equals $1/2$ package.*

Major Description	Minor Description	Serving Size	Calories	Grade
Cheese		¹/₄ pie	155	C–
Combination		¹/₄ pie	145	D–
Pepperoni		¹/₄ pie	270	C–
Sausage		¹/₄ pie	277	C–
Mexican Style		¹/₄ pie	190	D–
Brick Oven	3 Cheese	1 pie	320	B+
Brick Oven	Bianca	1 pie	330	B–+
Cheese		1 pie	300	B–
Combination		1 pie	330	B–
Pepperoni		1 pie	320	B–
Sausage		1 pie	320	B–
Cheese		6.9 oz	380	B
Hamburger		6.9 oz	330	B–
Cheese		9.7 oz	430	A–
Cheese		3 oz, 6 rolls	240	D–
Hamburger		3 oz, 6 rolls	240	D
Pepperoni & Cheese		3 oz, 6 rolls	230	D–
Sausage & Pepperoni		3 oz, 6 rolls	230	D–
Pepperoni & Cheese		3 oz, 6 rolls	240	D–
Sausage & Cheese		3 oz, 6 rolls	250	D–
Cheese		1 pie	430	D–
Deluxe		1 pie	440	D–
Pepperoni		1 pie	420	D–
Cheese		4.5 oz	310	B–
Deluxe		4.8 oz	330	C–
Pepperoni		4.5 oz	350	D–
Cheese		1 piece	290	A–
Deluxe		1 piece	330	B–
Italian Turkey Sausage		1 piece	330	A
Pepperoni		1 piece	310	B–
Combination		1 piece	430	D–
Extra Cheese		1 piece	360	C–
Pepperoni		1 piece	410	D–
Sausage		1 piece	410	C–
Cheese		1 piece	370	C–
Pepperoni		1 piece	430	C–
Sausage		1 piece	410	C–
Sausage & Pepperoni		1 piece	450	D–
Canadian-style Bacon		1 piece	360	C–
Cheese		1 piece	340	C–
Deluxe		1 piece	430	D–
Hamburger		1 piece	410	D–
Pepperoni		1 piece	410	D–
Pepperoni & Mushroom		1 piece	430	D–
Sausage		1 piece	420	D–
Sausage & Mushroom		1 piece	410	D–
Sausage & Pepperoni		1 piece	450	D–
Vegetable Deluxe		1 piece	420	D–
Cheese		1 piece	410	C–
Cheese		1 pkg	350	C–
Cheese		1 pkg	350	B–
Deluxe		1 pkg	330	B–
Pepperoni		1 pkg	330	B–

"+" indicates the food meets minimum fiber requirements; "–" indicates the food has a high sodium content.

Food	Processing Category	Brand
Pizza, French Bread	Frozen	Stouffer's Lean Cuisine
Pizza, French Bread	Frozen	Weight Watchers
Pizza, French Bread	Frozen	Weight Watchers
Pizza, Italian Bread	Frozen	Celeste
Pizza, Italian Bread	Frozen	Celeste
Pizza, Italian Bread	Frozen	Celeste
Pizza, Italian Bread	Frozen	Celeste
Pizza, Pocket Sandwich	Frozen	Hot Pockets
Pizza, Pocket Sandwich	Frozen	Hot Pockets
Pizza, Pocket Sandwich	Frozen	Lean Pockets
Pork Entree	Frozen or Refrigerated	John Morrell Pork Classics
Pork Entree	Frozen or Refrigerated	John Morrell Pork Classics
Pork Entree	Frozen or Refrigerated	John Morrell Pork Classics
Pork Entree	Frozen or Refrigerated	John Morrell Pork Classics
Pork Entree	Frozen or Refrigerated	John Morrell Pork Classics
Potato Dishes [6]	Frozen	Birds Eye for One
Potato Dishes	Frozen	Budget Gourmet Side Dish
Potato Dishes	Frozen	Budget Gourmet Side Dish
Potato Dishes	Frozen	Budget Gourmet Side Dish
Potato Dishes	Frozen	Budget Gourmet Side Dish
Potato Dishes	Frozen	Budget Gourmet Side Dish
Potato Dishes	Frozen	Freezer Queen Family Side Dish
Potato Dishes	Frozen	Freezer Queen Family Side Dish
Potato Dishes	Frozen	Green Giant
Potato Dishes	Frozen	Green Giant
Potato Dishes	Frozen	Green Giant One Serving
Potato Dishes	Frozen	Green Giant One Serving
Potato Dishes	Frozen	Oh Boy
Potato Dishes	Frozen	Oh Boy
Potato Dishes	Frozen	Oh Boy
Potato Dishes	Frozen	Stokely Singles
Potato Dishes	Frozen	Stokely Singles
Potato Dishes	Frozen	Stouffer's
Potato Dishes	Frozen	Stouffer's
Potato Entree	Frozen	Budget Gourmet Light & Healthy
Potato Entree	Frozen	Healthy Choice
Potato Entree	Frozen	Healthy Choice Quick Meals
Potato Entree	Frozen	Stouffer's Lean Cuisine
Potato Entree	Frozen	Weight Watchers
Potato Entree	Frozen	Weight Watchers
Potato Entree	Frozen	Weight Watchers
Potato Entree	Frozen	Weight Watchers
Ravioli	Canned	Buitoni
Ravioli	Canned	Buitoni

[6] *Potato dishes are usually a mix of potatoes and other components serving as side items. One package is approximately 5 ozs except where noted.*

Major Description	Minor Description	Serving Size	Calories	Grade
Sausage		1 pkg	350	B–
Deluxe		1 piece	330	C–
Pepperoni		1 piece	320	C–
Deluxe		1 piece	290	C–
Four Cheese		1 piece	300	C–
Garlic & Herb	Chicken	1 piece	260	B–
Pepperoni		1 piece	320	C–
Pepperoni		1 piece	380	D–
Sausage		1 piece	360	C–
Deluxe		1 piece	280	B–
Back Ribs	Barbecued	4.75 oz	240	D–
Chops, Center Cut	Barbecued	4.5 oz	230	C–
Loin, Thin Sliced	Barbecued	5 slices or 3 oz	150	C–
Spare Ribs	Barbecued	4.5 oz	250	D–
Tenderloin	Barbecued	3 oz	130	C–
au Gratin		1 pkg	240	D–
3 Cheese		1 pkg	230	D–
Cheddar Cheese & Broccoli		1 pkg	130	B–
Nacho		1 pkg	180	D–
New Potatoes	in Sour Cream Sauce	1 pkg	120	D–
Cheddar Cheese		1 pkg	230	C–
au Gratin		1 pkg	100	B–
Broccoli	with Cheese Sauce	1 pkg	140	B
Stuffed	Baked, with Cheese-flavored Topping	1 pkg	200	B–
Stuffed	Baked, with Sour Cream & Chives	1 pkg	230	C–
Au Gratin		1 pkg	200	D–
Broccoli	in Cheese Flavored Sauce	1 pkg	130	C–
Stuffed	Cheddar Cheese	1 pkg	142	B–
Stuffed	Real Bacon	1 pkg	116	B–
Stuffed	Sour Cream & Chives	1 pkg	129	C–
Shredded with Vegetables		1 pkg	130	C–
Sliced with Bacon	in Cheddar Cheese Sauce	1 pkg	150	B–
Au Gratin		$^1/_2$ pkg	165	D–
Scalloped		$^1/_2$ pkg	135	C–
Baked	Broccoli & Cheese	10.5 oz	300	B–
Baked, Wedges	Broccoli & Cheese	9.5 oz	240	A–
Garden Style	Casserole	9.25 oz	180	B–
Cheddar Cheese	Deluxe	$10^3/_8$ oz	270	C–
Stuffed	Baked, with Homestyle Turkey	12 oz	300	B–
Stuffed	Baked, with Chicken Divan	11 oz	280	A–
Stuffed	Baked, with Ham Lorraine	11 oz	250	A–
Stuffed	Broccoli & Cheese	10.5 oz	290	B–
Cheese	in Sauce	7.5 oz	190	B–
Meat	in Sauce	7.5 oz	180	B–

"+" indicates the food meets minimum fiber requirements; "–" indicates the food has a high sodium content.

Food	Processing Category	Brand
Ravioli	Canned	Chef Boyardee Microwave
Ravioli	Canned	Chef Boyardee Microwave
Ravioli	Canned	Estee
Ravioli	Canned	Franco-American RavioliOs
Ravioli	Canned	Hormel Microcup
Ravioli	Canned	Nalleys
Ravioli	Frozen	Buitoni
Ravioli	Frozen	Celentano
Ravioli	Frozen	Celentano
Ravioli	Frozen	Weight Watchers
Ravioli Dinner	Frozen	Kid Cuisine
Ravioli Dinner	Frozen	Ultra Slim-Fast
Ravioli Entree	Frozen	Budget Gourmet Light & Healthy
Ravioli Entree	Frozen	Budget Gourmet Slim
Ravioli Entree	Frozen	Healthy Choice
Ravioli Entree	Frozen	Marie Callender's
Ravioli Entree	Frozen	Stouffer's Lean Cuisine
Ravioli Entree	Frozen	Weight Watchers
Rice Dishes	Canned	Featherweight
Rice Dishes	Canned	Heinz
Rice Dishes	Canned	La Choy
Rice Dishes	Canned	Old El Paso
Rice Dishes	Canned	Van Camp's
Rice Dishes	Frozen	Birds Eye for One
Rice Dishes [7]	Frozen	Birds Eye International
Rice Dishes [7]	Frozen	Birds Eye International
Rice Dishes [7]	Frozen	Birds Eye International
Rice Dishes	Frozen	Budget Gourmet Side Dish
Rice Dishes	Frozen	Budget Gourmet Side Dish
Rice Dishes	Frozen	Chun King
Rice Dishes	Frozen	Chun King
Rice Dishes	Frozen	Green Giant Microwave
Rice Dishes	Frozen	Green Giant One Serving
Rice Dishes	Frozen	Green Giant One Serving
Rice Dishes	Frozen	Green Giant Rice Originals
Rice Dishes	Frozen	Green Giant Rice Originals
Rice Dishes	Frozen	Green Giant Rice Originals
Rice Dishes	Frozen	Green Giant Rice Originals
Rice Dishes	Frozen	Green Giant Rice Originals
Rice Entree	Freeze-dried	Mountain House
Rigatoni Entree	Frozen	Budget Gourmet Light & Healthy
Rigatoni Entree	Frozen	Healthy Choice
Rigatoni Entree	Frozen	Healthy Choice Quick Meals
Rigatoni Entree	Frozen	Marie Callender's
Rigatoni Entree	Frozen	Stouffer's Lean Cuisine
Rotini	Frozen	Portafino
Sandwich	Frozen	Weight Watchers
Sandwich	Frozen	Weight Watchers Sandwiches on the Run
Sandwich	Frozen	Weight Watchers Sandwiches on the Run
Sandwich	Frozen	Weight Watchers Sandwiches on the Run

[7] Serving size is approximate.

Major Description	Minor Description	Serving Size	Calories	Grade
Beef		7.5 oz	190	B–
Cheese	in Meat Sauce	7.5 oz	200	A–
Beef		7.5 oz	230	D
Beef	in Meat Sauce	7.5 oz	250	B–
Beef	in Tomato Sauce	7.5 oz	247	D–
Beef		7.5 oz	180	A–
Cheese		4 oz	360	B
		4 oz	234	B–
Cheese	Mini	4 oz	250	B
Cheese		4 oz	280	B–+
Mini, Cheese		8.75 oz	250	A–
Cheese		12 oz	330	A
Cheese		9.5 oz	210	C–
Cheese		10 oz	260	B–
Cheese	Baked	9 oz	250	A–
Marinara	with Garlic Bread	16 oz	370	C–
Cheese		8$^1/_2$ oz	250	B–+
Cheese	Baked	9 oz	290	B–
Spanish		$^1/_2$ cup	70	A
Spanish		$^1/_2$ cup	75	B–
Fried		$^1/_2$ cup	120	A–
Spanish		$^1/_2$ cup	70	A–
Spanish		$^1/_2$ cup	80	B–
Broccoli	au Gratin	1 pkg	180	B–
Country Style		$^1/_2$ cup	90	A–
French Style		$^1/_2$ cup	110	A–
Spanish Style		$^1/_2$ cup	110	A–
Oriental Style	Vegetables	5.75 oz	210	D–
Pilaf with Green Beans		5.5 oz	240	C–
Fried, with Chicken		1 pkg	260	A–
Fried, with Pork		1 pkg	270	B–
Wild Rice	with Sherry	1 pkg	210	B–
Broccoli	in Cheese Sauce	1 pkg	180	B–
Peas & Mushrooms		1 pkg	130	A–
Broccoli	in Cheese Sauce	$^1/_2$ cup	120	B–
Italian Blend White Rice	in Cheese Sauce	$^1/_2$ cup	140	B–
Medley		$^1/_2$ cup	100	A–
Pilaf		$^1/_2$ cup	110	A–
White & Wild Rice		$^1/_2$ cup	130	A–
Chicken		$^1/_2$ cup	200	B
Broccoli & Chicken	in Cream Sauce	10.8 oz	290	B–
Chicken & Vegetables		12.5 oz	360	A
Meat Sauce		9.5 oz	260	B–
Parmigiana		13 oz	300	C–
		9 oz	180	B–+
Pasta	Frozen	9.5 oz	150	A–+
Honey Dijon Turkey		1 sandwich	220	B–
Chicken & Broccoli		1 sandwich	250	B
Deluxe Pizza Pocket Sandwich		1 sandwich	300	A–
Grilled Chicken		1 sandwich	270	B–

"+" indicates the food meets minimum fiber requirements; "–" indicates the food has a high sodium content.

Food	Processing Category	Brand
Sandwich	Frozen	Weight Watchers Sandwiches on the Run
Sandwich	Frozen	Weight Watchers Sandwiches on the Run
Sandwich	Frozen	Weight Watchers Sandwiches on the Run
Sausage & Biscuit Breakfast	Frozen	Swanson Great Starts
Sausage & Biscuit Breakfast	Frozen	Weight Watchers Microwave
Sausage & Biscuit Breakfast	Refrigerated	Owens Border Breakfasts
Sausage & Biscuit Breakfast	Refrigerated	Owens Border Breakfasts
Sausage & Biscuit Breakfast	Refrigerated	Owens Border Breakfasts
Shrimp Dinner	Frozen	Armour Classics Lite
Shrimp Dinner	Frozen	Armour Classics Lite
Shrimp Dinner	Frozen	Healthy Choice
Shrimp Dinner	Frozen	Healthy Choice
Shrimp Dinner	Frozen	Ultra Slim-Fast
Shrimp Dinner	Frozen	Ultra Slim-Fast
Shrimp Entree	Canned	La Choy Bi-Pack
Shrimp Entree	Frozen	Booth
Shrimp Entree	Frozen	Booth
Shrimp Entree	Frozen	Booth
Shrimp Entree	Frozen	Booth
Shrimp Entree	Frozen	Booth
Shrimp Entree	Frozen	Budget Gourmet
Shrimp Entree	Frozen	Cajun Cookin'
Shrimp Entree	Frozen	Cajun Cookin'
Shrimp Entree	Frozen	Cajun Cookin'
Shrimp Entree	Frozen	Gordon's Specialty
Shrimp Entree	Frozen	Gorton's Microwave
Shrimp Entree	Frozen	Gorton's Microwave
Shrimp Entree	Frozen	La Choy Fresh & Lite
Shrimp Entree	Frozen	Mrs. Paul's
Shrimp Entree	Frozen	Mrs. Paul's Light
Shrimp Entree	Frozen	Mrs. Paul's Light
Shrimp Entree	Frozen	Mrs. Paul's Light
Shrimp Entree	Frozen	Right Course
Shrimp Entree	Frozen	Seapak
Shrimp Entree	Frozen	Seapak
Shrimp Entree	Frozen	Seapak
Shrimp Entree	Frozen	Seapak Mikado
Shrimp Entree	Frozen	Seapak Super Valu
Shrimp Entree	Frozen	Stouffer's Lean Cuisine
Sole Dinner	Frozen	Gorton's Microwave
Sole Dinner	Frozen	Healthy Choice
Sole Dinner	Frozen	Healthy Choice
Sole Dinner	Frozen	Mrs. Paul's Light
Sole Entree	Frozen	Van de Kamp's Light
Spaghetti Dinner	Frozen	Banquet
Spaghetti Dinner	Frozen	Kid Cuisine
Spaghetti Dinner	Frozen	Morton
Spaghetti Dinner	Frozen	Morton
Spaghetti Dinner	Frozen	Swanson

Major Description	Minor Description	Serving Size	Calories	Grade
Ham & Cheese Pocket Sandwich		1 sandwich	240	B–+
Hickory Smoked Ham & Cheddar		1 sandwich	260	B–
Reuben Pocket Sandwich		1 sandwich	220	B–
		4.7 oz	410	D–
		3 oz	220	D–
		2 oz	210	D–
Egg & Cheese		2.5 oz	250	D–
Smoked		2 oz	200	B–
Baby Bay Shrimp		9.75 oz	220	C–
Creole Style		11.25 oz	260	B–
Creole Style		11.25 oz	210	B–
Marinara		10.5 oz	260	B
Creole Style		12 oz	240	B–
Marinara		12 oz	290	B–
Chow Mein		³/₄ cup	50	C–+
Fettuccine Alfredo Style		10 oz	260	C–
in Garlic Butter Sauce		10 oz	400	D–
New Orleans Style	with Wild Rice	10 oz	230	C–
Oriental Style	with Pineapple Rice	10 oz	190	B–
Primavera	Fettuccine	10 oz	200	C–
Fettuccine		9.5 oz	375	D–
Creole Style		12 oz	390	C–
Étouffée		17 oz	360	C–
Jambalaya		12 oz	450	D–
Crisps		4 oz	280	D–
Crunchy, Whole		5 oz	380	D–
Scampi		5 oz	390	D–
with Lobster Sauce		10 oz	240	D–
Breaded	Fried	3 oz	200	D–
Cajun Style		9 oz	230	C–
Clams	Linguini	10 oz	240	C–
Primavera		9.5 oz	180	D–
Primavera		4 oz	240	C–
Breaded	Butterfly, Round	4 oz	150	D
in Batter		4 oz	260	D–
in Batter with Crab Meat Stuffing		4 oz	260	D–
Breaded	Butterfly	4 oz	160	D
Heat & Serve		4 oz	210	D–
Chicken Cantonese Style		10.13 oz	270	D–
in Lemon Butter		1 pkg	380	D–
au Gratin		11 oz	270	B–
in Lemon Butter Sauce		8.25 oz	230	B–
Fillets, Breaded		1 piece	240	C–
Fillets, Breaded		1 piece	250	D–
Meatballs		10 oz	290	C–
in Meat Sauce		9.25 oz	310	C–
in Meat Sauce		8.5 oz	170	A–
Meatballs		10 oz	200	A–
Meatballs		12.5 oz	390	C–

"+" indicates the food meets minimum fiber requirements; "–" indicates the food has a high sodium content.

Food	Processing Category	Brand
Spaghetti Dinner	Frozen	Ultra Slim-Fast
Spaghetti Entree	Canned	Buitoni
Spaghetti Entree	Canned	Chef Boyardee
Spaghetti Entree	Canned	Chef Boyardee
Spaghetti Entree	Canned	Chef Boyardee Beef-o-getti
Spaghetti Entree	Canned	Chef Boyardee Microwave
Spaghetti Entree	Canned	Estee
Spaghetti Entree	Canned	Featherweight
Spaghetti Entree	Canned	Franco-American
Spaghetti Entree	Canned	Franco-American
Spaghetti Entree	Canned	Franco-American SpaghettiOs
Spaghetti Entree	Canned	Franco-American SpaghettiOs
Spaghetti Entree	Canned	Franco-American SpaghettiOs
Spaghetti Entree	Canned	Nalley's
Spaghetti Entree	Canned	Van Camp's Spaghettee Weenee
Spaghetti Entree	Freeze-dried	Mountain House
Spaghetti Entree	Frozen	Banquet Casserole
Spaghetti Entree	Frozen	Budget Gourmet Light & Healthy
Spaghetti Entree	Frozen	Dining Lite
Spaghetti Entree	Frozen	Freezer Queen Single Serve
Spaghetti Entree	Frozen	Healthy Choice
Spaghetti Entree	Frozen	Le Menu Lightstyle
Spaghetti Entree	Frozen	Marie Callender's
Spaghetti Entree	Frozen	Marie Callender's
Spaghetti Entree	Frozen	Stouffer's
Spaghetti Entree	Frozen	Stouffer's
Spaghetti Entree	Frozen	Stouffer's Lean Cuisine
Spaghetti Entree	Frozen	Stouffer's Lean Cuisine
Spaghetti Entree	Frozen	Stouffer's Lean Cuisine
Spaghetti Entree	Frozen	Swanson Homestyle Recipe
Spaghetti Entree	Frozen	Weight Watchers
Spinach Soufflé	Frozen	Stouffer's
Tamale	Canned	Gebhardt
Tamale	Canned	Hormel
Tamale	Canned	Hormel Hot N Spicy
Tamale	Canned	Old El Paso
Tamale	Canned	Van Camp's
Tamale	Canned	Wolf Brand
Tamale	Frozen	Hormel
Tamale Dinner	Frozen	Patio
Tamatillo	Canned	Dennisons
Tofu Patty	Frozen	Natural Touch
Tofu Patty	Frozen	Natural Touch Okara
Tortellini	Refrigerated	Contadina Fresh
Tortellini	Refrigerated	Contadina Fresh
Tortellini	Refrigerated	Contadina Fresh
Tortellini	Refrigerated	Contadina Fresh
Tortellini	Refrigerated	Contadina Fresh
Tortellini	Refrigerated	Contadina Fresh
Tortellini Dinner	Frozen	Dinner Classics Lite
Tortellini Dishes	Canned	Hormel Top Shelf
Tortellini Dishes	Canned	Hormel Top Shelf
Tortellini Dishes	Frozen	Birds Eye for One

Major Description	Minor Description	Serving Size	Calories	Grade
Beef	in Mushroom Sauce	12 oz	370	B–
Meatballs	in Sauce	7.5 oz	190	C–
Beef	in Tomato Sauce	7.5 oz	240	C–
Meatballs	in Tomato Sauce	7.5 oz	230	C–
Beef		7.5 oz	220	C–
Meatballs		7.5 oz	230	C–
Meatballs		7.5 oz	240	D
Meatballs		7.5 oz	160	B–
in Tomato & Cheese Sauce		7.4 oz	180	A–
Meatballs	in Tomato Sauce	7.4 oz	220	C–
Franks, Sliced	in Tomato Sauce	7.5 oz	220	C–
in Tomato & Cheese Sauce		7.5 oz	170	A–
Meatballs	in Tomato Sauce	7.4 oz	220	C–
Meatballs		7.5 oz	190	B–
Franks		1 cup	243	B–
	in Meat Sauce	1 cup	260	B
	in Meat Sauce	8 oz	270	B–
Chunky Tomato	in Meat Sauce	10 oz	300	B–
with Beef		9 oz	220	C–
	in Meat Sauce	10 oz	350	C–
	in Meat Sauce	10 oz	310	B–
Beef & Mushrooms Sauce		9 oz	280	B–
in Meat Sauce	with Garlic Bread	17 oz	260	C–
Marinara		16 oz	270	C–
in Meat Sauce		12.87 oz	370	B–
Meatballs		12.87 oz	380	C–
	in Meat Sauce	11.5 oz	290	B–
Beef & Mushroom Sauce		11.5 oz	280	B–
Meatballs		9.5 oz	290	B–
Italian-style Meatballs		13 oz	490	C–
	in Meat Sauce	10.5 oz	280	B–
		4 oz	140	D–
Beef		4 oz	230	D–
Beef		2 pieces	280	D–
Beef		2 pieces	280	D–
		2 pieces	220	D–
in Sauce		1 cup	293	D–
		1 cup	328	D–
Beef		2 pieces	280	D–
		13 oz	470	D–
Chili Gravy		7.5 oz	310	D–
Garden		one 2.5 oz patty	90	C–
Okara		one 2.5 oz patty	160	D–
Egg	Cheese	4.5 oz	380	A–
Egg	Chicken & Prosciutto	4.5 oz	370	B–
Egg	Meat	4.5 oz	380	A–
Spinach	Cheese	4.5 oz	380	A–
Spinach	Chicken & Prosciutto	4.5 oz	340	B–
Spinach	Meat	4.5 oz	380	A–
Meat		10 oz	250	C–
	in Marinara Sauce	10 oz	211	A–
Cheese with Shrimp		10 oz	278	B–
Cheese	in Tomato Sauce	5.5 oz	210	B–

"+" indicates the food meets minimum fiber requirements; "–" indicates the food has a high sodium content.

Food	Processing Category	Brand
Tortellini Dishes	Frozen	Budget Gourmet Side Dish
Tortellini Dishes	Frozen	Green Giant Microwave
Tortellini Dishes	Frozen	Green Giant One Serving
Tortellini Dishes	Frozen	Le Menu Lightstyle
Tortellini Dishes	Frozen	Stouffer's
Tortellini Dishes	Frozen	Stouffer's
Tortellini Dishes	Frozen	Stouffer's
Tortellini Dishes	Frozen	Stouffer's
Tortellini Dishes	Frozen	Stouffer's
Tortellini Dishes	Frozen	Weight Watchers
Tortilla Entree	Frozen	Stouffer's Grande
Tuna Entree	Frozen	Banquet
Tuna Entree	Frozen	Stouffer's
Turkey Dinner	Frozen	Armour Classics
Turkey Dinner	Frozen	Banquet
Turkey Dinner	Frozen	Banquet Extra Helping
Turkey Dinner	Frozen	Budget Gourmet
Turkey Dinner	Frozen	Budget Gourmet
Turkey Dinner	Frozen	Freezer Queen
Turkey Dinner	Frozen	Healthy Choice
Turkey Dinner	Frozen	Healthy Choice
Turkey Dinner	Frozen	Le Menu
Turkey Dinner	Frozen	Le Menu Lightstyle
Turkey Dinner	Frozen	Le Menu Lightstyle
Turkey Dinner	Frozen	Morton
Turkey Dinner	Frozen	Stouffer's Dinner Supreme
Turkey Dinner	Frozen	Stouffer's Lean Cuisine
Turkey Dinner	Frozen	Swanson
Turkey Dinner	Frozen	Swanson Hungry-Man
Turkey Dinner	Frozen	Ultra Slim-Fast
Turkey Dinner	Frozen	Ultra Slim-Fast
Turkey Entree	Freeze-dried	Mountain House
Turkey Entree	Frozen	Banquet
Turkey Entree	Frozen	Banquet Cookin' Bags
Turkey Entree	Frozen	Banquet Family Entrees
Turkey Entree	Frozen	Banquet Microwave
Turkey Entree	Frozen	Budget Gourmet
Turkey Entree	Frozen	Budget Gourmet Light & Healthy
Turkey Entree	Frozen	Budget Gourmet Slim
Turkey Entree	Frozen	Freezer Queen Cook in Pouch
Turkey Entree	Frozen	Freezer Queen Deluxe Family
Turkey Entree	Frozen	Freezer Queen Family Suppers
Turkey Entree	Frozen	Freezer Queen Family Suppers
Turkey Entree	Frozen	Freezer Queen Single Serve
Turkey Entree	Frozen	Healthy Choice
Turkey Entree	Frozen	Healthy Choice
Turkey Entree	Frozen	Healthy Choice
Turkey Entree	Frozen	Le Menu Lightstyle
Turkey Entree	Frozen	Le Menu Lightstyle Traditional
Turkey Entree	Frozen	Morton
Turkey Entree	Frozen	On-Cor
Turkey Entree	Frozen	On-Cor
Turkey Entree	Frozen	Pillsbury Microwave

Major Description	Minor Description	Serving Size	Calories	Grade
Cheese		5.5 oz	180	D–
Provencale		1 pkg	260	B–
Cheese	Marinara	5.5 oz	260	C–
Cheese	in Meat Sauce	8 oz	250	B–
Beef	in Marinara Sauce	10 oz	360	B–
Cheese	in Alfredo Sauce	8.87 oz	600	D–
Cheese	in Tomato Sauce	9.63 oz	360	C–
Cheese	in Vinaigrette Dressing	6.87 oz	400	D–
Veal in Alfredo Sauce		8.63 oz	500	D–
Cheese		9 oz	310	B–
		9.63 oz	530	D–
Pie		7 oz	540	D–
Noodle Casserole		10 oz	310	C–
Dressing & Gravy		11.5 oz	320	C–
		10.5 oz	390	D–
		19 oz	750	D–
Breast	Dijon Style	11.2 oz	340	C–
Breast	Sliced	11.1 oz	290	B–
Sliced		10 oz	280	B–
Breast		10.5 oz	290	B–
Tetrazzini		12.6 oz	340	B–
Breast	Mushroom Gravy	10.5 oz	300	B–
Divan		10 oz	260	B–
Sliced		10 oz	210	B–
		10 oz	230	B–
Breast	Roast	10.75 oz	300	B–
Breast	in Mushroom Sauce	8 oz	240	B–
		11.5 oz	350	B–
		17 oz	550	B–
Glazed	Dressing	10.5 oz	340	A–
Medallions	in Herb Sauce	12 oz	280	B–
Tetrazzini		1 cup	200	C
Pie		7 oz	510	D–
Sliced	Gravy	5 oz	100	D
Sliced	Gravy	8 oz	150	D
Pie		7 oz	430	D–
à la King with Rice		10 oz	390	D–
Glazed		9 oz	260	B–
Glazed		9 oz	270	B–
Sliced	Gravy	5 oz	70	B–
Gravy	with Dressing	7 oz	160	B–
Croquettes	with Breaded Gravy	7 oz	250	D–
Sliced	Gravy	7 oz	110	D–
Sliced	Gravy & Dressing	9 oz	230	B–
Breast	Sliced, with Gravy	10 oz	270	A–
Homestyle	Vegetables	9.5 oz	260	A–
Roasted	Gravy	8.5 oz	200	A–
Glazed		8.25 oz	260	B–
White Meat	Gravy	8 oz	200	B–
Pie		7 oz	420	D–
Croquettes		8 oz	227	C–
Gravy		8 oz	129	D–
Casserole		1 pkg	430	D–

"+" indicates the food meets minimum fiber requirements; "–" indicates the food has a high sodium content.

Food	Processing Category	Brand
Turkey Entree	Frozen	Right Course
Turkey Entree	Frozen	Stouffer's
Turkey Entree	Frozen	Stouffer's
Turkey Entree	Frozen	Stouffer's Lean Cuisine
Turkey Entree	Frozen	Stouffer's Lean Cuisine
Turkey Entree	Frozen	Stouffer's Lean Cuisine
Turkey Entree	Frozen	Stouffer's Lean Cuisine
Turkey Entree	Frozen	Swanson Homestyle Recipe
Turkey Entree	Frozen	Swanson Hungry-Man
Turkey Entree	Frozen	Swanson Pot Pie
Turkey Entree	Frozen	Tyson Gourmet Selection
Turkey Entree	Frozen	Weight Watchers
Turkey Entree	Frozen	Weight Watchers
Turkey Entree	Frozen	Weight Watchers
Turkey Pocket Sandwich	Frozen	Hot Pockets
Veal Dinner	Frozen	Armour Classics
Veal Dinner	Frozen	Freezer Queen
Veal Dinner	Frozen	Freezer Queen
Veal Dinner	Frozen	Le Menu
Veal Dinner	Frozen	Le Menu Lightstyle
Veal Dinner	Frozen	Morton
Veal Dinner	Frozen	Stouffer's Dinner Supreme
Veal Dinner	Frozen	Swanson
Veal Dinner	Frozen	Swanson Hungry-Man
Veal Entree	Frozen	Banquet Cookin' Bags
Veal Entree	Frozen	Banquet Family Entrees
Veal Entree	Frozen	Freezer Queen Cook in Pouch
Veal Entree	Frozen	Freezer Queen Deluxe Family
Veal Entree	Frozen	Hormel
Veal Entree	Frozen	Hormel
Veal Entree	Frozen	On-Cor
Veal Entree	Frozen	Stouffer's Lean Cuisine
Veal Entree	Frozen	Swanson Homestyle Recipe
Veal Entree	Frozen	Weight Watchers
Vegetable Entree	Canned	Dinty Moore
Vegetable Entree	Canned	La Choy
Vegetable Entree	Freeze-dried	Mountain House
Vegetable Sticks	Frozen	Farm Rich
Vegetable Sticks	Frozen	Stilwell Quickkrisp
Vegetables, Mixed	Frozen	Green Giant American Mixtures
Vegetables, Mixed	Frozen	Green Giant American Mixtures
Waffle Breakfast	Frozen	Kid Cuisine
Waffle Breakfast	Frozen	Swanson Great Starts
Waffle Breakfast	Frozen	Swanson Great Starts
Waffle Breakfast	Frozen	Swanson Great Starts
Welsh Rarebit	Canned	Snow's
Welsh Rarebit	Frozen	Stouffer's
Western Dinner	Frozen	Banquet
Western Dinner	Frozen	Mortons
Western Dinner	Frozen	Swanson
Ziti	Frozen	The Budget Gourmet Side Dish

Major Description	Minor Description	Serving Size	Calories	Grade
Sliced	in Mild Curry Sauce with Rice Pilaf	8.75 oz	320	B–
Pie		10 oz	540	D–
Tetrazzini		10 oz	380	D–
Breast	Roasted	9.75 oz	290	A–
Dijon Style		9.5 oz	270	C–
Homestyle		9.4 oz	230	B–
Pie		9.5 oz	300	B–
Dressing & Potatoes		9 oz	290	C–
Pie		16 oz	650	D–
		7 oz	380	D–
		11.5 oz	380	B–
Breast, Stuffed		8.5 oz	260	C–
Breast	Stuffed	4 oz	110	B–
Medallions	Roast	4 oz	89	A–
Ham & Cheese		5 oz	320	C–
Parmigiana		11.25 oz	400	D–
Parmigiana		5 oz	220	D–
Parmigiana	Platter	10 oz	400	D–
Parmigiana		11.5 oz	390	C–
Marsala		10 oz	230	A–.
Parmigiana		10 oz	260	B–
Parmigiana		11.25 oz	350	C–
Parmigiana		12.25 oz	430	D–
Parmigiana		18.25 oz	590	C–
Parmigiana		4 oz	230	D
Parmigiana	Patty	8 oz	370	D
Parmigiana		5 oz	220	D–
Parmigiana		7 oz	300	D–
Steak		4 oz	130	B
Steak	Breaded	4 oz	240	D
Parmigiana		8 oz	350	D–
Primavera		9.13 oz	250	C–
Parmigiana		10 oz	330	C–
Parmigiana	Patty	8.44 oz	190	B–
Stew		8 oz	170	D–
Meatless Chow Mein		3/4 cup	35	A–+
Stew	with Beef	1 cup	230	B
Breaded		4 oz	240	C–
Breaded		3 oz	240	B–
Manhattan Style		1/2 cup	25	A+
Western Style		1/2 cup	60	B+
		1 piece	160	B–
Belgian Style	with Sausage	1 piece	280	D–
Belgian Style	with Strawberries	1 piece	210	C
with Bacon		1 piece	230	D–
		1/2 cup	170	D–
		4 oz	140	D–
		11 oz	630	D
		10 oz	290	D–
Style		11.5 oz	430	C–
in Marinara Sauce		6.25 oz	220	C–

"+" indicates the food meets minimum fiber requirements; "–" indicates the food has a high sodium content.

Fruits and Vegetables

The Fruits and Vegetables section contains all legumes, such as beans, and all nuts. Additonally, all canned, frozen, and otherwise processed fruits and vegetables will also be found in this section, including vegetables with added sauces, spices, etc.

The A- and B-rated foods in this section should supplement foods from the Cereals and Grains section as your *major* calorie and fiber source.

Food	Processing Category	Brand
Acerola	Fresh	Generic
Acorn	Bulk	Generic
Acorn	Bulk	Generic
Adzuki Bean	Bulk	Generic
Adzuki Bean	Bulk	Generic
Adzuki Bean	Canned	Generic
Alfalfa Seeds Sprouted	Fresh	
Almond	Bulk	Generic
Almond	Bulk	Generic
Almond	Bulk	Generic
Almond	Bulk	Generic
Almond	Bulk	Generic
Almond Powder	Dry	Generic
Almond Powder	Dry	Generic
Amaranth	Fresh	
Amaranth	Fresh	
Anasazi Bean	Bulk	Arrowhead Mills
Apple	Fresh	
Apple	Fresh	
Apple	Canned	All Brands
Apple	Canned	All Brands
Apple	Canned	All Brands
Apple	Canned	All Brands
Apple	Canned	All Brands
Apple	Canned	White House
Apple, Dehydrated	Dehydrated	Generic
Apple, Dehydrated	Dehydrated	Generic
Apple, Dehydrated	Dehydrated	Weight Watchers
Apple, Dried	All Forms	Del Monte
Apple, Dried	All Forms	Sun-Maid/Sunsweet
Applesauce	Canned or in Jars	All Brands
Applesauce	Canned or in Jars	All Brands
Applesauce	Canned or in Jars	All Brands
Applesauce	Canned or in Jars	All Brands
Applesauce	Canned or in Jars	All Brands
Apricot	Fresh	Generic
Apricot	Fresh	Generic
Apricot	Canned	Generic
Apricot	Canned	Generic
Apricot	Canned	Generic
Apricot	Canned	Generic
Apricot	Canned	S & W
Apricot	Canned	S & W/Nutradiet
Apricot, Dehydrated	All Forms	Generic
Apricot, Dehydrated	All Forms	Generic
Apricot, Dried	All Forms	Generic
Apricot, Dried	All Forms	Generic
Apricot, Dried	All Forms	Generic
Arrowhead	Fresh	Generic
Arrowhead	Fresh	Generic
Artichoke	Fresh	Generic
Artichoke Hearts	Canned	S & W
Artichoke Hearts	Frozen	Birds Eye Deluxe

Major Description	Minor Description	Serving Size	Calories	Grade
		1 medium, 2 oz	2	A+
Dried	Shelled	1 oz	145	D–
Raw	Shelled	1 oz	105	D–
Dry	Boiled	$^1/_2$ cup	145	A+
Dry	Raw	$^1/_2$ cup	323	A+
Sweetened		$^1/_2$ cup	351	A
Raw		$^1/_2$ cup	5	B+
Dried	Whole Kernels	$^1/_2$ cup	420	D
Dried, Blanched	Whole Kernels	$^1/_2$ cup	425	D
Dry Roasted		$^1/_2$ cup	405	D
Oil Roasted	Blanched or Regular	$^1/_2$ cup	485	D+
Oil Roasted	Salted	$^1/_2$ cup	485	D–+
Full Fat		$^1/_2$ cup	193	D
Partially Defatted		$^1/_2$ cup	128	C
Boiled		$^1/_2$ cup	14	A+
Raw		$^1/_2$ cup	4	A+
Raw		$^1/_2$ cup	300	A+
Raw, Cored, Unpeeled		1 medium, 5.5 oz	81	A+
Raw, Peeled		1 medium, 5.5 oz	70	A+
Baked, Whole		1 medium	110	A+
Dessert	Sliced	$^1/_2$ cup	70	A
in Syrup	Sliced	$^1/_2$ cup	50	A
in Water	Sliced	$^1/_2$ cup	40	A
Sweetened	Sliced	$^1/_2$ cup	68	A+
Spiced Rings		1 ring	25	A+
Cooked		$^1/_2$ cup	71	A
Uncooked		$^1/_2$ cup	104	A
Chips		.75 oz pkg	70	A–+
Sliced, Uncooked		2 oz	140	A
Chunks		2 oz	150	A
Diet		$^1/_2$ cup	50	A
Natural		$^1/_2$ cup	50	A+
Sweetened		$^1/_2$ cup	95	A+
Sweetened	with Cinnamon	$^1/_2$ cup	95	A
Unsweetened		$^1/_2$ cup	50	A+
		3 medium, 4 oz	51	A+
Halves		$^1/_2$ cup	37	A+
in Extra-Light Syrup	Unpeeled	4 oz	56	A+
in Heavy Syrup	Peeled	4 oz	94	A+
in Light Syrup	Unpeeled	4 oz	71	A+
in Water	Unpeeled	4 oz	31	A+
in Water	Halves	4 oz	35	A+
in Water	Halves	4 oz	35	A+
Cooked		$^1/_2$ cup	156	A+
Uncooked		$^1/_2$ cup	192	A+
Sulfured, Cooked	Sweetened, Halves	$^1/_2$ cup	153	A
Sulfured, Cooked	Unsweetened, Halves	$^1/_2$ cup	106	A
Sulfured, Uncooked	Halves	$^1/_2$ cup	155	A+
Boiled		1 medium, .6 oz	9	A+
Raw		1 medium, .6 oz	28	A
Boiled	Trimmed or Hearts	$^1/_2$ cup	45	A–+
Marinated		3.5 oz	225	D
		3 oz	30	A–+

"+" indicates the food meets minimum fiber requirements; "–" indicates the food has a high sodium content.

Food	Processing Category	Brand
Artichoke Hearts	Frozen	Generic
Artichoke Hearts	Frozen	Seabrook
Asparagus	Fresh	
Asparagus	Fresh	
Asparagus	Canned	Del Monte
Asparagus	Canned	Del Monte
Asparagus	Canned	Green Giant
Asparagus	Canned	Green Giant
Asparagus	Canned	Green Giant 50% Less Salt
Asparagus	Canned	S & W Fancy
Asparagus	Canned	S & W Fancy
Asparagus	Canned	S & W/Nutradiet
Asparagus	Canned	Stokely
Asparagus	Canned	Stokely No Salt or Sugar Added
Asparagus	Frozen	Generic
Asparagus	Frozen	Birds Eye
Asparagus	Frozen	Green Giant Harvest Fresh
Avocado	Fresh	
Avocado Dip	Packaged	Kraft
Avocado, California	Fresh	
Avocado, Florida	Fresh	
Baked Beans	Canned	Generic
Baked Beans	Canned	Generic
Baked Beans	Canned	Generic
Baked Beans	Canned	Generic
Baked Beans	Canned	Generic
Baked Beans	Canned	Generic
Baked Beans	Canned	Allen's
Baked Beans	Canned	Allen's
Baked Beans	Canned	Allen's
Baked Beans	Canned	Allen's Extra Fancy
Baked Beans	Canned	B & M
Baked Beans	Canned	B & M
Baked Beans	Canned	B & M
Baked Beans	Canned	B & M
Baked Beans	Canned	B & M
Baked Beans	Canned	B & M
Baked Beans	Canned	B & M
Baked Beans	Canned	B & M
Baked Beans	Canned	B & M
Baked Beans	Canned	B & M
Baked Beans	Canned	Campbell's
Baked Beans	Canned	Campbell's
Baked Beans	Canned	Campbell's
Baked Beans	Canned	Campbell's
Baked Beans	Canned	Campbell's Home Style
Baked Beans	Canned	Campbell's Old Fashioned
Baked Beans	Canned	Friends
Baked Beans	Canned	Friends
Baked Beans	Canned	Friends
Baked Beans	Canned	Friends

Major Description	Minor Description	Serving Size	Calories	Grade
Boiled		3 oz	35	A+
		3 oz	25	A+
Boiled		4 spears	15	A+
Raw		4 spears	15	A+
in Liquid	Green Tipped	$^1/_2$ cup	20	A–
in Liquid	Spears, All Green, & Tips	$^1/_2$ cup	20	A–
in Liquid	Green	$^1/_2$ cup	20	A–+
In Liquid	White	$^1/_2$ cup	16	A–+
in Liquid		$^1/_2$ cup	20	A–+
in Liquid	Spears, All Green	$^1/_2$ cup	18	A–
in Liquid	Spears, All Green, Colossal	$^1/_2$ cup	20	A–
Points, All Green		$^1/_2$ cup	17	A
		$^1/_2$ cup	20	A–
		$^1/_2$ cup	20	A
Cuts & Spears		$^1/_2$ cup	32	A+
Spears		$^1/_2$ cup	25	A
Cuts		3.3 oz	25	A–+
All Varieties		1 medium, 9.6 oz	324	D
		2 Tbsp	50	D–
All Varieties	Trimmed	1 medium, 8 oz	306	D+
All Varieties	Trimmed	1 medium, 16 oz	339	D+
Beef		$^1/_2$ cup	161	B–+
Franks		$^1/_2$ cup	182	D–+
Plain or Vegetarian		$^1/_2$ cup	118	A–+
Pork		$^1/_2$ cup	133	A–+
Pork	in Sweet Sauce	$^1/_2$ cup	140	A–+
Pork	in Tomato Sauce	$^1/_2$ cup	123	A–+
		$^1/_2$ cup	170	C–+
Pork		$^1/_2$ cup	90	A–+
Vegetarian		$^1/_2$ cup	110	A–+
Pork		$^1/_2$ cup	125	A–+
Barbecue		$^1/_2$ cup	130	B–+
Honey		$^1/_2$ cup	120	A–+
Hot & Spicy		$^1/_2$ cup	120	A–+
Maple		$^1/_2$ cup	120	A–+
Pea		$^1/_2$ cup	135	B–+
Plain		$^1/_2$ cup	115	A–+
Pork	in Tomato Sauce	$^1/_2$ cup	115	A–+
Red Kidney		$^1/_2$ cup	150	A–+
Vegetarian	99% Fat Free	$^1/_2$ cup	160	A–+
Yellow Eye		$^1/_2$ cup	125	B–+
Barbecue		$^1/_2$ cup	100	B–+
Hot Chili		$^1/_2$ cup	96	B–+
Plain or Vegetarian		$^1/_2$ cup	170	A–+
in Tomato Sauce	Pork	$^1/_2$ cup	100	A–+
		$^1/_2$ cup	110	B–+
in Molasses & Brown Sugar		$^1/_2$ cup	115	A–+
Maple		$^1/_2$ cup	120	A–+
Pea	Pork	$^1/_2$ cup	140	A–+
Pea, Small		$^1/_2$ cup	180	A–+
Red Kidney	Pork	$^1/_2$ cup	140	A–+

"+" indicates the food meets minimum fiber requirements; "–" indicates the food has a high sodium content.

Food	Processing Category	Brand
Baked Beans	Canned	Grandma Brown's
Baked Beans	Canned	Grandma Brown's Saucepan
Baked Beans	Canned	Green Giant
Baked Beans	Canned	Hain
Baked Beans	Canned	Hain
Baked Beans	Canned	Hain
Baked Beans	Canned	Hain
Baked Beans	Canned	Hain
Baked Beans	Canned	Hain 99% Fat Free
Baked Beans	Canned	Hain Fat Free
Baked Beans	Canned	Health Valley
Baked Beans	Canned	Health Valley No Salt Added
Baked Beans	Canned	Health Valley Vegetarian
Baked Beans	Canned	Hormel Micro-Cup
Baked Beans	Canned	Hunts
Baked Beans	Canned	Las Palmas
Baked Beans	Canned	Las Palmas
Baked Beans	Canned	Old El Paso
Baked Beans	Canned	Old El Paso
Baked Beans	Canned	Old El Paso
Baked Beans	Canned	S & W
Baked Beans	Canned	S & W Brick Oven
Baked Beans	Canned	Van Camp's
Baked Beans	Canned	Van Camp's
Baked Beans	Canned	Van Camp's
Baked Beans	Canned	Van Camp's Beanee Weenee
Baked Beans	Canned	Van Camp's Deluxe
Baked Beans	Canned	Van Camp's Vegetarian Style
Bamboo Shoots	Fresh	
Bamboo Shoots	Canned	All Brands
Banana	Fresh	
Banana Chip	Freeze Dried	Mountain House
Banana, Dehydrated	All Forms	Generic
Banana, Red	Fresh	
Bean Salad	Canned	Green Giant
Bean Salad	Canned	Joan of Arc
Bean Salad	Canned	Joan of Arc
Bean Salad	Canned	Joan of Arc
Bean Sprouts	Fresh	
Bean Sprouts	Fresh	
Bean Sprouts	Fresh	
Bean Sprouts	Fresh	
Bean Sprouts	Fresh	
Bean Sprouts	Fresh	
Beechnut	Bulk	Generic
Beet	Fresh	
Beet	Fresh	
Beet	Canned	Generic
Beet	Canned	Generic
Beet	Canned	Generic
Beet	Canned	Generic
Beet	Canned	Del Monte

Major Description	Minor Description	Serving Size	Calories	Grade
		$^1/_2$ cup	150	A–+
		$^1/_2$ cup	153	A–+
		$^1/_2$ cup	150	A–+
Black Turtle		$^1/_2$ cup	70	A–+
Great Northern		$^1/_2$ cup	80	A–+
Pinto		$^1/_2$ cup	70	A–+
Red Kidney		$^1/_2$ cup	80	A–+
Refried	Vegetarian	$^1/_2$ cup	70	A–+
Black, Refried	Vegetarian	$^1/_2$ cup	110	A–+
Refried	Vegetarian	$^1/_2$ cup	90	A–+
Boston		$^1/_2$ cup	213	A+
Boston		$^1/_2$ cup	213	A+
Plain or Vegetarian	Miso	$^1/_2$ cup	90	A–+
Pork		$^1/_2$ cup	127	B–+
Pork		$^1/_2$ cup	140	A–+
Refried		$^1/_2$ cup	110	B–+
Refried	No Fat	$^1/_2$ cup	110	A–+
Garbanzo		$^1/_2$ cup	190	A–+
Refried	Fat Free	$^1/_2$ cup	90	A–+
Refried	Spicy	$^1/_2$ cup	100	A+
Pork		$^1/_2$ cup	130	A+
		$^1/_2$ cup	160	A–+
		$^1/_2$ cup	130	A–+
Brown Sugar		$^1/_2$ cup	142	B–+
Pork		$^1/_2$ cup	118	A–+
Franks		$^1/_2$ cup	163	B–+
		$^1/_2$ cup	160	A–+
		$^1/_2$ cup	103	A–+
Boiled	Slices	$^1/_2$ cup	8	A+
Plain	Slices	$^1/_2$ cup	13	B+
		1 medium, 6.2 oz	105	A+
		$^1/_2$ cup	248	B
		$^1/_2$ cup	175	A
Sliced		$^1/_2$ cup	68	A
3 Bean		$^1/_2$ cup	70	A–+
3 Bean		$^1/_2$ cup	90	A–+
4 Bean		$^1/_2$ cup	100	A–+
Green Bean, German Style		$^1/_2$ cup	90	C–+
Kidney	Raw	$^1/_2$ cup	26	A+
Navy	Raw	$^1/_2$ cup	35	A+
Pinto	Raw	$^1/_2$ cup	72	A–+
Soy	Raw	$^1/_2$ cup	45	D+
Soy	Steamed	$^1/_2$ cup	38	D+
Soy	Stir-fried in Oil	4 oz	142	D+
Dried	Shelled	1 oz	164	D
Boiled		$^1/_2$ cup	35	A–+
Raw	Trimmed	$^1/_2$ cup	48	A–+
in Liquid		$^1/_2$ cup	36	A–+
in Liquid	Sliced	$^1/_2$ cup	27	A+–
in Liquid	Low Sodium	$^1/_2$ cup	36	A–+
Pickled	in Liquid	$^1/_2$ cup	74	A–
Pickled	Crinkle Sliced, in Liquid	$^1/_2$ cup	80	A–

"+" indicates the food meets minimum fiber requirements; "–" indicates the food has a high sodium content.

Food	Processing Category	Brand
Beet	Canned	Del Monte
Beet	Canned	Del Monte No Salt Added
Beet	Canned	Featherweight
Beet	Canned	S & W
Beet	Canned	S & W
Beet	Canned	S & W
Beet	Canned	S & W/Nutradiet
Beet	Canned	S & W Premium
Beet	Canned	S & W Regular or Party
Beet	Canned	Stokely
Beet	Canned	Stokely
Beet	Canned	Stokely
Beet	Canned	Stokely
Beet	Canned	Stokely No Salt or Sugar Added
Black Beans	Bulk	Generic
Black Beans	Bulk	Generic
Black Beans	Canned	Green Giant
Black Beans	Canned	Joan of Arc
Black Beans	Canned	Progresso
Black Beans	Mix	Fantastic Foods
Black Beans Dinner	Canned	Health Valley Fast Menu
Black Turtle Beans	Bulk	Arrowhead Mills
Black Turtle Soup Beans	Bulk	Generic
Black Turtle Soup Beans	Bulk	Generic
Black Turtle Soup Beans	Canned	Generic
Black-eyed Peas	Canned	Allen's
Black-eyed Peas	Canned	Allen's
Black-eyed Peas	Canned	Allen's
Black-eyed Peas	Canned	Joan of Arc
Black-eyed Peas	Canned	Joan of Arc/Green Giant
Black-eyed Peas	Canned	Luck's
Black-eyed Peas	Frozen	Frosty Acres
Black-eyed Peas	Frozen	Seabrook
Black-eyed Peas	Frozen	Southern
Blackberry	Fresh	
Blackberry	Canned	Generic
Blackberry	Canned	Generic
Blackberry	Frozen	Generic
Blueberry	Fresh	
Blueberry	Canned	Generic
Blueberry	Canned	Generic
Blueberry	Frozen	Generic
Blueberry	Frozen	Generic
Blueberry Syrup	Jar	Estee
Blueberry Syrup	Jar	Featherweight
Bok-choy	*See* Cabbage, Chinese	
Borage	Fresh	
Boysenberry	Canned	Generic
Boysenberry	Frozen	Generic
Boysenberry	*See* Blackberry	
Brazil Nut	Bulk	Generic

Major Description	Minor Description	Serving Size	Calories	Grade
Whole	Tiny or Sliced, in Liquid	¹/₂ cup	35	A−
Sliced	in Liquid	¹/₂ cup	35	A−
Sliced		¹/₂ cup	45	A
Diced or Julienne		¹/₂ cup	40	A−
Pickled	Whole, Extra Small	¹/₂ cup	70	A−
Whole	Small	¹/₂ cup	40	A−
Sliced		¹/₂ cup	35	A
Sliced	Small, Tender	¹/₂ cup	40	A−
Pickled	in Red Wine Vinegar, Sliced	¹/₂ cup	70	A−
Diced		¹/₂ cup	35	A−
Harvard		¹/₂ cup	70	A−
Pickled		¹/₂ cup	100	A−
Whole	Sliced or Cut	¹/₂ cup	40	A−
in Liquid		¹/₂ cup	40	A
Boiled		¹/₂ cup	113	A+
Pre-Cooked		¹/₂ cup	330	A+
in Brine		¹/₂ cup	90	A−+
in Brine		¹/₂ cup	90	A−+
		¹/₂ cup	90	A−+
Instant		¹/₂ cup	157	A−
Western Style	Garden Vegetables	7.5 oz	120	A−+
Pre-Cooked		2 oz	190	A+
Boiled		¹/₂ cup	120	A+
Pre-Cooked		¹/₂ cup	312	A+
with Liquid		¹/₂ cup	103	A−
Fresh		¹/₂ cup	100	A−+
Mature		¹/₂ cup	105	A−+
Mature	Pork	¹/₂ cup	105	A−+
in Brine		¹/₂ cup	70	A−+
Mature		¹/₂ cup	90	A−+
Mature	Pork	7.5 oz	200	B−+
		3.3 oz	130	A
		3.3 oz	130	A
		3.5 oz	136	A
		¹/₂ cup	37	A+
in Heavy Syrup		¹/₂ cup	118	A+
in Water		¹/₂ cup	25	A+
Unsweetened		¹/₂ cup	49	A+
		¹/₂ cup	41	A+
in Heavy Syrup		¹/₂ cup	100	A+
in Water		¹/₂ cup	40	A+
Sweetened		¹/₂ cup	94	A+
Unsweetened		¹/₂ cup	39	A+
		1 Tbsp	4	A−
		1 Tbsp	16	A−
Raw	1" Pieces	¹/₂ cup	9	B−+
in Heavy Syrup		¹/₂ cup	113	A+
Unsweetened		¹/₂ cup	33	A+
Raw		¹/₂ cup or 16 nuts	460	D

"+" indicates the food meets minimum fiber requirements; "−" indicates the food has a high sodium content.

Food	Processing Category	Brand
Breadfruit	Fresh	
Breadfruit Seeds	Bulk	Generic
Breadfruit Seeds	Bulk	Generic
Breadfruit Seeds	Bulk	Generic
Breadnut Tree Seeds	Bulk	Generic
Breadnut Tree Seeds	Bulk	Generic
Broad Beans	Bulk	Generic
Broad Beans	Bulk	Generic
Broad Beans	Canned	Generic
Broccoli	Fresh	
Broccoli	Fresh	
Broccoli	Frozen	Birds Eye
Broccoli	Frozen	Birds Eye
Broccoli	Frozen	Birds Eye
Broccoli	Frozen	Birds Eye Butter Sauce Combination
Broccoli	Frozen	Birds Eye Cheese Sauce Combination
Broccoli	Frozen	Birds Eye Deluxe
Broccoli	Frozen	Birds Eye Deluxe
Broccoli	Frozen	Birds Eye Farm Fresh
Broccoli	Frozen	Birds Eye Portion Pack
Broccoli	Frozen	Freezer Queen Family Size Dish
Broccoli	Frozen	Frosty Acres
Broccoli	Frozen	Frosty Acres
Broccoli	Frozen	Frosty Acres
Broccoli	Frozen	Frosty Acres
Broccoli	Frozen	Generic
Broccoli	Frozen	Generic
Broccoli	Frozen	Generic
Broccoli	Frozen	Green Giant
Broccoli	Frozen	Green Giant
Broccoli	Frozen	Green Giant
Broccoli	Frozen	Green Giant Harvest Fresh
Broccoli	Frozen	Green Giant Harvest Fresh
Broccoli	Frozen	Green Giant One Serving
Broccoli	Frozen	Green Giant One Serving
Broccoli	Frozen	Green Giant Polybag
Broccoli	Frozen	Seabrook
Broccoli	Frozen	Seabrook
Broccoli	Frozen	Seabrook
Broccoli	Frozen	Southern
Broccoli	Frozen	Stokely Singles
Broccoli	Frozen	Stokely Singles
Broccoli & Cheese	Frozen	Pepperidge Farm
Broccoli Combinations	Frozen	Birds Eye Butter Sauce Combination
Broccoli Combinations	Frozen	Birds Eye Cheese Sauce Combination
Broccoli Combinations	Frozen	Birds Eye Farm Fresh
Broccoli Combinations	Frozen	Birds Eye Farm Fresh
Broccoli Combinations	Frozen	Birds Eye Farm Fresh
Broccoli Combinations	Frozen	Birds Eye Farm Fresh
Broccoli Combinations	Frozen	Birds Eye Farm Fresh
Broccoli Combinations	Frozen	Birds Eye Farm Fresh
Broccoli Combinations	Frozen	Birds Eye For One

Major Description	Minor Description	Serving Size	Calories	Grade
		1/2 cup	114	A
Boiled	Shelled	1 oz	48	A
Raw	Shelled	1 oz	54	B
Roasted	Shelled	1 oz	59	A
Dried		1 oz	104	A+
Raw		8–14 seeds or 1 oz	62	A
Dried		1/2 cup	256	A+
Pre-Cooked		1/2 cup	40	A+
in Liquid		1/2 cup	91	A–
Boiled		1/2 cup	22	A+
Raw		1 spear, 9 oz	42	A+
Chopped		3.3 oz	25	A+
Cuts		3.3 oz	25	A+
Spears		3.3 oz	25	A+
in Butter Sauce	Spears	3.3 oz	45	C–+
in Cheese Sauce		5 oz	130	D–+
Florets		3.3 oz	25	A+
Spears, Baby		3.3 oz	30	A+
Spears, Whole		4 oz	30	A+
Cuts		3 oz	20	A+
in Cheese Sauce		4.5 oz	48	B–
Chopped		3.3 oz	25	A+
Cuts		3.3 oz	25	A–+
Florets		3.3 oz	30	A+
Spears		3.3 oz	25	A+
Boiled, Drained, Spears or Chopped		4 oz	32	A+
Chopped		4 oz	30	A+
Spears		4 oz	33	A+
in Butter Sauce	Spears	1/2 cup	40	C–+
in Cheese-Flavored Sauce		1/2 cup	60	B–+
Spears, Mini		1/2 cup	18	A–+
Cuts		1/2 cup	16	A–+
Spears		1/2 cup	20	A–+
in Butter Sauce	Cuts	4.5 oz	45	C–+
in Cheese Sauce	Cuts	5 oz	70	C–+
Cuts		1/2 bag	12	A–+
Chopped or Cuts		3.3 oz	25	A+
Spears		3.3 oz	25	A+
Spears, Baby		3.3 oz	30	A+
Chopped or Spears		3.5 oz	28	A
Cuts		3 oz	25	C
in Cheese Sauce	Cuts	4 oz	80	D–
in Pastry		1 piece	230	D–
Cauliflower & Carrots	in Butter Sauce	3.3 oz	45	C–+
Cauliflower & Carrots	in Cheese Sauce	4.5 oz	110	D–+
Baby Carrots	Water Chestnuts	4 oz	45	A+
Cauliflower & Carrots		4 oz	35	A+
Cauliflower & Red Peppers		4 oz	30	A+
Corn & Red Peppers		4 oz	60	A+
Green Beans & Pearl Onions		4 oz	35	A+
Red Peppers & Bamboo Shoots	Straw Mushrooms	4 oz	30	A+
Cauliflower & Carrots	in Cheese Sauce	5 oz	110	D–+

"+" indicates the food meets minimum fiber requirements; "–" indicates the food has a high sodium content.

Food	Processing Category	Brand
Broccoli Combinations	Frozen	Frosty Acres Swiss Mix
Broccoli Combinations	Frozen	Green Giant
Broccoli Combinations	Frozen	Green Giant
Broccoli Combinations	Frozen	Green Giant One Serving
Broccoli Combinations	Frozen	Green Giant One Serving
Broccoli Combinations	Frozen	Green Giant One Serving
Broccoli Combinations	Frozen	Green Giant Valley
Broccoli Combinations	Frozen	Green Giant Valley
Broccoli Combinations	Frozen	Stokely Singles
Broccoli Combinations	Frozen	Stokely Singles
Broccoli Combinations	Frozen	Stokely Singles
Broccoli Combinations	Frozen	Stokely Singles
Brussels Sprouts	Fresh	
Brussels Sprouts	Frozen	Birds Eye
Brussels Sprouts	Frozen	Birds Eye Cheese Sauce Combination
Brussels Sprouts	Frozen	Birds Eye Farm Fresh
Brussels Sprouts	Frozen	Frosty Acres
Brussels Sprouts	Frozen	Green Giant
Brussels Sprouts	Frozen	Green Giant Polybag
Brussels Sprouts	Frozen	Seabrook
Brussels Sprouts	Frozen	Seabrook
Brussels Sprouts	Frozen	Southern
Brussels Sprouts	Frozen	Stokely Singles
Brussels Sprouts	Frozen	Stokely Singles
Burdock Root	Fresh	
Butterbur	Fresh	
Butterbur	Canned	Generic
Butter Beans	Canned	Joan of Arc
Butter Beans	See Lima Beans	
Butternut	Bulk	Generic
Cabbage	Fresh	
Cabbage	Fresh	
Cabbage, Chinese	Fresh	
Cabbage, Chinese	Fresh	
Cabbage, Chinese	Fresh	
Cabbage, Entree	Frozen	Stouffer's Lean Cuisine
Cabbage, Red	Fresh	
Cabbage, Savoy	Fresh	
Cabbage, Swamp	Fresh	
Cabbage, Swamp	Fresh	
Cantaloupe	Fresh	
Carambola	Fresh	
Caraway Seed	Bulk	Generic
Cardoon	Fresh	
Carissa	Fresh	
Carrot	Fresh	
Carrot	Canned	Generic
Carrot	Canned	Generic
Carrot	Canned	Generic
Carrot	Canned	Generic
Carrot	Canned	Allen's
Carrot	Canned	Allen's
Carrot	Canned	Del Monte

Major Description	Minor Description	Serving Size	Calories	Grade
& Cauliflower		3 oz	25	A–+
Cauliflower & Carrots	in Butter Sauce	4 oz	30	B–+
Cauliflower & Carrots	in Cheese-Flavored Sauce	4 oz	60	B–+
Cauliflower & Carrots	in Cheese Sauce	5 oz	70	C–+
Cauliflower & Carrots	No Sauce	4 oz	25	A–+
with Rotini	in Cheese Sauce	5.5 oz	120	B–
& Cauliflower	Medley	4 oz	30	B–+
Fanfare		4 oz	70	B–+
& Baby Carrots	with Water Chestnuts	3 oz	30	B
& Cauliflower		3 oz	20	D
Cauliflower & Baby Carrots		3 oz	25	C
Cauliflower & Baby Carrots	in Cheese Sauce	4 oz	70	C–
Raw		1 sprout, .7 oz	8	A+
		3.3 oz	35	A+
	in Cheese Sauce	4.5 oz	130	D–+
	Cauliflower & Carrots	4 oz	40	A+
		3.3 oz	35	A+
	in Butter Sauce	4 oz	40	B–+
		4 oz	25	A+
		3.3 oz	35	A+
	Baby	3.3 oz	40	A+
		3.5 oz	37	A+
		3 oz	35	A+
	in Butter Sauce	4 oz	50	B+
Raw	Pieces	$^1/_2$ cup	43	A+
Raw		1 stalk, .2 oz	1	A+
		4 oz	12	A+
	in Brine	$^1/_2$ cup	90	A–+
Dried	Shelled	1 oz	174	D
Raw		6" head, 40 oz	215	A+
Raw	Shredded	$^1/_2$ cup	8	A+
Bok-choy	Raw, Shredded	$^1/_2$ cup	5	A–+
Pe-tsai		1 leaf, .5 oz	2	A+
Pe-tsai	Raw, Shredded	$^1/_2$ cup	6	A+
Stuffed		9.5 oz	220	B–+
Raw	Shredded	$^1/_2$ cup	10	A+
Raw	Shredded	$^1/_2$ cup	10	A+
Raw	Chopped	$^1/_2$ cup	6	A+
Trimmed	Chopped	$^1/_2$ cup	6	A–+
Raw		$^1/_2$ cup	94	A+
Raw		1 medium, 5 oz	48	A+
Dry		1 Tbsp	22	D+
Raw	Shredded	$^1/_2$ cup	18	A–
Trimmed		1 oz	18	B+
Raw		1 medium, 2.8 oz	31	A+
		$^1/_2$ cup	26	A–+
Low Sodium		$^1/_2$ cup	26	A–+
in Liquid		$^1/_2$ cup	26	A–+
in Liquid	Low Sodium	$^1/_2$ cup	26	A–+
Diced or Sliced		$^1/_2$ cup	30	A–
Whole	Baby	$^1/_2$ cup	30	A–
Whole, Sliced or Diced	in Liquid	$^1/_2$ cup	30	A–

"+" indicates the food meets minimum fiber requirements; "–" indicates the food has a high sodium content.

Food	Processing Category	Brand
Carrot	Canned	Featherweight
Carrot	Canned	S & W Fancy
Carrot	Canned	S & W Fancy
Carrot	Canned	S & W/Nutradiet
Carrot	Canned	Stokely
Carrot	Canned	Stokely No Salt or Sugar Added
Carrot	Frozen	Generic
Carrot	Frozen	Birds Eye
Carrot	Frozen	Birds Eye Deluxe
Carrot	Frozen	Birds Eye Deluxe
Carrot	Frozen	Frosty Acres
Carrot	Frozen	Green Giant Harvest Fresh
Carrot	Frozen	Seabrook
Carrot	Frozen	Southern
Carrot	Frozen	Stokely Singles
Carrot Chip	Packaged	Hain
Carrot Chip	Packaged	Hain
Carrot Chip	Packaged	Hain No Salt Added
Casaba	Fresh	
Cashew	Bulk	Generic
Cashew	Canned or in Jars	Beer Nuts
Cashew	Canned or in Jars	Planters
Cashew	Canned or in Jars	Planters
Cashew	Canned or in Jars	Planters
Cashew	Canned or in Jars	Planters Unsalted
Cassava	Fresh	
Cauliflower	Fresh	
Cauliflower	Canned or in Jars	Vlasic Hot & Spicy
Cauliflower	Canned or in Jars	Vlasic Hot & Spicy
Cauliflower	Frozen	Birds Eye
Cauliflower	Frozen	Birds Eye Cheese Sauce Combination
Cauliflower	Frozen	Budget Gourmet Side Dish
Cauliflower	Frozen	Frosty Acres
Cauliflower	Frozen	Green Giant
Cauliflower	Frozen	Green Giant
Cauliflower	Frozen	Kohl's
Cauliflower	Frozen	Seabrook
Cauliflower	Frozen	Southern
Cauliflower	Frozen	Stokely Singles
Cauliflower	Frozen	Stokely Singles
Cauliflower Combinations	Frozen	Birds Eye Farm Fresh
Cauliflower Combinations	Frozen	Birds Eye Farm Fresh
Cauliflower Combinations	Frozen	Freezer Queen Family Side Dishes
Celeriac	Fresh	
Celery	Fresh	
Celery Flakes	Jars	Tone's
Celery Root Juice	Bottled	Biotta
Celtus	Fresh	
Chayote	Fresh	
Cherimoya	Fresh	
Cherry, Maraschino	Jars	Generic
Cherry, Sour, Red	Fresh	
Cherry, Sour, Red	Canned	Generic

Major Description	Minor Description	Serving Size	Calories	Grade
Sliced		1/2 cup	30	A
Sliced, Diced or Julienne		1/2 cup	30	A–
Whole	Tiny	1/2 cup	30	A–
Sliced		1/2 cup	30	A–
		1/2 cup	35	A–
		1/2 cup	35	A
		4 oz	45	A–+
Sliced		3.2 oz	35	A+
Parisienne		2.6 oz	30	A+
Whole	Baby	3.3 oz	40	A+
Sliced		3.3 oz	40	A+
Whole	Baby	4 oz	18	A–+
		3.3 oz	40	A+
Whole		3.5 oz	42	A–
Whole	Baby	3 oz	35	A–
		1 oz	150	D
Barbecue		1 oz	140	D
		1 oz	150	D
	Cubed	1/2 cup	23	A
Dry or Oil Roasted	Salted	1 oz	163	D
		1 oz	170	D
Dry Roasted		1 oz	160	D–
Honey Roasted		1 oz	170	D
Honey Roasted	Peanuts	1 oz	170	D
Dry Roasted		1 oz	160	D
Trimmed		1 oz	34	A+
Raw		1/2 cup	15	A+
Pickled		1 oz	4	A–
Sweet		1 oz	35	A–
		3.3 oz	25	A+
in Cheese Sauce		5 oz	130	D–+
in Cheddar Cheese Sauce		5 oz	110	D–
		3.3 oz	25	A+
Cuts		1/2 cup	12	A–+
in Cheese-Flavored Sauce		1/2 cup	60	B–+
		3 oz	20	A
		3.3 oz	25	A+
		3.5 oz	26	A
		3 oz	20	A
in Cheese Sauce		4 oz	70	C–
Carrots, Baby, & Snow Pea Pods		4 oz	40	A+
Zucchini, Carrots & Red Peppers		4 oz	30	A+
Broccoli & Carrots		5 oz	60	A–
Raw		1/2 cup	30	A–+
Raw		1 stalk or 1.6 oz	6	A–+
Dry		1 tsp	9	D+
		6 fl oz	67	A–
		1 leaf, .4 oz	2	A
Raw	Trimmed	1 oz	7	A+
Trimmed		1 oz	27	A+
with Liquid		1 oz	33	A
Trimmed	with Pits	1/2 cup	26	A+
in Heavy Syrup		1/2 cup	116	A

"+" indicates the food meets minimum fiber requirements; "–" indicates the food has a high sodium content.

Food	Processing Category	Brand
Cherry, Sour, Red	Canned	Generic
Cherry, Sour, Red	Canned	Lucky Leaf/Musselman's
Cherry, Sour, Red	Canned	Stokely
Cherry, Sour, Red	Canned	White House
Cherry, Sour, Red	Frozen	Generic
Cherry, Sour, Red	Frozen	Generic
Cherry, Sweet	Fresh	
Cherry, Sweet	Canned	Generic
Cherry, Sweet	Canned	Generic
Cherry, Sweet	Canned	Generic
Cherry, Sweet	Canned	Generic
Chervil	All Forms	Generic
Chestnut, Chinese	Bulk	Generic
Chestnut, Chinese	Bulk	Generic
Chestnut, Chinese	Bulk	Generic
Chestnut, Chinese	Bulk	Generic
Chestnut, European	Bulk	Generic
Chestnut, European	Bulk	Generic
Chestnut, European	Bulk	Generic
Chestnut, European	Bulk	Generic
Chestnut, Japanese	Bulk	Generic
Chestnut, Japanese	Bulk	Generic
Chestnut, Japanese	Bulk	Generic
Chestnut, Japanese	Bulk	Generic
Chickpea	Fresh	
Chickpea	Fresh	
Chickpea	Canned	Generic
Chickpea	Canned	Progresso
Chickpea	Canned	S & W Lite
Chicory Greens	Fresh	
Chicory Root	Fresh	
Chili Bean	Canned	Allen's
Chili Bean	Canned	Allen's
Chili Bean	Canned	Campbell's
Chili Bean	Canned	Dennison's
Chili Bean	Canned	Gebhardt
Chili Bean	Canned	Green Giant/Joan of Arc
Chili Bean	Canned	Hormel
Chili Bean	Canned	Hunt's
Chili Bean	Canned	S & W
Chili Bean	Canned	Van Camp's
Chives	Fresh	
Cloves	Fresh	
Coconut	Fresh	
Coconut Cream	Fresh	
Coconut Milk	Fresh	
Coconut Water	Fresh	
Coconut, Dried	All Forms	Generic
Coconut, Dried	All Forms	Generic
Coconut, Dried	All Forms	Generic
Coleslaw	Fresh	Generic
Collard Greens	Fresh	
Collard Greens	Fresh	

Major Description	Minor Description	Serving Size	Calories	Grade
in Light Syrup		¹/₂ cup	94	A
	Pitted, Tart	¹/₂ cup	50	A
	Pitted, in Water	¹/₂ cup	45	A
	Pitted	¹/₂ cup	43	A
Sweetened		¹/₂ cup	116	A
Unsweetened		¹/₂ cup	36	A
		¹/₂ cup	52	A+
in Heavy Syrup		¹/₂ cup	107	A
in Juice		¹/₂ cup	68	A
in Light Syrup		¹/₂ cup	85	A
in Water		¹/₂ cup	57	A
Dried		1 Tbsp	4	A+
Boiled or Steamed		1 oz	44	A
Dried		1 oz	103	A
Raw		1 oz	64	A
Roasted		1 oz	68	A
Boiled or Steamed		1 oz	37	A
Dried	Shelled	1 oz	105	A
Raw		1 oz	56	A+
Roasted		1 oz	70	A+
Boiled or Steamed		1 oz	16	A
Dried		1 oz	102	A
Raw		1 oz	44	A
Roasted		1 oz	57	A
Boiled		¹/₂ cup	134	A+
Raw		¹/₂ cup	364	A+
in Liquid		¹/₂ cup	143	A–+
		¹/₂ cup	130	B–+
	50% Less Salt	¹/₂ cup	110	A–+
Chopped		¹/₂ cup	21	A–+
Chopped		¹/₂ cup	33	A+
Hot		1 cup	180	A–
Mexican Style		1 cup	270	A–
Baked, Hot		1 cup	180	B–
Chili Gravy		1 cup	180	A–+
Spiced		1 cup	211	A–+
Caliente Style		1 cup	200	A–+
in Sauce		1 cup	195	B–
		1 cup	191	A–
		1 cup	260	A–
Mexican Style		1 cup	210	A–
Raw	Chopped	¹/₄ cup	4	A+
Ground		1 tsp	7	D+
Shelled	Shredded	¹/₂ cup	140	D+
		¹/₂ cup	390	D
Raw		¹/₂ cup	275	D
		¹/₂ cup	23	B–+
Creamed		¹/₂ cup	240	D
Sweetened	Flaked	¹/₂ cup	170	D
Sweetened	Shredded	¹/₂ cup	233	D
		¹/₂ cup	41	C
Boiled, Drained	Chopped	¹/₂ cup	6	A+
Raw	Chopped	¹/₂ cup	17	A+

"+" indicates the food meets minimum fiber requirements; "–" indicates the food has a high sodium content.

Food	Processing Category	Brand
Collard Greens	Canned	Allen's
Collard Greens	Canned	Luck's
Coriander	Fresh	
Coriander Leaf	Jars	Generic
Coriander Seed	Bulk	Generic
Corn	Fresh	
Corn	Canned	Del Monte
Corn	Canned	Del Monte
Corn	Canned	Del Monte
Corn	Canned	Del Monte
Corn	Canned	Del Monte
Corn	Canned	Del Monte No Salt Added
Corn	Canned	Del Monte No Salt Added
Corn	Canned	Del Monte No Salt Added
Corn	Canned	Featherweight
Corn	Canned	Green Giant
Corn	Canned	Green Giant
Corn	Canned	Green Giant
Corn	Canned	Green Giant 50% Less Salt
Corn	Canned	Green Giant 50% Less Salt & No Sugar
Corn	Canned	Green Giant Deli Corn
Corn	Canned	Green Giant Mexicorn
Corn	Canned	Green Giant Niblets
Corn	Canned	Green Giant No Salt or Sugar
Corn	Canned	Green Giant Pantry Express
Corn	Canned	Green Giant Pantry Express
Corn	Canned	Green Giant Sweet Select
Corn	Canned	S & W Premium
Corn	Canned	S & W Premium Homestyle
Corn	Canned	S & W Premium Homestyle Starch
Corn	Canned	S & W/Nutradiet
Corn	Canned	S & W/Nutradiet
Corn	Canned	Stokely
Corn	Canned	Stokely
Corn	Canned	Stokely
Corn	Canned	Stokely
Corn	Canned	Stokely No Salt or Sugar Added
Corn	Canned	Vacuum Pack Green Giant
Corn	Canned	Vacuum Pack Green Giant
Corn	Canned	Vacuum Pack Stokely
Corn	Freeze Dried	Mountain House
Corn	Frozen	Birds Eye
Corn	Frozen	Birds Eye Big Ears
Corn	Frozen	Birds Eye Butter Combination
Corn	Frozen	Birds Eye Deluxe
Corn	Frozen	Birds Eye Deluxe
Corn	Frozen	Birds Eye Little Ears
Corn	Frozen	Birds Eye Portion Pack
Corn	Frozen	Birds Eye Sweet
Corn	Frozen	Birds Eye Tender Sweet Deluxe
Corn	Frozen	Budget Gourmet Dish
Corn	Frozen	Budget Gourmet Dish

Major Description	Minor Description	Serving Size	Calories	Grade
Chopped		$^1/_2$ cup	20	C
Chopped	Pork	$^1/_2$ cup	40	D–
Trimmed		1 oz	6	B–+
Dried		1 oz	79	A+
Dried		1 oz	84	D+
Sweet, Yellow or White	Kernels, Cooked	1 ear, 2.7 oz	83	A+
Kernel	Cream Style in Golden	$^1/_2$ cup	80	A–+
Kernel	Cream Style in White	$^1/_2$ cup	90	A–+
Kernel	Golden in Liquid	$^1/_2$ cup	70	A–+
Kernel	Vacuum Pack in Liquid	$^1/_2$ cup	90	A–+
Kernel	White, in Liquid	$^1/_2$ cup	70	A–+
Kernel	Cream Style in Golden	$^1/_2$ cup	80	A+
Kernel	Golden	$^1/_2$ cup	80	A+
Kernel	Vacuum Pack in Liquid	$^1/_2$ cup	90	A+
Kernel		$^1/_2$ cup	80	A+
	in Brine	$^1/_2$ cup	70	A–+
Kernel		$^1/_2$ cup	80	A–+
Kernel	Cream Style	$^1/_2$ cup	100	A–+
Kernel	Golden	$^1/_2$ cup	70	A–+
Kernel		$^1/_2$ cup	50	B–+
		$^1/_2$ cup	80	A–+
Kernel	Peppers	$^1/_2$ cup	80	A–+
Kernel	Vacuum Pack	$^1/_2$ cup	80	A–+
Kernel	Golden	$^1/_2$ cup	80	A+
Kernel	Beans, Carrots & Pasta	$^1/_2$ cup	80	B–+
Kernel	Golden	$^1/_2$ cup	80	A–+
Kernel	Sweet	$^1/_2$ cup	60	A–+
Kernel	Young, Tender	$^1/_2$ cup	90	A–+
Kernel	Cream Style	$^1/_2$ cup	120	A–+
Kernel	Cream Style	$^1/_2$ cup	105	A–+
Kernel		$^1/_2$ cup	80	A+
Kernel	Cream Style	$^1/_2$ cup	100	A+
Kernel	Cream Style, Golden	$^1/_2$ cup	100	A–+
Kernel	Cream Style, White	$^1/_2$ cup	100	A–+
Kernel	Golden	$^1/_2$ cup	90	A–+
Kernel	White	$^1/_2$ cup	90	A–+
Kernel	Golden	$^1/_2$ cup	80	A+
Kernel	Golden	$^1/_2$ cup	80	A–+
Kernel	White	$^1/_2$ cup	80	A–+
Kernel	Golden	$^1/_2$ cup	90	A–+
		$^1/_2$ cup	90	A+
On the Cob		1 ear	120	A+
On the Cob		1 ear	160	A+
Kernels	in Butter Sauce	3.3 oz	90	B–+
On the Cob	Baby	2.6 oz	25	A+
Petite		2.6 oz	70	A+
On the Cob		2 ears	130	A+
Cut		3 oz	70	A+
Kernel		3.3 oz	80	A+
Kernel		3.3 oz	80	A+
in Butter Sauce		5.5 oz	190	B–+
in Sauce, Country Style		5.75 oz	140	C–+

"+" indicates the food meets minimum fiber requirements; "–" indicates the food has a high sodium content.

Food	Processing Category	Brand
Corn	Frozen	Frosty Acres
Corn	Frozen	Frosty Acres
Corn	Frozen	Green Giant
Corn	Frozen	Green Giant
Corn	Frozen	Green Giant
Corn	Frozen	Green Giant
Corn	Frozen	Green Giant Harvest Fresh
Corn	Frozen	Green Giant Harvest Fresh
Corn	Frozen	Green Giant Nibblers
Corn	Frozen	Green Giant Nibblers
Corn	Frozen	Green Giant Niblet Ears Super Sweet
Corn	Frozen	Green Giant Niblets
Corn	Frozen	Green Giant Niblets
Corn	Frozen	Green Giant Niblets
Corn	Frozen	Health Valley
Corn	Frozen	Ore-Ida
Corn	Frozen	Ore-Ida Mini Gold
Corn	Frozen	Seabrook
Corn	Frozen	Seabrook
Corn	Frozen	Seabrook
Corn	Frozen	Southern
Corn	Frozen	Southern
Corn	Frozen	Stokely Singles
Corn	Frozen	Stokely Singles
Corn	Frozen	Stokely Singles
Cowpea	Fresh	
Cowpea	Fresh	
Cowpea	Fresh	
Cowpea	Canned	Generic
Cowpea	Canned	Generic
Cowpea	Frozen	*See also* Black-eyed Peas
Cowpea, Dried	Bulk	Generic
Cowpea, Dried	Bulk	Generic
Crabapple	Fresh	
Cranberry	Fresh	
Cranberry Bean	Fresh	
Cranberry Bean	Canned	Generic
Cress	Fresh	
Cucumber	Fresh	
Currant, Black European	Fresh	
Currant, Red or White	Fresh	
Currant, Zante	Bulk	
Dandelion Greens	Fresh	
Dandelion Greens	Fresh	
Date	Fresh	
Date	Fresh	All Brands
Dock	Fresh	
Eggplant	Fresh	
Eggplant	Fresh	
Eggplant Appetizer	Canned	Progresso
Eggplant Entree	Frozen	*See* Frozen Foods Section
Elderberry	Fresh	
Endive	Fresh	

Major Description	Minor Description	Serving Size	Calories	Grade
Cut		1/2 cup	80	A+
On the Cob		1 ear	120	A+
Cream Style		1/2 cup	110	A−+
in Butter Sauce	White	1/2 cup	100	B+−
in Butter Sauce	White or Golden	1/2 cup	100	B−+
White		1/2 cup	90	A+
Kernel		1/2 cup	80	A+
Kernel	White	1/2 cup	90	A+
On the Cob		1 ear	90	A+
On the Cob		1 ear	111	A+
On the Cob		1 ear	111	A+
in Butter Sauce		1/2 cup	100	B−+
Kernel		1/2 cup	60	A+
Kernel	White	1/2 cup	90	A+
		1/2 cup	76	A+
On the Cob		1 ear	180	A+
On the Cob	Mini	2 ears	180	A+
Cut		3.3 oz	80	A+
On the Cob		1 ear	120	A+
White		3.3 oz	80	A+
		3.5 oz	98	A+
On the Cob		5" ear	140	A+
Cut		3 oz	75	A+
in Butter Sauce		4 oz	110	A−+
in Butter Sauce	on Cob	1 ear	70	A−+
Leafy Tips, Raw		1/2 cup	5	A+
Raw	in Pods	1/2 cup	65	A+
Young Pods with Seeds	Raw	1/2 cup	21	A+
Plain	in Liquid	1/2 cup	92	A−
with Pork		1/2 cup	99	B−
Boiled		1/2 cup	100	A+
Raw		1/2 cup	283	A+
Whole	Sliced	1/2 cup	42	A
Whole		1/2 cup	23	A+
Raw		1/2 cup	328	A+
in Liquid		1/2 cup	108	A−
Raw	Trimmed	1 oz	9	B+
Ends Trimmed		1 medium, 8" × 2"	40	A+
Trimmed		1/2 cup	36	A+
Trimmed		1/2 cup	31	A+
Dried		1/2 cup	204	A
Boiled		1/2 cup	13	B−+
Raw	Trimmed and Chopped	1/2 cup	17	A−+
Domestic, Natural & Dry	Pitted, Chopped	1/2 cup	245	A+
Imported	Chopped	1/2 cup	260	A+
Raw	Trimmed, Chopped	1/2 cup	15	B+
Boiled, Drained	Cubed	1/2 cup	13	A+
Raw	Trimmed	1 medium, 4.5 oz	27	A+
Caponata		1/2 can	70	D−
Trimmed		1/2 cup	53	A+
Trimmed	Chopped	1/2 cup	4	A+

"+" indicates the food meets minimum fiber requirements; "−" indicates the food has a high sodium content.

Food	Processing Category	Brand
Eppaw	Fresh	
Fava Bean	Canned	Generic
Fennel	Fresh	Frieda of California
Fig	Fresh	
Fig	Canned	Generic
Fig	Canned	Generic
Fig	Canned	Generic
Fig	Canned	Generic
Fig, Dried	All Forms	Blue Ribbon/Sun-Maid
Fig, Dried	All Forms	Blue Ribbon/Sun-Maid
Fig, Dried	All Forms	Generic
Fig, Dried	All Forms	Generic
Filbert	Bulk	Generic
Filbert	Bulk	Generic
Filbert	Bulk	Generic
Filbert	Bulk	Generic
French Bean	Bulk	Generic
French Bean	Bulk	Generic
Fruit & Nut Mix	Packaged	Planters Fruit N Nut
Fruit, Mixed	Canned	Generic
Fruit, Mixed	Canned	Generic
Fruit, Mixed	Canned	Generic
Fruit, Mixed	Canned	Generic
Fruit, Mixed	Canned	Generic
Fruit, Mixed	Canned	Generic
Fruit, Mixed	Canned	Generic
Fruit, Mixed	Canned	Generic
Fruit, Mixed	Canned	Generic
Fruit, Mixed	Canned	Generic
Fruit, Mixed	Canned	Generic
Fruit, Mixed	Canned	Del Monte
Fruit, Mixed	Canned	Del Monte
Fruit, Mixed	Canned	Del Monte
Fruit, Mixed	Canned	Del Monte Fruit Cup
Fruit, Mixed	Canned	Del Monte Lite
Fruit, Mixed	Canned	Del Monte Lite
Fruit, Mixed	Canned	Featherweight
Fruit, Mixed	Canned	Libby Lite
Fruit, Mixed	Canned	Libby Lite
Fruit, Mixed	Canned	S & W
Fruit, Mixed	Canned	S & W
Fruit, Mixed	Canned	S & W
Fruit, Mixed	Canned	S & W/Nutradiet
Fruit, Mixed	Canned	S & W/Nutradiet Regular/Unsweetened
Fruit, Mixed	Packaged	Birds Eye Quick Thaw Pouch
Fruit, Mixed	Packaged	Del Monte
Fruit, Mixed	Packaged	Sun-Maid/Sunsweet
Fruit, Mixed	Packaged	Sun-Maid/Sunsweet
Garbanzo	Canned	Joan of Arc
Garbanzo	Canned	Joan of Arc
Garlic	Fresh	
Ginkgo Nut	Canned	Generic
Ginkgo Nut	Bulk	Generic

Major Description	Minor Description	Serving Size	Calories	Grade
Trimmed		¹/₂ cup	75	A
		¹/₂ cup	90	A−+
		1 oz	4	A−
Raw		1 medium, 1.8 oz	37	A+
in Extra-Heavy Syrup		¹/₂ cup	279	A+
in Heavy Syrup		¹/₂ cup	114	A+
in Light Syrup		¹/₂ cup	90	A+
in Water		¹/₂ cup	65	A+
Calimyrna		¹/₂ cup	250	A
Mission Style		¹/₂ cup	210	A
All Varieties	Cooked	¹/₂ cup	140	A+
All Varieties	Uncooked	¹/₂ cup	254	A+
Dried, Blanched	Shelled	1 oz	191	D
Dry Roasted, Unblanched	Shelled	1 oz	188	D
Dry, Unblanched	Shelled	1 oz	179	D
Oil Roasted Unblanched	Shelled	1 oz	187	D
Dried	Boiled	¹/₂ cup	111	A+
Raw		¹/₂ cup	316	A+
		1 oz	150	D
Fruit Cocktail	in Extra-Heavy Syrup	¹/₂ cup	115	A
Fruit Cocktail	in Extra-Light Syrup	¹/₂ cup	55	A
Fruit Cocktail	in Heavy Syrup	¹/₂ cup	93	A
Fruit Cocktail	in Juice	¹/₂ cup	56	A
Fruit Cocktail	in Light Syrup	¹/₂ cup	72	A
Fruit Cocktail	in Water	¹/₂ cup	40	A
Fruit Salad	in Extra-Heavy Syrup	¹/₂ cup	100	A
Fruit Salad	in Heavy Syrup	¹/₂ cup	83	A
Fruit Salad	in Juice	¹/₂ cup	57	A
Fruit Salad	in Light Syrup	¹/₂ cup	66	A
Fruit Salad	in Water	¹/₂ cup	34	A+
Chunky		¹/₂ cup	80	A
Fruit Cocktail		¹/₂ cup	80	A
Fruit Salad	Tropical	¹/₂ cup	90	A
		¹/₂ cup	50	A
Chunky		¹/₂ cup	50	A
Fruit Cocktail		¹/₂ cup	50	A
Fruit Cocktail	in Juice	¹/₂ cup	50	A
Chunky	in Juice	¹/₂ cup	50	A
Fruit Cocktail	in Juice	¹/₂ cup	50	A
Chunky	in Juice	¹/₂ cup	90	A
Fruit Cocktail	in Heavy Syrup	¹/₂ cup	90	A
Fruit Cocktail	in Juice, Sweetened	¹/₂ cup	90	A
Chunky		¹/₂ cup	40	A
Fruit Cocktail		¹/₂ cup	40	A
in Syrup		4 oz	96	A
Dried		4 oz	260	A
Dried		4 oz	300	A
Dried	Bits	4 oz	300	A
in Brine		¹/₂ cup	90	B−+
in Brine	50% Less Salt	¹/₂ cup	80	B−+
Trimmed		1 oz	42	A
Drained		1 cup	173	A−
Raw	Shelled	1 oz	52	A

"+" indicates the food meets minimum fiber requirements; "−" indicates the food has a high sodium content.

Food	Processing Category	Brand
Gooseberry	Fresh	
Gooseberry	Canned	Generic
Gourd, Dishcloth	Fresh	
Gourd, Wax	Fresh	
Gourd, White Floured	Fresh	
Grape	Canned	Generic
Grape	Canned	Generic
Grape	Canned	S & W
Grape, American	Fresh	
Grape, European	Fresh	
Grapefruit	Fresh	
Grapefruit	Fresh	
Grapefruit	Fresh	
Grapefruit	Fresh	
Grapefruit	Fresh	
Grapefruit	Canned	Generic
Grapefruit	Canned	Generic
Grapefruit	Canned	Generic
Grapefruit	Canned	S & W Nutradiet
Grapefruit	Canned	S & W Unsweetened
Great Northern Bean	Fresh	
Great Northern Bean	Canned	Allen's
Great Northern Bean	Canned	Allen's
Great Northern Bean	Canned	Green Giant/Joan of Arc
Great Northern Bean	Canned	Luck's
Green Bean	Fresh	
Green Bean	Fresh	
Green Bean	Canned	Generic
Green Bean	Canned	Generic
Green Bean	Canned	Generic
Green Bean	Canned	Generic
Green Bean	Canned	Allen's
Green Bean	Canned	Allen's
Green Bean	Canned	Allen's
Green Bean	Canned	Del Monte
Green Bean	Canned	Del Monte
Green Bean	Canned	Del Monte No Salt Added
Green Bean	Canned	Del Monte
Green Bean	Canned	Featherweight
Green Bean	Canned	Green Giant
Green Bean	Canned	Green Giant
Green Bean	Canned	Green Giant
Green Bean	Canned	Green Giant
Green Bean	Canned	Green Giant
Green Bean	Canned	Green Giant Pantry Express
Green Bean	Canned	Green Giant Pantry Express
Green Bean	Canned	S & W
Green Bean	Canned	S & W
Green Bean	Canned	S & W Premium Blue Lake
Green Bean	Canned	S & W Premium Golden
Green Bean	Canned	S & W Vertical Pack
Green Bean	Canned	S & W/Nutradiet
Green Bean	Canned	Stokeley

Major Description	Minor Description	Serving Size	Calories	Grade
	Trimmed	¹/₂ cup	34	A+
in Light Syrup		4 oz	83	A+
Raw	Trimmed and Sliced	¹/₂ cup	10	A+
Boiled	Cubed	¹/₂ cup	11	A–+
	Trimmed and Sliced	¹/₂ cup	8	A+
Thompson	in Heavy Syrup	¹/₂ cup	95	A+
Thompson	Seedless	¹/₂ cup	100	A+
Thompson	in Water	¹/₂ cup	45	A+
Concord, Niagara, Delaware		¹/₂ cup	29	A+
Thompson, Muscat, Tokay		¹/₂ cup	57	A+
Pink & Red, California	Sections	¹/₂ cup	43	A+
Red, Florida	Sections	¹/₂ cup	34	A+
White, California		¹/₂ cup	40	A+
White, California	Sections	¹/₂ cup	42	A+
White, Florida	Sections	¹/₂ cup	38	A+
in Juice		¹/₂ cup	42	A+
in Light Syrup		¹/₂ cup	68	A+
in Water		¹/₂ cup	41	A+
		¹/₂ cup	40	A+
		¹/₂ cup	40	A+
Boiled		¹/₂ cup	104	A+
		¹/₂ cup	105	A–+
Pork		¹/₂ cup	100	A–+
		¹/₂ cup	80	A–+
Pork		¹/₂ cup	110	B–+
Boiled		¹/₂ cup	22	A+
Raw		¹/₂ cup	17	A+
Drained		¹/₂ cup	23	A–+
in Liquid		¹/₂ cup	17	A+–
Low Sodium	in Liquid	¹/₂ cup	17	A+
Seasoned, in Liquid		¹/₂ cup	18	A–+
Cut or French Style		¹/₂ cup	20	A–+
Italian Style		¹/₂ cup	18	A–+
Shelly Beans		¹/₂ cup	35	B–+
Seasoned, in Liquid	French Style	¹/₂ cup	20	A–+
Whole, Cut or French Style		¹/₂ cup	20	A–+
Cut	in Liquid	¹/₂ cup	20	A+
Cut	Italian Style	¹/₂ cup	25	A–+
Cut		¹/₂ cup	25	A+
	50% Less Salt	¹/₂ cup	18	A–+
Almondine		¹/₂ cup	45	D–+
Cut		¹/₂ cup	16	A–+
French Style		¹/₂ cup	16	A–+
Kitchen Sliced		¹/₂ cup	16	A–+
Cut		¹/₂ cup	12	A–+
Potatoes & Mushrooms		¹/₂ cup	50	C–+
Dilled		¹/₂ cup	60	A–+
Whole, Cut or French Style	Stringless	¹/₂ cup	20	A–+
French Style or Cut		¹/₂ cup	20	A–+
Cut		¹/₂ cup	20	A–+
Whole		¹/₂ cup	20	A–+
Cut		¹/₂ cup	20	A+
		¹/₂ cup	20	A–+

"+" indicates the food meets minimum fiber requirements; "–" indicates the food has a high sodium content.

Food	Processing Category	Brand
Green Bean	Canned	Stokeley No Salt or Sugar
Green Bean	Freeze-dried	Mountain House
Green Bean	Frozen	Birds Eye
Green Bean	Frozen	Birds Eye Deluxe
Green Bean	Frozen	Birds Eye Deluxe
Green Bean	Frozen	Birds Eye Farm Fresh
Green Bean	Frozen	Birds Eye Portion Pack
Green Bean	Frozen	Birds Eye
Green Bean	Frozen	Frosty Acres
Green Bean	Frozen	Frosty Acres
Green Bean	Frozen	Frosty Acres
Green Bean	Frozen	Green Giant
Green Bean	Frozen	Green Giant
Green Bean	Frozen	Green Giant
Green Bean	Frozen	Green Giant Harvest Fresh
Green Bean	Frozen	Seabrook
Green Bean	Frozen	Seabrook
Green Bean	Frozen	Seabrook
Green Bean	Frozen	Seabrook
Green Bean	Frozen	Southern
Green Bean	Frozen	Southern
Green Bean	Frozen	Stokely Singles
Green Bean Combinations	Frozen	Birds Eye Combinations
Green Bean Combinations	Frozen	Birds Eye International
Green Bean Combinations	Frozen	Green Giant Garden Gourmet
Green Bean Combinations	Frozen	Stouffer's
Guava, Common	Fresh	
Guava, Strawberry	Fresh	
Hickory Nut	Bulk	
Hominy	Canned	Generic
Hominy	Canned	Generic
Honey	Canned or Jarred	All Varieties
Honeydew	Fresh	
Horse Bean	See Fava Bean	
Hyacinth Bean	Bulk	
Hyacinth Bean	Bulk	
Jackfruit	Fresh	
Java Plum	Fresh	
Jerusalem Artichoke	Fresh	
Jew's-Ear	Fresh	
Jujube	Fresh	
Jute	Fresh	
Kale, Scotch	Fresh	
Kale, Scotch	Fresh	
Kale	Fresh	
Kale	Fresh	
Kale	Canned	Allen's
Kale	Frozen	Frosty Acres
Kale	Frozen	Seabrook
Kale	Frozen	Southern
Kidney Bean	Fresh	
Kidney Bean	Fresh	
Kidney Bean	Canned	Generic

Major Description	Minor Description	Serving Size	Calories	Grade
		1/2 cup	20	A+
		1/2 cup	35	A+
Italian Style		3 oz	30	A+
Petite		3 oz	20	A+
Whole		3 oz	25	A+
Whole		3 oz	30	A+
Cut		3 oz	25	A+
Cut or French Style		3 oz	25	A+
Cut		3 oz	25	A+
French Style		3 oz	25	A+
Italian Style		3 oz	30	A+
		1/2 cup	14	A+
in Butter Sauce		1 serving, 5.5 oz	60	B−+
in Butter Sauce, Cut		1/2 cup	30	B−+
Cut		1/2 cup	16	A−+
Cut		3 oz	25	A+
French Style		3 oz	25	A+
Italian Style		3 oz	30	A+
Whole		3 oz	25	A+
French Style		3.5 oz	34	A+
Whole		3.5 oz	33	A+
Cut		1/2 cup	30	A+
French Style		3 oz	50	C−+
Bavarian Style		3 oz	100	D−+
& Mushroom, Creamy		1 pkg	220	D−+
Mushroom Casserole		1/2 cup	130	D−+
		1 medium, 4 oz	45	A+
		1 medium, 2 oz	4	B+
Dried	Shelled	1 oz	187	D
Golden		1/2 cup	64	A−
Mexican Style	White	1/2 cup	57	A−
		1 Tbsp	Approx 60	A
	Cubed	1/2 cup	30	A+
Dried	Raw	1/2 cup	362	A+
Raw	Trimmed	1/2 cup	19	A+
Trimmed		1 oz	27	A
Seeded		1/2 cup	41	A
Trimmed	Sliced	1/2 cup	57	A
Trimmed	Sliced	1/2 cup	13	A+
Raw	with Seeds	1 oz	21	A+
Raw	Trimmed	1/2 cup	5	A+
Boiled, Drained	Chopped	1/2 cup	18	A−+
Raw	Chopped	1/2 cup	14	A−+
Boiled, Drained	Chopped	1/2 cup	36	A+
Raw	Chopped	1/2 cup	17	A+
Chopped		1/2 cup	25	B
Chopped		3 oz	25	A+
Chopped		3 oz	25	A+
Chopped		3.5 oz	30	A
All Varieties	Boiled	1/2 cup	Approx 112	A+
All Varieties	Raw	1/2 cup	Approx 306	A+
All Varieties	in Liquid	1/2 cup	104	A−

"+" indicates the food meets minimum fiber requirements; "−" indicates the food has a high sodium content.

Food	Processing Category	Brand
Kidney Bean	Canned	B & M
Kidney Bean	Canned	Friends
Kidney Bean	Canned	S & W/Nutradiet
Kidney Bean, Sprouted	Fresh	
Kiwifruit	Fresh	
Kohlrabi	Fresh	
Kumquat	Fresh	
Leek	Fresh	
Leek	Fresh	
Leek	Freeze Dried	All Brands
Lemon	Fresh	
Lentil	Fresh	
Lentil	Fresh	
Lentil Dinner	Canned	Health Valley Fast Menu
Lentil Dinner	Canned	Health Valley Fast Menu
Lentil Pilaf	Mix	Casbah
Lentil Rice Loaf	Frozen	Harvest Bake
Lentil Sprouted	Fresh	
Lettuce	Fresh	
Lettuce	Fresh	
Lettuce	Fresh	
Lettuce	Fresh	
Lima Bean	Fresh	
Lima Bean	Fresh	
Lima Bean	Canned	Dennison's
Lima Bean	Canned	Featherweight
Lima Bean	Canned	Green Giant/Joan of Arc
Lima Bean	Canned	Joan of Arc
Lima Bean	Canned	Luck's
Lima Bean	Canned	Luck's
Lima Bean	Canned	S & W
Lima Bean	Canned	Stokely
Lima Bean	Canned	Stokely No Salt or Sugar Added
Lima Bean	Canned	Van Camp's
Lima Bean	Frozen	Generic
Lima Bean	Frozen	Generic
Lima Bean	Frozen	A & P
Lima Bean	Frozen	Birds Eye
Lima Bean	Frozen	Frosty Acres
Lima Bean	Frozen	Green Giant
Lima Bean	Frozen	Seabrook
Lima Bean	Frozen	Seabrook
Lima Bean	Frozen	Southern
Lima Bean	Frozen	Stokely Singles
Lime	Fresh	
Litchi	Bulk	Generic
Litchi	Bulk	Generic
Loganberry	Fresh	
Loganberry	Frozen	Generic

Major Description	Minor Description	Serving Size	Calories	Grade
Red, Baked		$^1/_2$ cup	125	B–+
Red, Baked		$^1/_2$ cup	170	A–+
		$^1/_2$ cup	90	A
Mature Seeds	Raw	$^1/_2$ cup	27	A
Trimmed		1 medium, 3 oz	46	A+
Raw	Trimmed, Sliced	$^1/_2$ cup	19	A+
Raw		1 medium, .7 oz	12	A+
Boiled	Chopped	$^1/_2$ cup	16	A+
Raw	Trimmed	1 medium, 10 oz	76	A+
		$^1/_4$ cup	3	A+
		1 medium, 2" diameter	22	A+
Boiled	Green or Red	$^1/_2$ cup	115	A+
Raw	Green or Red	$^1/_2$ cup	324	A+
Garden Style Vegetables		$7^1/_2$ oz	160	B–+
Vegetables		5 oz	80	A–+
Cooked		$^1/_2$ cup	100	A
		4 oz	190	D–
Raw		$^1/_2$ cup	40	A+
Bib, Boston or Butterhead		2 inner leaves or .5 oz	2	A+
Cob or Romaine		1 inner leaf or .4 oz	2	A+
Iceberg		1 leaf or .7 oz	3	A+
Loose-leaf		1 leaf or .4 oz	2	A+
All Varieties	Boiled	$^1/_2$ cup	104	A+
All Varieties	Raw	$^1/_2$ cup	88	A+
with Ham		Approx $^1/_2$ cup	133	B–+
		$^1/_2$ cup	80	A+
		$^1/_2$ cup	80	A–+
Butter Beans	in Brine	$^1/_2$ cup	90	A–+
Green, with Pork		Approx $^1/_2$ cup	117	B–+
with Pork		Approx $^1/_2$ cup	120	B–+
		$^1/_2$ cup	100	A–+
		$^1/_2$ cup	80	A–+
		$^1/_2$ cup	80	A+
Butter Beans		$^1/_2$ cup	81	A–+
Baby	Boiled	$^1/_2$ cup	95	A+
Fordhook	Boiled	$^1/_2$ cup	85	A+
Baby		3.3 oz	130	A+
Baby		3.3 oz	110	A+
Baby		3.3 oz	130	A+
	in Butter Sauce	$^1/_2$ cup	100	B–+
Baby		3.3 oz	130	A+
Baby	in Butter Sauce	3.3 oz	140	A–+
Baby		3.5 oz	135	A+
	in Butter Sauce	4 oz	140	A–+
Raw		1 medium, 2" diameter	20	A
Dried		1 oz	79	A
Raw		1 medium, .6 oz	6	A
Trimmed		$^1/_2$ cup	45	A
		$^1/_2$ cup	40	A

"+" indicates the food meets minimum fiber requirements; "–" indicates the food has a high sodium content.

Food	Processing Category	Brand
Longan	Fresh	
Longan, Dried	Bulk	Generic
Longbean	Fresh	
Longbean, Dried	Bulk	Generic
Loquat	Fresh	
Lotus Root	Fresh	
Lotus Seed	Bulk	Generic
Lupin	Fresh	
Macadamia Nut	Bulk	Generic
Mango	Fresh	
Miso	Packaged	Generic
Miso	Packaged	Generic
Miso	Packaged	Generic
Miso	Packaged	Generic
Miso	Packaged	Generic
Moth Bean	Fresh	
Moth Bean	Fresh	
Mulberry	Fresh	
Mung Bean	Fresh	
Mung Bean	Fresh	
Mung Bean Sprouted	Fresh	
Mung Bean Sprouted	Canned	Generic
Mungo Bean	Fresh	
Mushroom	Canned	Generic
Mushroom	Canned	Allen's
Mushroom	Canned	B in B
Mushroom	Canned	B in B
Mushroom	Canned	Empress
Mushroom	Canned	Green Giant
Mushroom	Canned	Green Giant
Mushroom, Oriental Straw	Canned	All Brands
Mushroom, Oyster	Fresh	
Mushroom, Shiitake	Fresh	
Mushroom, Shiitake	Fresh	
Mushroom, White	Fresh	
Mushroom, White	Frozen	Birds Eye Deluxe
Mushroom, White	Frozen	Stilwell Quick Krisp
Mustard Greens	Fresh	
Mustard Greens	Fresh	
Mustard Greens	Canned	Generic
Mustard Greens	Frozen	Generic
Mustard Greens	Frozen	Frosty Acres
Mustard Greens	Frozen	Seabrook
Mustard Seed	Dry	All Brands
Navy Bean	Fresh	
Navy Bean	Fresh	
Navy Bean	Canned	Generic
Nectarine	Fresh	
Oheloberry	Fresh	
Okra	Fresh	
Okra	Fresh	
Okra	Frozen	Generic
Okra	Frozen	Seabrook

Major Description	Minor Description	Serving Size	Calories	Grade
Raw	Shelled & Seeded	1 oz	17	A
Raw		1 oz	81	A
Boiled		$^1/_2$ cup	25	A+
Boiled		$^1/_2$ cup	102	A+
Raw		1 medium, .6 oz	5	A
Raw	Trimmed	1 oz	16	A
Dried		1 oz	94	A
Raw		$^1/_2$ cup	98	B+
Roasted	Whole	$^1/_2$ cup	480	D
Peeled, Seeded	Sliced	$^1/_2$ cup	54	A+
		1 oz	58	B—+
Kome-koji Dark Yellow	Rice Malt	1 oz	53	B—
Kome-koji Sweet	Rice Malt	1 oz	62	A—
Mame-koji	Soybean Malt	1 oz	62	D—
Mugi-koji	Barley Malt	1 oz	56	B—
Boiled		$^1/_2$ cup	103	A+
Raw		$^1/_2$ cup	337	A+
		$^1/_2$ cup	31	A+
Boiled		$^1/_2$ cup	107	A+
Raw		$^1/_2$ cup	361	A+
Raw		$^1/_2$ cup	16	A+
Stir-fry		$^1/_2$ cup	31	A+
Raw		$^1/_2$ cup	365	A
Pieces		$^1/_2$ cup	36	A
Pieces & Stems		$^1/_2$ cup	20	A—
		$^1/_2$ cup	24	A—+
Garlic		$^1/_2$ cup	24	A—+
Pieces & Stems		$^1/_2$ cup	28	A—
in Butter Sauce		$^1/_2$ cup	30	B—+
Whole, Pieces & Stems		$^1/_2$ cup	24	A—+
		$^1/_2$ cup	24	A—+
		1 oz	7	A+
Cooked		1 oz	16	A+
Dried		1 oz	84	A+
Raw	Pieces	$^1/_2$ cup	9	B+
Whole		2.6 oz	20	A+
Battered		2 oz	140	D—
Boiled		$^1/_2$ cup	10	B+
Raw, Trimmed	Chopped	$^1/_2$ cup	7	A+
		$^1/_2$ cup	20	D—
		1 oz	7	A—+
		3.3 oz	20	A+
Chopped		3.3 oz	20	A+
Yellow		1 tsp	15	D
Boiled		$^1/_2$ cup	129	A+
Raw		$^1/_2$ cup	348	A+
in Liquid		$^1/_2$ cup	150	A—+
Pitted		1 medium, 2"	67	A+
		$^1/_2$ cup	39	A+
Boiled		4 oz	36	A+
Raw	Trimmed	4 oz	44	A+
Boiled, Drained		4 oz	42	A+
Whole		3.3 oz	30	A+

"+" indicates the food meets minimum fiber requirements; "–" indicates the food has a high sodium content.

Food	Processing Category	Brand
Olive	Pickled, Canned or Bottled	All Brands
Olive, Green	Pickled, Canned or Bottled	All Brands
Olive, Green	Pickled, Canned or Bottled	All Brands
Olive, Ripe	Pickled Canned or Bottled	All Brands
Onion	Fresh	
Onion	Canned	Generic
Onion Ring	Frozen	
Onion Ring	Frozen	Farm-Rich Batter Dipt
Onion Ring	Frozen	Farm-Rich Onion O
Onion Ring	Frozen	Ore-Ida Onion Ringers
Onion Ring	Frozen	Stillwell
Onion, Dried or Dehydrated	All Forms	All Brands
Onion, Green	See Scallion	
Onion, Welsh	Fresh	
Orange	Fresh	
Papaya	Fresh	
Parsley	Fresh	
Parsley Root	Fresh	
Parsley, Dried	All Forms	Generic
Parsnip	Fresh	
Passion Fruit	Fresh	
Peach	Fresh	
Peach	Canned	All Brands
Peach	Canned	All Brands
Peach	Canned	All Brands
Peach	Canned	All Brands
Peach	Canned	All Brands
Peach	Canned	All Brands
Peach	Canned	All Brands
Peach	Frozen	All Brands
Peach, Dehydrated	All Forms	All Brands
Peach, Dried	All Forms	All Brands
Peach, Dried	All Forms	All Brands
Peach, Dried	All Forms	All Brands
Peanut	Fresh	All Varieties
Pear	Fresh	
Pear, Bartlett	Canned	All Brands
Pear, Bartlett	Canned	All Brands
Pear, Bartlett	Canned	All Brands
Pear, Bartlett	Canned	All Brands
Pear, Bartlett	Canned	All Brands
Pear, Bartlett	Canned	Del Monte Lite
Pear, Bartlett	Canned	S & W/Nutradiet
Pear, Bartlett	Canned	S & W/Nutradiet
Pear, Bartlett, Dried	All Forms	All Brands
Pear, Bartlett, Dried	All Forms	All Brands
Peas & Onions	Canned	Generic
Peas & Carrots	Canned	All Brands
Peas & Carrots	Canned	All Brands
Peas & Onions	Canned	Green Giant

Major Description	Minor Description	Serving Size	Calories	Grade
All Varieties & Sizes		1 oz	46	D–
Pitted		1 oz	33	D–+
with Pits		10 large or 1.6 oz	45	D–+
All Sizes		10 large or 1.6 oz	51	D–+
Raw, All Varieties	Chopped	$^1/_2$ cup	30	A+
in Liquid		4 oz	22	A–+
Breaded		2 oz	231	D
Battered, Precooked		2 oz	130	D–
Crispy		5 rings	190	D–
		2 oz	140	D–
Battered		2 oz	165	D
Flakes		$^1/_4$ cup	45	A
Trimmed		1 oz	10	A+
All Commercial Varieties		1 medium, 2$^1/_2$" diameter	62	A+
Trimmed	Cubed	$^1/_2$ cup	27	A+
Raw	Trimmed	1 oz	9	A+
		1 oz	3	D–+
		1 tsp	1	B–+
Raw	Trimmed	1 oz	21	A+
Trimmed		1 medium, 1.2 oz	27	A+
Whole		1 medium, 2$^1/_2$" diameter	37	A+
Freestone or Yellow Cling	Diet	$^1/_2$ cup	30	A
in Extra-Heavy Syrup	Halves or Slices	$^1/_2$ cup	126	A
in Extra-Light Syrup, Yellow Cling	Halves or Slices	$^1/_2$ cup	52	A
in Heavy Syrup	Halves or Slices	$^1/_2$ cup	95	A
in Juice	Halves or Slices	$^1/_2$ cup	55	A
in Light Syrup, Yellow Cling	Halves or Slices	$^1/_2$ cup	68	A
in Water, Yellow Cling	Halves or Slices	$^1/_2$ cup	29	A
Sliced	Sweetened	$^1/_2$ cup	107	A
Uncooked		$^1/_2$ cup	188	A
Sulfured	Halves, Sweetened	$^1/_2$ cup	139	A
Sulfured	Halves, Unsweetened	$^1/_2$ cup	91	A
Sulfured	Uncooked	$^1/_2$ cup	192	A+
		1 oz	160	D
Whole	3$^1/_2$" × 2$^1/_2$"	1 medium, 3$^1/_2$ × 2$^1/_2$	98	A+
in Extra-heavy Syrup	Halves	$^1/_2$ cup	127	A+
in Extra-light Syrup	Halves	$^1/_2$ cup	58	A+
in Heavy Syrup	Halves	$^1/_2$ cup	94	A+
in Juice	Halves	$^1/_2$ cup	62	A+
in Light Syrup	Halves	$^1/_2$ cup	72	A+
Bartlett	Halves or Slices	$^1/_2$ cup	50	A+
Bartlett	Peeled, Unsweetened	$^1/_2$ cup	35	A
in Water	Halves	$^1/_2$ cup	36	A+
Sulfured	Halves, Sweetened	$^1/_2$ cup	196	A+
Sulfured	Halves, Unsweetened	$^1/_2$ cup	163	A+
		$^1/_2$ cup	30	A–+
in Liquid		$^1/_2$ cup	48	A–+
in Liquid	Low Sodium	$^1/_2$ cup	48	A+
Pearl Onions		$^1/_2$ cup	50	A–+

"+" indicates the food meets minimum fiber requirements; "–" indicates the food has a high sodium content.

Food	Processing Category	Brand
Peas & Onions	Canned	S & W
Peas & Carrots	Frozen	Generic
Peas & Onions	Frozen	Generic
Peas & Carrots	Frozen	Frosty Acres
Peas & Carrots	Frozen	Seabrook
Peas & Carrots	Frozen	Southern
Peas & Onions	Frozen	Birds Eye
Peas & Onions	Frozen	Birds Eye
Peas & Onions	Frozen	Frosty Acres
Peas, Green or Sweet	Fresh	
Peas, Green or Sweet	Fresh	
Peas, Green or Sweet	Canned	Generic
Peas, Green or Sweet	Canned	Generic
Peas, Green or Sweet	Canned	Del Monte
Peas, Green or Sweet	Canned	Del Monte No Salt Added
Peas, Green or Sweet	Canned	Featherweight
Peas, Green or Sweet	Canned	Green Giant
Peas, Green or Sweet	Canned	Green Giant
Peas, Green or Sweet	Canned	Green Giant
Peas, Green or Sweet	Canned	Green Giant 50% Less Salt
Peas, Green or Sweet	Canned	S & W Perfection
Peas, Green or Sweet	Canned	S & W Petit Pois
Peas, Green or Sweet	Canned	S & W/Nutradiet
Peas, Green or Sweet	Canned	Stokely
Peas, Green or Sweet	Canned	Stokely
Peas, Green or Sweet	Canned	Stokely No Salt or Sugar Added
Peas, Green or Sweet	Freeze-dried	Mountain House
Peas, Green or Sweet	Frozen	Generic
Peas, Green or Sweet	Frozen	Birds Eye
Peas, Green or Sweet	Frozen	Birds Eye Combinations
Peas, Green or Sweet	Frozen	Birds Eye Deluxe
Peas, Green or Sweet	Frozen	Birds Eye Portion Pack
Peas, Green or Sweet	Frozen	Frosty Acres
Peas, Green or Sweet	Frozen	Frosty Acres
Peas, Green or Sweet	Frozen	Green Giant
Peas, Green or Sweet	Frozen	Green Giant
Peas, Green or Sweet	Frozen	Green Giant Harvest Fresh
Peas, Green or Sweet	Frozen	Green Giant Harvest Fresh
Peas, Green or Sweet	Frozen	Green Giant One Serving
Peas, Green or Sweet	Frozen	Health Valley
Peas, Green or Sweet	Frozen	Seabrook
Peas, Green or Sweet	Frozen	Seabrook
Peas, Green or Sweet	Frozen	Southern
Peas, Green or Sweet	Frozen	Southern
Peas, Green or Sweet	Frozen	Stokely Singles
Peas, Green or Sweet	Frozen	Stokely Singles
Peas, Green, Combinations	Frozen	Birds Eye Combinations
Peas, Green, Combinations	Frozen	Budget Gourmet Side Dish
Peas, Green, Combinations	Frozen	Budget Gourmet Side Dish
Peas, Green, Combinations	Frozen	Green Giant Valley
Peas, Green, Combinations	Frozen	Le Sueur
Peas, Green, Combinations	Frozen	Le Sueur

Major Description	Minor Description	Serving Size	Calories	Grade
Pearl Onions, Tiny		1/2 cup	60	A–
Boiled, Drained		4 oz	54	A–+
Boiled, Drained		4 oz	51	A
Boiled, Drained		3.3 oz	60	A–+
Boiled, Drained		3.3 oz	60	A–+
Boiled, Drained		3.5 oz	64	A–
Pearl Onions		3.3 oz	70	A–+
Pearl Onions	in Cheese Sauce	5 oz	140	C–+
Pearl Onions		3.3 oz	70	A
Boiled, Drained		1/2 cup	67	A+
Raw	Shelled	1/2 cup	58	A+
in Liquid		1/2 cup	61	A–+
in Liquid	Low Sodium	1/2 cup	61	A+
in Liquid		1/2 cup	60	A–
in Liquid		1/2 cup	60	A
Sweet		1/2 cup	70	A
Drained	Early Peas	1/2 cup	50	A–+
Sweet		1/2 cup	50	A–+
Sweet	Mini, in Brine	1/2 cup	60	A–+
Drained		1/2 cup	50	A–+
Sweet		1/2 cup	70	A–
Drained	Early Peas	1/2 cup	70	A–
Sweet		1/2 cup	40	A
Drained	Early Peas	1/2 cup	60	A–
Sweet		1/2 cup	60	A–
Drained		1/2 cup	50	A
		1/2 cup	70	A
Boiled, Drained		4 oz	88	A+
		3.3 oz	80	A–+
in Cream Sauce		5 oz	180	D–+
Tender, Tiny		3.3 oz	60	A–+
		3 oz	70	A–+
		3.3 oz	80	A+
Tiny		3.3 oz	60	A–+
Sweet		3.3 oz	50	A–+
Sweet	in Butter Sauce	3.3 oz	80	B–+
Early June		3.3 oz	60	A–+
Sweet		3.3 oz	50	A–+
Early	in Butter Sauce	4.5 oz	90	B–+
		3.3 oz	65	A+
		3.3 oz	80	A+
Tiny		3.3 oz	60	A–+
		3.5 oz	79	A–
Tiny		3.5 oz	64	A
		4 oz	87	A–
Sweet	in Butter Sauce	4 oz	90	A–
Potatoes	in Cream Sauce	5 oz	190	D–
and Water Chestnuts		5 oz	120	B–
Carrots & Cauliflower	Cream Sauce	5 oz	147	C–
Le Sueur Style		1/2 cup	70	B–+
Mini, with Pea Pods & Water Chestnuts	in Butter Sauce	1/2 cup	80	B–+
Onions & Carrots		1/2 cup	80	C–+

"+" indicates the food meets minimum fiber requirements; "–" indicates the food has a high sodium content.

Food	Processing Category	Brand
Peas, Snow	Fresh	
Peas, Snow	Fresh	
Peas, Snow	Frozen	Generic
Peas, Snow	Frozen	Birds Eye Deluxe
Peas, Snow	Frozen	Birds Eye Deluxe
Peas, Snow	Frozen	Chun King
Pecan	Bulk	Generic
Pecan	Bulk	Generic
Pepper, Cherry	Jar	Progresso
Pepper, Cherry	Jar	Progresso
Pepper, Cherry	Jar	Vlasic
Pepper, Cherry	Jar	Vlasic
Pepper, Hot Chili	Fresh	
Pepper, Hot Chili	Canned	Del Monte
Pepper, Hot Chili	Canned	Old El Paso
Pepper, Hot Chili	Canned	Ortega
Pepper, Jalapeño	Canned or in Jars	Del Monte
Pepper, Jalapeño	Canned or in Jars	La Victoria
Pepper, Jalapeño	Canned or in Jars	La Victoria
Pepper, Jalapeño	Canned or in Jars	Old El Paso
Pepper, Jalapeño	Canned or in Jars	Ortega
Pepper, Jalapeño	Canned or in Jars	Vlasic
Pepper, Pepperoncini	Canned or in Jars	Progresso
Pepper, Pepperoncini	Canned or in Jars	Vlasic
Pepper, Stuffed	Frozen	Celetano
Pepper, Stuffed	Frozen	Stouffer's
Pepper, Sweet	Fresh	
Pepper, Sweet	Fresh	
Pepper, Sweet	Canned	Progresso
Pepper, Sweet	Canned	Progresso
Pepper, Sweet	Frozen	Seabrook
Pepper, Sweet	Frozen	Seabrook
Persimmon	Fresh	
Persimmon	Fresh	
Pickle	Jar	All Brands
Pickle	Jar	All Brands
Pickle	Jar	All Brands
Pickle	Jar	All Brands
Pickle	Jar	All Brands
Pickle	Jar	All Brands
Pigeon Pea	Fresh	
Pigeon Pea, Dried	Bulk	Generic
Pigeon Pea, Dried	Bulk	Generic
Pimiento	Canned or in Jars	All Brands
Pine Nut	Bulk	Generic
Pineapple	Fresh	
Pineapple	Canned or in Jars	
Pineapple	Canned or in Jars	All Brands
Pineapple	Canned or in Jars	All Brands
Pineapple	Canned or in Jars	All Brands
Pineapple	Canned or in Jars	All Brands
Pineapple	Canned or in Jars	All Brands

Major Description	Minor Description	Serving Size	Calories	Grade
Boiled, Drained		$^1/_2$ cup	34	A+
Raw		$^1/_2$ cup	30	A+
Boiled, Drained		4 oz	59	A+
Chinese Style		4 oz	46	A+
Sugar Snap		4 oz	69	A+
Chinese Style		4 oz	53	A
Honey Roasted		1 oz	200	D–
Raw or Roasted	Unsalted	1 oz	190	D
	Drained	1 oz	30	D
Hot		1 oz	15	A–
Hot		1 oz	10	A–
Mild		1 oz	8	A–
Green & Red, Raw	Chopped	$^1/_2$ cup	30	A+
Green	Whole or Diced, with Liquid	2 Tbsp	3	A–
Chopped		2 Tbsp	4	A–
Diced, Sliced or Strips		2 Tbsp	7	A–
Whole or Sliced	in Liquid	4 oz	30	B–
Marinated		4 oz	40	A–
Nacho		4 oz	4	A–
Whole	Pickled	4 oz	20	A–
Whole	or Diced	4 oz	40	A–
Mexican Style, Hot		4 oz	32	A–
Tuscan		1 oz	10	A+
Greek Style, Mild		1 oz	4	A–
Sweet Red		13 oz	350	D–
Green	Beef & Tomato	7.95 oz	200	C–
Green & Red	Boiled, Drained	$^1/_2$ cup	19	A+
Green & Red	Chopped, Raw	$^1/_2$ cup	13	A+
Fried		1 oz	60	D+
Roasted		1 oz	10	A–+
Green		1 oz	6	A
Red		1 oz	8	A
Japanese Style	Trimmed	1 oz	20	A+
Native	Trimmed	1 oz	36	A
Dill		1 oz	5	A–+
Dill	Low Sodium	1 oz	5	A+
Sour		1 oz	3	A–+
Sour	Low Sodium	1 oz	3	A–+
Sweet		1 oz	33	A–
Sweet	Low Sodium	1 oz	33	A
Raw	Shelled	$^1/_2$ cup	105	A+
Boiled		$^1/_2$ cup	102	A+
Raw		$^1/_2$ cup	350	A+
		2 oz	13	A+
Dried		1 oz	14	A+
	Diced or Sliced	$^1/_2$ cup	39	A+
in Extra-Heavy Syrup		$^1/_2$ cup	109	A
in Heavy Syrup		$^1/_2$ cup	100	A
in Juice	All Cuts	$^1/_2$ cup	70	A
in Light Syrup		$^1/_2$ cup	66	A
in Water	Slices	$^1/_2$ cup	40	A+
Trimmed	Diced	$^1/_2$ cup	39	A+

"+" indicates the food meets minimum fiber requirements; "–" indicates the food has a high sodium content.

Food	Processing Category	Brand
Pineapple	Canned or in Jars	S & W/Nutradiet
Pineapple	Frozen	Generic
Pink Bean	Fresh	
Pink Bean	Fresh	
Pinto Bean	Fresh	
Pinto Bean	Fresh	
Pinto Bean	Canned	Generic
Pinto Bean	Canned	Allen's
Pinto Bean	Canned	Gebhardt
Pinto Bean	Canned	Green Giant/Joan of Arc
Pinto Bean	Canned	Luck's 15 oz
Pinto Bean	Canned	Old El Paso
Pinto Bean	Canned	Progresso
Pinto Bean	Frozen	Generic
Pistachio Nut	Bulk	Generic
Plantain	Fresh	
Plantain	Fresh	
Plum	Fresh	
Plum	Canned	All Brands
Plum	Canned	All Brands
Plum	Canned	All Brands
Plum	Canned	All Brands
Plum	Canned	All Brands
Pokeberry Shoots	Fresh	
Pomegrante	Fresh	
Poppy Seed	Bulk	Generic
Potato	Fresh	
Potato	Fresh	
Potato	Fresh	
Potato	Fresh	
Potato	Fresh	
Potato	Fresh	
Potato	Fresh	
Potato	Fresh	
Potato	Fresh	
Potato	Fresh	
Potato	Fresh	
Potato	Canned	Generic
Potato	Freeze-dried	Mountain House
Potato	Frozen	Generic
Potato	Frozen	Generic
Potato	Frozen	Generic
Potato	Frozen	Generic
Potato	Frozen	Generic
Potato	Frozen	Generic
Potato	Frozen	Generic
Potato	Frozen	Heinz Deep Fries
Potato	Frozen	Heinz Deep Fries
Potato	Frozen	Heinz Deep Fries
Potato	Frozen	Heinz Deep Fries
Potato	Frozen	Micro Magic
Potato	Frozen	Ore-Ida
Potato	Frozen	Ore-Ida

Major Description	Minor Description	Serving Size	Calories	Grade
Slices, Unsweetened		¹/₂ cup	60	A
Sweetened		¹/₂ cup	104	A
Boiled		¹/₂ cup	125	A+
Raw		¹/₂ cup	361	A+
Boiled		¹/₂ cup	117	A+
Raw		¹/₂ cup	326	A+
in Liquid		¹/₂ cup	93	A–+
		¹/₂ cup	105	A–
		¹/₂ cup	100	A–
		¹/₂ cup	90	A–+
Baked	Pork	¹/₂ can	220	B–+
		¹/₂ cup	100	A–+
		¹/₂ cup	110	A–+
Boiled		4 oz	184	A
Dried		¹/₂ cup	370	D+
Cooked	Slices	¹/₂ cup	89	A
Raw	Slices	¹/₂ cup	91	A
with Pits		1 whole, 2¹/₂ oz	36	A+
in Extra-Heavy Syrup		¹/₂ cup	133	A+
in Heavy Syrup		¹/₂ cup	115	A+
in Juice		¹/₂ cup	73	A+
in Light Syrup		¹/₂ cup	79	A+
in Water		¹/₂ cup	51	A+
Raw, Trimmed		¹/₂ cup	18	A
		1 medium, 10 oz	100	A
Raw		1 tsp	15	D
Baked in Skin		4 oz	124	A
Baked in Skin	Pulp Only	4 oz	105	A+
Baked in Skin	Skin Only	4 oz	224	A+
Boiled in Skin		4 oz	99	A+
Boiled without Skin		4 oz	98	A
Hash Brown		4 oz	237	D
Mashed with Whole Milk		4 oz	87	A–
Mashed with Whole Milk	& Margarine or Butter	4 oz	120	C–
Scalloped	with Butter	4 oz	98	C–
Scalloped	with Margarine	4 oz	98	C–
		4 oz	45	A–
Hash Brown		1 cup	150	A
Cottage Cut		3 oz	186	C
French & French Fried		3 oz	189	C+
Hash Brown		3 oz	80	A
Hash Brown	Prepared in Butter Sauce	3 oz	151	D
Hash Brown	Prepared in Vegetable Oil	3 oz	186	D
Puffs	Prepared	3 oz	189	D–
Whole	Peeled	10 oz	221	A
Crinkle Cut or Regular		3 oz	150	C
French Fried		3 oz	160	C
Hash Brown	Butter & Onions	3 oz	110	D
Shoestring		3 oz	200	D
French Fried		3 oz	290	D
Cottage Cut		3 oz	120	C
French & French Fried	Golden Fries	3 oz	120	B

"+" indicates the food meets minimum fiber requirements; "–" indicates the food has a high sodium content.

Food	Processing Category	Brand
Potato	Frozen	Ore-Ida
Potato	Frozen	Ore-Ida
Potato	Frozen	Ore-Ida
Potato	Frozen	Ore-Ida Cheddar Browns
Potato	Frozen	Seabrook
Potato	Frozen	Seabrook
Potato	Frozen	Seabrook
Potato	Frozen	Weight Watchers
Potato	Frozen	Weight Watchers
Prickly Pear	Fresh	
Prune	Canned	Generic
Prune, Dehydrated	Bulk or Packaged	Generic
Prune, Dried	Bulk or Packaged	Generic
Prune, Dried	Bulk or Packaged	Generic
Prune, Dried	Bulk or Packaged	Generic
Pummelo	Fresh	
Pumpkin	Fresh	
Pumpkin	Canned	Del Monte
Pumpkin	Canned	Libby's
Pumpkin	Canned	Stokely
Pumpkin Seed	Fresh	
Pumpkin Seed	Fresh	
Quince	Fresh	
Quinoa	Fresh	
Radish	Fresh	
Radish, Black	Fresh	
Radish, Oriental	Fresh	
Radish, White Icicle	Fresh	
Raisin	Bulk	All Brands
Raspberry	Fresh	
Raspberry	Canned	Generic
Raspberry	Frozen	Generic
Red Bean	Canned	Allen's
Red Bean	Canned	B & M
Red Bean	Canned	Green Giant/Joan of Arc
Red Bean	Canned	Hunt's
Red Bean	Canned	Van Camp's
Red Kidney, Dark	Canned	Joan of Arc
Red Kidney, Light	Canned	Joan of Arc
Red Kidney, Light	Canned	Joan of Arc
Refried Beans	Canned	Bearitos Organic
Refried Beans	Canned	Bearitos Organic
Refried Beans	Canned	Bearitos Organic No Salt
Refried Beans	Canned	Del Monte
Refried Beans	Canned	Del Monte
Refried Beans	Canned	Gebhardt
Refried Beans	Canned	Gebhardt
Refried Beans	Canned	Old El Paso
Refried Beans	Canned	Old El Paso
Refried Beans	Canned	Old El Paso
Refried Beans	Canned	Old El Paso
Refried Beans	Canned	Old El Paso
Refried Beans	Canned	Old El Paso

Major Description	Minor Description	Serving Size	Calories	Grade
Hash Brown	Microwave	3 oz	195	D–
Hash Brown	Shredded	3 oz	70	A
Shoestring		3 oz	140	C
Hash Brown	with Cheddar Cheese	3 oz	90	B–
Cottage Cut		3 oz	120	C
Crinkle Cut or Regular		3 oz	120	B
Shoestring		3 oz	140	C
Baked	Broccoli & Cheese	3 oz	69	B–+
Vegetable Primavera		3 oz	66	B–+
Trimmed		1 medium, 5 oz	12	A+
	in Heavy Syrup	¹/₂ cup	123	A+
Uncooked		¹/₂ cup	224	A+
Cooked, Stewed	Sweetened, with Pits	¹/₂ cup	147	A
Cooked, Stewed	Unsweetened, with Pits	¹/₂ cup	113	A+
Uncooked		¹/₂ cup	193	A+
Trimmed	Sections	¹/₂ cup	36	A
Cooked	Mashed	¹/₂ cup	24	A+
		¹/₂ cup	35	A
		¹/₂ cup	42	A+
		¹/₂ cup	40	A
Roasted Whole in Shell		¹/₂ cup	142	C+
Roasted Whole in Shell	Salted	¹/₂ cup	142	C–+
Trimmed		1 medium, 5 oz	53	A+
		¹/₂ cup	635	A
Trimmed	Sliced	¹/₂ cup	10	B–+
Trimmed	Sliced	¹/₂ cup	10	A+
Trimmed	Sliced	¹/₂ cup	8	A+
Trimmed	Sliced	¹/₂ cup	7	A–+
Seedless	All Varieties	¹/₂ cup	219	A+
Trimmed		¹/₂ cup	31	A+
Red, in Heavy Syrup		¹/₂ cup	117	A
Sweetened		¹/₂ cup	128	A+
		¹/₂ cup	115	A–+
Small, Baked Style		¹/₂ cup	111	B–+
		¹/₂ cup	90	A–+
Small		¹/₂ cup	91	A–
		¹/₂ cup	97	A–
in Brine		¹/₂ cup	90	A–+
in Brine		¹/₂ cup	90	A–+
in Brine	50% Less Salt	¹/₂ cup	90	A–+
		4 oz	120	A–
Spicy		4 oz	121	B–+
		4 oz	116	B
		¹/₂ cup	130	A–
Spicy		¹/₂ cup	130	A–
		¹/₂ cup	143	A–
Jalapeño Pepper		¹/₂ cup	120	B–
		¹/₂ cup	110	A–+
Cheese		¹/₂ cup	72	B–+
Green Chile		¹/₂ cup	98	A–+
Sausage		¹/₂ cup	360	C–
Spicy		¹/₂ cup	70	B–+
Vegetarian		¹/₂ cup	140	A–+

"+" indicates the food meets minimum fiber requirements; "–" indicates the food has a high sodium content.

Food	Processing Category	Brand
Refried Beans	Canned	Rosarita
Refried Beans	Mix	Fantastic Foods
Rhubarb	Fresh	
Rhubarb	Frozen	Generic
Roman Bean	Canned	Progresso
Rutabaga	Fresh	
Salsify (Oyster Plant)	Fresh	
Sapote	Fresh	
Scallion	Fresh	
Seaweed, Agar	Fresh	
Seaweed, Irish Moss	Fresh	
Seaweed, Kelp	Fresh	
Seaweed, Laver	Fresh	
Seaweed, Spirulina	Fresh	
Seaweed, Wakame	Fresh	
Shallot	Fresh	
Shallot	Freeze-dried	Generic
Soursop	Fresh	
Soy Protein	Bulk or Packaged	Generic
Soy Protein	Bulk or Packaged	Generic
Soy Protein	Bulk or Packaged	Generic
Soybean [1]	Fresh	
Soybean, Dried	Bulk	Generic
Soybean, Dried	Bulk	Generic
Soybean, Dried	Bulk	Generic
Soybean, Green	Fresh	
Soybean, Green	Fresh	
Soybean, Sprouted	Fresh	
Soybean, Sprouted	Fresh	
Spinach	Fresh	
Spinach	Fresh	
Spinach	Canned	Allen's
Spinach	Canned	Allen's Low Sodium
Spinach	Canned	Del Monte
Spinach	Canned	Del Monte No Salt Added
Spinach	Canned	Featherweight
Spinach	Canned	S & W Premium Northwest
Spinach	Canned	Stokely
Spinach	Frozen	Generic
Spinach	Frozen	Birds Eye
Spinach	Frozen	Birds Eye Combinations
Spinach	Frozen	Birds Eye Portion Pack
Spinach	Frozen	Frosty Acres
Spinach	Frozen	Green Giant
Spinach	Frozen	Green Giant
Spinach	Frozen	Green Giant Harvest Fresh
Spinach	Frozen	Green Giant Polybag
Spinach	Frozen	Seabrook
Spinach	Frozen	Southern
Spinach	Frozen	Stouffer's
Spinach, Mustard	Fresh	

[1] *Soybeans have high fat content but there is strong evidence that they provide cardiovascular benefits that make them a desirable food.*

Major Description	Minor Description	Serving Size	Calories	Grade
		¹/₂ cup	132	A–
Instant		¹/₂ cup	157	A–
Trimmed	Diced	¹/₂ cup	13	A+
		¹/₂ cup	14	A
		¹/₂ cup	110	A–+
Raw	Trimmed and Cubed	¹/₂ cup	25	A+
Raw	Sliced	¹/₂ cup	55	A+
Trimmed		1 medium, 11 oz	301	A
Chopped		¹/₂ cup	16	A+
Raw		1 oz	7	A
Raw		1 oz	14	A–
Raw		1 oz	12	A–+
Raw		1 oz	10	A–
Raw		1 oz	8	A–
Raw		1 oz	13	A–+
Trimmed	Chopped	¹/₄ cup	28	A
		¹/₄ cup	13	A
Trimmed	Chopped	¹/₂ cup	75	A+
Concentrate		1 oz	94	A–
Isolate		1 oz	96	A–
Isolate	No Sodium	1 oz	96	A
Raw		¹/₂ cup	387	D+
Boiled		¹/₂ cup	149	D
Dry Roasted		¹/₂ cup	387	D
Roasted		¹/₂ cup	405	D
Boiled		¹/₂ cup	127	D
Raw	Shelled	¹/₂ cup	188	D
Raw		¹/₂ cup	45	D+
Steamed		¹/₂ cup	38	D+
Boiled		¹/₂ cup	21	A–+
Raw	Trimmed	¹/₂ cup	6	A–+
Leaf	Sliced or Chopped, Curly	¹/₂ cup	28	B–+
No Salt Added		¹/₂ cup	28	B–+
Leaf	Whole or Chopped	¹/₂ cup	25	A–+
Leaf	in Liquid	¹/₂ cup	25	A–+
Leaf		¹/₂ cup	35	B+
		¹/₂ cup	25	A–+
		¹/₂ cup	30	A–+
		¹/₂ cup	22	A–+
Chopped		¹/₂ cup	20	A–+
Creamed		¹/₂ cup	60	D–+
Leaf		¹/₂ cup	20	A–+
Chopped		¹/₂ cup	20	A–+
Creamed		¹/₂ cup	70	C–+
in Butter Sauce	Cut	¹/₂ cup	40	D–+
Boiled		¹/₂ cup	25	A–+
Boiled		¹/₂ cup	25	A–+
Chopped or Leaf		¹/₂ cup	20	A–+
Chopped or Leaf		¹/₂ cup	25	A–+
Creamed		¹/₂ cup	170	D–+
Raw	Chopped	¹/₂ cup	16	A+

"+" indicates the food meets minimum fiber requirements; "–" indicates the food has a high sodium content.

Food	Processing Category	Brand
Spinach, New Zealand	Fresh	
Spinach, New Zealand	Fresh	
Spinach, Vine	Fresh	
Split Peas	Bulk	Generic
Squash	Frozen	Frosty Acres
Squash, Acorn	Fresh	
Squash, Acorn	Fresh	
Squash, Banana	Fresh	Frieda of California
Squash, Butternut	Fresh	
Squash, Butternut	Fresh	
Squash, Butternut	Frozen	Generic
Squash, Crookneck	Fresh	
Squash, Crookneck	Canned	Generic
Squash, Crookneck	Canned	Allen's
Squash, Crookneck	Frozen	Generic
Squash, Crookneck	Frozen	Generic
Squash, Hubbard	Fresh	
Squash, Hubbard	Fresh	
Squash, Marrow	Fresh	
Squash, Scallop	Fresh	
Squash, Spaghetti	Fresh	
Squash, Summer	Fresh	
Squash, Summer	Fresh	
Squash, Winter	Fresh	
Squash, Winter	Frozen	All Brands
Strawberry	Fresh	
Strawberry	Canned	Generic
Strawberry	Freeze-dried	Mountain House
Strawberry	Frozen	Generic
Strawberry	Frozen	Generic
Strawberry	Frozen	Birds Eye
Strawberry	Frozen	Birds Eye Quick Thaw Pouch
Strawberry	Frozen	Birds Eye Quick Thaw Pouch
Succotash	Fresh	
Succotash	Canned	Generic
Succotash	Canned	Generic
Succotash	Canned	S & W Country Style
Succotash	Canned	Stokely
Succotash	Frozen	Frosty Acres
Succotash	Frozen	Seabrook
Sugar Apple	Fresh	
Sunflower Seed	Bulk	Generic
Sunflower Seed	Bulk	Generic
Sweet Potato	Fresh	
Sweet Potato	Fresh	
Sweet Potato	Canned	Generic
Sweet Potato	Canned	Allen's
Sweet Potato	Frozen	Generic
Sweet Potato	Frozen	Mrs. Paul's
Sweet Potato	Frozen	Mrs. Paul's Sweets 'n Apples
Swiss Chard	Fresh	
Tamarind	Fresh	

Major Description	Minor Description	Serving Size	Calories	Grade
Boiled	Chopped	$^1/_2$ cup	11	A–+
Raw, Trimmed	Chopped	$^1/_2$ cup	4	B–+
Raw		$^1/_2$ cup	7	A+
Boiled	Green or Yellow	$^1/_2$ cup	116	A+
Cooked		$^1/_2$ cup	45	A+
Baked	Cubed	$^1/_2$ cup	57	A+
Boiled	Mashed	$^1/_2$ cup	41	A+
Baked		4 oz	72	A
Baked	Cubes	$^1/_2$ cup	41	A+
Raw	Cubes	$^1/_2$ cup	32	A+
	Mashed	$^1/_2$ cup	47	A+
Raw	Slices	$^1/_2$ cup	12	A+
No Salt Added		$^1/_2$ cup	15	A+
Yellow, Cut		$^1/_2$ cup	16	A–
Boiled	Slices	$^1/_2$ cup	18	A+
Yellow	Slices	$^1/_2$ cup	24	A
Baked	Cubes	$^1/_2$ cup	51	A+
Raw	Cubes	$^1/_2$ cup	23	A+
Raw	Trimmed	4 oz	16	B+
Raw	Trimmed and Sliced	$^1/_2$ cup	12	A+
Raw	Trimmed	$^1/_2$ cup	17	B+
Boiled	Sliced	$^1/_2$ cup	18	B+
Raw	Sliced	$^1/_2$ cup	13	A+
Baked	Sliced	$^1/_2$ cup	39	A+
Cooked		4 oz	44	A+
Trimmed		$^1/_2$ cup	23	A+
in Heavy Syrup		$^1/_2$ cup	117	A
		$^1/_2$ cup	90	A
Sweetened		$^1/_2$ cup	100	A
Unsweetened		$^1/_2$ cup	26	A+
in Light Syrup	Whole	$^1/_2$ cup	45	A+
in Light Syrup	Halves	$^1/_2$ cup	45	A
in Syrup	Halves	$^1/_2$ cup	60	A+
Boiled, Drained		$^1/_2$ cup	79	A
Cream-style Corn		$^1/_2$ cup	102	A–+
Whole Kernel Corn, in Liquid		$^1/_2$ cup	81	A–
		$^1/_2$ cup	80	A–
		$^1/_2$ cup	90	A–
Boiled, Drained		$^1/_2$ cup	100	A
Boiled, Drained		$^1/_2$ cup	100	A
		1 medium	146	A
Dried	Kernels	1 Tbsp	50	D
Dry or Oil Roasted	Kernels	1 Tbsp	50	D
Baked		1 medium, 5 oz	118	A+
Candied	with Butter or Margarine	4 oz	155	B
in Syrup	with Liquid	$^1/_2$ cup	90	A+
in Water, Cut		$^1/_2$ cup	70	A
Baked		4 oz	113	A+
Candied		4 oz	170	A
Candied, with Apples		4 oz	160	A
Trimmed	Chopped	$^1/_2$ cup	3	B–+
Trimmed		1 medium, .2 oz	5	A+

"+" indicates the food meets minimum fiber requirements; "–" indicates the food has a high sodium content.

Food	Processing Category	Brand
Tangerine	Fresh	
Tapioca, Pearl	Bulk	
Taro	Fresh	
Taro Chips	Bulk	Generic
Taro Leaf	Fresh	
Taro Shoots	Fresh	
Tempeh	Bulk	Generic
Tofu	Fresh	Generic
Tofu	Fresh	Generic
Tofu	Fresh	Generic
Tofu	Fresh	Generic
Tofu	Fresh	Generic
Tofu	Fresh	Generic
Tofu	Fresh	Generic
Tofu	All Forms	Azumaya
Tofu	All Forms	Azumaya
Tofu	All Forms	Azumaya
Tofu	All Forms	Azumaya
Tofu	All Forms	Jaclyn's
Tofu	All Forms	Jaclyn's
Tofu	All Forms	Mori-Nu Silken
Tofu	All Forms	Mori-Nu Silken
Tofu	All Forms	Mori-Nu Silken
Tofu	All Forms	Mori-Nu Silken
Tofu	All Forms	Nasoya
Tofu	All Forms	Nasoya
Tofu	All Forms	Spring Creek
Tofu	All Forms	Spring Creek
Tofu	All Forms	Spring Creek
Tomatillo	Fresh	Frieda of California
Tomato Pickled	in Jars	Claussen
Tomato Powder	Fresh	
Tomato, Green	Fresh	
Tomato, Peeled	Canned	Hunt's
Tomato, Peeled	Canned	Progresso
Tomato, Peeled	Canned	Progresso
Tomato, Red	Fresh	
Turnip	Fresh	
Turnip	Canned	Allen's
Turnip	Canned	Stokely
Turnip	Frozen	Generic
Turnip	Frozen	Generic
Turnip	Frozen	Southern Style
Turnip Greens	Fresh	
Turnip Greens	Fresh	
Turnip Greens	Canned	Generic
Turnip Greens	Frozen	
Turnip Greens	Frozen	Frosty Acres
Turnip Greens	Frozen	Seabrook
Turnip Greens	Frozen	Southern
Vegetables, Mixed	Canned	Del Monte
Vegetables, Mixed	Canned	Featherweight
Vegetables, Mixed	Canned	Green Giant Garden Medley

Major Description	Minor Description	Serving Size	Calories	Grade
		1 medium, 4 oz	37	A+
Dry		$^1/_2$ cup	260	A
Raw	Sliced	$^1/_2$ cup	56	A
		$^1/_2$ cup	57	D
Steamed		$^1/_2$ cup	18	B+
Raw	Trimmed	$^1/_2$ cup	5	A+
from Soybean		$^1/_2$ cup	165	C
	"Okara"	1 oz	22	B+
Dried, Frozen	"Koyadofu"	1 oz	136	D
Fried		1 oz	77	D
Grilled	"Yakidofu"	1 oz	25	D
Raw		1 oz	22	D
Salted, Fermented	"Fuyu"	1 oz	33	D–
Blue Label		1 oz	13	B
Green Label		1 oz	19	B
Name Age		1 oz	41	B
Red Label		1 oz	19	A
Black Bean Sauce		1 oz	25	B
Peanut Sauce		1 oz	24	C
Extra Firm		1 oz	17	B–
Firm		1 oz	17	C
Lite		1 oz	11	B–
Soft		1 oz	15	D
Flavored	Chinese Style, 5 Spice	1 oz	30	D
Firm Block		1 oz	25	D
Baked Barbeque		1 oz	13	D–
Baked Cajun		1 oz	12	D–
Baked Teriyaki		1 oz	11	D–
	Chopped	$^1/_2$ cup	21	B
Kosher		1 piece	9	A–
		1 oz	86	A+
Whole		1 medium, 4.75 oz	30	A+
Italian Style	Whole	$^1/_2$ cup	25	A–
Italian Style	Crushed	$^1/_2$ cup	40	A–
Italian Style	Whole	$^1/_2$ cup	20	A–
Boiled		$^1/_2$ cup	32	A+
Raw	Cubed	$^1/_2$ cup	18	A–+
Diced		$^1/_2$ cup	16	D–
		$^1/_2$ cup	20	A–
Boiled, Drained		1 oz	7	A–+
Mashed		1 oz	4	A–+
Diced		$^1/_2$ cup	17	A–
Boiled		$^1/_2$ cup	6	A–+
Raw, Trimmed		$^1/_2$ cup	7	A–+
in Liquid		$^1/_2$ cup	17	B–+
Boiled		$^1/_2$ cup	34	A+
Chopped		3.3 oz	20	A+
Chopped		3.3 oz	20	A+
Chopped		3.5 oz	25	A–
		$^1/_2$ cup	40	A–
		$^1/_2$ cup	40	A–
		$^1/_2$ cup	40	B–+

"+" indicates the food meets minimum fiber requirements; "–" indicates the food has a high sodium content.

Food	Processing Category	Brand
Vegetables, Mixed	Canned	Green Giant Pantry Express
Vegetables, Mixed	Canned	La Choy
Vegetables, Mixed	Canned	La Choy
Vegetables, Mixed	Canned	S & W Old Fashioned Harvest
Vegetables, Mixed	Canned	Stokely
Vegetables, Mixed	Canned	Stokely No Salt or Sugar Added
Vegetables, Mixed	Frozen	Birds Eye
Vegetables, Mixed	Frozen	Birds Eye Custom Cuisine
Vegetables, Mixed	Frozen	Birds Eye Custom Cuisine
Vegetables, Mixed	Frozen	Birds Eye Custom Cuisine
Vegetables, Mixed	Frozen	Birds Eye Custom Cuisine
Vegetables, Mixed	Frozen	Birds Eye Custom Cuisine
Vegetables, Mixed	Frozen	Birds Eye Custom Cuisine
Vegetables, Mixed	Frozen	Birds Eye Custom Cuisine
Vegetables, Mixed	Frozen	Birds Eye Custom Cuisine
Vegetables, Mixed	Frozen	Birds Eye International
Vegetables, Mixed	Frozen	Birds Eye International
Vegetables, Mixed	Frozen	Birds Eye International
Vegetables, Mixed	Frozen	Birds Eye International
Vegetables, Mixed	Frozen	Birds Eye International
Vegetables, Mixed	Frozen	Birds Eye International
Vegetables, Mixed	Frozen	Birds Eye International
Vegetables, Mixed	Frozen	Birds Eye Portion Pack
Vegetables, Mixed	Frozen	Birds Eye Stir-Fry
Vegetables, Mixed	Frozen	Birds Eye Stir-Fry
Vegetables, Mixed	Frozen	Frosty Acres
Vegetables, Mixed	Frozen	Frosty Acres
Vegetables, Mixed	Frozen	Frosty Acres
Vegetables, Mixed	Frozen	Frosty Acres
Vegetables, Mixed	Frozen	Frosty Acres
Vegetables, Mixed	Frozen	Frosty Acres
Vegetables, Mixed	Frozen	Green Giant
Vegetables, Mixed	Frozen	Green Giant
Vegetables, Mixed	Frozen	Green Giant American Mixtures
Vegetables, Mixed	Frozen	Green Giant American Mixtures
Vegetables, Mixed	Frozen	Green Giant American Mixtures
Vegetables, Mixed	Frozen	Green Giant American Mixtures
Vegetables, Mixed	Frozen	Green Giant American Mixtures
Vegetables, Mixed	Frozen	Green Giant American Mixtures
Vegetables, Mixed	Frozen	Green Giant American Mixtures
Vegetables, Mixed	Frozen	Green Giant American Mixtures
Vegetables, Mixed	Frozen	Green Giant Harvest Fresh
Vegetables, Mixed	Frozen	Health Valley
Vegetables, Mixed	Frozen	Kohl's
Vegetables, Mixed	Frozen	Ore-Ida
Vegetables, Mixed	Frozen	Seabrook
Vegetables, Mixed	Frozen	Southern
Vegetables, Mixed	Frozen	Stokely Singles
Vegetables, Mixed	Frozen	Stokely Singles
Vegetables, Mixed	Frozen	Stokely Singles
Vegetables, Mixed	Frozen	Stokely Singles
Vegetables, Mixed	Frozen	Stokely Singles
Walnut, Black	Bulk	Generic

Major Description	Minor Description	Serving Size	Calories	Grade
		¹/₂ cup	35	B–+
Chinese Style		¹/₂ cup	12	A–+
Chop Suey		¹/₂ cup	9	A–+
		¹/₂ cup	35	A–
		¹/₂ cup	40	A–
		¹/₂ cup	40	A
		3.3 oz	60	A+
Chow Mein	in Oriental Sauce	4.6 oz	80	B–
in Herb Sauce for Chicken		4.6 oz	90	D–+
in Mushroom Sauce, Creamy		4.6 oz	60	B–+
in Mustard Dijon Sauce		4.6 oz	70	C–
in Tomato Basil Sauce		4.6 oz	110	B–
Wild Rice in White Wine Sauce	Chicken	4.6 oz	100	A–
Oriental Style	in Sauce	4.6 oz	90	C–+
Chow Mein Style	in Seasoned Sauce	3.3 oz	90	C–
Italian Style	in Seasoned Sauce	3.3 oz	100	D–+
Japanese Style	in Seasoned Sauce	3.3 oz	90	D–+
New England Style		3.3 oz	130	D–+
Oriental Style	in Seasoned Sauce	3.3 oz	70	D–
Primavera		3.3 oz	120	C–+
San Francisco Style		3.3 oz	100	D–
		3 oz	50	A+
Chinese Style		3.3 oz	35	A–+
Japanese Style		3.3 oz	30	A–+
		3.2 oz	65	A+
Dutch Style		3.2 oz	30	A
Italian Style		3.2 oz	40	A
Oriental Style		3.2 oz	25	A
Soup, Mix		3 oz	45	A
Stew		3 oz	42	A
		¹/₂ cup	40	A+
in Butter Sauce		¹/₂ cup	60	B–+
California Style		¹/₂ cup	25	A–+
Heartland Style		¹/₂ cup	25	A–+
Manhattan Style		¹/₂ cup	25	A+
New England Style		¹/₂ cup	70	A+
San Francisco Style		¹/₂ cup	25	A–+
Santa Fe Style		¹/₂ cup	70	A+
Seattle Style		¹/₂ cup	25	A–+
Western Style		¹/₂ cup	60	B+
		¹/₂ cup	40	A–+
		¹/₂ cup	68	A+
Stew		3.3 oz	50	A
Stew		3 oz	60	A
		3.3 oz	65	A+
		3.5 oz	69	A
		3 oz	60	A
Rice	in Teriyaki Sauce	4 oz	100	A–
Rotini	in Cheddar Cheese Sauce	4 oz	100	B–
Shells	in Italian Style Sauce	4 oz	170	D–
White & Wild Rice Pilaf		4 oz	80	A–
Dried	Chopped	¹/₂ cup	380	D

"+" indicates the food meets minimum fiber requirements; "–" indicates the food has a high sodium content.

Food	Processing Category	Brand
Walnut, English	Bulk	Generic
Watercress	Fresh	
Watermelon	Fresh	
Watermelon Seed	Bulk	Generic
Water Chestnut, Chinese	Fresh	
Water Chestnut, Chinese	Canned	Generic
Wax Bean	Fresh	See Green Bean
Wax Bean	Canned	Del Monte
Wax Bean	Canned	Stokely
Wax Bean	Canned	Stokely No Salt or Sugar Added
Wax Bean	Frozen	Frosty Acres
Wax Bean	Frozen	Seabrook
White Bean	Fresh	
White Bean	Canned	Generic
Winged Bean	Fresh	
Winged Bean	Fresh	
Winged Bean, Dried	Bulk	Generic
Yam	Fresh	
Yam, Mountain (or Hawaiian)	Fresh	
Yardlong Bean	Fresh	
Yardlong Bean	Fresh	
Yardlong Bean, Dried	Bulk	Generic
Yellow Bean	Fresh	
Yellow Bean, Dried	Bulk	Generic
Yokan	Packaged	Generic
Zucchini	Fresh	
Zucchini	Fresh	
Zucchini	Canned	Generic
Zucchini	Canned	Del Monte
Zucchini	Canned	Progresso
Zucchini	Frozen	Generic
Zucchini	Frozen	Stilwell Quickkrisp
Zucchini Combinations	Frozen	Birds Eye Farm Fresh

Major Description	Minor Description	Serving Size	Calories	Grade
Dried	Chopped	$^1/_2$ cup	365	D
Trimmed	Chopped	$^1/_2$ cup	2	A–+
Trimmed	Cubes	$^1/_2$ cup	25	A
Dried	Kernels	$^1/_4$ cup	125	D
Trimmed	Sliced	$^1/_2$ cup	66	A
in Liquid	Sliced	$^1/_2$ cup	35	A
Golden Cut or French Style		$^1/_2$ cup	20	A–+
		$^1/_2$ cup	20	A–+
		$^1/_2$ cup	20	A+
		$^1/_2$ cup	25	A+
Cut		$^1/_2$ cup	25	A+
Raw		$^1/_2$ cup	336	A+
		$^1/_2$ cup	153	A–+
Boiled	Mature Seeds	$^1/_2$ cup	126	A+
Raw	Mature Seeds	$^1/_2$ cup	372	B+
Boiled		$^1/_2$ cup	126	C+
Baked or Boiled		$^1/_2$ cup	79	A
Steamed	Trimmed and Cubed	$^1/_2$ cup	59	A
Boiled	Sliced & Drained	$^1/_2$ cup	25	A+
Raw	Trimmed & Sliced	$^1/_2$ cup	22	A+
Boiled		$^1/_2$ cup	102	A+
Boiled		$^1/_2$ cup	27	A+
Boiled		$^1/_2$ cup	126	A
		1 oz	74	A
Boiled	Sliced	$^1/_2$ cup	14	A+
Raw	Sliced	$^1/_2$ cup	9	A+
in Tomato Juice		$^1/_2$ cup	33	A–+
in Tomato Sauce		$^1/_2$ cup	30	A–+
Italian Style		$^1/_2$ cup	50	C–+
Boiled Drained		4 oz	19	A+
Breaded		3.3 oz	200	D–+
Carrots, Pearl Onions & Mushrooms		4 oz	30	A+

"+" indicates the food meets minimum fiber requirements; "–" indicates the food has a high sodium content.

Meat, Poultry, Seafood, and Meat Products

It's from the foods in this section of the book that most Americans—regardless of what I or anyone else advises—will satisfy the majority of their protein requirements. It's also from this section that most of the cholesterol and saturated fat in the American diet originates. (The other major sources are the milk and dairy products.) By not eating excessive amounts of protein and following the A-B-C-D ratings when selecting these foods, you can't get too much saturated fat and cholesterol.

How Much Protein Do You Need?

There's a simple way to figure this out:

Your Daily Limit of A or B Foods in This Section

Your weight:	100 lb	120 lb	140 lb	160 lb	180 lb	200 lb	220 lb
Red meat:	3 oz	$3^3/_4$ oz	$4^1/_2$ oz	5 oz	$5^2/_3$ oz	$6^1/_4$ oz	7 oz
Fish or fowl:	$3^1/_2$ oz	$4^1/_2$ oz	$5^1/_4$ oz	6 oz	$6^3/_4$ oz	$7^1/_2$ oz	$8^1/_3$ oz

Personal Adjustments: For people participating in moderate regular exercise add 25% of the value in chart. Heavy exercise add 50%. This equals your final meat requirement in ounces of A or B red meat, poultry, or seafood.

This section of the book has been divided into four parts: Meats, Poultry, Seafood, with the fourth part, Meat Products, containing luncheon meats, packaged, canned, and processed meats. One will find all deli-type foods in the Meat Products part as well as items such as frankfurters, sausages, vegetarian, and imitation meat and seafood products. All listings are alphabetical.

For all *red meats*, the "Food" column of this section will identify the cut of meat. The grade of meat, when applicable, will be listed under "Brand." The "Major Description" will describe how it was butchered and eaten. *Trim to 0" or*

Food	Processing Category	Brand
MEAT		
Antelope	Fresh	Generic
Bacon	All Forms	All Brands
Bacon Bits	All Forms	Hormel
Bacon Bits	All Forms	Libby's Bacon Crumbles
Bacon Bits	All Forms	Oscar Mayer
Bacon Bits, Imitation	All Forms	McCormick/Shilling Bacon Piece
Bacon Bits, Imitation	All Forms	Tone's
Bacon Substitute	All Forms	Generic
Bacon Substitute	All Forms	Generic
Bacon Substitute	All Forms	JM
Bacon Substitute	All Forms	Louis Rich
Bacon Substitute	All Forms	Louis Rich
Bacon Substitute	All Forms	Sizzlean
Bacon Substitute	All Forms	Sizzlean
Bacon, Canadian Style	All Forms	Generic
Bacon, Canadian Style	All Forms	Hormel
Bacon, Canadian Style	All Forms	Light & Lean
Bacon, Canadian Style	All Forms	Oscar Mayer
Bacon, Vegetarian	All Forms	Heart Line
Bacon, Vegetarian	Frozen	Morningstar Farms Breakfast
Bacon, Vegetarian	Frozen	Worthington Stripples
Bear	Fresh	
Beaver	Fresh	
Beef, All Cuts	Fresh-cut	
Beef, All Cuts	Fresh-cut	
Beef, All Cuts	Fresh-cut	
Beef, Brisket, Flat Half	Fresh-cut	All Grades
Beef, Brisket, Whole	Fresh-cut	All Grades
Beef, Brisket, Whole	Fresh-cut	All Grades
Beef, Brisket, Ponit Half	Fresh-cut	All Grades
Beef, Canned or Processed	*See* Luncheon and Packaged Meat	
Beef, Chuck Arm Pot Roast	Fresh-cut	Choice Grade
Beef, Chuck Arm Pot Roast	Fresh-cut	Choice Grade
Beef, Chuck Arm Pot Roast	Fresh-cut	Select Grade
Beef, Chuck Arm Pot Roast	Fresh-cut	Select Grade

[1] *10% fat by weight.*
[2] *7% fat by weight.*
[3] *3% fat by weight.*

$^1/_4$" *fat* refers to the amount of fat remaining along the edges of the cut before cooking. *Lean and Fat* refers to cooked meat eaten *without* removing visual fat on the edges and within the meat. *Lean Only* means all visual fat has been removed *after* cooking. The "Minor Description" will describe how the meat was prepared. Most listings are for meat cooked several different ways. The manner of preparation impacts on final calorie content and sometimes the grade a cut of meat receives.

Seafood values are for uncooked products unless otherwise specified.

Major Description	Minor Description	Serving Size	Calories	Grade
Meat Only	Roasted	4 oz	170	B
All Varieties	Smoked	1 oz slice	Approx 160	D–
Dried		1 Tbsp	30	D–
Dried		1 Tbsp	25	C
Dried		1 Tbsp	5	D–
Dried		1 Tbsp	78	A–
Dried		1 Tbsp	21	C–
Beef		1 oz slice	115	D–
Pork		1 oz slice	110	D–
Beef		1 slice	50	D–
Pork	80% Fat Free	1 slice	35	D–
Turkey		1 slice	32	D–
Pork		1 slice	45	D–
Pork	Brown Sugar Cured	1 slice	55	D–
Smoked		1 oz slice	45	C–
Sliced, Smoked		1 oz slice	45	C–
Smoked		1 slice	17	B
Smoked	93% Lean	1 oz slice	35	B–
Canadian Style	Lite	1 oz slice	44	A–
		1 slice	27	D–
		1 slice	30	D–
Meat Only	Roasted	4 oz	294	D
Meat Only	Roasted	4 oz	188	B
90% Lean Meat [1]		4 oz	262	C
93% Lean Meat [2]		4 oz	233	B
97% Lean Meat [3]		4 oz	218	A
Lean Meat & Fat, Trim to 0" Fat	Braised	4 oz	217	B
Lean Meat & Fat, Trim to 0" Fat	Braised	4 oz	330	D
Lean Meat Only, Trim to 0" Fat	Braised	4 oz	247	D
Lean Meat Only, Trim to 0" Fat	Braised	4 oz	277	D
Lean Meat & Fat, Trim to 0" Fat	Braised	4 oz	332	D
Lean Meat Only, Trim to 0" Fat	Braised	4 oz	255	C
Lean Meat & Fat, Trim to 0" Fat	Braised	4 oz	295	D
Lean Meat Only, Trim to 0" Fat	Braised	4 oz	225	B

"+" indicates the food meets minimum fiber requirements; "–" indicates the food has a high sodium content.

Food	Processing Category	Brand
Beef, Chuck Blade Pot Roast	Fresh-cut	Choice Grade
Beef, Chuck Blade Pot Roast	Fresh-cut	Choice Grade
Beef, Chuck Blade Pot Roast	Fresh-cut	Select Grade
Beef, Chuck Blade Pot Roast	Fresh-cut	Select Grade
Beef, Flank	Fresh-cut	Choice Grade
Beef, Flank	Fresh-cut	Choice Grade
Beef, Ground	Fresh-cut	
Beef, Ground	Fresh-cut	
Beef, Ground	Fresh-cut	
Beef, Ground	Fresh-cut	
Beef, Ground	Fresh-cut	
Beef, Ground	Fresh-cut	
Beef, Ground	Fresh-cut	
Beef, Ground	Fresh-cut	
Beef, Luncheon Meat	*See* Luncheon and Packaged Meat	
Beef, Porterhouse Steak	Fresh-cut	Choice Grade
Beef, Porterhouse Steak	Fresh-cut	Choice Grade
Beef, Rib Eye	Fresh-cut	Choice Grade
Beef, Rib Eye	Fresh-cut	Choice Grade
Beef, Rib, Large End	Fresh-cut	Choice Grade
Beef, Rib, Large End	Fresh-cut	Choice Grade
Beef, Rib, Large End	Fresh-cut	Prime Grade
Beef, Rib, Large End	Fresh-cut	Prime Grade
Beef, Rib, Large End	Fresh-cut	Select Grade
Beef, Rib, Large End	Fresh-cut	Select Grade
Beef, Rib, Shortrib	Fresh-cut	Choice Grade
Beef, Rib, Shortrib	Fresh-cut	Choice Grade
Beef, Rib, Small End	Fresh-cut	Choice Grade
Beef, Rib, Small End	Fresh-cut	Choice Grade
Beef, Rib, Small End	Fresh-cut	Prime Grade
Beef, Rib, Small End	Fresh-cut	Prime Grade
Beef, Rib, Small End	Fresh-cut	Select Grade
Beef, Rib, Small End	Fresh-cut	Select Grade
Beef, Rib, Whole	Fresh-cut	Choice Grade
Beef, Rib, Whole	Fresh-cut	Choice Grade
Beef, Rib, Whole	Fresh-cut	Choice Grade
Beef, Rib, Whole	Fresh-cut	Choice Grade
Beef, Rib, Whole	Fresh-cut	Prime Grade
Beef, Rib, Whole	Fresh-cut	Prime Grade
Beef, Rib, Whole	Fresh-cut	Prime Grade
Beef, Rib, Whole	Fresh-cut	Prime Grade
Beef, Rib, Whole	Fresh-cut	Select Grade
Beef, Rib, Whole	Fresh-cut	Select Grade
Beef, Rib, Whole	Fresh-cut	Select Grade
Beef, Rib, Whole	Fresh-cut	Select Grade
Beef, Round, Bottom	Fresh-cut	Choice Grade
Beef, Round, Bottom	Fresh-cut	Choice Grade
Beef, Round, Bottom	Fresh-cut	Choice Grade
Beef, Round, Bottom	Fresh-cut	Choice Grade
Beef, Round, Bottom	Fresh-cut	Select Grade

[4] *Percentage fat in ground beef is by weight.*

Major Description	Minor Description	Serving Size	Calories	Grade
Lean Meat & Fat, Trim to 0" Fat	Braised	4 oz	395	D
Lean Meat Only, Trim to 0" Fat	Braised	4 oz	270	D
Lean Meat & Fat, Trim to 0" Fat	Braised	4 oz	355	D
Lean Meat Only, Trim to 0" Fat	Braised	4 oz	301	D
Lean Meat & Fat, Trim to 0" Fat	Braised	4 oz	256	D
Lean Meat Only, Trim to 0" Fat	Braised	4 oz	235	D
15% Fat [4]	Baked	4 oz	298	D
15% Fat	Broiled	4 oz	301	D
15% Fat	Panfried	4 oz	311	D
23% Fat	Broiled	4 oz	308	D
23% Fat	Panfried	4 oz	324	D
7% Fat	Baked	4 oz	284	B
7% Fat	Broiled	4 oz	290	B
7% Fat	Panfried	4 oz	289	B
Lean Meat & Fat, Trim to 1/4" Fat	Broiled	4 oz	346	D
Lean Meat Only, Trim to 1/4" Fat	Broiled	4 oz	247	D
Lean Meat & Fat, Trim to 1/4" Fat	Broiled	4 oz	348	D
Lean Meat Only, Trim to 1/4" Fat	Broiled	4 oz	255	D
Lean Meat & Fat, Trim to 0" Fat	Roasted	4 oz	422	D
Lean Meat Only, Trim to 0" Fat	Roasted	4 oz	287	D
Lean Meat & Fat, Trim to 1/4" Fat	Roasted	4 oz	456	D
Lean Meat Only, Trim to 1/4" Fat	Roasted	4 oz	321	D
Lean Meat & Fat, Trim to 0" Fat	Roasted	4 oz	375	D
Lean Meat Only, Trim to 0" Fat	Roasted	4 oz	249	D
Lean Meat & Fat, Untrimmed	Braised	4 oz	534	D
Lean Meat Only, Untrimmed	Braised	4 oz	335	D
Lean Meat & Fat, Trim to 0" Fat	Roasted	4 oz	354	D
Lean Meat Only, Trim to 0" Fat	Roasted	4 oz	255	D
Lean Meat & Fat, Trim to 1/4" Fat	Roasted	4 oz	473	D
Lean Meat Only, Trim to 1/4" Fat	Roasted	4 oz	345	D
Lean Meat & Fat, Trim to 0" Fat	Roasted	4 oz	323	D
Lean Meat Only, Trim to 0" Fat	Roasted	4 oz	225	C
Lean Meat & Fat, Trim to 1/4" Fat	Broiled	4 oz	408	D
Lean Meat & Fat, Trim to 1/4" Fat	Roasted	4 oz	426	D
Lean Meat Only, Trim to 1/4" Fat	Broiled	4 oz	269	D
Lean Meat Only, Trim to 1/4" Fat	Roasted	4 oz	276	D
Lean Meat & Fat, Trim to 1/4" Fat	Broiled	4 oz	445	D
Lean Meat & Fat, Trim to 1/4" Fat	Roasted	4 oz	464	D
Lean Meat Only, Trim to 1/4" Fat	Broiled	4 oz	318	D
Lean Meat Only, Trim to 1/4" Fat	Roasted	4 oz	331	D
Lean Meat & Fat, Trim to 1/4" Fat	Broiled	4 oz	366	D
Lean Meat & Fat, Trim to 1/4" Fat	Roasted	4 oz	381	D
Lean Meat Only, Trim to 1/4" Fat	Broiled	4 oz	234	D
Lean Meat Only, Trim to 1/4" Fat	Roasted	4 oz	242	D
Lean Meat & Fat, Trim to 0" Fat	Braised	4 oz	257	D
Lean Meat & Fat, Trim to 0" Fat	Roasted	4 oz	230	C
Lean Meat Only, Trim to 0" Fat	Braised	4 oz	242	C
Lean Meat Only, Trim to 0" Fat	Roasted	4 oz	219	C
Lean Meat & Fat, Trim to 0" Fat	Braised	4 oz	228	C

"+" indicates the food meets minimum fiber requirements; "–" indicates the food has a high sodium content.

Food	Processing Category	Brand
Beef, Round, Bottom	Fresh-cut	Select Grade
Beef, Round, Bottom	Fresh-cut	Select Grade
Beef, Round, Bottom	Fresh-cut	Select Grade
Beef, Round, Eye	Fresh-cut	Choice Grade
Beef, Round, Eye	Fresh-cut	Choice Grade
Beef, Round, Eye	Fresh-cut	Select Grade
Beef, Round, Eye	Fresh-cut	Select Grade
Beef, Round, Full Cut	Fresh-cut	Choice Grade
Beef, Round, Full Cut	Fresh-cut	Choice Grade
Beef, Round, Full Cut	Fresh-cut	Select Grade
Beef, Round, Full Cut	Fresh-cut	Select Grade
Beef, Round, Tip	Fresh-cut	Choice Grade
Beef, Round, Tip	Fresh-cut	Choice Grade
Beef, Round, Tip	Fresh-cut	Prime Grade
Beef, Round, Tip	Fresh-cut	Prime Grade
Beef, Round, Tip	Fresh-cut	Select Grade
Beef, Round, Tip	Fresh-cut	Select Grade
Beef, Round, Top	Fresh-cut	Choice Grade
Beef, Round, Top	Fresh-cut	Choice Grade
Beef, Round, Top	Fresh-cut	Choice Grade
Beef, Round, Top	Fresh-cut	Choice Grade
Beef, Round, Top	Fresh-cut	Choice Grade
Beef, Round, Top	Fresh-cut	Choice Grade
Beef, Round, Top	Fresh-cut	Choice Grade
Beef, Round, Top	Fresh-cut	Choice Grade
Beef, Round, Top	Fresh-cut	Prime Grade
Beef, Round, Top	Fresh-cut	Prime Grade
Beef, Round, Top	Fresh-cut	Select Grade
Beef, Round, Top	Fresh-cut	Select Grade
Beef, Round, Top	Fresh-cut	Select Grade
Beef, Round, Top	Fresh-cut	Select Grade
Beef, Round, Top	Fresh-cut	Select Grade
Beef, Shank, Crosscut	Fresh-cut	Choice Grade
Beef, Shank, Crosscut	Fresh-cut	Choice Grade
Beef, Sirloin	Fresh-cut	Choice Grade
Beef, Sirloin	Fresh-cut	Choice Grade
Beef, Sirloin	Fresh-cut	Select Grade
Beef, Sirloin	Fresh-cut	Select Grade
Beef, T-bone Steak	Fresh-cut	Choice Grade
Beef, T-bone Steak	Fresh-cut	Choice Grade
Beef, Tenderloin	Fresh-cut	Choice Grade
Beef, Tenderloin	Fresh-cut	Choice Grade
Beef, Tenderloin	Fresh-cut	Choice Grade
Beef, Tenderloin	Fresh-cut	Choice Grade
Beef, Tenderloin	Fresh-cut	Choice Grade
Beef, Tenderloin	Fresh-cut	Prime Grade
Beef, Tenderloin	Fresh-cut	Prime Grade
Beef, Tenderloin	Fresh-cut	Select Grade
Beef, Tenderloin	Fresh-cut	Select Grade
Beef, Tenderloin	Fresh-cut	Select Grade
Beef, Tenderloin	Fresh-cut	Select Grade
Beef, Tenderloin	Fresh-cut	Select Grade
Beef, Top Loin	Fresh-cut	Choice Grade

Major Description	Minor Description	Serving Size	Calories	Grade
Lean Meat & Fat, Trim to 0" Fat	Roasted	4 oz	201	B
Lean Meat Only, Trim to 0" Fat	Braised	4 oz	218	B
Lean Meat Only, Trim to 0" Fat	Roasted	4 oz	194	B
Lean Meat & Fat, Trim to 0" Fat	Roasted	4 oz	204	C
Lean Meat Only, Trim to 0" Fat	Roasted	4 oz	198	B
Lean Meat & Fat, Trim to 0" Fat	Roasted	4 oz	183	B
Lean Meat Only, Trim to 0" Fat	Roasted	4 oz	176	B
Lean Meat & Fat, Trim to $1/4$" Fat	Broiled	4 oz	272	D
Lean Meat Only, Trim to $1/4$" Fat	Broiled	4 oz	217	C
Lean Meat & Fat, Trim to $1/4$" Fat	Broiled	4 oz	253	D
Lean Meat Only, Trim to $1/4$" Fat	Broiled	4 oz	195	B
Lean Meat & Fat, Trim to 0" Fat	Roasted	4 oz	227	D
Lean Meat Only, Trim to 0" Fat	Roasted	4 oz	204	C
Lean Meat & Fat, Trim to $1/4$" Fat	Roasted	4 oz	311	D
Lean Meat Only, Trim to $1/4$" Fat	Roasted	4 oz	242	D
Lean Meat & Fat, Trim to 0" Fat	Roasted	4 oz	211	C
Lean Meat Only, Trim to 0" Fat	Roasted	4 oz	193	B
Lean Meat & Fat, Trim to 0" Fat	Braised	4 oz	245	B
Lean Meat & Fat, Trim to $1/4$" Fat	Braised	4 oz	295	D
Lean Meat & Fat, Trim to $1/4$" Fat	Broiled	4 oz	254	D
Lean Meat & Fat, Trim to $1/4$" Fat	Fried	4 oz	314	D
Lean Meat Only, Trim to 0" Fat	Braised	4 oz	235	B
Lean Meat Only, Trim to $1/4$" Fat	Braised	4 oz	242	B
Lean Meat Only, Trim to $1/4$" Fat	Broiled	4 oz	214	B
Lean Meat Only, Trim to $1/4$" Fat	Fried	4 oz	257	C
Lean Meat & Fat, Trim to $1/4$" Fat	Broiled	4 oz	260	D
Lean Meat Only, Trim to $1/4$" Fat	Broiled	4 oz	244	C
Lean Meat & Fat, Trim to 0" Fat	Braised	4 oz	227	B
Lean Meat & Fat, Trim to $1/4$" Fat	Broiled	4 oz	234	C
Lean Meat Only, Trim to 0" Fat	Braised	4 oz	215	B
Lean Meat Only, Trim to $1/4$" Fat	Braised	4 oz	222	B
Lean Meat Only, Trim to $1/4$" Fat	Broiled	4 oz	192	B
Lean Meat & Fat, Trim to $1/4$" Fat	Simmered	4 oz	298	D
Lean Meat Only, Trim to $1/4$" Fat	Simmered	4 oz	228	B
Lean Meat & Fat, Trim to 0" Fat	Broiled	4 oz	260	D
Lean Meat Only, Trim to 0" Fat	Broiled	4 oz	227	C
Lean Meat & Fat, Trim to 0" Fat	Broiled	4 oz	221	C
Lean Meat Only, Trim to 0" Fat	Broiled	4 oz	204	B
Lean Meat & Fat, Trim to $1/4$" Fat	Broiled	4 oz	338	D
Lean Meat Only, Trim to $1/4$" Fat	Broiled	4 oz	243	D
Lean Meat & Fat, Trim to 0" Fat	Broiled	4 oz	277	D
Lean Meat & Fat, Trim to $1/4$" Fat	Broiled	4 oz	345	D
Lean Meat Only, Trim to 0" Fat	Broiled	4 oz	240	D
Lean Meat Only, Trim to $1/4$" Fat	Roasted	4 oz	262	B
Lean Meat & Fat, Trim to $1/4$" Fat	Roasted	4 oz	400	D
Lean Meat Only, Trim to $1/4$" Fat	Roasted	4 oz	289	D
Lean Meat & Fat, Trim to 0" Fat	Broiled	4 oz	260	D
Lean Meat & Fat, Trim to $1/4$" Fat	Broiled	4 oz	307	D
Lean Meat & Fat, Trim to $1/4$" Fat	Roasted	4 oz	367	D
Lean Meat Only, Trim to 0" Fat	Broiled	4 oz	227	C
Lean Meat Only, Trim to $1/4$" Fat	Roasted	4 oz	239	D
Lean Meat & Fat, Trim to 0" Fat	Broiled	4 oz	259	D

"+" indicates the food meets minimum fiber requirements; "−" indicates the food has a high sodium content.

Food	Processing Category	Brand
Beef, Top Loin	Fresh-cut	Choice Grade
Beef, Top Loin	Fresh-cut	Prime Grade
Beef, Top Loin	Fresh-cut	Prime Grade
Beef, Top Loin	Fresh-cut	Select Grade
Beef, Top Loin	Fresh-cut	Select Grade
Bison	Fresh	
Boar, Wild	Fresh	
Brain	Fresh	
Brain	Fresh	
Brain	Fresh	
Brain	Fresh	
Brain	Fresh	
Brain	Fresh	
Brain	Fresh	
Buffalo	Fresh	
Caribou	Fresh	
Chitterlings	Fresh	
Elk	Fresh	
Frogs Legs	Fresh	
Goat	Fresh	
Ham	Canned	Generic
Ham	Canned	Generic
Ham	Canned	Black Label 1$^1/_2$ lb
Ham	Canned	Black Label Refrigerated
Ham	Canned	Black Label Shelf
Ham	Canned	EXL
Ham	Canned	Holiday Glaze 3 lb
Ham	Canned	Hormel
Ham	Canned	Hormel
Ham	Canned	Hormel
Ham	Canned	Hormel 8 lb
Ham	Canned	Hormel Bone-In
Ham	Canned	Hormel Cure 81
Ham	Canned	Hormel Curemaster
Ham	Canned	JM 95% Fat Free
Ham	Canned	Light & Lean Boneless
Ham	Canned	Oscar Mayer Jubilee
Ham	Canned	Rath Black Hawk
Ham, Boneless	Cured	
Ham, Boneless	Cured	
Ham, Boneless	Cured	
Ham, Boneless	Cured	
Ham, Boneless	Cured	
Ham, Boneless	Cured	
Ham, Boneless	Cured	Oscar Mayer Jubilee
Ham, Boneless	Fresh	

[5] Percentage fat in ham is by weight.

Major Description	Minor Description	Serving Size	Calories	Grade
Lean Meat Only, Trim to 0" Fat	Broiled	4 oz	237	D
Lean Meat & Fat, Trim to 1/4" Fat	Broiled	4 oz	366	D
Lean Meat Only, Trim to 1/4" Fat	Broiled	4 oz	278	D
Lean Meat & Fat, Trim to 0" Fat	Broiled	4 oz	226	C
Lean Meat Only, Trim to 0" Fat	Broiled	4 oz	209	C
Meat Only	Roasted	4 oz	162	A
Meat Only	Roasted	4 oz	181	B
Beef	Panfried in Vegetable Oil	4 oz	222	D
Beef	Simmered	4 oz	181	D
Lamb	Braised	4 oz	164	D
Lamb	Panfried in Vegetable Oil	4 oz	310	D
Pork	Braised	4 oz	156	D
Veal	Braised	4 oz	154	D
Veal	Panfried in Vegetable Oil	4 oz	242	D
Meat Only	Roasted	4 oz	213	B
Meat Only	Roasted	4 oz	189	B
Pork		4 oz	280	D
Meat Only	Roasted	4 oz	166	A
Meat Only		4 oz	80	A
Meat Only	Roasted	4 oz	162	B
Extra Lean 4% Fat [5]	Baked	4 oz	154	C−
Regular 13% Fat	Baked	4 oz	256	D−
		4 oz	150	D−
		4 oz	135	D−
		4 oz	145	D−
		4 oz	120	B−
		4 oz	130	B
Chunk		4 oz	183	D−
Roll		4 oz	170	D−
Spiced		4 oz	320	D−
Chopped		4 oz	320	D−
		4 oz	210	D
		4 oz	160	D−
		4 oz	140	C−
		4 oz	120	B−
		4 oz	120	B−
		4 oz	116	B−
Hickory Smoked		4 oz	120	B−
Center Slice	Lean Meat & Fat, Roasted	4 oz	128	D−
Center Slice	Lean Meat, Roasted	4 oz	120	C
Steak		4 oz	140	C−
Whole	Extra Lean Meat, Roasted	4 oz	148	B−
Whole	Lean Meat & Fat, Roasted	4 oz	272	D−
Whole	Lean Meat, Roasted	4 oz	178	C−
Steak		4 oz	114	B−
Leg, Whole	Lean Meat & Fat, Roasted	4 oz	333	D

"+" indicates the food meets minimum fiber requirements; "−" indicates the food has a high sodium content.

Food	Processing Category	Brand
Ham, Boneless	Fresh	
Ham, Boneless	Fresh	
Ham, Boneless	Fresh	
Ham, Boneless	Fresh	
Ham, Boneless	Fresh	
Heart	Fresh	
Heart	Fresh	
Heart	Fresh	
Heart	Fresh	
Heart	Fresh	
Heart	Fresh	
Jowl	Fresh	
Kidneys	Fresh	
Kidneys	Fresh	
Kidneys	Fresh	
Kidneys	Fresh	
Lamb, Foreshank	Fresh-cut	Choice
Lamb, Foreshank	Fresh-cut	Choice
Lamb, Leg, Shank	Fresh-cut	Choice
Lamb, Leg, Shank	Fresh-cut	Choice
Lamb, Leg, Sirloin	Fresh-cut	Choice
Lamb, Leg, Sirloin	Fresh-cut	Choice
Lamb, Leg, Whole	Fresh-cut	Choice
Lamb, Leg, Whole	Fresh-cut	Choice
Lamb, Loin	Fresh-cut	Choice
Lamb, Loin	Fresh-cut	Choice
Lamb, Loin	Fresh-cut	Choice
Lamb, Rib	Fresh-cut	Choice
Lamb, Rib	Fresh-cut	Choice
Lamb, Shoulder & Leg	Fresh-cut	Choice
Lamb, Shoulder, Arm	Fresh-cut	Choice
Lamb, Shoulder, Arm	Fresh-cut	Choice
Lamb, Shoulder, Arm	Fresh-cut	Choice
Lamb, Shoulder, Arm	Fresh-cut	Choice
Lamb, Shoulder, Blade	Fresh-cut	Choice
Lamb, Shoulder, Blade	Fresh-cut	Choice
Lamb, Shoulder, Blade	Fresh-cut	Choice
Lamb, Shoulder, Blade	Fresh-cut	Choice
Lamb, Shoulder, Whole	Fresh-cut	Choice
Lamb, Shoulder, Whole	Fresh-cut	Choice
Lamb, Shoulder, Whole	Fresh-cut	Choice
Lamb, Shoulder, Whole	Fresh-cut	Choice
Lard	All Forms	
Liver	Fresh	
Liver	Fresh	
Liver	Fresh	
Liver	Fresh	

Major Description	Minor Description	Serving Size	Calories	Grade
Leg, Whole	Lean Meat Only, Roasted	4 oz	249	D
Rump, Half	Lean Meat & Fat, Roasted	4 oz	311	D
Rump, Half	Lean Meat Only, Roasted	4 oz	251	D
Shank	Lean Meat & Fat, Roasted	4 oz	344	D
Shank	Lean Meat Only, Roasted	4 oz	244	D
Beef	Simmered	4 oz	198	B
Chicken	Simmered	4 oz	210	C
Lamb	Simmered	4 oz	210	C
Pork	Simmered	4 oz	168	C
Turkey	Simmered	4 oz	201	C
Veal	Simmered	4 oz	211	C
Pork		4 oz	744	D
Beef	Braised	4 oz	163	D
Lamb	Braised	4 oz	155	D
Pork	Braised	4 oz	171	D
Veal	Braised	4 oz	185	D
Lean Meat & Fat	Braised or Stewed	4 oz	276	D
Lean Meat Only	Braised or Stewed	4 oz	212	B
Lean Meat & Fat	Roasted	4 oz	255	D
Lean Meat Only	Roasted	4 oz	204	C
Lean Meat & Fat	Roasted	4 oz	331	D
Lean Meat Only	Roasted	4 oz	231	C
Lean Meat & Fat	Roasted	4 oz	293	D
Lean Meat Only	Roasted	4 oz	217	C
Lean Meat & Fat	Broiled	4 oz	358	D
Lean Meat Only	Broiled	4 oz	245	D
Lean Meat Only	Roasted	4 oz	229	D
Lean Meat & Fat	Roasted or Broiled	4 oz	409	D
Lean Meat Only	Roasted or Broiled	4 oz	266	D
Lean Meat Only	Cubed, Broiled	4 oz	253	C
Lean Meat & Fat	Roasted	4 oz	315	D
Lean Meat & Fat	Stewed	4 oz	392	D
Lean Meat Only	Roasted	4 oz	227	C
Lean Meat Only	Stewed	4 oz	319	D
Lean Meat & Fat	Broiled	4 oz	315	D
Lean Meat & Fat	Stewed	4 oz	391	D
Lean Meat Only	Broiled	4 oz	238	D
Lean Meat Only	Stewed	4 oz	327	D
Lean Meat & Fat	Roasted or Broiled	4 oz	313	D
Lean Meat & Fat	Stewed	4 oz	390	D
Lean Meat Only	Roasted or Broiled	4 oz	235	D
Lean Meat Only	Stewed	4 oz	321	D
All Varieties		1 Tbsp	115	D
Beef	Braised	4 oz	183	C
Beef	Panfried in Vegetable Oil	4 oz	246	D
Chicken	Simmered	4 oz	178	D
Lamb	Braised	4 oz	249	D

"+" indicates the food meets minimum fiber requirements; "−" indicates the food has a high sodium content.

Food	Processing Category	Brand
Liver	Fresh	
Liver	Fresh	
Liver	Fresh	
Liver	Fresh	
Liver	Fresh	
Lungs	Fresh	
Lungs	Fresh	
Lungs	Fresh	
Lungs	Fresh	
Opossum	Fresh	
Pancreas	Fresh	
Pancreas	Fresh	
Pancreas	Fresh	
Pancreas	Fresh	
Pig's Ear	Frozen	
Pig's Feet	Fresh	
Pig's Feet	Pickled	Generic
Pig's Knuckles	Pickled	Penrose
Pig's Tail	Fresh	
Pork Fat	All Forms	
Pork Rind Snack	Packaged	Baken-ets
Pork Shoulder	Cured	
Pork Shoulder	Cured	
Pork, All Cuts	Fresh-cut	Choice
Pork, All Cuts	Fresh-cut	Choice
Pork, All Cuts	Fresh-cut	Choice
Pork, Back Rib	Fresh-cut	Choice
Pork, Loin, Blade	Fresh-cut	Choice
Pork, Loin, Blade	Fresh-cut	Choice
Pork, Loin, Blade	Fresh-cut	Choice
Pork, Loin, Blade	Fresh-cut	Choice
Pork, Loin, Blade	Fresh-cut	Choice
Pork, Loin, Blade	Fresh-cut	Choice
Pork, Loin, Blade	Fresh-cut	Choice
Pork, Loin, Blade	Fresh-cut	Choice
Pork, Loin, Center	Fresh-cut	Choice
Pork, Loin, Center	Fresh-cut	Choice
Pork, Loin, Center	Fresh-cut	Choice
Pork, Loin, Center	Fresh-cut	Choice
Pork, Loin, Center	Fresh-cut	Choice
Pork, Loin, Center	Fresh-cut	Choice
Pork, Loin, Center	Fresh-cut	Choice
Pork, Loin, Center	Fresh-cut	Choice
Pork, Loin, Center Rib	Fresh-cut	Choice
Pork, Loin, Center Rib	Fresh-cut	Choice
Pork, Loin, Center Rib	Fresh-cut	Choice
Pork, Loin, Center Rib	Fresh-cut	Choice
Pork, Loin, Center Rib	Fresh-cut	Choice
Pork, Loin, Center Rib	Fresh-cut	Choice
Pork, Loin, Center Rib	Fresh-cut	Choice
Pork, Loin, Center Rib	Fresh-cut	Choice

[6] *Percentage fat in pork is by weight.*

Major Description	Minor Description	Serving Size	Calories	Grade
Lamb	Panfried in Vegetable Oil	4 oz	270	D
Pork	Braised	4 oz	187	C
Turkey	Simmered	4 oz	192	D
Veal	Braised	4 oz	187	D
Veal	Panfried in Vegetable Oil	4 oz	278	D
Beef	Braised	4 oz	136	D
Lamb	Braised	4 oz	128	D
Pork	Braised	4 oz	112	D
Veal	Braised	4 oz	118	D
Meat Only	Roasted	4 oz	251	D
Beef	Braised	4 oz	307	D
Lamb	Braised	4 oz	265	D
Pork	Braised	4 oz	248	D
Veal	Braised	4 oz	290	D
	Simmered	4 oz	188	D
	Simmered	4 oz	220	D
		4 oz	232	D
		1 piece or 6 oz	290	D–
	Simmered	4 oz	449	D
Roasted		1 oz	167	D
		1 oz	160	D–
Lean Meat & Fat	Roasted	4 oz	318	D–
Lean Meat Only	Roasted	4 oz	193	C–
Lean Meat Only	10% Fat [6]	4 oz	262	C
Lean Meat Only	3% Fat	4 oz	218	A
Lean Meat Only	7% Fat	4 oz	238	B
		4 oz	160	D
Lean Meat & Fat	Braised	4 oz	465	D
Lean Meat & Fat	Broiled	4 oz	446	D
Lean Meat & Fat	Panfried	4 oz	469	D
Lean Meat & Fat	Roasted	4 oz	413	D
Lean Meat Only	Braised	4 oz	355	D
Lean Meat Only	Broiled	4 oz	340	D
Lean Meat Only	Panfried	4 oz	321	D
Lean Meat Only	Roasted	4 oz	316	D
Lean Meat & Fat	Braised	4 oz	401	D
Lean Meat & Fat	Broiled	4 oz	358	D
Lean Meat & Fat	Panfried	4 oz	425	D
Lean Meat & Fat	Roasted	4 oz	346	D
Lean Meat Only	Braised	4 oz	308	D
Lean Meat Only	Broiled	4 oz	262	D
Lean Meat Only	Panfried	4 oz	302	D
Lean Meat Only	Roasted	4 oz	272	D
Lean Meat & Fat	Braised	4 oz	416	D
Lean Meat & Fat	Broiled	4 oz	389	D
Lean Meat & Fat	Panfried	4 oz	442	D
Lean Meat & Fat	Roasted	4 oz	361	D
Lean Meat Only	Braised	4 oz	314	D
Lean Meat Only	Broiled	4 oz	293	D
Lean Meat Only	Panfried	4 oz	291	D
Lean Meat Only	Roasted	4 oz	278	D

"+" indicates the food meets minimum fiber requirements; "–" indicates the food has a high sodium content.

Food	Processing Category	Brand
Pork, Loin, Sirloin	Fresh-cut	Choice
Pork, Loin, Sirloin	Fresh-cut	Choice
Pork, Loin, Sirloin	Fresh-cut	Choice
Pork, Loin, Sirloin	Fresh-cut	Choice
Pork, Loin, Sirloin	Fresh-cut	Choice
Pork, Loin, Sirloin	Fresh-cut	Choice
Pork, Loin, Top	Fresh-cut	Choice
Pork, Loin, Top	Fresh-cut	Choice
Pork, Loin, Top	Fresh-cut	Choice
Pork, Loin, Top	Fresh-cut	Choice
Pork, Loin, Top	Fresh-cut	Choice
Pork, Loin, Top	Fresh-cut	Choice
Pork, Loin, Top	Fresh-cut	Choice
Pork, Loin, Top	Fresh-cut	Choice
Pork, Loin, Whole	Fresh-cut	Choice
Pork, Loin, Whole	Fresh-cut	Choice
Pork, Loin, Whole	Fresh-cut	Choice
Pork, Loin, Whole	Fresh-cut	Choice
Pork, Loin, Whole	Fresh-cut	Choice
Pork, Loin, Whole	Fresh-cut	Choice
Pork, Shoulder	Fresh-cut	Choice
Pork, Shoulder	Fresh-cut	Choice
Pork, Shoulder, Whole	Fresh-cut	Choice
Pork, Shoulder, Whole	Fresh-cut	Choice
Pork, Spareribs	Fresh-cut	Choice
Pork, Tenderloin	Fresh-cut	Choice
Rabbit, Domesticated	Fresh	
Rabbit, Domesticated	Fresh	
Rabbit, Wild	Fresh	
Salt Pork	All Forms	
Spleen	Fresh	
Spleen	Fresh	
Spleen	Fresh	
Spleen	Fresh	
Stomach	Fresh	
Thymus	Fresh	
Thymus	Fresh	
Tongue	Fresh	
Tongue	Fresh	
Tongue	Fresh	
Tongue	Fresh	
Tongue	Fresh	
Veal, Ground	Fresh-cut	Choice
Veal, Leg & Shoulder	Fresh-cut	Choice
Veal, Leg, Top Round	Fresh-cut	Choice
Veal, Leg, Top Round	Fresh-cut	Choice
Veal, Leg, Top Round	Fresh-cut	Choice
Veal, Leg, Top Round	Fresh-cut	Choice
Veal, Leg, Top Round	Fresh-cut	Choice
Veal, Leg, Top Round	Fresh-cut	Choice
Veal, Leg, Top Round	Fresh-cut	Choice
Veal, Leg, Top Round	Fresh-cut	Choice
Veal, Leg, Top Round	Fresh-cut	Choice
Veal, Loin	Fresh-cut	Choice

Major Description	Minor Description	Serving Size	Calories	Grade
Lean Meat & Fat	Braised	4 oz	399	D
Lean Meat & Fat	Broiled	4 oz	375	D
Lean Meat & Fat	Roasted	4 oz	330	D
Lean Meat Only	Braised	4 oz	296	D
Lean Meat Only	Broiled	4 oz	276	D
Lean Meat Only	Roasted	4 oz	268	D
Lean Meat & Fat	Braised	4 oz	432	D
Lean Meat & Fat	Broiled	4 oz	408	D
Lean Meat & Fat	Panfried	4 oz	445	D
Lean Meat & Fat	Roasted	4 oz	374	D
Lean Meat Only	Braised	4 oz	314	D
Lean Meat Only	Broiled	4 oz	293	D
Lean Meat Only	Panfried	4 oz	291	D
Lean Meat Only	Roasted	4 oz	278	D
Lean Meat & Fat	Braised	4 oz	417	D
Lean Meat & Fat	Broiled	4 oz	392	D
Lean Meat & Fat	Roasted	4 oz	362	D
Lean Meat Only	Braised	4 oz	310	D
Lean Meat Only	Broiled	4 oz	291	D
Lean Meat Only	Roasted	4 oz	272	D
Lean Meat & Fat	Roasted	4 oz	375	D
Lean Meat Only	Roasted	4 oz	259	D
Lean Meat & Fat	Roasted	4 oz	270	D
Lean Meat Only	Roasted	4 oz	277	D
with Bone		4 oz	324	D
Lean Meat Only	Roasted	4 oz	188	B
Meat Only	Roasted	4 oz	175	C
Meat Only	Stewed	4 oz	234	C
Meat Only	Stewed	4 oz	196	B
		1 oz	212	D–
Beef	Braised	4 oz	164	D
Lamb	Braised	4 oz	177	D
Pork	Braised	4 oz	169	D
Veal	Braised	4 oz	146	D
Pork		4 oz	176	D
Beef	Braised	4 oz	362	D
Veal	Braised	4 oz	197	B
Beef	Braised	4 oz	321	D
Lamb	Braised	4 oz	312	D
Pork	Braised	4 oz	307	D
Pork	Cured	4 oz	253	D–
Veal	Braised	4 oz	229	D
Mixed Cuts	Broiled	4 oz	195	C
Lean Meat Only	Braised or Stewed	4 oz	213	B
Lean Meat & Fat	Braised or Stewed	4 oz	239	B
Lean Meat & Fat	Panfried in Vegetable Oil	4 oz	239	C
Lean Meat & Fat	Panfried, Breaded	4 oz	259	C–
Lean Meat & Fat	Roasted	4 oz	181	B
Lean Meat Only	Braised or Stewed	4 oz	230	B
Lean Meat Only	Panfried in Vegetable Oil	4 oz	208	B
Lean Meat Only	Panfried, Breaded	4 oz	234	B–
Lean Meat Only	Roasted	4 oz	170	B
Lean Meat & Fat	Braised or Stewed	4 oz	322	D

"+" indicates the food meets minimum fiber requirements; "–" indicates the food has a high sodium content.

Food	Processing Category	Brand
Veal, Loin	Fresh-cut	Choice
Veal, Loin	Fresh-cut	Choice
Veal, Loin	Fresh-cut	Choice
Veal, Rib	Fresh-cut	Choice
Veal, Rib	Fresh-cut	Choice
Veal, Rib	Fresh-cut	Choice
Veal, Rib	Fresh-cut	Choice
Veal, Shoulder Blade	Fresh-cut	Choice
Veal, Shoulder Blade	Fresh-cut	Choice
Veal, Shoulder Blade	Fresh-cut	Choice
Veal, Shoulder Blade	Fresh-cut	Choice
Veal, Shoulder, Arm	Fresh-cut	Choice
Veal, Shoulder, Arm	Fresh-cut	Choice
Veal, Shoulder, Arm	Fresh-cut	Choice
Veal, Shoulder, Arm	Fresh-cut	Choice
Veal, Shoulder, Whole	Fresh-cut	Choice
Veal, Shoulder, Whole	Fresh-cut	Choice
Veal, Shoulder, Whole	Fresh-cut	Choice
Veal, Shoulder, Whole	Fresh-cut	Choice
Veal, Sirloin	Fresh-cut	Choice
Veal, Sirloin	Fresh-cut	Choice
Veal, Sirloin	Fresh-cut	Choice
Veal, Sirloin	Fresh-cut	Choice
Venison	Fresh	
Water Buffalo	Fresh	
POULTRY		
Chicken	Fresh	
Chicken	Fresh	
Chicken	Fresh	
Chicken Broiler or Fryer	Fresh	
Chicken Broiler or Fryer	Fresh	
Chicken Broiler or Fryer	Fresh	
Chicken Broiler or Fryer	Fresh	
Chicken Broiler or Fryer	Fresh	
Chicken Broiler or Fryer	Fresh	
Chicken Broiler or Fryer	Fresh	
Chicken Broiler or Fryer	Fresh	
Chicken Broiler or Fryer	Fresh	
Chicken Broiler or Fryer	Fresh	
Chicken Broiler or Fryer	Fresh	
Chicken Broiler or Fryer	Fresh	
Chicken Broiler or Fryer	Fresh	
Chicken Broiler or Fryer	Fresh	
Chicken Broiler or Fryer	Fresh	
Chicken Broiler or Fryer	Fresh	
Chicken Broiler or Fryer	Fresh	
Chicken Broiler or Fryer	Fresh	
Chicken Broiler or Fryer	Fresh	
Chicken Broiler or Fryer	Fresh	
Chicken Broiler or Fryer	Fresh	
Chicken Broiler or Fryer	Fresh	
Chicken Broiler or Fryer	Fresh	

[7] Percentage fat in chicken is by weight.

Major Description	Minor Description	Serving Size	Calories	Grade
Lean Meat & Fat	Roasted	4 oz	246	D
Lean Meat Only	Braised or Stewed	4 oz	256	C
Lean Meat Only	Roasted	4 oz	198	C
Lean Meat & Fat	Braised or Stewed	4 oz	285	D
Lean Meat & Fat	Roasted	4 oz	259	D
Lean Meat Only	Braised or Stewed	4 oz	247	C
Lean Meat Only	Roasted	4 oz	201	C
Lean Meat & Fat	Braised or Stewed	4 oz	255	D
Lean Meat & Fat	Roasted	4 oz	211	D
Lean Meat Only	Braised or Stewed	4 oz	224	C
Lean Meat Only	Roasted	4 oz	194	C
Lean Meat & Fat	Braised	4 oz	268	C
Lean Meat & Fat	Roasted	4 oz	208	C
Lean Meat Only	Braised	4 oz	228	B
Lean Meat Only	Roasted	4 oz	186	B
Lean Meat & Fat	Braised or Stewed	4 oz	259	C
Lean Meat & Fat	Roasted	4 oz	209	D
Lean Meat Only	Braised or Stewed	4 oz	226	B
Lean Meat Only	Roasted	4 oz	193	C
Lean Meat & Fat	Braised or Stewed	4 oz	286	D
Lean Meat & Fat	Roasted	4 oz	229	D
Lean Meat Only	Braised or Stewed	4 oz	231	B
Lean Meat Only	Roasted	4 oz	191	B
Meat Only	Roasted	4 oz	179	B
Meat Only	Roasted	4 oz	149	A
White Meat without Skin	2% Fat [7]	3.5 oz	150	A
White Meat without Skin	6% Fat	3.5 oz	170	B
White Meat without Skin	8% Fat	3.5 oz	180	C
Back	Fried, Batter Dipped	4 oz	375	D
Back	Fried, Flour Coated	4 oz	375	D
Back Meat Only	Roasted	4 oz	271	D
Back Meat Only	Stewed	4 oz	237	D
Back Meat with Skin	Roasted	4 oz	340	D
Back Meat with Skin	Stewed	4 oz	293	D
Breast	Fried, Batter Dipped	4 oz	295	D
Breast	Fried, Flour Coated	4 oz	252	C
Breast Meat Only	Roasted	4 oz	187	B
Breast Meat Only	Stewed	4 oz	169	B
Breast Meat with Skin	Roasted	4 oz	223	C
Breast Meat with Skin	Stewed	4 oz	209	C
Dark Meat	Fried, Batter Dipped	4 oz	338	D
Dark Meat	Fried, Flour Coated	4 oz	323	D
Dark Meat Only	Roasted	4 oz	232	D
Dark Meat Only	Stewed	4 oz	218	D
Dark Meat with Skin	Roasted	4 oz	287	D
Dark Meat with Skin	Stewed	4 oz	264	D
Drumstick	Fried, Batter Dipped	4 oz	304	D
Drumstick	Fried, Flour Coated	4 oz	278	D
Drumstick Meat Only	Roasted	4 oz	195	B
Drumstick Meat Only	Stewed	4 oz	196	C
Drumstick Meat with Skin	Roasted	4 oz	245	D
Drumstick Meat with Skin	Stewed	4 oz	231	D

"+" indicates the food meets minimum fiber requirements; "–" indicates the food has a high sodium content.

Food	Processing Category	Brand
Chicken Broiler or Fryer	Fresh	
Chicken Broiler or Fryer	Fresh	
Chicken Broiler or Fryer	Fresh	
Chicken Broiler or Fryer	Fresh	
Chicken Broiler or Fryer	Fresh	
Chicken Broiler or Fryer	Fresh	
Chicken Broiler or Fryer	Fresh	
Chicken Broiler or Fryer	Fresh	
Chicken Broiler or Fryer	Fresh	
Chicken Broiler or Fryer	Fresh	
Chicken Broiler or Fryer	Fresh	
Chicken Broiler or Fryer	Fresh	
Chicken Broiler or Fryer	Fresh	
Chicken Broiler or Fryer	Fresh	
Chicken Broiler or Fryer	Fresh	
Chicken Broiler or Fryer	Fresh	
Chicken Broiler or Fryer	Fresh	
Chicken Broiler or Fryer	Fresh	
Chicken Broiler or Fryer	Fresh	
Chicken Broiler or Fryer	Fresh	
Chicken Broiler or Fryer	Fresh	
Chicken Broiler or Fryer	Fresh	
Chicken Broiler or Fryer	Fresh	
Chicken Broiler or Fryer	Fresh	
Chicken Broiler or Fryer	Fresh	
Chicken Broiler or Fryer	Fresh	
Chicken Broiler or Fryer	Fresh	
Chicken Broiler or Fryer	Fresh	
Chicken Broiler or Fryer	Fresh	
Chicken Broiler or Fryer	Fresh	
Chicken Broiler or Fryer	Fresh	
Chicken Broiler or Fryer	Fresh	
Chicken Broiler or Fryer	Fresh	
Chicken Broiler or Fryer	Fresh	
Chicken Capon	Fresh	
Chicken Fat	Fresh	
Chicken Giblets	Fresh	
Chicken Giblets	Fresh	
Chicken Giblets	Fresh	
Chicken Gizzard	Fresh	
Chicken Roaster	Fresh	
Chicken Roaster	Fresh	
Chicken Roaster	Fresh	
Chicken Roaster	Fresh	
Chicken, Boneless & Luncheon Meat	*See* under Luncheon & Packaged Meats	
Chicken, Canned or Processed	*See* under Luncheon & Packaged Meats	
Cornish Game Hen	Frozen	Tyson
Duck, Domesticated	Fresh	
Duck, Domesticated	Fresh	
Duck, Domesticated	Fresh	

Major Description	Minor Description	Serving Size	Calories	Grade
Leg	Fried, Batter Dipped	4 oz	310	D
Leg Meat Only	Roasted	4 oz	214	C
Leg Meat Only	Stewed	4 oz	210	C
Leg Meat with Skin	Roasted	4 oz	265	D
Leg Meat with Skin	Stewed	4 oz	249	D
Light Meat	Fried, Batter Dipped	4 oz	312	D
Light Meat	Fried, Flour Coated	4 oz	279	D
Light Meat Only	Roasted	4 oz	196	B
Light Meat Only	Stewed	4 oz	180	B
Light Meat with Skin	Roasted	4 oz	252	D
Light Meat with Skin	Stewed	4 oz	228	D
Mixed Meat Only	Roasted	4 oz	215	C
Mixed Meat Only	Stewed	4 oz	201	C
Mixed Meat with Skin	Roasted	4 oz	271	D
Mixed Meat with Skin	Stewed	4 oz	248	D
Neck	Fried, Batter Dipped	4 oz	374	D
Neck	Fried, Flour Coated	4 oz	376	D
Neck Meat Only	Simmered Neck	1 neck, .6 oz	32	D
Neck Meat with Skin	Simmered Neck	1 neck, 1.3 oz	94	D
Skin Only	Roasted	4 oz	516	D
Thigh	Fried, Batter Dipped	4 oz	314	D
Thigh	Fried, Flour Coated	4 oz	297	D
Thigh Meat Only	Roasted	2 thighs, 4 oz	240	D
Thigh Meat Only	Stewed	4 oz	221	D
Thigh Meat with Skin	Roasted	2 thighs, 4 oz	278	D
Thigh Meat with Skin	Roasted	4 oz	280	D
Thigh Meat with Skin	Stewed	4 oz	263	D
Wing	Fried, Batter Dipped	4 oz	367	D
Wing	Fried, Flour Coated	4 oz	364	D
Wing Meat Only	Roasted	4 wings or 4 oz	240	C
Wing Meat Only	Roasted	4 oz	230	C
Wing Meat Only	Stewed	4 oz	205	C
Wing Meat with Skin	Roasted	4 oz	329	D
Wing Meat with Skin	Stewed	4 oz	282	D
Wing Meat with Skin 1 Wing	Roasted	4 wings or 4 oz	332	D
Meat with Skin	Roasted	4 oz	260	D
		1 oz	178	D
Broiler Fryer	Fried, Flour Coated	4 oz	314	D
Broiler Fryer	Simmered	4 oz	178	B
Capon	Simmered	4 oz	186	B
	Simmered	.8 oz	34	B
Dark Meat Only	Roasted	4 oz	202	D
Light Meat Only	Roasted	4 oz	174	B
Meat Only	Roasted	4 oz	189	C
Meat with Skin	Roasted	4 oz	253	D
		3.5 oz	240	D
Meat Only	Roasted	4 oz	228	D
Meat with Separable Fat	Roasted	1/2 duck	445	D
Meat with Skin	Roasted	4 oz	381	D

"+" indicates the food meets minimum fiber requirements; "−" indicates the food has a high sodium content.

Food	Processing Category	Brand
Duck, Wild	Fresh	
Duck, Wild	Fresh	
Duck, Wild	Fresh	
Goose	Fresh	
Goose	Fresh	
Guinea Hen	Fresh	
Guinea Hen	Fresh	
Pheasant	Fresh	
Pheasant	Fresh	
Pheasant	Fresh	
Quail	Fresh	
Quail	Fresh	
Quail	Fresh	
Squab	Fresh	
Squab	Fresh	
Squab	Fresh	
Turkey	Fresh or Frozen	Generic
Turkey	Fresh or Frozen	Generic
Turkey	Fresh or Frozen	Generic
Turkey	Fresh or Frozen	Land O Lakes
Turkey	Fresh or Frozen	Land O Lakes
Turkey	Fresh or Frozen	Land O Lakes
Turkey	Fresh or Frozen	Land O Lakes
Turkey	Fresh or Frozen	Land O Lakes
Turkey	Fresh or Frozen	Land O Lakes
Turkey	Fresh or Frozen	Land O Lakes
Turkey	Fresh or Frozen	Land O Lakes
Turkey	Fresh or Frozen	Longacre Cook N Bag
Turkey	Fresh or Frozen	Longacre Ready to Cook
Turkey	Fresh or Frozen	Louis Rich
Turkey	Fresh or Frozen	Louis Rich
Turkey	Fresh or Frozen	Louis Rich
Turkey	Fresh or Frozen	Louis Rich
Turkey	Fresh or Frozen	Louis Rich
Turkey	Fresh or Frozen	Louis Rich
Turkey	Fresh or Frozen	Louis Rich
Turkey	Fresh or Frozen	Louis Rich
Turkey	Fresh or Frozen	Louis Rich
Turkey	Fresh or Frozen	Louis Rich
Turkey	Fresh or Frozen	Louis Rich
Turkey	Fresh or Frozen	Louis Rich
Turkey	Fresh or Frozen	Louis Rich
Turkey	Fresh or Frozen	Louis Rich
Turkey	Fresh or Frozen	Louis Rich
Turkey	Fresh or Frozen	Louis Rich
Turkey	Fresh or Frozen	Louis Rich Drumettes
Turkey	Fresh or Frozen	Mr. Turkey Chub
Turkey	Fresh or Frozen	Mr. Turkey Chub
Turkey	Fresh or Frozen	Mr. Turkey Chub
Turkey	Fresh or Frozen	Norbest
Turkey	Fresh or Frozen	Norbest
Turkey	Fresh or Frozen	Norbest
Turkey	Fresh or Frozen	Norbest

Major Description	Minor Description	Serving Size	Calories	Grade
Breast Meat Only	Roasted	4 oz	140	C
Breast with Bone & Skin	Fat Roasted	4 oz	240	C
Mixed Cuts with Bone & Skin	Roasted	4 oz	260	D
Meat Only	Roasted	4 oz	270	D
Meat with Skin	Roasted	4 oz	346	D
Meat Only		4 oz	125	B
Meat with Skin		4 oz	179	C
Breast, Meat Only		4 oz	152	B
Leg, Meat Only		4 oz	152	B
Mixed Meat with Skin		4 oz	204	D
Breast Meat Only		4 oz	140	B
Meat Only		4 oz	152	C
Meat with Skin		4 oz	216	D
Breast Meat Only		4 oz	152	C
Mixed Meat Only		4 oz	160	D
Mixed Meat with Skin		4 oz	332	D
Breast with Skin	Roasted	4 oz	143	B–
Thigh with Skin	Roasted	4 oz	178	D–
White & Dark Meat	Roasted	4 oz	176	C–
Breast, Cooked		4 oz	133	A
Drumsticks		4 oz	160	C
Hindquarter, Roasted		4 oz	187	D
Thigh		4 oz	200	D
Wings		4 oz	160	C
Young		4 oz	173	D
Young	Butter Basted	4 oz	187	D
Young	Self-Basting Broth	4 oz	160	C
Breast		4 oz	108	C–
Breast		4 oz	156	B–
Breast, Cooked		4 oz	188	B
Breast, Cooked	Barbecue	4 oz	132	B–
Breast, Cooked	Hen without Wing	4 oz	20	C
Breast, Cooked	Hickory Smoked	4 oz	132	B–
Breast, Cooked	Honey Roasted	4 oz	132	B–
Breast, Cooked	Oven Roasted	4 oz	124	B–
Breast, Cooked	Roast	4 oz	168	B
Breast, Cooked	Slices	4 oz	156	A
Breast, Cooked	Smoked	4 oz	132	B–
Breast, Cooked	Steaks	4 oz	156	A
Breast, Cooked	Tenderloins	4 oz	156	A
Drumsticks	Cooked	4 oz	224	D
Thigh	Cooked	4 oz	256	D
Whole Cooked	without Giblets	4 oz	208	C
Wings	Cooked	4 oz	216	D
Wings	Portions	4 oz	216	D
Wings		4 oz	204	C
Breast, Cooked	Barbecue, Quarter	4 oz	136	B–
Breast, Cooked	Oven Prepared, Quarter	4 oz	136	B–
Breast, Cooked	Smoked, Quarter	4 oz	132	B–
Breast, Pre-Cooked	Steaks Cubed	4 oz	135	A
Breast, Pre-Cooked	with Gravy	4 oz	115	B–
with Gravy, Pre-Cooked		4 oz	115	B–
Whole, Cooked	Boneless	4 oz	168	C–

"+" *indicates the food meets minimum fiber requirements; "–" indicates the food has a high sodium content.*

Food	Processing Category	Brand
Turkey	Fresh or Frozen	Norbest
Turkey	Fresh or Frozen	Norbest Tastilean
Turkey	Fresh or Frozen	Norbest Tastilean
Turkey	Fresh or Frozen	Norbest Tastilean Tenders
Turkey	Fresh or Frozen	Swift Butterball
Turkey	Fresh or Frozen	Swift Butterball
Turkey	Fresh or Frozen	Swift Butterball
Turkey Fat	All Forms	
Turkey Giblets	Fresh or Frozen	
Turkey Gizzard	Fresh or Frozen	
Turkey, All Classes	Fresh or Frozen	
Turkey, All Classes	Fresh or Frozen	
Turkey, All Classes	Fresh or Frozen	
Turkey, All Classes	Fresh or Frozen	
Turkey, All Classes	Fresh or Frozen	
Turkey, All Classes	Fresh or Frozen	
Turkey, All Classes	Fresh or Frozen	
Turkey, All Classes	Fresh or Frozen	
Turkey, All Classes	Fresh or Frozen	
Turkey, All Classes	Fresh or Frozen	
Turkey, All Classes	Fresh or Frozen	
Turkey, All Classes	Fresh or Frozen	
Turkey, All Classes	Fresh or Frozen	
Turkey, All Classes	Fresh or Frozen	
Turkey, All Classes	Fresh or Frozen	
Turkey, Boneless & Luncheon Meat	*See* Luncheon & Packaged Meats	
Turkey, Canned or Processed	*See* Luncheon & Packaged Meats	
Turkey, Fryer-Roaster	Fresh	
Turkey, Fryer-Roaster	Fresh	
Turkey, Fryer-Roaster	Fresh	
Turkey, Fryer-Roaster	Fresh	
Turkey, Fryer-Roaster	Fresh	
Turkey, Fryer-Roaster	Fresh	
Turkey, Fryer-Roaster	Fresh	
Turkey, Fryer-Roaster	Fresh	
Turkey, Fryer-Roaster	Fresh	
Turkey, Fryer-Roaster	Fresh	
Turkey, Fryer-Roaster	Fresh	
Turkey, Fryer-Roaster	Fresh	
Turkey, Fryer-Roaster	Fresh	
Turkey, Ground	Packaged	Generic
Turkey, Ground	Packaged	Hudson's
Turkey, Ground	Packaged	Longacre
Turkey, Ground	Packaged	Louis Rich
Turkey, Ground	Packaged	Louis Rich
Turkey, Ground	Packaged	Louis Rich
Turkey, Ground	Packaged	Mr. Turkey
Turkey, Ground	Packaged	Norbest
Turkey, Young Hen	Fresh	
Turkey, Young Hen	Fresh	

[8] *Percentage fat turkey is by weight.*

Major Description	Minor Description	Serving Size	Calories	Grade
Whole, Cooked	Boneless Smoked	4 oz	168	C–
Breast, Pre-Cooked	Strips & Tips	4 oz	135	A
Cutlets, Pre-Cooked		4 oz	135	A
Breast, Pre-Cooked	Tenderloin	4 oz	135	A
Dark Meat without Skin	Roasted	4 oz	223	D
White & Dark Meat with Skin		4 oz	223	D
White Meat without Skin	Roasted	4 oz	183	B
		1 oz	255	D
	Simmered	4 oz	189	D
	Simmered	2.4 oz	109	D
Back Meat with Skin	Roasted	4 oz	276	D
Breast Meat with Skin	Roasted	4 oz	214	C
Dark Meat Only	Roasted	4 oz	212	C
Dark Meat with Skin	Roasted	4 oz	251	D
Leg Meat with Skin	Roasted	4 oz	236	D
Light Meat Only	Roasted	4 oz	178	B
Light Meat with Skin	Roasted	4 oz	223	C
Mixed Meat Only	Roasted	4 oz	193	B
Mixed Meat with Skin	Roasted	4 oz	236	D
Neck Meat Only	Simmered	4 oz	204	C
Neck Meat with Bone & Skin	Simmered	4 oz	274	C
Skin Only	Roasted	4 oz	500	D
White Meat without Skin	2% Fat [8]	3.5 oz	150	A
White Meat without Skin	6% Fat	3.5 oz	170	B
White Meat without Skin	8% Fat	3.5 oz	180	C
Wing Meat with Skin	Roasted	4 oz	260	D
Back Meat with Skin	Roasted	4 oz	231	D
Breast Meat Only	Roasted	4 oz	153	A
Breast Meat with Skin	Roasted	4 oz	174	B
Dark Meat Only	Roasted	4 oz	184	B
Dark Meat with Skin	Roasted	4 oz	206	C
Leg Meat Only	Roasted	4 oz	180	B
Leg Meat with Skin	Roasted	4 oz	193	B
Light Meat Only	Roasted	4 oz	159	A
Light Meat with Skin	Roasted	4 oz	186	B
Meat Only	Roasted	4 oz	170	B
Meat with Skin	Roasted	4 oz	195	B
Wing Meat Only	Roasted	4 oz	185	B
Wing Meat with Skin	Roasted	4 oz	235	D
Cooked		4 oz	260	D
Cooked		4 oz	220	D
Cooked		4 oz	240	D
Cooked		4 oz	240	C
Cooked		4 oz	208	D
Cooked	with Natural Flavor	4 oz	200	C
Cooked		4 oz	216	D
Raw		4 oz	180	D
Back Meat with Skin	Roasted	4 oz	288	D
Breast Meat with Skin	Roasted	4 oz	220	C

"+" indicates the food meets minimum fiber requirements; "–" indicates the food has a high sodium content.

Food	Processing Category	Brand
Turkey, Young Hen	Fresh	
Turkey, Young Hen	Fresh	
Turkey, Young Hen	Fresh	
Turkey, Young Hen	Fresh	
Turkey, Young Hen	Fresh	
Turkey, Young Hen	Fresh	
Turkey, Young Hen	Fresh	
Turkey, Young Hen	Fresh	
Turkey, Young Hen	Fresh	
Turkey, Young Tom	Fresh	
Turkey, Young Tom	Fresh	
Turkey, Young Tom	Fresh	
Turkey, Young Tom	Fresh	
Turkey, Young Tom	Fresh	
Turkey, Young Tom	Fresh	
Turkey, Young Tom	Fresh	
Turkey, Young Tom	Fresh	
Turkey, Young Tom	Fresh	
Turkey, Young Tom	Fresh	
LUNCHEON AND PACKAGED MEATS AND POULTRY		
Barbecue Loaf	All Forms	Most Brands
Beef Corned Hashed	Canned Or Packaged	Armour
Beef Corned Hashed	Canned Or Packaged	Libby's
Beef Corned Hashed	Canned Or Packaged	Mary Kitchen
Beef Corned Hashed	Canned Or Packaged	Nalleys
Beef Jerky	All Forms	Frito-Lay's
Beef Jerky	All Forms	Frito-Lay's Tender
Beef Jerky	All Forms	Hickory Farms
Beef Jerky	All Forms	Hormel Lumberjack
Beef Jerky	All Forms	Pemmican
Beef Jerky	All Forms	Pemmican
Beef Jerky	All Forms	Pemmican
Beef Jerky	All Forms	Pemmican Arrowhead
Beef Jerky	All Forms	Pemmican Steakers
Beef Jerky	All Forms	Pemmican Steakers
Beef Jerky	All Forms	Pemmican Tender Brave Chief
Beef Jerky	All Forms	Pemmican Tender Tomahawk
Beef Jerky	All Forms	Slim Jim
Beef Jerky	All Forms	Slim Jim Big Jerk
Beef Jerky	All Forms	Slim Jim Super Jerk
Beef Luncheon Meat	All Forms	Generic
Beef Luncheon Meat	All Forms	Boar's Head
Beef Luncheon Meat	All Forms	Boar's Head Deluxe
Beef Luncheon Meat	All Forms	Eckrich Slender Sliced
Beef Luncheon Meat	All Forms	Healthy Deli
Beef Luncheon Meat	All Forms	Healthy Deli
Beef Luncheon Meat	All Forms	Hillshire Farm Deli Select
Beef Luncheon Meat	All Forms	Hillshire Farm Deli Select
Beef Luncheon Meat	All Forms	Hormel
Beef Luncheon Meat	All Forms	Hormel
Beef Luncheon Meat	All Forms	Hormel Perma-fresh
Beef Luncheon Meat	All Forms	Oscar Mayer
Beef Luncheon Meat	All Forms	Oscar Mayer Deli-Thin

Major Description	Minor Description	Serving Size	Calories	Grade
Dark Meat Only	Roasted	4 oz	218	C
Dark Meat with Skin	Roasted	4 oz	263	D
Leg Meat with Skin	Roasted	4 oz	242	D
Light Meat Only	Roasted	4 oz	183	B
Light Meat with Skin	Roasted	4 oz	235	D
Mixed Meat Only	Roasted	4 oz	198	B
Mixed Meat with Skin	Roasted	4 oz	247	D
Skin Only	Roasted	4 oz	548	D
Wing Meat with Skin	Roasted	4 oz	270	D
Back Meat with Skin	Roasted	4 oz	270	D
Breast Meat with Skin	Roasted	4 oz	214	C
Dark Meat Only	Roasted	4 oz	210	C
Dark Meat with Skin	Roasted	4 oz	245	D
Leg Meat with Skin	Roasted	4 oz	234	D
Light Meat Only	Roasted	4 oz	175	B
Light Meat with Skin	Roasted	4 oz	217	C
Mixed Meat Only	Roasted	4 oz	191	B
Mixed Meat with Skin	Roasted	4 oz	229	D
Wing Meat with Skin	Roasted	4 oz	251	D
		1 oz slice	49	D–
		1 oz	55	D–
		1 oz	53	D–
		1 oz	48	D–
		1 oz	53	D–
		.21 oz	25	C–
		.7 oz	120	D–
		1 oz	100	B–
		1 oz	101	D–
Natural Style		1 oz	80	B–
Peppered, Natural Style	Tabasco	1.1 oz	90	B–
Teriyaki Natural Style		1 oz	80	B–
		.7 oz	70	C–
		1.1 oz	80	A–
		.37 oz	40	B–
		1 oz	80	B–
		.25 oz	20	D–
		.14 oz	20	D–
		.25 oz	25	C–
Regular or Tabasco		.31 oz	30	B–
Beef Loaf		1 oz slice	87	D–
Roast Beef	Top Round, Roasted	1 oz slice	40	B
Roast Beef	Top Round, Roasted	1 oz slice	45	C
Roast Beef		1 oz slice	35	B–
Roast Beef		1 oz slice	30	A–
Roast Beef	Italian Style	1 oz slice	31	B–
Roast Beef	Roasted, Cured	1 oz slice	31	A–
Smoked Beef		1 oz slice	31	A–
Smoked	Cured	1 oz slice	50	C–
Smoked	Cured, Dried	1 oz slice	45	B–
Loaf, Jellied		1 slice	45	C–
Smoked		.5 oz slice	14	B–
Roast Beef		1 slice	15	B–

"+" indicates the food meets minimum fiber requirements; "–" indicates the food has a high sodium content.

Food	Processing Category	Brand
Beef Luncheon Meat	All Forms	Oscar Mayer Thin Sliced
Beef Luncheon Meat	All Forms	Steak-umms
Beef Tallow	All Forms	Generic
Beef, Corned	Canned Or Packaged	Generic
Beef, Corned	Canned Or Packaged	Generic
Beef, Corned	Canned Or Packaged	Dinty Moore
Beef, Corned	Canned Or Packaged	Eckrich Slender Sliced
Beef, Corned	Canned Or Packaged	Healthy Deli
Beef, Corned	Canned Or Packaged	Healthy Deli St. Paddys
Beef, Corned	Canned Or Packaged	Hillshire Farm
Beef, Corned	Canned Or Packaged	Libby's
Beef, Corned	Canned Or Packaged	Oscar Mayer
Beef, Corned	Cured	Generic
Beef, Vegetarian	Canned	Worthington Country Stew
Beef, Vegetarian	Canned	Worthington Prime Steaks
Beef, Vegetarian	Canned	Worthington Savory Slices
Beef, Vegetarian	Canned	Worthington Vegetable Steaks
Beef, Vegetarian	Frozen	Worthington
Beef, Vegetarian	Frozen	Worthington
Beef, Vegetarian	Frozen	Worthington
Beef, Vegetarian	Frozen	Worthington
Beef, Vegetarian	Frozen	Worthington Stakelets
Beerwurst	All Forms	Generic
Beerwurst	All Forms	Generic
Berliner	All Forms	Generic
Blood Sausage	All Forms	Generic
Bockwurst	All Forms	All Brands
Bologna	All Forms	Generic
Bologna	All Forms	Generic
Bologna	All Forms	Generic
Bologna	All Forms	Generic
Bologna	All Forms	Boar's Head
Bologna	All Forms	Boar's Head
Bologna	All Forms	Boar's Head
Bologna	All Forms	Boar's Head Lower Salt
Bologna	All Forms	Eckrich
Bologna	All Forms	Eckrich
Bologna	All Forms	Eckrich
Bologna	All Forms	Eckrich
Bologna	All Forms	Eckrich German Brand
Bologna	All Forms	Eckrich Lean Supreme
Bologna	All Forms	Eckrich Sandwich
Bologna	All Forms	Eckrich Smorgas Pac
Bologna	All Forms	Eckrich Thick Sliced
Bologna	All Forms	Healthy Deli
Bologna	All Forms	Hebrew National Original Deli
Bologna	All Forms	Hillshire Farm Large
Bologna	All Forms	Hillshire Farm Ring
Bologna	All Forms	Hormel Coarse Ground 1 lb
Bologna	All Forms	Hormel Perma-fresh
Bologna	All Forms	Hormel Perma-fresh
Bologna	All Forms	
Bologna	All Forms	JM

Major Description	Minor Description	Serving Size	Calories	Grade
Roast Beef		.4 oz slice	14	B–
Sandwich Steak		2 oz	180	D
		1 oz	256	D
		1 oz	71	D–
Loaf	Jellied	1 oz slice	46	C–
		1 oz	65	D
		1 oz	40	B–
		1 oz	35	B–
		1 oz	24	A–
		1 oz	31	A–
Canned		1 oz	67	D–
		.6 oz	17	B–
Brisket	Cooked	1 oz	71	D–
		9.5 oz	220	C–
		3.25 oz	160	D–
		1 oz	100	D–
Steak		1.3 oz	44	B–
	Pie	8 oz	360	C–
Roll		.6 oz	33	D–
Roll	Corned	1 oz	60	D–
Roll	Smoked	1 slice	40	D–
		2.5oz	150	D–
Beef		.8 oz slice	75	D–
Pork		.8 oz slice	55	D–
Beef & Pork		1 oz slice	65	D–
		1 oz	107	D
		1 oz slice	87	D
Beef		1 oz slice	90	D–
Beef & Pork		1 oz slice	89	D–
Lebanese Style		1 oz slice	64	D–
Pork		1 oz slice	70	D–
Beef		1 oz slice	74	D–
Ham		1 oz slice	40	D
Pork & Beef		1 oz slice	80	D–
		1 oz slice	80	D–
		1 oz slice	100	D–
Beef		1 oz slice	90	D–
Cheese		1 oz slice	90	D–
Garlic		1 oz slice	90	D–
		1 oz slice	80	D–
		1 oz slice	70	D–
		1 oz slice	100	D–
		1 oz slice	100	D–
Beef		1.5 oz slice	130	D–
Regular German		1 oz slice	35	C–
Beef		1 oz slice	90	D–
		1 oz slice	90	D
		1 oz slice	89	D
Beef		1 oz slice	80	D–
		1 slice	90	D–
Beef		1 slice	85	D–
		1 oz slice	90	D–
Beef		1 oz slice	90	D–

"+" indicates the food meets minimum fiber requirements; "–" indicates the food has a high sodium content.

Food	Processing Category	Brand
Bologna	All Forms	JM
Bologna	All Forms	JM German Brand
Bologna	All Forms	Kahn's
Bologna	All Forms	Kahn's
Bologna	All Forms	Kahn's
Bologna	All Forms	Kahn's Deluxe Club
Bologna	All Forms	Kahn's Family Pack
Bologna	All Forms	Kahn's Giant Deluxe
Bologna	All Forms	Kahn's Giant Thick Deluxe
Bologna	All Forms	Kahn's Pounder
Bologna	All Forms	Kahn's Thick Deluxe
Bologna	All Forms	Kahn's Thin-Sliced Deluxe
Bologna	All Forms	Kahn's/Kahn's Giant
Bologna	All Forms	Light & Lean
Bologna	All Forms	Light & Lean Thin Sliced
Bologna	All Forms	OHSE
Bologna	All Forms	OHSE
Bologna	All Forms	OHSE 15% Chicken
Bologna	All Forms	Oscar Mayer
Bologna	All Forms	Oscar Mayer
Bologna	All Forms	Oscar Mayer
Bologna	All Forms	Oscar Mayer
Bologna	All Forms	Oscar Mayer
Bologna	All Forms	Oscar Mayer Fat Free
Bologna	All Forms	Oscar Mayer Fun Pack
Bologna	All Forms	Oscar Mayer Healthy Favorites
Bologna	All Forms	Oscar Mayer Light
Bologna	All Forms	Pilgrims Pride
Bologna, Vegetarian	Frozen	Worthington Bolono
Bratwurst	All Forms	Generic
Bratwurst	All Forms	Generic
Bratwurst	All Forms	Eckrich
Bratwurst	All Forms	Hickory Farms Bratwurst
Bratwurst	All Forms	Hickory Farms Cheddy Brots
Bratwurst	All Forms	Hickory Farms Hot Brots
Bratwurst	All Forms	Hillshire Farm
Bratwurst	All Forms	Hillshire Farm
Bratwurst	All Forms	Hillshire Farm
Bratwurst	All Forms	Hillshire Farm Fully Cooked
Bratwurst	All Forms	Kahn's
Braunschweiger	All Forms	Generic
Braunschweiger	All Forms	Hormel
Braunschweiger	All Forms	JM
Braunschweiger	All Forms	Oscar Mayer German Brand
Braunschweiger	All Forms	Oscar Mayer Slices
Braunschweiger	All Forms	Oscar Mayer Slices
Braunschweiger	All Forms	Oscar Mayer Tube
Burger, Vegetarian	Canned	Worthington Vegetarian Burger
Burger, Vegetarian	Canned	Worthington Vegetarian Burger
Burger, Vegetarian	Frozen	Morningstar Farms Grillers
Burger, Vegetarian	Frozen	Worthington Fripats
Burger, Vegetarian	Mix	Fantastic Foods
Burger, Vegetarian	Mix	Love Natural Foods Loveburger

Major Description	Minor Description	Serving Size	Calories	Grade
Garlic		1 oz slice	90	D–
		1 oz slice	70	D–
Beef & Cheddar		1 slice	90	D–
Garlic		1 slice	90	D–
Ham		1 slice	90	D–
		1 slice	90	D–
Beef		1 slice	70	D–
		1 slice	90	D–
		1 slice	110	D–
Beef		1 slice	90	D–
		1 slice	140	D–
		1 slice	60	D–
Beef		1 slice	90	D–
		1 slice	70	D
		1 slice	35	D
		1 oz slice	75	D–
Beef		1 oz slice	85	D–
		1 oz slice	90	D–
		1 oz slice	90	D–
		1.6 oz slice	144	D–
Beef		1 oz slice	89	D–
Beef	Garlic Flavor	1 oz slice	90	D–
Cheese		.8 oz slice	74	D–
		.8 oz slice	18	A–
Wild Cherry		1 oz slice	50	D–
		2 slices	45	B–
Beef		1 oz slice	64	D–
		1 oz slice	59	D–
		.6 oz slice	30	B–
Pork	Cooked	1 oz slice	85	D–
Pork & Beef		1 oz slice	92	D–
		1 link	310	D–
		1 oz slice	90	D–
Cheddar Cheese		1 oz slice	98	D–
Hot		1 oz slice	96	D–
Fresh		1 oz slice	95	D–
Smoked		1 oz slice	95	D–
Spicy		1 oz slice	90	D
		1 oz slice	85	D–
		1 link	190	D–
Pork		1 oz slice	102	D–
		1 oz slice	80	D–
		1 oz slice	80	D–
		1 oz slice	96	D–
		1 oz slice	96	D–
		.9 oz slice	89	D–
		1 oz slice	97	D–
		$^1/_2$ cup	150	B–
No Salt		$^1/_2$ cup	160	C–
	Patty	1 patty	180	D–
		1 patty	180	D–
	with Tofu	1 patty	133	C–
	2 oz Mix	1 patty	245	C+

"+" indicates the food meets minimum fiber requirements; "–" indicates the food has a high sodium content.

Food	Processing Category	Brand
Burger, Vegetarian	Mix	Nature's Burger
Burger, Vegetarian	Mix	Nature's Burger
Burger, Vegetarian	Mix	Nature's Burger
Burger, Vegetarian	Mix	Worthington Granburger
Cheddarwurst	All Forms	Generic
Chicken Bologna	All Forms	Health Valley
Chicken Canned	Canned	Generic
Chicken Canned	Canned	Featherweight
Chicken Canned	Canned	Hormel
Chicken Canned	Canned	Hormel
Chicken Canned	Canned	Hormel
Chicken Canned	Canned	Hormel
Chicken Canned	Canned	Hormel
Chicken Canned	Canned	Swanson
Chicken Canned	Canned	Swanson
Chicken Canned	Canned	Swanson Mixin' Chicken
Chicken Frankfurter	All Forms	Generic
Chicken Frankfurter	All Forms	Health Valley Weiners
Chicken Frankfurter	All Forms	Longacre
Chicken Frankfurter	All Forms	Tyson Corn Dogs
Chicken Ham	All Forms	Pilgrims Pride
Chicken Luncheon Meat	All Forms	Generic
Chicken Luncheon Meat	All Forms	Hillshire Farm Deli Select
Chicken Luncheon Meat	All Forms	Longacre Premium
Chicken Luncheon Meat	All Forms	Louis Rich
Chicken Luncheon Meat	All Forms	Louis Rich
Chicken Luncheon Meat	All Forms	Louis Rich Deluxe
Chicken Luncheon Meat	All Forms	Louis Rich Thin Sliced
Chicken Luncheon Meat	All Forms	Mr. Turkey
Chicken Luncheon Meat	All Forms	Oscar Mayer
Chicken Luncheon Meat	All Forms	Oscar Mayer
Chicken Luncheon Meat	All Forms	Oscar Mayer Deli-Thin
Chicken Luncheon Meat	All Forms	Oscar Mayer Healthy Favorites
Chicken Luncheon Meat	All Forms	Oscar Mayer Thin Sliced
Chicken Luncheon Meat	All Forms	Pilgrims Pride
Chicken Salad	Packaged	Longacre
Chicken Salad	Packaged	Longacre Saladfest
Chicken Spread	Canned	Generic
Chicken Spread	Canned	Hormel
Chicken Spread	Canned	Underwood
Chicken Spread	Canned	Underwood
Chicken Spread	Canned	Underwood Light
Chicken Vegetarian	Canned	Worthington
Chicken Vegetarian	Canned	Worthington Frichik
Chicken Vegetarian	Frozen	Morningstar Farm Country Crisps
Chicken Vegetarian	Frozen	Morningstar Farm Country Crisps
Chicken Vegetarian	Frozen	Morningstar Farm Country Crisps
Chicken Vegetarian	Frozen	Worthington
Chicken Vegetarian	Frozen	Worthington Chicketts
Chicken Vegetarian	Frozen	Worthington Chik Stiks
Chicken Vegetarian	Frozen	Worthington Crispy Chik
Chicken Vegetarian	Frozen	Worthington Crispy Chik
Chicken Vegetarian	Frozen	Worthington Meatless Chicken

Major Description	Minor Description	Serving Size	Calories	Grade
	Barbeque	1 patty	117	A–+
	Original	1 patty	152	B–+
	Pizza	1 patty	121	A–
		1 patty	110	A–
		1 oz slice	95	D–
		1 slice	85	D–
Boned	in Broth	4 oz	188	D–
Chunk		4 oz	120	B
Chunk	Breast	4 oz	210	D–
Chunk	Dark	4 oz	194	D–
Chunk	White & Dark	4 oz	200	D–
Chunk	White & Dark, Unsalted	4 oz	195	D
Loaf		4 oz	260	D–
White		4 oz	160	C–
White & Dark		4 oz	160	C–
Chunk	Style	4 oz	108	D–
		1 link (1.6 oz)	116	D–
		1 link	96	D
		1 oz	63	D–
Battered		3.5 oz	280	D
		1 oz slice	35	D–
Light Meat	Roll	1 oz slice	45	D–
Breast	Smoked	1 oz slice	31	A–
Breast		1 oz slice	45	D–
Breast	Hickory Smoked	1 oz slice	30	B–
White Meat	Roasted	1 oz slice	35	D–
Breast	Roasted	1 oz slice	30	B–
Breast	Roasted	.4 oz slice	12	B–
Breast		1 oz slice	32	C–
Breast	Roasted	1 oz slice	29	B–
Breast	Smoked	1 oz slice	25	A–
Breast	Honey Glazed	.5 oz slice	15	A–
Breast	Roasted	1 slice	10	A–
Breast	Roasted	.4 oz slice	13	B–
Roll		1 oz slice	35	C–
		1 oz	64	D–
		1 oz	47	D–
		1 oz	55	D
		1 oz	60	D
Chunk		1 oz	70	D–
Smoky		1 oz	70	D–
		1 oz	38	C–
	Sliced	2 slices (c. 2.1 oz)	90	D–
		2 pieces (c. 3.2 oz)	180	D–
	Nuggets Homestyle	3 oz	250	D–
	Nuggets Zesty	3 oz	280	D–
	Patty	2.5 oz patty	220	D–
	Pie	8 oz pie	380	D–
	Roll	1/2 cup	160	C–
	Sticks	1 piece (c. 1.7 oz)	110	D–
		3 oz	280	D–
	Patty	2.5 oz patty	220	D–
	Diced	1/2 cup	190	D–

"+" indicates the food meets minimum fiber requirements; "–" indicates the food has a high sodium content.

Food	Processing Category	Brand
Chicken Vegetarian	Frozen	Worthington Meatless Chicken
Chicken Vegetarian	Frozen	Worthington Meatless Chicken
Chili	Canned	Generic
Chili	Canned	Chef Boyardee
Chili	Canned	Chef Boyardee Chili Mac
Chili	Canned	Dennison's
Chili	Canned	Dennison's 15 oz
Chili	Canned	Dennison's 19 oz
Chili	Canned	Dennison's Cook Off
Chili	Canned	Estee
Chili	Canned	Featherweight
Chili	Canned	Gebhardt
Chili	Canned	Gebhardt
Chili	Canned	Hain
Chili	Canned	Hain
Chili	Canned	Hain
Chili	Canned	Hain Reduced Sodium
Chili	Canned	Healthy Valley Fat Free
Chili	Canned	Healthy Valley Fat Free
Chili	Canned	Healthy Valley Fat Free
Chili	Canned	Heinz
Chili	Canned	Heinz Chili Con Carne
Chili	Canned	Heinz Chili Mac
Chili	Canned	Hormel 15 oz
Chili	Canned	Hormel 15 oz
Chili	Canned	Hormel 15 oz
Chili	Canned	Hormel Micro-Cup
Chili	Canned	Libby's
Chili	Canned	Libby's 15 oz
Chili	Canned	Nalley's
Chili	Canned	Nalley's
Chili	Canned	Nalley's Big Chunk
Chili	Canned	Nalley's Thick
Chili	Canned	Natural Touch
Chili	Canned	Van Camp's
Chili	Canned	Van Camp's
Chili	Canned	Van Camp's Chilee Weenee
Chili	Canned	Wolf Brand
Chili	Canned	Wolf Brand
Chili	Canned	Wolf Brand
Chili	Canned	Wolf Brand
Chili	Canned	Wolf Brand Chili-Mac
Chili	Canned	Worthington
Chorizo	Canned	Generic
Dutch Brand Loaf	All Forms	Generic
Dutch Brand Loaf	All Forms	Eckrich
Dutch Brand Loaf	All Forms	Eckrich Smorgas Pac
Dutch Brand Loaf	All Forms	Erkrich Lean Supreme
Dutch Brand Loaf	All Forms	Kahn's
Frankfurter	All Forms	All Brands Except as Noted
Frankfurter	All Forms	Ball Park
Frankfurter	All Forms	Healthy Choice
Frankfurter	All Forms	Healthy Favorites

Major Description	Minor Description	Serving Size	Calories	Grade
	Roll	2.5 oz	150	D–
	Slices	2 oz slice	130	D–
Beans		7.5 oz	238	D–+
Beans	Beef	7.5 oz	330	D–
		7.5 oz	230	D–
Beans	Chunky	7.5 oz	310	D–+
Beans	Hot	7.5 oz	310	D–+
without Beans		7.5 oz	300	D–
Beans		7.5 oz	340	D–+
Beans		7.5 oz	370	D
Beans		7.5 oz	280	C–
Beans	Hot	7.5 oz	354	D–
Vegetarian		7.5 oz	410	D–
Chicken Spicy		7.5 oz	130	A–
Vegetarian	Spicy	7.5 oz	160	A–
Vegetarian	Tempeh Spicy	7.5 oz	160	B–
Vegetarian	Spicy	7.5 oz	170	A
3 Bean	Mild Vegetarian	7.5 oz	105	A–+
Beans	Mild Vegetarian	7.5 oz	105	A–+
Beans	Spicy Vegetarian	7.5 oz	105	A–+
Beans	Hot	7.75 oz	330	D–
		7.75 oz	350	D–
		7.5 oz	250	D–
Beans		7.5 oz	310	D–
Beans	Hot	7.5 oz	310	D–
without Beans	Hot	7.5 oz	370	D–
Beans		7.5 oz	250	C–
without Beans		7.5 oz	390	D–
Beans		7.5 oz	270	D–
Beans		7.5 oz	280	C–
Beans	Jalapeño	7.5 oz	260	C–
without Beans		7.5 oz	270	D–
Beans		7.5 oz	260	C–
Vegetarian	Spicy	1 cup	345	D–
Beans		1 cup	352	D–
without Beans		1 cup	412	D–
without Beans	Franks	1 cup	309	D–
Beans		7.5 oz	325	D–
Beans	Extra Spicy	7.75 oz	324	D–
without Beans		7.5 oz	363	D–
without Beans	Extra Spicy	7.5 oz	363	D–
without Beans		7.75 oz	317	D–
Vegetarian		1 cup	285	D–
Beef & Pork		1 oz	125	D
Pork & Beef		1 oz slice	68	D–
		1 oz slice	70	D–
		1 oz slice	70	D–
		1 oz slice	60	D–
		1 slice	80	D–
All Varieties		1 oz frank	c. 90	D–
	Fat Free	1 frank	40	A–
Turkey, Pork & Beef	Low Fat	1 frank	70	B–
with Turkey		1 frank	57	B–

"+" indicates the food meets minimum fiber requirements; "–" indicates the food has a high sodium content.

Food	Processing Category	Brand
Frankfurter	All Forms	Hormel Light & Lean
Frankfurter	All Forms	John Morell Lite
Frankfurter	All Forms	Kahn's
Frankfurter	All Forms	Oscar Mayer
Frankfurter	All Forms	Oscar Mayer Healthy Favorites
Frankfurter, Vegetarian	Canned	Worthington Super-Links
Frankfurter, Vegetarian	Canned	Worthington Veja-Links
Frankfurter, Vegetarian	Frozen	Worthington Dixie Dogs
Frankfurter, Vegetarian	Frozen	Worthington Leanies
German Sausage	All Forms	Hickory Farms
Ham Luncheon Meat	All Forms	Generic
Ham Luncheon Meat	All Forms	Generic
Ham Luncheon Meat	All Forms	Generic
Ham Luncheon Meat	All Forms	Boar's Head Deluxe
Ham Luncheon Meat	All Forms	Boar's Head Lower Salt
Ham Luncheon Meat	All Forms	Eckrich
Ham Luncheon Meat	All Forms	Eckrich
Ham Luncheon Meat	All Forms	Eckrich Slender Sliced
Ham Luncheon Meat	All Forms	Erkrich Lean Supreme
Ham Luncheon Meat	All Forms	Healthy Deli
Ham Luncheon Meat	All Forms	Healthy Deli
Ham Luncheon Meat	All Forms	Healthy Deli
Ham Luncheon Meat	All Forms	Healthy Deli
Ham Luncheon Meat	All Forms	Healthy Deli Deluxe
Ham Luncheon Meat	All Forms	Healthy Deli Honey Valley
Ham Luncheon Meat	All Forms	Healthy Deli Lessalt
Ham Luncheon Meat	All Forms	Healthy Deli Lessalt
Ham Luncheon Meat	All Forms	Healthy Deli Light AM
Ham Luncheon Meat	All Forms	Healthy Deli Taverne
Ham Luncheon Meat	All Forms	Hillshire Farm Deli Select
Ham Luncheon Meat	All Forms	Hillshire Farm Deli Select
Ham Luncheon Meat	All Forms	Hillside Farm Deli Select
Ham Luncheon Meat	All Forms	Hormel Perma-fresh
Ham Luncheon Meat	All Forms	J&M
Ham Luncheon Meat	All Forms	J&M
Ham Luncheon Meat	All Forms	J&M
Ham Luncheon Meat	All Forms	J&M
Ham Luncheon Meat	All Forms	J&M Slice 'n Eat 93% Fat Free
Ham Luncheon Meat	All Forms	J&M Slice 'n Eat 95% Fat Free
Ham Luncheon Meat	All Forms	Jones Dairy Farm
Ham Luncheon Meat	All Forms	Jones Dairy Farm Family Ham
Ham Luncheon Meat	All Forms	Kahn's
Ham Luncheon Meat	All Forms	Kahn's
Ham Luncheon Meat	All Forms	Kahn's Low Salt
Ham Luncheon Meat	All Forms	Light & Lean
Ham Luncheon Meat	All Forms	Light & Lean
Ham Luncheon Meat	All Forms	Light & Lean
Ham Luncheon Meat	All Forms	Light & Lean
Ham Luncheon Meat	All Forms	Light & Lean
Ham Luncheon Meat	All Forms	Light & Lean
Ham Luncheon Meat	All Forms	Light & Lean
Ham Luncheon Meat	All Forms	Louis Rich Carving Board
Ham Luncheon Meat	All Forms	Louis Rich Carving Board

Major Description	Minor Description	Serving Size	Calories	Grade
		1 frank	45	B–
	50% Less Fat	1 frank	45	D–
	Fat Free	1 frank	40	A–
	Fat Free	1 frank	40	A–
Turkey & Beef		1 frank	60	B–
		1 frank	100	D–
		1 frank	70	D–
on a Stick		1 frank	200	D–
		1 frank	100	D–
		1 oz	100	D–
Chopped		1 oz slice	65	D–
Cooked	Regular Sliced	1 oz slice	52	D–
Minced		1 oz slice	75	D–
Boiled		1 oz slice	28	C–
		1 oz slice	28	C–
Chopped		1 oz slice	45	C–
Loaf		1 oz slice	50	D–
Smoked		1 oz slice	40	D–
Chopped		1 oz slice	35	D–
Black Forest	Baked	1 oz slice	32	B–
Fresh	Cooked	1 oz slice	33	B–
Jalapeño Pepper		1 oz slice	25	B–
Virginia	Baked	1 oz slice	34	B–
		1 oz slice	31	B–
Honey		1 oz slice	31	B
		1 oz slice	32	B–
Virginia	Baked	1 oz slice	32	B
		1 oz slice	27	B–
		1 oz slice	31	B–
Honey		1 oz slice	31	B–
Smoked		1 oz slice	31	B–
Cajun Style		1 oz slice	31	B–
Chopped		1 oz slice	44	D–
Chopped		1 oz slice	80	D–
Cooked		1 oz slice	30	B–
Golden Smoked		1 oz slice	40	D–
Golden Smoked	with Water	1 oz slice	35	B–
		1 oz slice	35	C–
		1 slice	30	B–
		1 slice	50	B–
		1 oz slice	35	C–
Chopped		1 slice	50	D–
Cooked		1 slice	30	B–
		1 slice	30	B–
Barbecue		1 slice	25	C
Chopped		1 slice	25	D
Cooked		1 slice	25	C
Glazed		1 slice	25	C
Peppered	Black	1 slice	25	C
Peppered	Red	1 slice	25	C
Smoked	Cooked	1 slice	25	C
Baked	in Natural Juice	1 oz slice	28	B–
Honey	in Natural Juice	1 oz slice	31	B–

"+" indicates the food meets minimum fiber requirements; "–" indicates the food has a high sodium content.

Food	Processing Category	Brand
Ham Luncheon Meat	All Forms	Louis Rich Carving Board
Ham Luncheon Meat	All Forms	Louis Rich Dinner Slices
Ham Luncheon Meat	All Forms	OHSE
Ham Luncheon Meat	All Forms	OHSE
Ham Luncheon Meat	All Forms	OHSE 95% Fat Free
Ham Luncheon Meat	All Forms	Oscar Mayer
Ham Luncheon Meat	All Forms	Oscar Mayer
Ham Luncheon Meat	All Forms	Oscar Mayer
Ham Luncheon Meat	All Forms	Oscar Mayer
Ham Luncheon Meat	All Forms	Oscar Mayer
Ham Luncheon Meat	All Forms	Oscar Mayer
Ham Luncheon Meat	All Forms	Oscar Mayer
Ham Luncheon Meat	All Forms	Oscar Mayer
Ham Luncheon Meat	All Forms	Oscar Mayer Breakfast Ham
Ham Luncheon Meat	All Forms	Oscar Mayer Deli-Thin
Ham Luncheon Meat	All Forms	Oscar Mayer Deli-Thin
Ham Luncheon Meat	All Forms	Oscar Mayer Deli-Thin
Ham Luncheon Meat	All Forms	Oscar Mayer Healthy Favorites
Ham Luncheon Meat	All Forms	Oscar Mayer Healthy Favorites
Ham Luncheon Meat	All Forms	Oscar Mayer Healthy Favorites
Ham Luncheon Meat	All Forms	Oscar Mayer Jubilee
Ham Luncheon Meat	All Forms	Oscar Mayer Lower Salt
Ham Luncheon Meat	All Forms	Oscar Mayer Thin Sliced
Ham Luncheon Meat	All Forms	Oscar Mayer Lean Meats
Ham Luncheon Meat	All Forms	Oscar Mayer Lean Meats
Ham Luncheon Meat	All Forms	Oscar Mayer Lean Meats
Ham Luncheon Meat	All Forms	Oscar Mayer Lean Meats
Ham Luncheon Meat	All Forms	Oscar Mayer Lean Meats
Ham Luncheon Meat	All Forms	Swift Premium Hostess
Ham Luncheon Meat	All Forms	Swift Premium Sugar Plum
Ham Patty	All Forms	Swift Premium Brown 'n Serve
Ham Patty	Canned	Hormel
Ham, Vegetarian	Frozen	Worthington Wham
Honey Loaf	All Forms	Eckrich
Honey Loaf	All Forms	Eckrich Smorgas Pac
Honey Loaf	All Forms	Hormel Perma-fresh
Honey Loaf	All Forms	Kahn's
Honey Loaf	All Forms	Oscar Mayer
Honey Roll Sausage	All Forms	Generic
Italian Sausage	All Forms	Generic
Italian Sausage	All Forms	Generic
Italian Sausage	All Forms	Hillshire Farm Flavorseal
Italian Sausage	All Forms	Hillshire Farm Links
Italian Sausage	All Forms	Hillshire Farm Links
Jalapeño Loaf	All Forms	Kahn's
Kielbasa	All Forms	All Brands
Kielbasa	All Forms	Healthy Choice
Kielbasa	All Forms	Hillshire Farm
Knockwurst	All Forms	All Brands
Liver Cheese	All Forms	Generic
Liver Loaf	All Forms	Kahn's
Liverwurst	All Forms	Generic
Luncheon Meat, Spiced	All Forms	Light & Lean

Major Description	Minor Description	Serving Size	Calories	Grade
Smoked	in Natural Juice	1 oz slice	31	B–
Baked		1 slice	80	B–
Chopped		1 oz slice	65	D–
Cooked		1 oz slice	30	B–
Smoked		1 oz slice	30	B–
Baked		.75 oz slice	21	B–
Boiled		.75 oz slice	23	B–
Boiled	Thin Sliced	1 oz slice	13	B–
Chopped		1 oz slice	41	D–
Honey		.75 oz slice	23	B–
Peppered	Black	.75 oz slice	22	C–
Peppered	Chopped	1 oz	55	D–
Smoked	Cooked	.75 oz slice	22	B–
		1.5 oz slice	47	B–
	Boiled	1 slice	13	C–
	Honey	1 slice	15	B–
	Smoked	1 slice	13	C–
	Baked	1 slice	13	B–
	Honey	1 slice	13	B–
	Smoked	1 slice	13	B–
		1 oz slice	43	D–
		.7 oz slice	23	B–
Honey		.4 oz slice	13	B–
Baked		1 slice	20	A–
Boiled		1 slice	20	C–
Cooked		1 slice	20	C–
Honey		1 slice	23	C–
Low Sodium		1 slice	23	C–
		1 oz slice	30	B–
		1 oz slice	30	B–
		1 patty	130	D–
		1 patty	180	D–
Roll or Sliced		3 slices (2.4 oz)	120	D–
		1 oz slice	35	B–
		1 oz slice	35	B–
		1 slice	45	D–
		1 slice	40	D–
		1 oz slice	34	B–
Beef		1 oz	52	D–
All Varieties Except as Noted	Cooked	1 oz	92	D–
Pork	Cooked	1 oz	98	D–
Smoked		1 oz	100	D–
Hot		1 oz	90	D
Mild		1 oz	95	D
		1 slice	70	D–
Pork or Beef	All Varieties	1 oz	88	D–
Low Fat		1 oz	35	B–
Low Fat		1 oz	35	B–
Pork & Beef	All Varieties	1 oz	87	D–
Pork		1 oz	86	D–
		1 slice	170	D–
All Varieties		1 oz	92	D
		1 slice	60	D

"+" indicates the food meets minimum fiber requirements; "–" indicates the food has a high sodium content.

Food	Processing Category	Brand
Luncheon Meat, Spiced	Canned	Hormel
Luncheon Meat, Spiced	Canned	Hormel Perma-fresh
Luncheon Meat, Spiced	Canned	JM
Luncheon Meat, Spiced	Canned	Kahn's Luncheon Loaf
Luncheon Meat, Vegetarian	Canned	Worthington Numete
Luncheon Meat, Vegetarian	Canned	Worthington Protose
Meat Spread	Canned	Hormel
Meat Spread	Canned	Underwood
Meat Spread	Canned	Underwood
Meat Spread	Canned	Underwood
Meat Spread	Canned	Underwood
Meat Spread	Canned	Underwood
Meat Spread	Canned	Underwood
Meat Spread	Canned	Underwood
Meat Spread	Canned	Underwood
Meat Spread	Canned	Underwood
Meat Spread	Canned	Underwood
Meat Spread	Canned	Underwood Light
New England Brand Sausage	All Forms	Generic
New England Brand Sausage	All Forms	Eckrich
New England Brand Sausage	All Forms	Light & Lean
New England Brand Sausage	All Forms	Oscar Mayer
Olive Loaf	All Forms	Generic
P & B Loaf	All Forms	J&M
P & B Loaf	All Forms	Kahn's
Pastrami	All Forms	Generic
Pastrami	All Forms	Boar's Head Round
Pastrami	All Forms	Healthy Deli Round
Pastrami	All Forms	Hillshire Farm Deli Select
Pastrami	All Forms	Oscar Mayer
Pâté	Canned	Generic
Pâté	Canned	Generic
Peppered Loaf	All Forms	Generic
Peppered Loaf	All Forms	Eckrich
Peppered Loaf	All Forms	Kahn's
Peppered Loaf	All Forms	Oscar Mayer
Pepperoni	All Forms	All Brands
Pepperoni Bits	All Forms	Hormel
Pickle Loaf	All Forms	Eckrich
Pickle Loaf	All Forms	Eckrich Smorgas Pac
Pickle Loaf	All Forms	Hormel Perma-fresh
Pickle Loaf	All Forms	Kahn's
Pickle Loaf	All Forms	Kahn's Family Pack
Pickle Loaf	All Forms	Kahn's Family Pack
Pickle Loaf	All Forms	Light & Lean
Pickle Loaf	All Forms	OHSE
Polish Sausage	All Forms	All Brands
Pork Luncheon Meat	All Forms	Eckrich Slender Sliced
Prosciutto	All Forms	All Brands
Roast Beef Hash	Canned	Mary Kitchen
Roast Beef Hash	Frozen	Stouffer's
Salami	All Forms	All Brands Except as Noted
Salami	All Forms	All Brands Except as Noted

Major Description	Minor Description	Serving Size	Calories	Grade
		1 oz	93	D–
		1 slice	59	D–
Loaf, Spiced		1 oz slice	70	D–
Spiced		1 slice	80	D–
		1 oz slice	67	D–
		1 oz slice	67	C–
Roast Beef		1 oz	62	D
Chunky Chicken		1 oz	70	D–
Chunky Chicken	Light	1 oz	47	D–
Chunky Turkey	Light	1 oz	35	B–
Deviled Ham		1 oz	103	D–
Deviled Ham	Light	1 oz	56	D–
Honey Ham		1 oz	76	D–
Liver Pâté		1 oz	84	D–
Liverwurst		1 oz	84	D–
Roast Beef		1 oz	66	D–
Roast Beef	Mesquite Smoked	2.13 oz	126	D–
Roast Beef		1 oz	42	D–
Pork & Beef		1 oz slice	46	D–
		1 oz slice	35	B–
		1 slice	45	D
		1 slice	35	D–
Pork		1 oz slice	67	D–
		1 oz slice	70	D–
		1 slice	40	D–
Beef		1 oz slice	99	D–
		1 oz slice	40	C–
		1 oz slice	34	B–
		1 oz slice	31	A–
		1 oz slice	22	B–
Chicken Liver		1 oz	57	D
Goose Liver, Foie Gras	Smoked	1 oz	131	D
Pork & Beef		1 oz slice	42	C–
		1 oz slice	35	B–
		1 oz slice	40	D–
		1 oz slice	39	C–
All Varieties		1 oz	140	D–
		1 Tbsp	35	D
		1 oz slice	80	D–
		1 oz slice	80	D–
		1 slice	50	D–
		1 slice	80	D–
		1 slice	70	D–
Beef		1 slice	60	D–
		1 slice	50	D
		1 oz slice	60	D–
All Varieties		1 oz slice	92	D–
		1 oz slice	45	C–
All Varieties		1 oz	90	D–
		1 oz	47	D–
		1 oz	38	D–
Beef		1 oz slice	70	D–
Genoa		1 oz slice	110	D–

"+" indicates the food meets minimum fiber requirements; "–" indicates the food has a high sodium content.

Food	Processing Category	Brand
Salami	All Forms	All Brands Except as Noted
Salami	All Forms	All Brands Except as Noted
Salami	All Forms	Boar's Head
Salami	All Forms	Kahn's
Salami, Vegetarian	Frozen	Worthington
Sandwich Spread	All Forms	Generic
Sandwich Spread	All Forms	Generic
Sandwich Spread	All Forms	Hellmann's/Best Foods
Sandwich Spread	All Forms	Kraft
Sandwich Spread	All Forms	Oscar Mayer Chub
Sausage	All Forms	Eckrich Lean Supreme
Sausage	All Forms	Eckrich Lean Supreme
Sausage	All Forms	OHSE Hot Links
Sausage Stick	All Forms	Hickory Farms Sportsman Stick
Sausage, Vegetarian	All Forms	Generic
Spam	All Forms	OHSE
Spam	Canned	Spam
Spam	Canned	Spam
Spam	Canned	Spam
Souse Loaf	All Forms	Kahn's
Spice Loaf	All Forms	Kahn's Family Pack
Spice Loaf	All Forms	Kahn's Family Pack
Summer Sausage	All Forms	Eckrich
Summer Sausage	All Forms	Lean & Lite
Thuringer Cervelat	*See also* Summer Sausage	Hormel Viking Club Cervelat
Tuna Salad	Fresh	Generic
Tuna Salad	Packaged	Longacre
Turkey	Canned	Generic
Turkey	Canned	Hormel
Turkey	Canned	Swanson
Turkey Ham Salad	Canned	Longacre
Turkey Ham Salad	Canned	Longacre Saladfest
Turkey Salad	Canned	Longacre
Turkey Salad	Canned	Longacre Saladfest
Turkey & Corned Beef Sandwich	Packaged	Healthy Deli Doubledecker
Turkey & Ham Sandwich	Packaged	Healthy Deli Doubledecker
Turkey Bologna	All Forms	All Brands
Turkey Frankfurter	All Forms	All Brands
Turkey Frankfurter	All Forms	Healthy Choice
Turkey Ham	All Forms	Generic
Turkey Ham	All Forms	Butterball Cold Cuts
Turkey Ham	All Forms	Butterball Cold Cuts
Turkey Ham	All Forms	Butterball Cold Cuts
Turkey Ham	All Forms	Butterball Deli Thin
Turkey Ham	All Forms	Butterball Slice N Serve
Turkey Ham	All Forms	Butterball Slice N Serve
Turkey Ham	All Forms	Longacre
Turkey Ham	All Forms	Longacre
Turkey Ham	All Forms	Longacre Deli
Turkey Ham	All Forms	Louis Rich
Turkey Ham	All Forms	Louis Rich
Turkey Ham	All Forms	Louis Rich

Major Description	Minor Description	Serving Size	Calories	Grade
Pork		1 oz slice	115	D–
Pork & Beef		1 oz slice	120	D–
Beef		1 oz slice	60	D–
Beef		1 oz slice	60	D–
Roll		1.5 oz slice	90	D–
Meatless		1 oz	110	D
Pork & Beef		1 oz	67	D–
Meatless		1 Tbsp	50	D–
Meatless		1 Tbsp	50	D–
Meat		1 oz	67	D–
Heat & Serve		1 oz	60	D–
Smoked	Beef	1 oz	80	D–
Hot		1 oz	80	C–
		1 oz	138	D–
		1 oz	73	D–
Loaf		1 oz slice	75	D–
Cheese Chunks		1 oz	85	D–
Deviled		1 Tbsp	35	D–
Smoked Flavor		1 oz	85	D–
		1 slice	90	D–
		1 slice	70	D–
Beef		1 slice	60	D–
		1 oz slice	80	D–
		1 oz slice	43	D
		1 oz slice	90	D–
		4 oz	212	D–
		1 oz	52	D–
Boned with Broth		4 oz	184	C–
Chunk		6.75 oz	230	C–
White		2.5 oz	80	A–
		1 oz	53	D–
		1 oz	58	D–
		1 oz	70	D–
		1 oz	68	D–
		1 oz	30	B–
		1 oz	30	B–
All Varieties		1 oz slice	60	D–
All Varieties		1 oz frank	60	D–
Turkey	Low Fat	1 frank	50	B–
Thigh Meat	Cured	1 oz slice	36	C–
		1 oz slice	35	B–
Honey Cured		1 oz slice	35	B–
Honey Cured	Chopped	1 oz slice	35	B–
Sliced		1 oz slice	35	B–
		1 oz slice	35	D–
Honey Cured		1 oz slice	40	D–
Chunk		1 oz slice	37	D–
Sliced		1 oz slice	33	B–
Lean & Lite		1 oz slice	37	D–
Chopped		1 oz slice	46	D–
Honey Cured		1 oz slice	25	B–
Smoked	Water Added	1 oz	33	C–

"+" indicates the food meets minimum fiber requirements; "–" indicates the food has a high sodium content.

Food	Processing Category	Brand
Turkey Ham	All Forms	Louis Rich Round
Turkey Ham	All Forms	Louis Rich Round
Turkey Ham	All Forms	Louis Rich Square
Turkey Ham	All Forms	Louis Rich Square
Turkey Ham	All Forms	Louis Rich Thin Sliced
Turkey Ham	All Forms	Mr. Turkey
Turkey Ham	All Forms	Mr. Turkey
Turkey Ham	All Forms	Mr. Turkey
Turkey Ham	All Forms	Mr. Turkey
Turkey Ham	All Forms	Mr. Turkey Chub
Turkey Ham	All Forms	Norbest
Turkey Ham	All Forms	Norbest
Turkey Ham	All Forms	Norbest Gold Label
Turkey Ham	All Forms	Norbest Tavern 2–2.5 lb Half
Turkey Ham	All Forms	Norbest Tavern 5–6 lb Whole
Turkey Ham	All Forms	OHSE
Turkey Kielbasa, see, Kielbasa, Turkey		
Turkey Luncheon Meat	All Forms	Generic
Turkey Luncheon Meat	All Forms	Generic
Turkey Luncheon Meat	All Forms	Generic
Turkey Luncheon Meat	All Forms	Generic
Turkey Luncheon Meat	All Forms	Blue Label, Norbest Salt-free
Turkey Luncheon Meat	All Forms	Blue Label, Norbest Salt-free
Turkey Luncheon Meat	All Forms	Boar's Head
Turkey Luncheon Meat	All Forms	Boar's Head
Turkey Luncheon Meat	All Forms	Butterball Cold Cuts
Turkey Luncheon Meat	All Forms	Butterball Cold Cuts
Turkey Luncheon Meat	All Forms	Butterball Cold Cuts
Turkey Luncheon Meat	All Forms	Butterball Deli No Salt Added
Turkey Luncheon Meat	All Forms	Butterball Slice N Serve
Turkey Luncheon Meat	All Forms	Butterball Slice N Serve BBQ
Turkey Luncheon Meat	All Forms	Butterball Turkey Variety Pak
Turkey Luncheon Meat	All Forms	Glazed Longacre Gourmet
Turkey Luncheon Meat	All Forms	Glazed Longacre Premium
Turkey Luncheon Meat	All Forms	Healthy Deli
Turkey Luncheon Meat	All Forms	Healthy Deli
Turkey Luncheon Meat	All Forms	Healthy Deli 3 lb.
Turkey Luncheon Meat	All Forms	Healthy Deli Gourmet
Turkey Luncheon Meat	All Forms	Healthy Deli Gourmet
Turkey Luncheon Meat	All Forms	Healthy Deli Less Salt
Turkey Luncheon Meat	All Forms	Hickory Butterball Slice
Turkey Luncheon Meat	All Forms	Hillshire Farm Deli Select
Turkey Luncheon Meat	All Forms	Hillshire Farm Deli Select
Turkey Luncheon Meat	All Forms	Hormel Perma-fresh
Turkey Luncheon Meat	All Forms	Hormel Perma-fresh
Turkey Luncheon Meat	All Forms	Light & Lean
Turkey Luncheon Meat	All Forms	Longacre Catering
Turkey Luncheon Meat	All Forms	Longacre
Turkey Luncheon Meat	All Forms	Longacre
Turkey Luncheon Meat	All Forms	Longacre
Turkey Luncheon Meat	All Forms	Longacre Catering
Turkey Luncheon Meat	All Forms	Longacre Deli

Major Description	Minor Description	Serving Size	Calories	Grade
Smoked		1 oz slice	34	C–
Smoked	Water Added	1 oz slice	35	B–
Smoked		.75 oz slice	24	B–
Smoked	Water Added	1 oz	31	B–
Smoked		.4 oz sliced	12	B–
Breakfast Smoked		1 oz	33	C–
Buffet Style, Smoked		1 oz	32	C–
Chopped		1 oz	37	C–
Smoked		1 oz	32	B–
Smoked		1 oz	32	C–
Canadian Style Thigh Meat	Cured	1 oz	35	C–
Roll		1 oz	31	C–
Thigh Meat	Cured	1 oz	27	B–
Thigh Meat	Cured	1 oz	29	B–
Thigh Meat	Cured	1 oz	27	B–
		1 oz	30	B–
Breast		1 oz slice	31	A–
Light & Dark Meat	Roll	1 oz slice	42	D–
Light Meat	Roll	1 oz slice	42	D–
White & Dark Meat	Diced	1 oz slice	39	C–
Breast	without Skin	1 oz slice	33	A
Breast	with Skin	1 oz slice	35	A
Breast	Golden	1 oz slice	35	B–
Breast	Golden without Skin	1 oz slice	30	B
	Smoked	1 oz slice	35	B–
Breast		1 oz slice	30	B–
Breast	Smoked	1 oz slice	35	B–
Breast		1 oz slice	45	C
Breast		1 oz slice	35	B–
Breast	Barbecue	1 oz slice	40	D–
	Smoked	1 oz slice	33	C–
Breast	Browned	1 oz slice	35	B–
Breast	Browned	1 oz slice	30	B–
Breast	Honey Roasted	1 oz slice	28	B–
Breast	Oven Roasted	1 oz slice	26	A–
Breast	Smoked	1 oz slice	29	B–
Breast		1 oz slice	28	B–
Breast	Smoked	1 oz slice	31	A–
Breast		1 oz slice	25	B–
Breast	Smoked	1 oz slice	35	B–
Breast	Roasted	1 oz slice	31	A–
Breast	Smoked	1 oz slice	31	A–
Breast		1 slice	30	B–
Breast	Smoked	1 slice	30	B–
Breast		1 slice	30	B
Breast	without Skin	1 oz slice	35	B–
Breast	Sliced	1 oz slice	30	B–
Breast	Smoked	1 oz slice	35	B–
Breast	Smoked	1 oz slice	26	C–
Breast		1 oz slice	35	B–
Breast		1 oz slice	35	B–

"+" indicates the food meets minimum fiber requirements; "–" indicates the food has a high sodium content.

Food	Processing Category	Brand
Turkey Luncheon Meat	All Forms	Longacre Deli
Turkey Luncheon Meat	All Forms	Longacre Deli
Turkey Luncheon Meat	All Forms	Longacre Deli Chef
Turkey Luncheon Meat	All Forms	Longacre Deli Chef
Turkey Luncheon Meat	All Forms	Longacre Deli Chef
Turkey Luncheon Meat	All Forms	Longacre Gourmet
Turkey Luncheon Meat	All Forms	Longacre Gourmet
Turkey Luncheon Meat	All Forms	Longacre Gourmet Low Salt
Turkey Luncheon Meat	All Forms	Longacre Premium
Turkey Luncheon Meat	All Forms	Longacre Premium
Turkey Luncheon Meat	All Forms	Longacre Salt Watchers
Turkey Luncheon Meat	All Forms	Louis Rich
Turkey Luncheon Meat	All Forms	Louis Rich
Turkey Luncheon Meat	All Forms	Louis Rich
Turkey Luncheon Meat	All Forms	Louis Rich
Turkey Luncheon Meat	All Forms	Louis Rich
Turkey Luncheon Meat	All Forms	Louis Rich Carving Board
Turkey Luncheon Meat	All Forms	Louis Rich Deli-Thin
Turkey Luncheon Meat	All Forms	Louis Rich Deli-Thin
Turkey Luncheon Meat	All Forms	Louis Rich Dinner Slices
Turkey Luncheon Meat	All Forms	Louis Rich Dinner Slices
Turkey Luncheon Meat	All Forms	Louis Rich Dinner Slices
Turkey Luncheon Meat	All Forms	Louis Rich Fat Free Cold Cuts
Turkey Luncheon Meat	All Forms	Louis Rich Fat Free Cold Cuts
Turkey Luncheon Meat	All Forms	Mr. Turkey
Turkey Luncheon Meat	All Forms	Mr. Turkey
Turkey Luncheon Meat	All Forms	Mr. Turkey
Turkey Luncheon Meat	All Forms	Norbest
Turkey Luncheon Meat	All Forms	Norbest Blue Label
Turkey Luncheon Meat	All Forms	Norbest Blue Label
Turkey Luncheon Meat	All Forms	Norbest Blue Label
Turkey Luncheon Meat	All Forms	Norbest Gold Label
Turkey Luncheon Meat	All Forms	Norbest Gourmet Cured
Turkey Luncheon Meat	All Forms	Norbest Norfresh
Turkey Luncheon Meat	All Forms	Norbest Norfresh Blue Label
Turkey Luncheon Meat	All Forms	Norbest Norfresh Orange Label
Turkey Luncheon Meat	All Forms	Norbest Norfresh Yellow Label
Turkey Luncheon Meat	All Forms	Norbest Norfresh Yellow Label
Turkey Luncheon Meat	All Forms	Norbest Orange Label
Turkey Luncheon Meat	All Forms	Norbest Orange Label
Turkey Luncheon Meat	All Forms	Norbest Orange Label
Turkey Luncheon Meat	All Forms	Norbest Orange Label
Turkey Luncheon Meat	All Forms	Norbest Tan Label
Turkey Luncheon Meat	All Forms	Norbest Yellow Label
Turkey Luncheon Meat	All Forms	Norbest Yellow Label
Turkey Luncheon Meat	All Forms	OHSE
Turkey Luncheon Meat	All Forms	OHSE
Turkey Luncheon Meat	All Forms	Oscar Mayer
Turkey Luncheon Meat	All Forms	Oscar Mayer
Turkey Luncheon Meat	All Forms	Oscar Mayer Deli-Thin
Turkey Luncheon Meat	All Forms	Oscar Mayer Deli-Thin
Turkey Luncheon Meat	All Forms	Oscar Mayer Healthy Favorites

Major Description	Minor Description	Serving Size	Calories	Grade
Breast	Smoked	1 oz slice	35	B–
Breast	without Skin	1 oz slice	35	B–
Breast & White		1 oz slice	35	B–
Breast & White	Browned & Roasted	1 oz slice	40	D–
Breast & White	without Skin	1 oz slice	40	D–
Breast		1 oz slice	35	B–
Breast	without Skin	1 oz slice	30	B–
Breast		1 oz slice	30	B–
Breast		1 oz slice	30	B–
Breast	without Skin	1 oz slice	30	B–
Breast		1 oz slice	32	B
Breast	Barbecue	1 oz slice	30	A–
Breast	Hickory Smoked	1 oz slice	30	A–
Breast	Honey Roasted	1 oz slice	30	A–
Breast	Roasted	1 oz slice	25	A–
Breast	Roasted	1 oz slice	30	A–
Breast	Smoked	1 oz slice	27	A–
Breast	Roasted	.5 oz slice	10	A–
Breast	Smoked	.5 oz slice	13	A–
Breast	Hickory Smoked	1 oz slice	23	A–
Breast	Honey Roasted	1 oz slice	27	A–
Breast	Roasted	1 oz slice	23	A–
Breast	Hickory Smoked	1 oz slice	25	A–
Breast	Roasted	1 oz slice	25	A–
Breast		1 oz slice	31	B–
Breast	Smoked	1 oz slice	31	B–
Luncheon Loaf, Spiced		1 oz slice	51	D–
White Meat, Diced		1 oz slice	31	B–
Breast	without Skin	1 oz slice	26	A–
Breast	with Skin	1 oz slice	28	B–
Breast & Thigh		1 oz slice	31	B–
Breast	Smoked	1 oz slice	29	B–
	Ham Flavor, Hickory Smoked	1 oz slice	39	D–
Breast	without Skin	1 oz slice	27	A–
Breast	without Skin	1 oz slice	24	A–
Breast	without Skin	1 oz slice	26	A–
Breast	without Skin	1 oz slice	24	B–
Breast	without Skin	1 oz slice	25	B–
Breast	without Skin	1 oz slice	26	A–
Breast	without Skin	1 oz slice	28	A–
Roll	White & Dark Meat	1 oz slice	36	D–
Roll	White Meat	1 oz slice	29	B–
Breast	without Skin	1 oz slice	24	B–
Breast	without Skin	1 oz slice	26	B–
Breast	without Skin	1 oz slice	26	A–
		1 oz slice	30	B–
Breast	Smoked	1 oz slice	30	B–
Breast	Roasted	1 oz slice	23	B–
Breast	Smoked	.35 oz slice	20	A–
Turkey	Roasted	1 slice	13	B–
Turkey	Smoked	1 slice	16	A–
Turkey Breast	Roasted	1 slice	10	A–

"+" indicates the food meets minimum fiber requirements; "–" indicates the food has a high sodium content.

Food	Processing Category	Brand
Turkey Luncheon Meat	All Forms	Oscar Mayer Healthy Favorites
Turkey Luncheon Meat	All Forms	Prebrowned Norbest Orange
Turkey Luncheon Meat	All Forms	Roasted Longacre Gourmet
Turkey Luncheon Meat	All Forms	Roasted Longacre Premium
Turkey Luncheon Meat	All Forms	Smoked Norbest Orange Label
Turkey Pastrami	All Forms	Generic
Turkey Nuggets	All Forms	Louis Rich
Turkey Pastrami	All Forms	Butterball Cold Cuts
Turkey Pastrami	All Forms	Butterball Slice N Serve
Turkey Pastrami	All Forms	Longacre
Turkey Pastrami	All Forms	Louis Rich
Turkey Pastrami	All Forms	Louis Rich Round
Turkey Pastrami	All Forms	Louis Rich Square
Turkey Pastrami	All Forms	Louis Rich Square
Turkey Pastrami	All Forms	Louis Rich Thin Sliced
Turkey Pastrami	All Forms	Mr. Turkey
Turkey Pastrami	All Forms	Norbest
Turkey Patty	All Forms	
Turkey Patty	All Forms	Louis Rich
Turkey Salami	All Forms	All Brands
Turkey Sausage	All Forms	Butterball
Turkey Sausage	All Forms	Hudson's
Turkey Sausage	All Forms	Louis Rich
Turkey Sausage	All Forms	Louis Rich
Turkey Sausage	All Forms	Louis Rich
Turkey Sausage	All Forms	Louis Rich
Turkey Sausage	All Forms	Louis Rich Polish Kielbasa
Turkey Sausage	All Forms	Mr. Turkey
Turkey Sausage	All Forms	Mr. Turkey
Turkey Sausage	All Forms	Mr. Turkey Polish Kielbasa
Turkey Sausage	All Forms	Norbest Tasti Lean Chub or Links
Turkey Spread	All Forms	Underwood Light
Turkey Sticks	All Forms	Generic
Turkey Sticks	All Forms	Louis Rich
Turkey Summer Sausage	All Forms	Louis Rich
Turkey, Vegetarian	All Forms	Worthington
Turkey, Vegetarian	Canned	Worthington
Turkey, Vegetarian	Canned	Worthington Turkee Slices
Vienna Sausage	Canned	All Brands
SEAFOOD		
Abalone	Fresh	
Abalone	Fresh	
Anchovy	Canned	Generic
Anchovy	Fresh	
Barracuda	Fresh	
Bass, Freshwater	Fresh	
Bass, Striped	Fresh	
Bluefish	Fresh	
Bonito, Caribbean	Fresh	
Bonito, Japanese	Fresh	
Burbot	Fresh	
Butterfish	Fresh	
Carp	Fresh	

Major Description	Minor Description	Serving Size	Calories	Grade
Turkey Breast	Smoked	1 slice	10	A–
Breast	with Skin	1 oz slice	29	B–
Breast	Browned	1 oz slice	35	B–
Breast	Browned	1 oz slice	30	B–
Breast	with Skin	1 oz slice	30	A–
		1 oz slice	40	C–
		1 piece	62	D–
		1 oz slice	30	B–
		1 oz slice	35	B–
Sliced		1 oz slice	32	B–
		1 oz slice	35	B–
		1 oz slice	32	C–
		.8 oz slice	24	B–
		1 oz slice	28	B–
		.4 oz slice	11	C–
		1 oz slice	28	B–
		1 oz slice	29	B–
Breaded, Battered & Fried		3 oz patty	240	D–
		2.8 oz patty	209	D–
All Varieties		1 oz slice	50	D–
		1 oz slice	50	D–
Breakfast	Ground	1 oz slice	65	D–
Breakfast	Ground	1 oz slice	56	D–
Links		1 link	46	D–
Smoked		1 oz slice	43	D–
Smoked	Cheese	1 oz slice	47	D–
		1 oz slice	40	D–
Breakfast		1 oz slice	58	D–
Smoked		1 oz slice	47	D–
		1 oz slice	59	D–
		1 oz slice	53	D–
Chunky		1 oz slice	35	B–
Breaded, Battered & Fried		1 oz slice	79	D–
Cooked		1 stick	81	D–
		1 oz slice	55	D–
Frozen, Smoked, Roll or Slices		.7 oz slice	45	D–
Drained		1 slice	60	D
		1 oz slice	65	D–
Beef & Pork		1 oz	79	D–
Meat Only	Fried	4 oz	214	C–
Meat Only		4 oz	120	A–
in Olive Oil, Drained		1 oz	60	D–
Meat Only		1 oz	37	C
Meat Only		1 oz	27	A
Meat Only		4 oz	64	B
Meat Only		4 oz	110	B
Meat Only		4 oz	140	C
Meat Only		4 oz	157	B
Meat Only		4 oz	146	A
Meat Only		4 oz	104	A
Meat Only		4 oz	160	D
Meat Only		4 oz	184	C

"+" indicates the food meets minimum fiber requirements; "–" indicates the food has a high sodium content.

Food	Processing Category	Brand
Catfish	Fresh	
Catfish	Frozen	Booth
Catfish	Frozen	Delta Pride
Catjang	Fresh	
Caviar, Black & Red	All Forms	
Cisco	Fresh	
Cisco	Smoked	
Clam	Canned	Generic
Clam	Canned	Generic
Clam	Canned	Doxsee
Clam	Canned	Gorton's
Clam	Canned	Orleans
Clam	Canned	Progresso
Clam	Fresh	
Clam	Fresh	
Clam	Fresh	
Cod	Frozen	Booth
Cod	Frozen	Booth Individually
Cod	Frozen	Gorton's Fishmarket Fresh
Cod	Frozen	Seapak
Cod	Frozen	Van de Kamp's Light
Cod	Frozen	Van de Kamp's Natural
Cod, Atlantic	Canned	
Cod, Atlantic	Fresh	
Cod, Atlantic	Fresh	
Cod, Atlantic	Fresh	
Cod, Pacific	Fresh	
Crab, Alaska King	Fresh	
Crab, Alaska King	Fresh	
Crab, Blue	Canned	Generic
Crab, Blue	Fresh	
Crab, Blue	Fresh	
Crab, Blue	Fresh	
Crab, Deviled	Frozen	Mrs. Paul's
Crab, Deviled	Frozen	Mrs. Paul's
Crab, Dungeness	Canned	S & W
Crab, Dungeness	Fresh	
Crab, Imitation	All Forms	
Crab, Queen	Fresh	
Crab, Queen	Frozen	Wakefield
Crayfish	Fresh	
Crayfish	Fresh	
Croaker, Atlantic	Fresh	
Croaker, Atlantic	Fresh	
Cuttlefish	Fresh	
Dolphin Fish	Fresh	
Eel	Fresh	

Major Description	Minor Description	Serving Size	Calories	Grade
Meat Only		4 oz	132	C
Ocean		4 oz	115	D
Fillets		4 oz	132	C
Meat Only	Boiled	4 oz	133	A
Granular		1 oz	71	D–
Meat Only		4 oz	112	B
Meat Only		4 oz	200	D–
Mixed Species	Drained	1 cup	236	A
Mixed Species	in Liquid	1 cup	6	A–
Chopped or Minced	in Liquid	6.5 oz	100	A–
Chopped or Minced		1/2 can	70	A–
Chopped or Minced	in Liquid	6.5 oz	100	A–
Chopped or Minced		1/2 cup	70	A–
Meat Only, All Species	Boiled, Poached or Steamed	1 oz	42	A
Meat Only, All Species	Breaded, Fried	1 oz	57	D–
Meat Only, All Species		1 oz	21	A
Fillet		4 oz	89	A–
Fillet		4 oz	90	A
Fillet		5 oz	110	A
Fillet		4 oz	90	A–
Fillet		1 piece	250	C–
Fillet		4 oz	90	A
Meat Only	in Liquid	4 oz	119	A–
Meat Only	Baked, Broiled or Microwaved	4 oz	119	A
Meat Only	Dried, Salted	4 oz	324	A–
Meat Only		4 oz	92	A
Meat Only		4 oz	92	A
Meat Only		1 leg (6.1 oz)	144	A–
Meat Only	Boiled, Poached or Steamed	4 oz	110	A–
Meat Only		4 oz	112	A–
Meat Only	Boiled, Poached or Steamed	4 oz	116	B–
Meat Only	Cake, Fried	4 oz	176	D–
Meat Only		4 oz	100	A–
	Breaded	3 oz	180	D–
Mini	Breaded	4 oz	274	D–
Meat Only		4 oz	100	B–
Meat Only		4 oz	96	A–
		4 oz	116	A–
Meat Only		4 oz	104	A–
		4 oz	80	A–
Mixed Species, Meat Only	Boiled or Steamed	4 oz	129	A
Mixed Species, Meat Only		4 oz	100	A
Meat Only	Breaded, Fried	4 oz	251	D–
Meat Only		4 oz	116	B
Mixed Species, Meat Only		4 oz	88	A–
Meat Only		4 oz	96	A
Meat Only	Baked, Broiled or Microwaved	4 oz	268	D

"+" indicates the food meets minimum fiber requirements; "–" indicates the food has a high sodium content.

Food	Processing Category	Brand
Eel	Fresh	
Fish Paste Cake	Japanese Style	
Fish Paste Cake	Japanese Style	
Flounder	Fresh	
Flounder	Fresh	
Flounder	Frozen	Booth
Flounder	Frozen	Booth Individually Packed
Flounder	Frozen	Gorton's Fishmarket Fresh
Flounder	Frozen	Seapak
Flounder	Frozen	Van de Kamp's Natural
Flying Fish	Fresh	
Gefilte Fish	Jar	Mother's
Gefilte Fish	Jar	Mother's 12 oz
Gefilte Fish	Jar	Mother's 24 oz
Gefilte Fish	Jar	Mother's 24 oz
Gefilte Fish	Jar	Mother's 24 oz
Gefilte Fish	Jar	Mother's Old Fashioned, 12 oz
Gefilte Fish	Jar	Mother's Old Fashioned, 12 oz
Gefilte Fish	Jar	Mother's Old Fashioned, 24 oz
Gefilte Fish	Jar	Mother's Old Fashioned, 24 oz
Gefilte Fish	Jar	Mother's Old World
Gefilte Fish	Jar	Mother's Old World
Gefilte Fish	Jar	Rokeach Old Vienna
Gefilte Fish	Jar	Rokeach, Redi-jelled
Goatfish	Fresh	
Gorn	Fresh	Metrone Foods
Grouper	Fresh	
Haddock	Fresh	
Haddock	Fresh	
Haddock	Fresh	
Haddock	Frozen	Booth
Haddock	Frozen	Gorton's Fishmarket Fresh
Haddock	Frozen	Gorton's Microwave Entrees
Haddock	Frozen	Mrs. Paul's Crunchy
Haddock	Frozen	Mrs. Paul's Light
Haddock	Frozen	Seapak
Haddock	Frozen	Van de Kamp's
Haddock	Frozen	Van de Kamp's
Haddock	Frozen	Van de Kamp's
Haddock	Frozen	Van de Kamp's Light
Haddock	Frozen	Van de Kamp's Natural
Halibut	Frozen	Seapak
Halibut	Frozen	Van de Kamp's
Halibut, Atlantic & Pacific	Fresh	
Halibut, Atlantic & Pacific	Fresh	
Halibut, Greenland	fresh	
Herring, Atlantic	Fresh	

Major Description	Minor Description	Serving Size	Calories	Grade
Meat Only		4 oz	208	D
Block Kamaboko	Steamed	4 oz	111	A–
Stick Chikuwa	Grilled	4 oz	143	B–
Meat Only	Baked, Broiled or Microwaved	4 oz	133	A
Meat Only		4 oz	104	A
Atlantic		4 oz	90	A–
		4 oz	90	A
		5 oz	110	A–
		4 oz	90	A–
		4 oz	100	B
Meat Only		4 oz	104	A
Whitefish & Pike	in Liquid	1 ball	70	A–
Whitefish & Pike	in Jelled Broth	1 ball	46	A–
Whitefish	in Jelled Broth	1 ball	60	A–
Whitefish	in Liquid	1 ball	70	A–
Whitefish & Pike	in Jelled Broth	1 ball	60	A–
	in Jelled Broth	1 ball	54	A–
	in Liquid	1 ball	54	A–
	in Jelled Broth	1 ball	70	A–
	in Liquid	1 ball	70	A–
	in Jelled Broth	1 ball	70	A–
Whitefish & Pike	in Jelled Broth	1 ball	70	A–
	in Jelled Broth	4 oz	108	A
in Jelled Broth		4 oz	92	B–
Meat Only		4 oz	108	A
Meat with Scales	Phasered	4 oz	450	D
Mixed Species, Meat Only	Baked, Broiled or Microwaved	4 oz	134	A
Meat Only	Baked, Broiled or Microwaved	4 oz	127	A
Meat Only		4 oz	99	A
Meat Only	Smoked	4 oz	132	A–
Individually Wrapped Fillet		4 oz	90	A
Fillet		4 oz	88	A
in Lemon Butter		1 pkg	360	D–
Fillets, Battered		2 pieces	190	B–
Fillets, Breaded		1 piece	220	C–
Fillet		4 oz	90	A–
Fillet	Light	1 piece	240	D–
Fillets, Battered		2 pieces	250	D–
Fillets, Breaded		2 pieces	270	D
Fillets, Breaded		1 piece	240	D–
Fillet		4 oz	90	A–
Steaks		6 oz pkg	160	A
Fillets, Battered		2 pieces	150	C–
Meat Only	Baked, Broiled or Microwaved	4 oz	159	B
Meat Only		4 oz	124	B
Meat Only		4 oz	211	D
Meat Only	Baked, Broiled or Microwaved	4 oz	230	D

"+" indicates the food meets minimum fiber requirements; "–" indicates the food has a high sodium content.

Food	Processing Category	Brand
Herring, Atlantic	Fresh	
Herring, Atlantic	Fresh	
Herring, Atlantic	Fresh	
Herring, Pacific	Fresh	
Lobster Entree	Frozen	Stouffer's
Lobster, Northern	Fresh	
Lobster, Spiny	Fresh	
Mackerel, Atlantic	Fresh	
Mackerel, Atlantic	Fresh	
Mackerel, Jack	Canned	Generic
Mackerel, King	Fresh	
Mackerel, Pacific & Jack	Fresh	
Mackerel, Spanish	Fresh	
Mackerel, Spanish	Fresh	
Mahi Mahi	*See* Dolphin Fish	
Milkfish	Fresh	
Monkfish	Fresh	
Mullet, Striped	Fresh	
Mullet, Striped	Fresh	
Mussel, Blue	Fresh	
Mussel, Blue	Fresh	
Ocean Perch	Frozen	Booth
Ocean Perch	Frozen	Gorton's Fishmarket Fresh
Ocean Perch	Frozen	Van de Kamp's Natural
Ocean Perch Entree	Frozen	Van de Kamp's Light
Ocean Perch, Atlantic	Fresh	
Ocean Perch, Atlantic	Fresh	
Octopus	Fresh	
Oyster, Eastern	Fresh	
Oyster, Eastern	Fresh	
Oyster, Eastern	Fresh	
Oyster, Pacific	Fresh	
Parrot Fish	Fresh	
Perch	Fresh	
Perch	Fresh	
Perch	Frozen	Booth
Perch	Frozen	Seapak
Pike, Northern	Fresh	
Pike, Northern	Fresh	
Pike, Walleye	Fresh	
Pollack, Atlantic	Fresh	
Pollack, Walleye	Fresh	
Pollack, Walleye	Fresh	
Pompano, Florida	Fresh	
Pompano, Florida	Fresh	
Pout, Ocean	Fresh	
Rockfish, Pacific	Fresh	
Rockfish, Pacific	Fresh	
Roe	All Forms	

Major Description	Minor Description	Serving Size	Calories	Grade
Meat Only	Kippered	4 oz	246	D–
Meat Only	Pickled	4 oz	297	D–
Meat Only		4 oz	180	D
Meat Only		4 oz	221	D
Newburg		6½ oz	380	D–
Meat Only	Boiled, Poached or Steamed	4 oz	111	C–
Mixed Species, Meat Only		4 oz	127	D–
Meat Only	Baked, Broiled or Microwaved	4 oz	297	D
Meat Only		4 oz	232	D
Meat Only		4 oz	177	C–
Meat Only		4 oz	120	B–
Mixed Species, Meat Only		4 oz	180	D
Meat Only	Baked, Broiled or Microwaved	4 oz	179	C
Meat Only		4 oz	156	D
Meat Only		4 oz	168	D
Meat Only		4 oz	88	B
Meat Only		4 oz	132	B
Meat Only	Baked or Broiled	4 oz	170	B
Meat Only	Boiled or Steamed	4 oz	195	B–
Meat Only		4 oz	98	B–
		4 oz	100	A–
		4 oz	112	B
		4 oz	130	C
Fillet	Breaded	1 piece	280	D–
Meat Only	Baked or Broiled	4 oz	137	B
Meat Only		4 oz	108	B
Meat Only		1 oz	23	A
Meat Only	Boiled, Poached or Steamed	4 oz	155	C–
Meat Only	Breaded, Fried	4 oz	223	D–
Meat Only		4 oz	80	C–
Meat Only		4 oz	92	B–
Meat Only		4 oz	96	A
Meat Only	Baked or Broiled	4 oz	133	A
Meat Only		4 oz	104	A
		4 oz	100	A
		4 oz	100	B
Meat Only	Baked or Broiled	4 oz	128	A
Meat Only		4 oz	100	A
Meat Only		4 oz	104	A
Meat Only		4 oz	104	A
Meat Only	Baked or Broiled	4 oz	128	A
Meat Only		4 oz	92	A
Meat Only	Baked or Broiled	4 oz	239	D
Meat Only		4 oz	184	D
Meat Only		4 oz	88	A
Meat Only	Baked or Broiled	4 oz	137	B
Meat Only		4 oz	108	A
Mixed Species		1 oz	40	D

"+" indicates the food meets minimum fiber requirements; "–" indicates the food has a high sodium content.

Food	Processing Category	Brand
Sablefish	Fresh	
Sablefish	Fresh	
Salmon	Fresh	
Salmon	Fresh	
Salmon	Frozen	Seapak
Salmon, Atlantic	Fresh	
Salmon, Chinook	Fresh	
Salmon, Chinook	Fresh	
Salmon, Chum	Canned	Generic
Salmon, Chum	Fresh	
Salmon, Coho	Canned	Deming's
Salmon, Coho	Fresh	
Salmon, Coho	Fresh	
Salmon, Pink	Canned	Generic
Salmon, Pink	Canned	Bumble Bee
Salmon, Pink	Canned	Del Monte
Salmon, Pink	Canned	Deming's
Salmon, Pink	Canned	Deming's
Salmon, Pink	Canned	Featherweight
Salmon, Pink	Canned	Libby's
Salmon, Red	Canned	Del Monte
Salmon, Sockeye or Red	Canned	Generic
Salmon, Sockeye or Red	Canned	Bumble Bee
Salmon, Sockeye or Red	Canned	Deming's
Salmon, Sockeye or Red	Canned	Deming's
Salmon, Sockeye or Red	Canned	Libby's
Salmon, Sockeye or Red	Canned	S & W Fancy
Salmon, Sockeye or Red	Canned	S & W/Nutradiet
Salmon, Sockeye or Red	Canned	S & W/Nutradiet
Salmon, Sockeye or Red	Fresh	
Sardine, Atlantic	Canned	Generic
Sardine, Brisling	Canned	Underwood
Sardine, Maine	Canned	Beach Cliff
Sardine, Maine	Canned	Beach Cliff
Sardine, Mixed	Canned	Brunswick Kippered Snacks
Sardine, Mixed	Canned	Del Monte
Sardine, Mixed	Canned	Featherweight
Sardine, Mixed	Canned	Featherweight
Sardine, Mixed	Canned	Underwood
Sardine, Mixed	Canned	Underwood
Sardine, Mixed	Canned	Underwood
Sardine, Norway	Canned	Empress
Sardine, Norway	Canned	Empress
Sardine, Pacific	Canned	Generic
Scallop	Fresh	
Scallop	Fresh	
Scallop, Imitation	Canned	Generic
Scallop, Vegetarian	Canned	Worthington
Scrod	See Cod	

Major Description	Minor Description	Serving Size	Calories	Grade
Meat Only		4 oz	220	D
Meat Only	Smoked	4 oz	292	D–
Mixed Species, Meat Only	Baked, Broiled or Microwaved	4 oz	245	D
Mixed Species, Pink Meat Only		4 oz	132	B
Steaks with Seasoning Mix		4 oz	135	B
Meat Only		4 oz	160	C–
Meat Only		4 oz	204	D
Meat Only	Smoked	4 oz	132	C–
		4 oz	160	C–
Meat Only		4 oz	136	B
Alaskan		1/2 cup	140	C–
Meat Only	Boiled, Poached or Steamed	4 oz	210	C
Meat Only		4 oz	164	C
		4 oz	158	B–
		1/2 cup	155	C–
		1/2 cup	160	C–
	Alaskan Style	1/2 cup	140	C–
Chunk	without Skin, Boneless, in Liquid	4 oz	148	C–
		4 oz	140	C
		4 oz	172	C–
	in Liquid	1/2 cup	180	D–
		4 oz	174	D–
		1/2 cup	188	D–
Alaskan		1/2 cup	150	D–
Alaskan		1/2 cup	170	D–
		4 oz	196	D–
Blueback	Fancy	1/2 cup	190	D–
		1/2 cup	188	D
Blueback		1/2 cup	188	D
Meat Only		4 oz	48	D
in Soybean Oil		4 oz	236	D–
in Liquid		4 oz	277	D–
in Soybean Oil		4 oz	320	D–
in Water		4 oz	306	D–
Kippered		4 oz	211	D–
in Tomato Sauce		1/2 cup	360	B–
in Oil		4 oz	278	D
in Water		4 oz	203	D
Brisling, in Liquid		4 oz	277	D–
in Mustard Sauce		4 oz	234	D–
in Tabasco Sauce		4 oz	293	D–
in Sardine Oil		4 oz	490	D
in Sardine Oil		4 oz	277	D
in Tomato Sauce		4 oz	202	D–
Meat Only		4 oz	100	A–
Meat Only	Breaded, Fried	4 oz	244	D–
Made from Surimi		4 oz	112	A–
		1/2 cup	90	A–

"+" indicates the food meets minimum fiber requirements; "–" indicates the food has a high sodium content.

Food	Processing Category	Brand
Scrod Entree	Frozen	Gorton's Microwave
Sea Bass	Fresh	
Shark	Fresh	
Sheepshead	Fresh	
Sheepshead	Fresh	
Shrimp	Canned	Generic
Shrimp	Canned	Louisiana Brand
Shrimp	Fresh	
Shrimp	Fresh	
Shrimp	Fresh	
Shrimp, Imitation	Canned	Generic
Smelt, Rainbow	Fresh	
Smelt, Rainbow	Fresh	
Snapper	Fresh	
Snapper	Fresh	
Sole	Fresh	
Sole	Fresh	
Sole	Frozen	Gorton's Fishmarket Fresh
Sole	Frozen	Seapak
Sole	Frozen	Van de Kamp's Natural
Sole, Atlantic	Frozen	Booth
Squid	Fresh	
Squid	Fresh	
Squid	Fresh	
Sturgeon	Fresh	
Sturgeon	Fresh	
Sturgeon	Fresh	
Sucker	Fresh	
Sunfish	Fresh	
Swordfish	Fresh	
Swordfish	Fresh	
Swordfish	Frozen	Seapak
Tarpon, Atlantic	Fresh	
Tilefish	Fresh	
Tilefish	Fresh	
Trout	Fresh	
Trout, Rainbow	Fresh	
Trout, Rainbow	Fresh	
Tuna	Canned	Generic
Tuna	Canned	Generic
Tuna	Canned	Generic
Tuna	Canned	Generic
Tuna	Canned	Generic
Tuna	Canned	Generic
Tuna	Canned	Generic
Tuna	Canned	Generic
Tuna	Canned	A & P
Tuna	Canned	A & P

Major Description	Minor Description	Serving Size	Calories	Grade
Baked		1 pkg	320	D–
Meat Only		4 oz	108	B
Meat Only		1 oz	37	C
Meat Only	Baked or Broiled	4 oz	143	A
Meat Only		4 oz	124	B
		4 oz	136	D–
		4 oz	116	D
Meat Only	Boiled, Poached or Steamed	4 oz	112	D–
Meat Only	Breaded, Fried	4 oz	274	D–
Meat Only		4 oz	120	D–
Made from Surimi		4 oz	116	A–
Meat Only	Baked or Broiled	4 oz	141	B
Meat Only		4 oz	108	B
Meat Only	Baked or Broiled	4 oz	145	A
Meat Only		4 oz	112	A
Meat Only	Baked or Broiled	4 oz	133	A
Meat Only		4 oz	104	A
		4 oz	90	A–
Fillets		4 oz	90	A–
Fillets		4 oz	100	B
		4 oz	90	A–
Mixed Species, Meat Only	Dried	4 oz	344	A
Mixed Species, Meat Only	Fried	4 oz	198	C–
Mixed Species, Meat Only		4 oz	104	A
Meat Only	Baked, Broiled or Microwaved	4 oz	153	C
Meat Only		4 oz	120	C
Meat Only	Smoked	4 oz	196	B
White Meat Only		4 oz	104	B
Meat Only		4 oz	100	A
Meat Only		4 oz	136	B
Meat Only	Baked, Broiled or Microwaved	4 oz	176	B
Steaks with Seasoning Mix		4 oz	140	B
Meat Only		4 oz	104	A
Meat Only	Baked, Broiled or Microwaved	4 oz	167	B
Meat Only		4 oz	108	B
Meat Only		4 oz	168	D
Meat Only	Baked, Broiled or Microwaved	4 oz	171	B
Meat Only		4 oz	132	B
Light, in Vegetable Oil		2 oz	112	C–
Light, in Vegetable Oil	No Salt Added	2 oz	112	C
Light, in Water		2 oz	74	A–
Light, in Water	No Salt Added	2 oz	74	A
White, in Vegetable Oil		2 oz	106	C–
White, in Vegetable Oil	No Salt Added	2 oz	106	C
White, in Water		2 oz	78	B–
White, in Water	No Salt Added	2 oz	78	B
Light, in Water		2 oz	120	A–
White, in Vegetable Oil		2 oz	150	D–

"+" indicates the food meets minimum fiber requirements; "–" indicates the food has a high sodium content.

Food	Processing Category	Brand
Tuna	Canned	A & P
Tuna	Canned	A & P
Tuna	Canned	Bumble Bee
Tuna	Canned	Bumble Bee
Tuna	Canned	Bumble Bee
Tuna	Canned	Bumble Bee
Tuna	Canned	Bumble Bee
Tuna	Canned	Bumble Bee
Tuna	Canned	Empress
Tuna	Canned	Featherweight
Tuna	Canned	Finast
Tuna	Canned	Finast
Tuna	Canned	Finast
Tuna	Canned	Finast
Tuna	Canned	Pathmark
Tuna	Canned	Pathmark
Tuna	Canned	Progresso
Tuna	Canned	S & W Fancy
Tuna	Canned	S & W Fancy
Tuna	Canned	S & W Fancy
Tuna	Canned	Starkist
Tuna	Canned	Starkist
Tuna	Canned	Starkist
Tuna	Canned	Starkist
Tuna	Canned	Diet in Distilled Water Star Kist
Tuna	Canned	Diet Starkist
Tuna	Canned	Starkist Prime Catch
Tuna	Canned	Starkist Prime Catch
Tuna	Canned	Starkist Select 60% Less Salt
Tuna	Canned	Starkist Select in Spring Water
Tuna	Canned	Weight Watchers No Salt Added
Tuna	Canned	Weight Watchers No Salt Added
Tuna	Canned	Weight Watchers No Salt Added
Tuna	Frozen	Seapak
Tuna	Frozen	Weight Watchers
Tuna, Bluefin	Fresh	
Tuna, Bluefin	Fresh	
Tuna, Skipjack	Fresh	
Tuna, Vegetarian	Frozen	Worthington
Tuna, Yellowfin	Fresh	
Turbot, European	Fresh	
Whelk	Fresh	
Whitefish	Fresh	
Whitefish	Fresh	
Whiting	Fresh	
Whiting	Fresh	
Whiting	Frozen	Booth
Wolf Fish, Atlantic	Fresh	
Yellowtail	Fresh	

Major Description	Minor Description	Serving Size	Calories	Grade
White, in Water	Chunk	2 oz	100	D–
White, in Water	Solid	2 oz	70	A–
Light, in Vegetable Oil	Chunk	2 oz	110	D–
Light, in Water	Chunk	2 oz	50	B–
White, in Vegetable Oil	Chunk	2 oz	110	D–
White, in Vegetable Oil	Solid	2 oz	80	B–
White, in Water	Chunk	2 oz	60	B–
White, in Water	Solid	2 oz	60	B–
Light, in Water		2 oz	60	A–
Light, in Water	Chunk	2 oz	60	A
Light, in Vegetable Oil	Chunk	2 oz	150	D–
Light, in Water	Chunk	2 oz	60	A–
White, in Vegetable Oil	Solid	2 oz	145	D–
White, in Water	Solid	2 oz	70	A–
Light, in Water	Chunk	2 oz	70	B–
White, in Water	Solid	2 oz	70	B–
Light, in Vegetable Oil	Solid	2 oz	150	D–
Light, in Vegetable Oil	Chunk	2 oz	90	B–
Light, in Water	Chunk	2 oz	60	A–
White, in Vegetable Oil	Solid	2 oz	160	D–
		2 oz	60	A–
Light, in Vegetable Oil	Chunk	2 oz	150	D–
White, in Vegetable Oil	Chunk	2 oz	140	D–
White, in Vegetable Oil	Solid	2 oz	90	B–
White, in Water	Chunk	2 oz	70	A
Light, in Water	Chunk	2 oz	65	A
Light, in Water	Solid	2 oz	60	A–
Light, in Vegetable Oil	Solid	2 oz	150	D–
Light, in Water	Chunk	2 oz	65	A–
White, in Water	Chunk	2 oz	70	A–
		2 oz	70	A–
Light, in Water	Chunk	2 oz	60	A–
White, in Water	Solid	2 oz	70	A–
Steak without Seasoning Mix		2 oz	60	A
Noodle Casserole		9.5 oz	240	B–+
Meat Only	Baked, Broiled or Microwaved	4 oz	209	C
Meat Only		4 oz	164	C
Meat Only		4 oz	116	A
		4 oz	400	D–
Meat Only		4 oz	124	A
Meat Only		4 oz	112	B–
Meat Only		4 oz	156	A–
Meat Only		4 oz	152	C
Meat Only	Smoked	4 oz	124	A–
Meat Only	Baked or Broiled	4 oz	132	A
Meat Only		4 oz	104	A
		4 oz	100	A
Meat Only		4 oz	108	B
Meat Only		4 oz	164	C

"+" indicates the food meets minimum fiber requirements; "–" indicates the food has a high sodium content.

Milk and Dairy

Calcium

This section of foods will represent the major source of calcium in the diet. Even high potency vitamin-mineral supplements don't contain enough calcium for most people.

The normal daily requirement is 800 to 1,000 milligrams but post-menopausal women and pregnant and lactating women need at least 1,200 milligrams. Much of this can come from low fat milk and milk products. For those of you who must eat cheese, not all cheese has the same calcium density. You should choose cheeses that deliver the most calcium for the least amount of fat and calories. Hard cheeses are more calcium dense, but also carry D ratings, so be careful.

Cheese	Milligrams calcium per ounce
Cheddar	200
Goat (hard)	250
Gruyère	280

Milk	Milligrams calcium per 8 ounces (or 1 cup)
Whole	290
2%	296
2% protein fortified	350
1%	310
Skim	310

Natural and Processed Cheeses

I've chosen to list all natural cheeses together with their processed counterparts. I find this less confusing and more instructive since most people don't distinguish

Food	Processing Category	Brand
Butter	All Forms	All Brands
Butter	All Forms	All Brands
Butter	All Forms	All Brands
Butter	All Forms	All Brands
Cheese	Natural	Bel Paese Lite
Cheese, American	Natural	Generic
Cheese, American	Processed	Generic
Cheese, American	Processed	Alpine Lace
Cheese, American	Processed	Alpine Lace
Cheese, American	Processed	Alpine Lace
Cheese, American	Processed	Alpine Lace Fat Free
Cheese, American	Processed	Alpine Lace Free & Lean
Cheese, American	Processed	Borden Light
Cheese, American	Processed	Borden Singles
Cheese, American	Processed	Borden Singles
Cheese, American	Processed	Borden Singles
Cheese, American	Processed	Churny Delicia
Cheese, American	Processed	Churny Delicia
Cheese, American	Processed	Churny Delicia
Cheese, American	Processed	Churny Delicia
Cheese, American	Processed	Darigold
Cheese, American	Processed	Golden Image
Cheese, American	Processed	Harvest Moon
Cheese, American	Processed	Hoffman's
Cheese, American	Processed	Kraft
Cheese, American	Processed	Kraft Light Singles
Cheese, American	Processed	Kraft Light Singles
Cheese, American	Processed	Kraft Singles
Cheese, American	Processed	Kraft Singles
Cheese, American	Processed	Light n' Lively Singles
Cheese, American	Processed	Light n' Lively Singles
Cheese, American	Processed	Lite Line
Cheese, American	Processed	Lite Line Reduced Sodium
Cheese, American	Processed	Lite Line Sodium Lite
Cheese, American	Processed	Weight Watchers Low Sodium Slices

how cheese is processed when selecting a kind of cheese. However, I think, when reading a product label you should understand what you're getting:

1. Natural—made directly from milk.
2. Pasteurized Processed Cheese—natural cheese blended and mixed with emulsifier and pasteurized.
3. Pasteurized Processed Cheese Food—similar to number 2 but with more milk and/or nonmilk additives. These add bulk and texture while reducing actual cheese content.

When "processed" appears in the "Processing Category" column, the cheese item is produced as described in numbers 2 or 3.

Major Description	Minor Description	Serving Size	Calories	Grade
Regular, Salted		1 Tbsp	100	D
Regular, Sweet		1 Tbsp	100	D
Whipped		1 Tbsp	67	D
Whipped, Salted		1 Tbsp	67	D
		1 oz	76	D–
		1 oz	106	D–
		1 oz	93	D–
		1 oz	80	D–
		1 oz	90	D–
Hot Pepper		1 oz	80	D–
		1 oz	45	A–
		1 oz	40	A–
		1 oz	70	D–
		1 oz	90	D–
		1 oz	100	D–
Sharp		1 oz	90	D–
Caraway Seeds		1 oz	80	D–
Hickory Smoked		1 oz	80	D–
Hot Pepper		1 oz	80	D–
Salami		1 oz	80	D–
		1 oz	80	D–
		1 oz	90	D–
		1 oz	70	D–
Colored		1 oz	100	D–
Grated		1 oz	130	D–
		1 oz	70	D–
White		1 oz	70	D–
		1 oz	90	D–
White		1 oz	90	D–
		1 oz	70	D–
White		1 oz	70	D–
		1 oz	50	C–
		1 oz	70	D–
		1 oz	70	D–
		1 oz	50	C–

"+" indicates the food meets minimum fiber requirements; "–" indicates the food has a high sodium content.

Food	Processing Category	Brand
Cheese, American	Processed	Weight Watchers Slices
Cheese, American	Processed	Weight Watchers Slices
Cheese, American	Processed	Weight Watchers Slices
Cheese, Asiago Wheel	Natural	Frigo
Cheese, Babybel	Natural	Laughing Cow
Cheese, Bacon	Processed	Cracker Barrel
Cheese, Bacon	Processed	Hoffman's Chees N Bacon
Cheese, Bacon	Processed	Kaukauna Cup
Cheese, Bacon	Processed	Kraft Cheez'N Bacon
Cheese, Blue	Natural	Generic
Cheese, Bonbel	Natural	Laughing Cow
Cheese, Brick	Natural	Generic
Cheese, Brie	Natural	Generic
Cheese, Burger Cheese	Natural	Sargento
Cheese, Butternip	Natural	Hickory Farms
Cheese, Cajun Style	Natural	Sargento
Cheese, Caljack	Natural	Churney
Cheese, Camembert	Natural	Generic
Cheese, Caraway	Natural	Generic
Cheese, Caraway	Processed	Hoffman's Swiss on Rye
Cheese, Cheddar	Natural	Generic
Cheese, Cheddar	Natural	Alpine Lace
Cheese, Cheddar	Natural	Axelrod
Cheese, Cheddar	Natural	Cracker Barrel Light
Cheese, Cheddar	Natural	Dorman's Low Sodium
Cheese, Cheddar	Natural	Hickory Farms Light Choice Low Sodium
Cheese, Cheddar	Natural	Kraft Light Naturals
Cheese, Cheddar	Natural	Kraft Light Naturals
Cheese, Cheddar	Natural	Weight Watchers Natural
Cheese, Cheddar	Natural	Weight Watchers Natural
Cheese, Cheddar	Natural	Weight Watchers Natural
Cheese, Cheddar	Natural	Weight Watchers Natural Low
Cheese, Cheddar	Processed	Alpine Lace Free & Lean
Cheese, Cheddar	Processed	Cracker Barrel
Cheese, Cheddar	Processed	Cracker Barrel
Cheese, Cheddar	Processed	Cracker Barrel
Cheese, Cheddar	Processed	Frigo
Cheese, Cheddar	Processed	Kaukauna Cup
Cheese, Cheddar	Processed	Kaukauna Cup
Cheese, Cheddar	Processed	Kaukauna Lite
Cheese, Cheddar	Processed	Kraft Light
Cheese, Cheddar	Processed	Land O Lakes La Cheddar
Cheese, Cheddar	Processed	Light n' Lively Singles
Cheese, Cheddar	Processed	Lite Line
Cheese, Cheddar	Processed	Lite Line
Cheese, Cheddar	Processed	Spreadery
Cheese, Cheddar	Processed	Spreadery
Cheese, Cheddar	Processed	Spreadery
Cheese, Cheddar	Processed	Weight Watchers
Cheese, Cheddar	Processed	Weight Watchers Slices
Cheese, Cheddar	Processed	Wispride
Cheese, Cheddar Jack	Natural	Dorman's Chedda-Jack

Major Description	Minor Description	Serving Size	Calories	Grade
		1 oz	50	C–
White	Low Sodium	.75 oz	50	C–
Yellow	Low Sodium	.75 oz	50	C–
		1 oz	110	D–
		1 oz	91	D–
		1 oz	90	D–
		1 oz	90	D–
Bacon with Horseradish		1 oz	100	D–
		1 oz	90	D–
		1 oz	100	D–
		1 oz	100	D–
		1 oz	105	D–
		1 oz	95	D–
		1 oz	110	D–
		1 oz	110	D
		1 oz	110	D–
		1 oz	100	D
		1 oz	85	D–
		1 oz	114	D–
		1 oz	90	D–
		1 oz	114	D–
		1 oz	80	D–
Sharp or Extra Sharp		1 oz	110	D–
Sharp White, Reduced Fat		1 oz	80	D–
Reduced Fat		1 oz	80	D–
Raw Milk		1 oz	114	D
Reduced Fat		1 oz	80	D–
Sharp, Reduced Fat		1 oz	80	D–
Mild		1 oz	80	D–
Mild or Sharp		1 oz	80	D–
Shredded		1 oz	80	D–
Mild		1 oz	80	D
		1 oz	40	A–
Extra Sharp		1 oz	90	D–
Port Wine		1 oz	100	D–
Sharp		1 oz	100	D–
Imitation		1 oz	90	D–
Nacho, Cold Pack		1 oz	100	D–
Sharp, Extra Sharp, or Smokey		1 oz	100	D–
Sharp or Smoky		1 oz	70	D–
Sharp		1 oz	70	D–
		1 oz	90	D–
Sharp		1 oz	70	D–
Mild		1 oz	50	C–
Sharp		1 oz	50	C–
Medium		1 oz	70	D–
Sharp		1 oz	70	D–
Vermont, White		1 oz	70	D–
Sharp	Fat Free	.75 oz	30	A–
Sharp		1 oz	50	C–
Sharp, Cold Pack		1 oz	100	D–
		1 oz	90	D

"+" indicates the food meets minimum fiber requirements; "–" indicates the food has a high sodium content.

Food	Processing Category	Brand
Cheese, Cheese Food	Processed	Cheeztwin
Cheese, Cheese Food	Processed	Fisher Sandwich Mate
Cheese, Cheese Food	Processed	Lite Line Low Cholesterol
Cheese, Cheshire	Natural	Generic
Cheese, Chutter	Natural	Hickory Farms Cold Pack
Cheese, Colby	Natural	Generic
Cheese, Colby	Natural	Hickory Farms Light Choice
Cheese, Colby	Natural	Hickory Farms Light Choice Low Sodium
Cheese, Colby	Natural	Kraft Light Naturals
Cheese, Colby	Natural	Kraft Light Naturals
Cheese, Colby	Natural	Weight Watchers Natural
Cheese, Colby	Processed	Dorman's Lochol
Cheese, Colby	Processed	Golden Image
Cheese, Colby Jack	Natural	Sargento
Cheese, Cottage [1]	Natural	Generic
Cheese, Cottage	Natural	Generic
Cheese, Cottage	Natural	Generic
Cheese, Cottage	Natural	Generic
Cheese, Cottage	Natural	Generic
Cheese, Cottage	Natural	Generic
Cheese, Cottage	Natural	Generic
Cheese, Cottage	Natural	Generic
Cheese, Cottage	Natural	Bison
Cheese, Cottage	Natural	Bison
Cheese, Cottage	Natural	Bison
Cheese, Cottage	Natural	Bison 4% Fat
Cheese, Cottage	Natural	Borden
Cheese, Cottage	Natural	Borden 4% Fat
Cheese, Cottage	Natural	Borden Unsalted
Cheese, Cottage	Natural	Breakstone's
Cheese, Cottage	Natural	Breakstone's
Cheese, Cottage	Natural	Breakstone's
Cheese, Cottage	Natural	Crowley
Cheese, Cottage	Natural	Crowley
Cheese, Cottage	Natural	Crowley
Cheese, Cottage	Natural	Crowley 4% Fat
Cheese, Cottage	Natural	Crowley 4% Fat
Cheese, Cottage	Natural	Crowley 4% Fat
Cheese, Cottage	Natural	Crowley No Salt Added
Cheese, Cottage	Natural	Darigold
Cheese, Cottage	Natural	Darigold 4%
Cheese, Cottage	Natural	Darigold Trim
Cheese, Cottage	Natural	Friendship
Cheese, Cottage	Natural	Friendship
Cheese, Cottage	Natural	Friendship
Cheese, Cottage	Natural	Friendship
Cheese, Cottage	Natural	Friendship 4%
Cheese, Cottage	Natural	Friendship California Style
Cheese, Cottage	Natural	Friendship No Salt Added
Cheese, Cottage	Natural	Kemp's
Cheese, Cottage	Natural	Kemp's

[1] For all cottage cheese entries, $^1/_2$ cup serving equals approximately 4 oz.

Major Description	Minor Description	Serving Size	Calories	Grade
		1 oz	90	D–
		1 oz	90	D–
		1 oz	90	D–
		1 oz	110	D–
		1 oz	87	D–
		1 oz	112	D–
Low Fat, Calcium Enriched		1 oz	100	D–
		1 oz	100	D
Reduced Fat		1 oz	80	D–
Reduced Fat, Shredded		1 oz	80	D–
		1 oz	80	D–
		1 oz	90	D–
Imitation		1 oz	110	D–
		1 oz	110	D–
		¹/₂ cup	116	D–
Creamed		¹/₂ cup	117	C–
Dry Curd, Unsalted		¹/₂ cup	96	A
Fruit		¹/₂ cup	140	B–
Fruit		¹/₂ cup	140	B–
Low Fat, 1%		¹/₂ cup	80	A–
Low Fat, 1%		¹/₂ cup	80	A–
Low Fat, 2%		¹/₂ cup	100	B–
Garden Salad		¹/₂ cup	110	C–
Low Fat, 1%		¹/₂ cup	90	B–
with Pineapple		¹/₂ cup	140	B–
		¹/₂ cup	120	C–
		¹/₂ cup	80	A
		¹/₂ cup	120	C–
		¹/₂ cup	120	C
		¹/₂ cup	90	A
		¹/₂ cup	110	D–
Low Fat, 2%		¹/₂ cup	100	B–
Low Fat 1%		¹/₂ cup	90	A–
Low Fat with Pineapple, 1%		¹/₂ cup	110	A–
Low Fat, Calcium Fortified, 1%		¹/₂ cup	90	A–
		¹/₂ cup	120	C–
Peaches		¹/₂ cup	140	B–
Pineapple		¹/₂ cup	140	B–
Low Fat, 1%		¹/₂ cup	90	A
		¹/₂ cup	80	A
		¹/₂ cup	120	C–
Low Fat, 2%		¹/₂ cup	100	B–
Low Fat with Pineapple, 1%		¹/₂ cup	110	A–
Low Fat, 1%		¹/₂ cup	90	A–
Low Fat, Lactose Reduced, 1%		¹/₂ cup	90	A–
Pot Style, Large Curd, Low Fat, 2%		¹/₂ cup	100	B–
with Pineapple		¹/₂ cup	140	B–
		¹/₂ cup	120	C–
Low Fat, 1%		¹/₂ cup	90	A
Dry Curd		¹/₂ cup	80	A
Light, 1%		¹/₂ cup	90	A–

"+" indicates the food meets minimum fiber requirements; "–" indicates the food has a high sodium content.

Food	Processing Category	Brand
Cheese, Cottage	Natural	Kemp's
Cheese, Cottage	Natural	Kemp's
Cheese, Cottage	Natural	Knudsen
Cheese, Cottage	Natural	Knudsen
Cheese, Cottage	Natural	Knudsen
Cheese, Cottage	Natural	Knudsen
Cheese, Cottage	Natural	Knudsen
Cheese, Cottage	Natural	Knudsen
Cheese, Cottage	Natural	Knudsen
Cheese, Cottage	Natural	Knudsen
Cheese, Cottage	Natural	Knudsen
Cheese, Cottage	Natural	Knudsen
Cheese, Cottage	Natural	Knudson
Cheese, Cottage	Natural	Light n' Lively
Cheese, Cottage	Natural	Light n' Lively
Cheese, Cottage	Natural	Light n' Lively
Cheese, Cottage	Natural	Lite Line
Cheese, Cottage	Natural	Sealtest
Cheese, Cottage	Natural	Weight Watchers
Cheese, Cottage	Natural	Weight Watchers
Cheese, Country Style	Processed	Kaukauna Cup
Cheese, Cream	Natural	Generic
Cheese, Cream	Natural	Dorman's 65%
Cheese, Cream	Natural	Dorman's 70%
Cheese, Cream	Natural	Philadelphia Brand
Cheese, Cream	Natural	Philadelphia Brand
Cheese, Cream	Natural	Philadelphia Brand
Cheese, Cream	Processed	Kraft Free
Cheese, Cream	Processed	Philadelphia Brand Light
Cheese, Cream	Processed	Tofutti Better Than Cream Cheese
Cheese, Cream	Processed	Weight Watchers
Cheese, Cream	Processed	Weight Watchers
Cheese, Danbo	Natural	Dorman's 20%
Cheese, Danbo	Natural	Dorman's 45%
Cheese, Danbo	Natural	Dorman's Crema Dania 70%
Cheese, Edam	Natural	Generic
Cheese, Edam	Natural	Dorman's 45%
Cheese, Feta	Natural	Generic
Cheese, Feta	Natural	Dorman's 45%
Cheese, Farmer	Natural	Friendship
Cheese, Farmer	Natural	Hickory Farms Light Choice
Cheese, Fontina	Natural	Generic
Cheese, Garlic	Processed	Kraft
Cheese, Gjetost	Natural	Generic
Cheese, Gjetost	Natural	Generic
Cheese, Goat	Natural	Generic
Cheese, Goat	Natural	Generic
Cheese, Goat	Natural	Generic
Cheese, Gouda	Natural	Generic
Cheese, Gruyère	Natural	Generic
Cheese, Harvati	Natural	Dorman's 45%
Cheese, Harvati	Natural	Dorman's 60%

Major Description	Minor Description	Serving Size	Calories	Grade
Low Fat, 2%		¹/₂ cup	100	B–
Nonfat		¹/₂ cup	80	A–
Low Fat with Apple, 2%		¹/₂ cup	120	A–
Low Fat with Fruit Cocktail, 2%		¹/₂ cup	130	A–
Low Fat with Mandarin Orange		¹/₂ cup	110	B–
Low Fat with Peach, 2%		¹/₂ cup	113	A–
Low Fat with Pear, 2%		¹/₂ cup	110	B–
Low Fat with Pineapple, 2%		¹/₂ cup	113	A–
Low Fat with Strawberry, 2%		¹/₂ cup	113	A–
Low Fat, 2%		¹/₂ cup	100	B–
Nonfat		¹/₂ cup	70	A–
Pineapple, 4%		¹/₂ cup	140	C–
Large Curd		¹/₂ cup	120	C–
Low Fat Garden Salad, 1%		¹/₂ cup	90	A–
Low Fat with Peach & Pineapple, 1%		¹/₂ cup	100	A–
Low Fat, 1%		¹/₂ cup	90	A–
Low Fat, 1.5%		¹/₂ cup	90	B–
Low Fat, 2%		¹/₂ cup	100	B–
Low Fat, 1%		¹/₂ cup	90	A–
Low Fat, 2%		¹/₂ cup	100	B–
Cold Pack		1 oz	100	D–
		1 oz	99	D
		1 oz	90	D–
		1 oz	102	D–
		1 oz	100	D
Soft		1 oz	100	D
Whipped		1 oz	100	D
		1 oz	45	A–
		1 oz	60	D–
Imitation Cheese		1 oz	80	D–
		1 oz	35	D
		1 oz	35	D
		1 oz	62	D–
		1 oz	98	D–
		1 oz	134	D–
		1 oz	101	D–
		1 oz	91	D–
Sheep's Milk		1 oz	75	D–
		1 oz	91	D
		¹/₂ cup	160	D–
		1 oz	90	D–
		1 oz	110	D
		1 oz	90	D–
Goat's Milk		1 oz	132	D–
Goat's Milk Fresh		1 oz	82	D–
Hard		1 oz	128	D
Semi-soft		1 oz	103	D–
Soft		1 oz.	76	D–
		1 oz	101	D–
		1 oz	117	D
		1 oz	91	D–
		1 oz	118	D–

"+" indicates the food meets minimum fiber requirements; "–" indicates the food has a high sodium content.

Food	Processing Category	Brand
Cheese, Havarti	Natural	Casino
Cheese, Horseradish	Processed	Kaukauna Cup
Cheese, Hot Pepper	Natural	Hickory Farms
Cheese, Italian Style	Natural	Sargento
Cheese, Jalapeño Pepper	Processed	Hoffman's
Cheese, Jalapeño Pepper	Processed	Kraft
Cheese, Jalapeño Pepper	Processed	Kraft Singles
Cheese, Jalapeño Pepper	Processed	Land O Lakes
Cheese, Jalapeño Pepper	Processed	Spreadery
Cheese, Jalapeño Pepper	Processed	Velveeta Mexican
Cheese, Jalapeño Pepper	Processed	Velveeta Mexican
Cheese, Jarlsberg	Natural	Hickory Farms
Cheese, Jarlsberg	Natural	Norseland Jarlsberg
Cheese, Limburger	Natural	Generic
Cheese, Mexican	Processed	Velveeta
Cheese, Mexican	Processed	Velveeta
Cheese, Monterey Jack	Natural	Generic
Cheese, Monterey Jack	Natural	Alpine Lace Monti-Jack
Cheese, Monterey Jack	Natural	Dorman's
Cheese, Monterey Jack	Natural	Dorman's Low Sodium
Cheese, Monterey Jack	Natural	Hickory Farms Light Choice Low Sodium
Cheese, Monterey Jack	Natural	Kraft
Cheese, Monterey Jack	Natural	Kraft Light Naturals
Cheese, Monterey Jack	Natural	Kraft Light Naturals
Cheese, Monterey Jack	Natural	Kraft Light Naturals
Cheese, Monterey Jack	Natural	Weight Watchers Natural
Cheese, Monterey Jack	Processed	Kraft Singles
Cheese, Mozzarella	Natural	Generic
Cheese, Mozzarella	Natural	Generic
Cheese, Mozzarella	Natural	Generic
Cheese, Mozzarella	Natural	Dorman's
Cheese, Mozzarella	Natural	Dorman's Low Sodium
Cheese, Mozzarella	Natural	Frigo
Cheese, Mozzarella	Natural	Hickory Farms
Cheese, Mozzarella	Natural	Hickory Farms Light Choice Low Sodium
Cheese, Mozzarella	Natural	Kraft Light Naturals
Cheese, Mozzarella	Natural	Polly-O Fiordi Latte
Cheese, Mozzarella	Natural	Polly-O Lite
Cheese, Mozzarella	Natural	Weight Watchers Natural
Cheese, Mozzarella	Natural	Weight Watchers Natural
Cheese, Mozzarella	Processed	Alpine Lace Free & Lean
Cheese, Mozzarella	Processed	Frigo
Cheese, Mozzarella	Processed	Lite Line
Cheese, Mozzarella	Processed	Alpine Lace Fat Free
Cheese, Muenster	Natural	Generic
Cheese, Muenster	Natural	Dorman's 50%
Cheese, Muenster	Natural	Dorman's Low Sodium
Cheese, Muenster	Natural	Hickory Farms Light Choice Low Sodium
Cheese, Muenster	Processed	Dorman's Lochol
Cheese, Muenster	Processed	Lite Line

Major Description	Minor Description	Serving Size	Calories	Grade
		1 oz	120	D
Cold Pack		1 oz	100	D–
		1 oz	106	D–
		1 oz	110	D
		1 oz	90	D–
		1 oz	90	D–
		1 oz	90	D–
		1 oz	90	D–
Mexican Style		1 oz	70	D–
Hot		1 oz	100	D–
Mild		1 oz	100	D–
		1 oz	100	D–
		1 oz	97	D–
		1 oz	93	D–
Hot, Shredded		1 oz	100	D–
Mild, Shredded		1 oz	100	D–
		1 oz	106	D–
		1 oz	80	D
		1 oz	90	D
Reduced Fat		1 oz	80	D
		1 oz	110	D
Caraway Seeds		1 oz	100	D–
Reduced Fat		1 oz	80	D–
Reduced Fat, Shredded		1 oz	80	D–
with Peppers, Reduced Fat		1 oz	80	D–
		1 oz	80	D–
		1 oz	90	D–
Low Moisture		1 oz	79	D–
Part Skim Milk		1 oz	72	D–
Whole Milk		1 oz	80	D–
		1 oz	90	D–
Reduced Fat		1 oz	80	D
Reduced Fat		1 oz	60	D–
		1 oz	72	D–
		1 oz	80	D
Reduced Fat		1 oz	80	D–
	Fresh	1 oz	80	D
		1 oz	70	D–
		1 oz	70	D–
Shredded		1 oz	80	D–
		1 oz	40	A–
Imitation		1 oz	90	D–
		1 oz	50	C–
		1 oz	45	A–
		1 oz	104	D–
		1 oz	100	D–
Reduced Fat		1 oz	80	D–
		1 oz	110	D
		1 oz	100	D–
		1 oz	50	C–

"+" indicates the food meets minimum fiber requirements; "–" indicates the food has a high sodium content.

Food	Processing Category	Brand
Cheese, Nacho	Processed	Spreadery
Cheese, Neufchatel	Natural	Philadelphia Brand Light
Cheese, Neufchatel	Processed	Spreadery
Cheese, Neufchatel	Processed	Spreadery
Cheese, Neufchatel	Processed	Spreadery
Cheese, Neufchatel	Processed	Spreadery
Cheese, Neufchatel	Processed	Spreadery
Cheese, New Holland	Natural	Hickory Farms Light Choice
Cheese, Onion	Processed	Hoffman's Chees N Onion
Cheese, Onion	Processed	Land O Lakes
Cheese, Parmesan	Natural	Generic
Cheese, Parmesan	Natural	Generic
Cheese, Parmesan	Processed	Alpine Lace Free & Lean
Cheese, Parmesan	Processed	Weight Watchers
Cheese, Pepperoni	Processed	Kraft Singles
Cheese, Pepperoni	Processed	Land O Lakes
Cheese, Pimento	Natural	Generic
Cheese, Pizza	Natural	Frigo
Cheese, Pizza	Natural	Frigo
Cheese, Port Du Salut	Natural	Generic
Cheese, Port Wine	Natural	Hickory Farms
Cheese, Port Wine	Processed	Kaukauna Cup
Cheese, Port Wine	Processed	Spreadery
Cheese, Port Wine	Processed	Wispride
Cheese, Pot Cheese	Natural	Sargento
Cheese, Primavera	Natural	Bel Paese Lite
Cheese, Provolone	Natural	Generic
Cheese, Provolone	Natural	Alpine Lace Provo-lo
Cheese, Provolone	Natural	Hickory Farms Light Choice Low Sodium
Cheese, Pub	Natural	Hickory Farms
Cheese, Queso Blanco	Natural	Sargento
Cheese, Queso de Pasa	Natural	Sargento
Cheese, Queso de Taco	Natural	Hickory Farms
Cheese, Ricotta	Natural	Generic
Cheese, Ricotta	Natural	Generic
Cheese, Ricotta	Natural	Polly-O Lite
Cheese, Ricotta	Natural	Sargento Lite
Cheese, Romano	Natural	Generic
Cheese, Romano	Natural	Frigo
Cheese, Roquefort	Natural	Generic
Cheese, Salami	Processed	Hoffman's Chees N Salami
Cheese, Salami	Processed	Land O Lakes
Cheese, Sandwich Slices	Processed	Lunch Wagon
Cheese, Sharp	Processed	Kraft Singles
Cheese, Shredded	Processed	Velveeta
Cheese, Smoked	Natural	Hickory Farms Light Choice Low Sodium
Cheese, Smoked	Natural	Sargento Smokestick
Cheese, String	Natural	Frigo
Cheese, Swiss	Natural	Generic
Cheese, Swiss	Processed	Generic
Cheese, Swiss	Natural	Alpine Lace Swiss-lo

Major Description	Minor Description	Serving Size	Calories	Grade
		1 oz	70	D–
		1 oz	80	D–
French Onion		1 oz	70	D–
Garlic & Herb		1 oz	70	D–
Ranch Classic		1 oz	70	D–
Strawberries		1 oz	70	D–
Vegetable Garden		1 oz	70	D–
with Herbs		1 oz	90	D
		1 oz	100	D–
		1 oz	90	D–
Grated		1 oz	129	D–
Hard		1 oz	111	D–
Grated		1 oz	45	A–
Grated	Fat Free	1 Tbsp	15	A–
Pimento		1 oz	90	D–
		1 oz	90	D–
Processed		1 oz	106	D–
Shredded		1 oz	90	D–
Shredded, Low Fat		1 oz	65	D–
		1 oz	100	D–
		1 oz	97	D–
Cold Pack		1 oz	100	D–
		1 oz	70	D–
Cold Pack		1 oz	100	D–
		1 oz	25	A
		1 oz	68	D–
		1 oz	100	D–
		1 oz	70	D
		1 oz	90	D–
		1 oz	94	D–
		1 oz	100	D–
		1 oz	110	D–
		1 oz	106	D–
Part Skim Milk		1 oz	39	D
Whole Milk		1 oz	49	D
		1 oz	40	D
		1 oz	12	C
		1 oz	110	D–
Grated		1 oz	130	D–
Sheep's Milk		1 oz	105	D–
		1 oz	90	D–
		1 oz	100	D–
		1 oz	90	D–
		1 oz	100	D–
		1 oz	100	D–
		1 oz	80	D–
		1 oz	100	D–
		1 oz	80	D–
Processed		1 oz	95	D–
		1 oz	92	D–
		1 oz	100	D

"+" indicates the food meets minimum fiber requirements; "–" indicates the food has a high sodium content.

Food	Processing Category	Brand
Cheese, Swiss	Natural	Dorman's Reduced Fat
Cheese, Swiss	Natural	Hickory Farms Light Choice
Cheese, Swiss	Natural	Hickory Farms Light Choice Low Sodium
Cheese, Swiss	Natural	Kraft
Cheese, Swiss	Natural	Kraft Light Naturals
Cheese, Swiss	Natural	Kraft Light Naturals
Cheese, Swiss	Natural	Natural
Cheese, Swiss	Processed	Dorman's Lochol
Cheese, Swiss	Processed	Kaukauna Lite
Cheese, Swiss	Processed	Kraft Light
Cheese, Swiss	Processed	Kraft Singles
Cheese, Swiss	Processed	Light n' Lively Singles
Cheese, Swiss	Processed	Lite Line
Cheese, Swiss	Processed	Velveeta
Cheese, Swiss	Processed	Velveeta Light
Cheese, Swiss	Processed	Weight Watchers Slices
Cheese, Swiss	Processed	Weight Watchers Slices
Cheese, Tilsit	Natural	Generic
Cheese, White	Processed	Weight Watchers Slices
Cheese, Yellow	Processed	Weight Watchers
Cheese Ball or Log	All Forms	Cracker Barrel
Cheese Ball or Log	All Forms	Cracker Barrel
Cheese Ball or Log	All Forms	Cracker Barrel
Cheese Ball or Log	All Forms	Kaukauna
Cheese Ball or Log	All Forms	Kaukauna
Cheese Ball or Log	All Forms	Sargento
Cheese Ball or Log	All Forms	Sargento
Cheese Nuggets, Mozzarella	Frozen	Banquet Cheese Hot Bits
Cheese Sauce	All Forms	Contadina Fresh
Cheese Sauce	All Forms	Kaukauna
Cheese Sauce	All Forms	Lucky Leaf/Musselman's
Cheese Sauce	All Forms	Lucky Leaf/Musselman's
Cheese Sauce	All Forms	Stouffer's
Cheese Sauce	All Forms	White House
Cheese Sauce	All Forms	White House
Cheese Sauce	All Forms	White House
Cheese Sauce	Mix	French's
Cheese Sauce	Mix	Knorr
Cheese Sauce	Mix	Land O Lakes
Cheese Sauce	Mix	Land O Lakes
Cheese Sauce	Mix	McCormick/Schilling
Cheese Spread	All Forms	Alpine Lace Free & Lean
Cheese Spread	All Forms	Alpine Lace Free & Lean
Cheese Spread	All Forms	Alpine Lace Free & Lean
Cheese Spread	All Forms	Alpine Lace Free & Lean
Cheese Spread	All Forms	Alpine Lace Free & Lean
Cheese Spread	All Forms	Alpine Lace Free & Lean
Cheese Spread	All Forms	Cheez Whiz
Cheese Spread	All Forms	Cheez Whiz

Major Description	Minor Description	Serving Size	Calories	Grade
		1 oz	90	D
		1 oz	100	D
		1 oz	100	D
		1 oz	110	D
		1 oz	90	D
Reduced Fat		1 oz	90	D
		1 oz	107	D
		1 oz	100	D–
Country Style		1 oz	70	D–
		1 oz	70	C–
		1 oz	90	D–
		1 oz	70	C–
		1 oz	50	C–
		1 oz	100	D–
		1 oz	70	D–
		1 oz	50	C–
Fat Free		75 oz	30	A–
Whole Milk		1 oz	96	D–
Fat Free		.75 oz	30	A–
Fat Free		75 oz	30	A–
Cheddar with Almonds	Port Wine	1 oz	90	D–
Cheddar with Almonds	Sharp	1 oz	100	D–
Log	Sharp Cheddar or Smoky	1 oz	90	D–
Cheese Balls	All Flavors	1 oz	100	D–
Cheese Logs	All Flavors	1 oz	100	D–
Log	Sharp Cheddar or Port Wine	1 oz	100	D–
Log	Swiss Almond	1 oz	90	D–
Breaded		2.63 oz	240	D–
Four Cheese	Refrigerated	1 oz	78	D
Nacho		1 oz	80	D–
Cheddar		1 oz	55	D–
Nacho		1 oz	55	D–
Cheddar		1 oz	72	D–
Aged		1 oz	61	D–
Jalapeño Pepper		1 oz	55	D–
Nacho		1 oz	55	D–
		1/4 cup	80	D–
Parmesano	Prepared with Chicken	1/8 pkg	190	B–
Cheddar		1 oz	24	D–
Nacho		1 oz	46	D–
		1 Tbsp	40	D–
Cheddar		1 oz	30	A–
French Onion		1 oz	30	A–
Garden-style Vegetable		1 oz	30	A–
Garlic & Herb		1 oz	30	A–
Horseradish		1 oz	30	A–
Mexican-style Nacho		1 oz	30	A–
		1 oz	80	D–
Jalapeño Pepper		1 oz	80	D–

"+" indicates the food meets minimum fiber requirements; "–" indicates the food has a high sodium content.

Food	Processing Category	Brand
Cheese Spread	All Forms	Cheez Whiz
Cheese Spread	All Forms	Kraft
Cheese Spread	All Forms	Kraft
Cheese Spread	All Forms	Kraft
Cheese Spread	All Forms	Kraft
Cheese Spread	All Forms	Kraft
Cheese Spread	All Forms	Kraft
Cheese Spread	All Forms	Land O Lakes Golden Velvet
Cheese Spread	All Forms	Laughing Cow Cheezbits
Cheese Spread	All Forms	Micro Melt
Cheese Spread	All Forms	Mohawk Valley
Cheese Spread	All Forms	Old English
Cheese Spread	All Forms	Roka
Cheese Spread	All Forms	Sargento Cracker Snacks
Cheese Spread	All Forms	Sargento Cracker Snacks
Cheese Spread	All Forms	Squeez A Snak
Cheese Spread	All Forms	Velveeta
Cheese Spread	All Forms	Velveeta Slices
Cheese Spread	All Forms	Weight Watchers Cup
Cheese Spread	All Forms	Weight Watchers Cup
Cheese Sticks	Frozen	Farm Rich
Cheese Sticks	Frozen	Farm Rich
Cheese Sticks	Frozen	Farm Rich
Cheese Sticks	Frozen	Farm Rich
Cream	Canned	Generic
Cream	Fluid	Generic
Cream	Fluid	Generic
Cream	Fluid	Generic
Cream	Fluid	Generic
Cream	Fluid	Generic
Cream	Frozen	Kraft Real Cream
Creamer	Frozen, Liquid	Generic
Creamer	Powdered	Generic
Creamer	Liquid	Coffeemate
Creamer	Powdered	Coffeemate
Creamer	Powdered	Coffeemate Lite
Creamer	Powdered	Cremora
Creamer		Crowley
Creamer		Diehl
Creamer		N-rich
Creamer	Frozen, Liquid	Rich's Coffee Rich
Creamer	Frozen, Liquid	Rich's Farm Rich
Creamer	Frozen, Liquid	Rich's Poly Rich
Egg Breakfast	Freeze-dried	Mountain House
Egg Breakfast	Freeze-dried	Mountain House
Egg Breakfast	Freeze-dried	Mountain House
Egg Breakfast	Freeze-dried	Mountain House
Egg Substitute	Frozen	Generic
Egg Substitute	Powdered	Generic
Egg Substitute	Frozen	Morningstar Farms Scramblers
Egg Substitute	Frozen	Tofutti Egg Watchers
Egg Substitute	Mix	Tofu Scrambler
Egg Substitute	Mix	Tofu Scrambler

Major Description	Minor Description	Serving Size	Calories	Grade
Mexican Style	Mild	1 oz	80	D–
Bacon		1 oz	80	D–
Jalapeño Pepper		1 oz	70	D–
Jalapeño Pepper	Loaf	1 oz	80	D–
Olives & Pimento		1 oz	60	D–
Pimento		1 oz	70	D–
Pineapple		1 oz	70	D
		1 oz	80	D–
		0.17	13	D–
		1 oz	80	D–
Limburger		1 oz	70	D–
Sharp		1 oz	80	D–
Blue		1 oz	70	D–
Brick		1 oz	100	D–
Swiss		1 oz	100	D–
All Flavors		1 oz	80	D–
All Varieties		1 oz	80	D–
All Varieties		1 oz	90	D–
Cheddar, Sharp		1 oz	70	C–
Port Wine		1 oz	70	C–
Cheddar	Breaded	3 oz	300	D–
Hot Pepper	Breaded	3 oz	260	D–
Mozzarella	Breaded	3 oz	240	D–
Provolone	Breaded	3 oz	270	D–
Whipped Topping	Pressurized	1 oz	73	D
Half & Half		1 oz	37	D
Light, Coffee or Table		1 oz	55	D
Medium, 25% Fat		1 oz	69	D
Whipping, Heavy		1 oz	98	D
Whipping, Light		1 oz	83	D
Whipped Topping		1/4 cup	30	D
		1 oz	39	D
		1 oz	155	D
		1 Tbsp	16	D
		1 Tbsp	30	A
		1 Tbsp	24	A
		1 Tbsp	30	A
		1 Tbsp	16	D
		1 Tbsp	30	A
		1 Tbsp	30	D
		1 Tbsp	20	D
		1 Tbsp	20	D
		1 Tbsp	20	D
Bacon		1/2 pkg	170	D
Butter		1/2 pkg	160	D
Omelet	Cheese	1/2 pkg	180	D
Precooked, Bacon		1/2 pkg	180	D
		1 oz	45	D
		1 oz	126	B–
		1/4 cup	60	D
		1/4 cup	50	C–
	with Tofu	1/4 cup	35	A–
Butter Added	with Tofu	1/4 cup	80	D–

"+" indicates the food meets minimum fiber requirements; "–" indicates the food has a high sodium content.

Food	Processing Category	Brand
Egg Substitute	Refrigerated	Featherweight
Egg Substitute	Refrigerated	Fleischmann's Egg Beater Cheez
Egg Substitute	Refrigerated	Fleischmann's Egg Beaters
Egg Substitute	Refrigerated	Generic
Egg, Chicken	Fresh	All Brands
Egg, Chicken	Fresh	All Brands
Egg, Chicken	Fresh	All Brands
Egg, Chicken	Fresh	All Brands
Egg, Chicken	Fresh	All Brands
Egg, Chicken	Fresh	All Brands
Egg, Chicken	Fresh	All Brands
Egg, Chicken	Fresh	All Brands
Egg, Chicken	Fresh	All Brands
Egg, Chicken	Fresh	All Brands
Egg, Chicken	Fresh	All Brands
Egg, Chicken	Fresh	All Brands
Egg, Chicken	Fresh	All Brands
Egg, Chicken	Fresh	All Brands
Egg, Chicken	Dried	All Brands
Egg, Chicken	Dried	All Brands
Egg, Chicken	Dried	All Brands
Egg, Chicken	Dried	All Brands
Egg, Chicken	Pickled	Penrose
Egg, Duck	Fresh	All Brands
Egg, Goose	Fresh	All Brands
Egg, Quail	Fresh	All Brands
Egg, Turkey	Fresh	All Brands
Ice Cream	Fast and Frivolous Foods	
Milk	Fresh	All Brands
Milk	Fresh	All Brands
Milk	Fresh	All Brands
Milk	Fresh	All Brands
Milk	Fresh	All Brands
Milk	Fresh	All Brands
Milk	Fresh	All Brands
Milk	Fresh	All Brands
Milk	Canned	Generic
Milk	Canned	Generic
Milk	Canned	Generic
Milk	Canned	Borden
Milk	Canned	Carnation
Milk	Canned	Carnation
Milk	Canned	Carnation
Milk	Canned	Carnation
Milk	Canned	Pet
Milk	Canned	Diehl Jerzee
Milk	Dry	All Brands
Milk	Dry	All Brands
Milk	Dry	All Brands
Milk	Dry	All Brands
Milk	Dry	All Brands
Milk	Dry	Weight Watchers Dairy Creamer
Milk, Goat's	Fresh	Generic

Major Description	Minor Description	Serving Size	Calories	Grade
		2 eggs	120	D–
	with Cheese	$1/4$ cup	65	D–
		$1/4$ cup	25	A–
		1 oz	24	C–
White Only		1 egg	14	A–
White Only		1 large egg	17	A–
Whole	Fried	1 large egg	91	D–
Whole	Hard Boiled	1 large egg	77	D
Whole	Hard Boiled, Chopped	$1/2$ cup	105	D
Whole	Omelet	1 large egg	92	D–
Whole	Poached	1 large egg	74	D–
Whole		$1/2$ cup	180	D
Whole		1 large egg	75	D
Whole	Scrambled	$1/2$ cup	180	D–
Whole	Scrambled	1 large egg	101	D–
Yolk Only	Raw	$1/2$ cup	435	D
Yolk Only	Raw	1 large egg	59	D
White Only	Powdered	$1/2$ cup	200	A–
Whole	Powdered	$1/2$ cup	250	D
Whole	Stabilized, Glucose Reduced	$1/2$ cup	260	D
Yolk Only	Powdered	$1/2$ cup	230	D
		2 oz	80	D–
Whole		1 egg or 2.5 oz	130	D
Whole		1 egg or 5.1 oz	267	D
Whole		1 egg or 0.3 oz	14	D
Whole		1 egg or 2.8 oz	135	D
	3.3% Fat	1 cup	150	D–
Buttermilk, Cultured		1 cup	99	B–
Low Fat	1% Fat	1 cup	102	B–
Low Fat	1.5% Fat	1 cup	120	B–
Low Fat	2% Fat	1 cup	121	C–
Low Fat, Protein Fortified	1% Fat	1 cup	119	B–
Skim		1 cup	86	A–
Whole	3.7% Fat	1 cup	157	D
Condensed	Sweetened	1 cup	982	B
Whole		1 cup	338	D
Evaporated, Skim		1 cup	200	A
Condensed	Sweetened	1 cup	960	B
Condensed	Sweetened	1 cup	960	B
Evaporated		1 cup	340	D
Evaporated, Skim	"Lite"	1 cup	200	A
Whole	Low Fat	1 cup	200	A–
Evaporated, Skim	"Lite"	1 cup	200	A
Condensed	Sweetened	1 cup	960	B
Buttermilk, Sweet Cream		$1/2$ cup	230	A–
Nonfat		$1/2$ cup	217	A–
Nonfat	Instant	$1/2$ cup	163	A–
Skim		$1/2$ cup	120	A
Whole		$1/2$ cup	317	D
Nonfat	Instant	1 pkt	10	A–
Whole		1 cup	168	D

"+" indicates the food meets minimum fiber requirements; "–" indicates the food has a high sodium content.

Food	Processing Category	Brand
Milk, Imitation	Liquid	Generic
Milk, Sheep's	Fresh	Generic
Sour Cream	All Forms	Generic
Sour Cream	All Forms	Generic
Sour Cream	All Forms	Generic
Sour Cream	All Forms	Crowley
Sour Cream	All Forms	Friendship Lite Delite
Sour Cream	All Forms	Kemp's
Sour Cream	All Forms	Knudsen
Sour Cream	All Forms	Weight Watchers
Sour Cream	Non Dairy	Generic
Sour Cream	Non Dairy	Crowley
Sour Cream	Non Dairy	Pet
Whey	Dry	Generic
Whey	Dry	Generic
Whey	Fluid	Generic
Whey	Fluid	Generic
Yogurt [2]	Frozen	Ben & Jerry's
Yogurt	Frozen	Ben & Jerry's
Yogurt	Frozen	Ben & Jerry's
Yogurt	Frozen	Ben & Jerry's
Yogurt	Frozen	Ben & Jerry's
Yogurt	Frozen	Ben & Jerry's
Yogurt	Frozen	Ben & Jerry's
Yogurt	Frozen	Ben & Jerry's
Yogurt	Frozen	Ben & Jerry's
Yogurt	Frozen	Ben & Jerry's
Yogurt	Frozen	Ben & Jerry's
Yogurt	Frozen	Ben & Jerry's
Yogurt	Frozen	Ben & Jerry's
Yogurt	Frozen	Ben & Jerry's
Yogurt	Frozen	Ben & Jerry's
Yogurt	Frozen	Ben & Jerry's
Yogurt	Frozen	Ben & Jerry's
Yogurt	Frozen	Ben & Jerry's
Yogurt	Frozen	Ben & Jerry's
Yogurt	Frozen	Ben & Jerry's
Yogurt	Frozen	Ben & Jerry's
Yogurt	Frozen	Bison
Yogurt	Frozen	Breyers
Yogurt	Frozen	Breyers
Yogurt	Frozen	Breyers
Yogurt	Frozen	Breyers
Yogurt	Frozen	Breyers
Yogurt	Frozen	Breyers
Yogurt	Frozen	Breyers
Yogurt	Frozen	Colombo Gourmet
Yogurt	Frozen	Colombo Gourmet
Yogurt	Frozen	Colombo Gourmet
Yogurt	Frozen	Colombo Gourmet
Yogurt	Frozen	Colombo Gourmet
Yogurt	Frozen	Colombo Gourmet

[2] *Processed yogurts invariably contain a substantial amount of simple sugar. Intake should be limited to one serving per day.*

Major Description	Minor Description	Serving Size	Calories	Grade
		1 cup	150	D–
Whole		1 cup	264	D
		1 oz	61	D
Half & Half		1 oz	38	D
No Fat		1 oz	15	A
Light		1 oz	30	D
Low Fat		1 oz	35	D
	Light	1 oz	30	D
Light		1 oz	40	D
Light		1 oz	35	D
		1 oz	59	D
Dressing		1 oz	40	D
		1 Tbsp	25	D
Acid		1 oz	96	A–
Sweet		1 oz	100	A–
Acid		1 oz	7	A–
Sweet		1 oz	8	A–
Apple Pie		$^1/_2$ cup	170	B
Banana & Strawberry		$^1/_2$ cup	160	A
Banana & Strawberry		$^1/_2$ cup	140	A
Black Raspberry	Nonfat	$^1/_2$ cup	150	A
Blueberry		$^1/_2$ cup	130	A
Blueberry Cheesecake		$^1/_2$ cup	150	A
Bluesberry		$^1/_2$ cup	160	A
Bluesberry	Nonfat	$^1/_2$ cup	120	A
Cappuccino	Nonfat	$^1/_2$ cup	120	A
Cappuccino Express		$^1/_2$ cup	160	B
Cherry Garcia		$^1/_2$ cup	170	B
Chocolate	Nonfat	$^1/_2$ cup	120	A
Chocolate Chip Cookie Dough		$^1/_2$ cup	180	B
Chocolate Fudge Brownie		$^1/_2$ cup	180	B
Chocolate Raspberry Swirl		$^1/_2$ cup	170	A
Coffee Almond Fudge		$^1/_2$ cup	180	C
English Toffee Crunch		$^1/_2$ cup	180	B
Raspberry		$^1/_2$ cup	110	A
Strawberry	Nonfat	$^1/_2$ cup	120	A
Sweet Cream	Nonfat	$^1/_2$ cup	120	A
Vanilla	Nonfat	$^1/_2$ cup	120	A
Chocolate		$^1/_2$ cup	107	B
Black Cherry		$^1/_2$ cup	120	A
Chocolate		$^1/_2$ cup	120	A
Peach		$^1/_2$ cup	110	A
Raspberry		$^1/_2$ cup	120	A
Strawberry		$^1/_2$ cup	110	A
Strawberry & Banana		$^1/_2$ cup	110	A
Vanilla		$^1/_2$ cup	120	A
Caramel Pecan Chunk		$^1/_2$ cup	160	B–
Cheesecake, Wild Raspberry		$^1/_2$ cup	130	B
Chocolate	Bavarian Style	$^1/_2$ cup	160	B
Heath Bar Crunch		$^1/_2$ cup	173	C
Mocha Swiss Almond		$^1/_2$ cup	160	C
Peanut Butter Cup		$^1/_2$ cup	187	D

"+" indicates the food meets minimum fiber requirements; "–" indicates the food has a high sodium content.

Food	Processing Category	Brand
Yogurt	Frozen	Colombo Gourmet
Yogurt	Frozen	Colombo Gourmet
Yogurt	Frozen	Colombo Shoppe Style
Yogurt	Frozen	Colombo Shoppe Style
Yogurt	Frozen	Colombo Shoppe Style
Yogurt	Frozen	Colombo Shoppe Style
Yogurt	Frozen	Colombo Shoppe Style
Yogurt	Frozen	Colombo Shoppe Style
Yogurt	Frozen	Colombo Shoppe Style
Yogurt	Frozen	Colombo Shoppe Style
Yogurt	Frozen	Colombo Shoppe Style
Yogurt	Frozen	Colombo Shoppe Style
Yogurt	Frozen	Crowley
Yogurt	Frozen	Crowley
Yogurt	Frozen	Crowley
Yogurt	Frozen	Crowley
Yogurt	Frozen	Crowley
Yogurt	Frozen	Crowley
Yogurt	Frozen	Dannon Nonfat
Yogurt	Frozen	Dreyer's Inspirations
Yogurt	Frozen	Dreyer's Inspirations
Yogurt	Frozen	Dreyer's Inspirations
Yogurt	Frozen	Dreyer's Inspirations
Yogurt	Frozen	Dreyer's Inspirations
Yogurt	Frozen	Dreyer's Inspirations
Yogurt	Frozen	Dreyer's Inspirations
Yogurt	Frozen	Dreyer's Inspirations
Yogurt	Frozen	Dreyer's Inspirations
Yogurt	Frozen	Elan
Yogurt	Frozen	Häagen-Dazs
Yogurt	Frozen	Häagen-Dazs
Yogurt	Frozen	Häagen-Dazs
Yogurt	Frozen	Häagen-Dazs
Yogurt	Frozen	Häagen-Dazs
Yogurt	Frozen	Häagen-Dazs
Yogurt	Frozen	Häagen-Dazs
Yogurt	Frozen	Häagen-Dazs Extras
Yogurt	Frozen	Häagen-Dazs Extras
Yogurt	Frozen	Häagen-Dazs Extras
Yogurt	Frozen	Häagen-Dazs Extras
Yogurt	Frozen	Häagen-Dazs Extras
Yogurt	Frozen	Kemp's
Yogurt	Frozen	Kemp's
Yogurt	Frozen	Kemp's
Yogurt	Frozen	Sealtest Free
Yogurt	Frozen	Sealtest Free
Yogurt	Frozen	Sealtest Free
Yogurt	Frozen	Sealtest Free
Yogurt	Frozen	Sealtest Free
Yogurt	Frozen	Sealtest Free
Yogurt	Frozen	TCBY
Yogurt	Frozen	TCBY
Yogurt	Frozen	TCBY

Major Description	Minor Description	Serving Size	Calories	Grade
Strawberry		¹/₂ cup	130	B
Vanilla		¹/₂ cup	120	B
Banana Split		¹/₂ cup	140	A
Chocolate Cappuccino		¹/₂ cup	110	A
Chocolate Peanut Butter Twist		¹/₂ cup	140	B
Double Chocolate		¹/₂ cup	130	A
Old World Chocolate		¹/₂ cup	130	A
Piña Colada		¹/₂ cup	130	A
Simply Vanilla		¹/₂ cup	120	A
Strawberry Vanilla Twist		¹/₂ cup	110	A
Vanilla Cherry		¹/₂ cup	110	A
White & Dutch Chocolate		¹/₂ cup	110	A
Cherry		¹/₂ cup	106	A
Chocolate		¹/₂ cup	106	B
Peach		¹/₂ cup	106	A
Raspberry		¹/₂ cup	106	A
Strawberry		¹/₂ cup	106	A
Vanilla		¹/₂ cup	106	B
All Flavors		¹/₂ cup	90	A
Blueberry		3 oz	80	A
Cherry		3 oz	80	A
Chocolate		3 oz	80	A
Peach		3 oz	80	A
Raspberry		3 oz	80	A
Strawberry		3 oz	80	A
Strawberry & Banana		3 oz	80	A
Vanilla		3 oz	80	A
Vanilla & Raspberry Swirl		3 oz	80	A
Chocolate Almond		¹/₂ cup	160	C
Banana & Strawberry		¹/₂ cup	170	B
Chocolate		¹/₂ cup	170	B
Coffee		¹/₂ cup	180	B
Peach		¹/₂ cup	170	B
Strawberry		¹/₂ cup	170	B
Vanilla		¹/₂ cup	170	B
Vanilla Almond Crunch		¹/₂ cup	200	B
Brownie Nut		¹/₂ cup	220	C
Orange		¹/₂ cup	130	A
Praline		¹/₂ cup	240	C
Raspberry		¹/₂ cup	130	A
Strawberry Cheesecake		¹/₂ cup	210	B
Strawberry		4 oz	107	A
Strawberry	Nonfat	4 oz	93	A
Vanilla	Nonfat	4 oz	100	A
Black Cherry	Nonfat	¹/₂ cup	110	A
Chocolate	Nonfat	¹/₂ cup	110	A
Peach	Nonfat	¹/₂ cup	100	A
Raspberry	Nonfat	¹/₂ cup	100	A
Strawberry	Nonfat	¹/₂ cup	100	A
Vanilla	Nonfat	¹/₂ cup	100	A
Banana Pudding		¹/₂ cup	120	A
Classic Vanilla		¹/₂ cup	110	A
Cookies & Cream		¹/₂ cup	120	B

"+" indicates the food meets minimum fiber requirements; "–" indicates the food has a high sodium content.

Food	Processing Category	Brand
Yogurt	Frozen	TCBY
Yogurt	Frozen	TCBY
Yogurt	Frozen	TCBY
Yogurt	Frozen	TCBY
Yogurt	Frozen	TCBY
Yogurt	Frozen	TCBY
Yogurt	Frozen	TCBY Gourmet
Yogurt	Frozen	TCBY Gourmet
Yogurt	Frozen	TCBY Gourmet
Yogurt	Frozen	TCBY Gourmet
Yogurt	Frozen	TCBY Gourmet
Yogurt	Frozen	TCBY Gourmet
Yogurt	Frozen	TCBY Gourmet
Yogurt	Frozen	TCBY Gourmet
Yogurt	Frozen	TCBY Gourmet
Yogurt	Frozen	TCBY Traditional
Yogurt	Frozen	TCBY Traditional
Yogurt	Frozen	TCBY Traditional
Yogurt	Frozen Bar	Good Humor
Yogurt	Frozen Bars	Häagen-Dazs
Yogurt	Frozen Bars	Häagen-Dazs
Yogurt	Frozen Bars	Häagen-Dazs
Yogurt	Frozen Bars	Häagen-Dazs
Yogurt	Frozen Bars	Häagen-Dazs
Yogurt	Frozen Bars	Häagen-Dazs
Yogurt	Frozen Bars	Häagen-Dazs
Yogurt	Frozen Bars	Häagen-Dazs
Yogurt	Frozen Bars	Häagen-Dazs
Yogurt	Frozen Bars	Häagen-Dazs
Yogurt	Frozen Bars	Starburst
Yogurt	Frozen Bars	Starburst
Yogurt	Frozen Bars	TCBY Yog-a-Bar
Yogurt	Frozen Bars	TCBY Yog-a-Bar
Yogurt	Frozen Bars	TCBY Yog-a-Bar
Yogurt	Frozen Bars	TCBY Yog-a-Bar
Yogurt	Frozen Soft Serve	Bresler's Gourmet
Yogurt	Frozen Soft Serve	Bresler's Lite
Yogurt	Frozen Soft Serve	Breyers
Yogurt	Frozen Soft Serve	Colombo
Yogurt	Frozen Soft Serve	Colombo
Yogurt	Frozen Soft Serve	Colombo
Yogurt	Frozen Soft Serve	Crowley Peaks of Perfection
Yogurt	Frozen Soft Serve	Crowley Peaks of Perfection
Yogurt	Frozen Soft Serve	Crowley Peaks of Perfection
Yogurt	Frozen Soft Serve	Crowley Peaks of Perfection
Yogurt	Frozen Soft Serve	Crowley Peaks of Perfection
Yogurt	Frozen Soft Serve	Crowley Peaks of Perfection
Yogurt	Frozen Soft Serve	Crowley Peaks of Perfection
Yogurt	Frozen Soft Serve	Dannon
Yogurt	Frozen Soft Serve	Dannon
Yogurt	Frozen Soft Serve	Dannon
Yogurt	Frozen Soft Serve	Dannon
Yogurt	Frozen Soft Serve	Dannon

Major Description	Minor Description	Serving Size	Calories	Grade
Dutch Chocolate		$^1/_2$ cup	100	A
Peach		$^1/_2$ cup	110	A
Peanut Butter Fudge		$^1/_2$ cup	110	A
Pecan Praline		$^1/_2$ cup	120	B
Summertime Strawberry		$^1/_2$ cup	100	A
Yogwich		1 piece	200	B–
Blueberry Cheesecake		$^1/_2$ cup	140	A
Brazil & Cashew Nut		$^1/_2$ cup	160	A
Chocolate & Cherry		$^1/_2$ cup	150	B
French Milk Chocolate		$^1/_2$ cup	150	B
Homestyle Peanut Butter		$^1/_2$ cup	160	B
Honey Almond Vanilla		$^1/_2$ cup	150	B
Strawberry with Chocolate		$^1/_2$ cup	130	A
Triple Chocolate Brownie		$^1/_2$ cup	150	A
Vanilla Chocolate Flake		$^1/_2$ cup	150	B
All Flavors	Light	$^1/_2$ cup	50	A–
All Flavors	Low Fat	$^1/_2$ cup	105	A
Plain		$^1/_2$ cup	70	A
Raspberry	Creamsicle	1.76 oz	60	A
Cherry Chocolate Fudge		1 bar	230	D
Coffee Chocolate Crunch		1 bar	210	D
Daiquiri		1 bar	100	A
Peach		1 bar	90	A
Piña Colada		1 bar	100	A
Raspberry		1 bar	100	A
Raspberry & Vanilla		1 bar	90	A
Strawberry Daiquiri		1 bar	90	A
Tropical Orange		1 bar	100	A
Vanilla Chocolate Crunch		1 bar	210	D
Raspberry	Low Fat	1.5 oz	60	A
Strawberry	Low Fat	1.5 oz	60	A
Raspberry Swirl		1 bar	200	B–
Vanilla	Sugar Free	1 bar	120	D
Vanilla & Almonds		1 bar	190	D
Vanilla & Heath Toffee		1 bar	190	D
All Flavors		4 oz	116	B
All Flavors		4 oz	108	A
All Flavors	Nonfat	4 oz	120	A
All Flavors	Diet	4 oz	60	A
All Flavors	Low Fat	4 oz	110	B
All Flavors	Nonfat	4 oz	100	A
Banana		$^1/_2$ cup	100	B
Chocolate		$^1/_2$ cup	100	B
Lemon		$^1/_2$ cup	100	B
Plain		$^1/_2$ cup	90	A
Raspberry		$^1/_2$ cup	100	B
Strawberry		$^1/_2$ cup	100	B
Vanilla		$^1/_2$ cup	100	B
All Flavors	Low Fat	$^1/_2$ cup	100	B
All Flavors	Nonfat	$^1/_2$ cup	90	A
Blueberry		$^1/_2$ cup	100	B
Butter Pecan		$^1/_2$ cup	100	B
Cappuccino		$^1/_2$ cup	100	B

"+" indicates the food meets minimum fiber requirements; "–" indicates the food has a high sodium content.

Food	Processing Category	Brand
Yogurt	Frozen Soft Serve	Dannon
Yogurt	Frozen Soft Serve	Dannon
Yogurt	Frozen Soft Serve	Dannon
Yogurt	Frozen Soft Serve	Dannon
Yogurt	Frozen Soft Serve	Dannon
Yogurt	Frozen Soft Serve	Dannon
Yogurt	Frozen Soft Serve	Dannon
Yogurt	Frozen Soft Serve	Dannon
Yogurt	Frozen Soft Serve	Dannon Nonfat
Yogurt	Frozen Soft Serve	Gise
Yogurt	Frozen Soft Serve	Häagen-Dazs
Yogurt	Frozen Soft Serve	Häagen-Dazs
Yogurt	Frozen Soft Serve	Häagen-Dazs
Yogurt	Frozen Soft Serve	Häagen-Dazs
Yogurt	Frozen Soft Serve	Häagen-Dazs
Yogurt	Frozen Soft Serve	Hawthorne Melody
Yogurt	Frozen Soft Serve	Hawthorne Melody
Yogurt	Frozen Soft Serve	Honey Hill
Yogurt	Frozen Soft Serve	Honey Hill
Yogurt	Frozen Soft Serve	Just 10
Yogurt	Frozen Soft Serve	Kemp's
Yogurt	Frozen Soft Serve	Skinny Dip
Yogurt	Frozen Soft Serve	Sugar Creek
Yogurt	Frozen Soft Serve	Sugar Creek
Yogurt	Frozen Soft Serve	TCBY
Yogurt	Frozen Soft Serve	TCBY
Yogurt	Frozen Soft Serve	TCBY
Yogurt	Frozen Soft Serve	TCBY
Yogurt	Frozen Soft Serve	TCBY
Yogurt	Frozen Soft Serve	TCBY
Yogurt	Frozen Soft Serve	TCBY
Yogurt	Ready to Eat	Bison Low Fat
Yogurt	Ready to Eat	Bison Low Fat
Yogurt	Ready to Eat	Bison Low Fat
Yogurt	Ready to Eat	Bison Low Fat
Yogurt	Ready to Eat	Bison Nonfat
Yogurt	Ready to Eat	Breyers Low Fat
Yogurt	Ready to Eat	Breyers Low Fat
Yogurt	Ready to Eat	Breyers Low Fat
Yogurt	Ready to Eat	Breyers Low Fat
Yogurt	Ready to Eat	Breyers Low Fat
Yogurt	Ready to Eat	Breyers Low Fat
Yogurt	Ready to Eat	Breyers Low Fat
Yogurt	Ready to Eat	Breyers Low Fat
Yogurt	Ready to Eat	Breyers Low Fat
Yogurt	Ready to Eat	Breyers Low Fat
Yogurt	Ready to Eat	Colombo
Yogurt	Ready to Eat	Colombo
Yogurt	Ready to Eat	Colombo Nonfat Lite
Yogurt	Ready to Eat	Colombo Nonfat Lite
Yogurt	Ready to Eat	Colombo Nonfat Lite Minipack
Yogurt	Ready to Eat	Colombo
Yogurt	Ready to Eat	Colombo Fruit on the Bottom

Major Description	Minor Description	Serving Size	Calories	Grade
Cheesecake		¹/₂ cup	100	B
Chocolate		¹/₂ cup	120	A
Lemon Meringue		¹/₂ cup	100	B
Peach		¹/₂ cup	100	B
Piña Colada		¹/₂ cup	100	B
Raspberry		¹/₂ cup	100	B
Strawberry		¹/₂ cup	100	B
Strawberry & Banana		¹/₂ cup	100	B
Raspberry	Red	¹/₂ cup	90	A
All Flavors	Diet	4 oz	38	A
Chocolate		¹/₂ cup	120	A
Coffee		¹/₂ cup	140	B
Raspberry		¹/₂ cup	140	B
Strawberry		¹/₂ cup	120	A
Vanilla		¹/₂ cup	110	A
All Flavors	Low Fat	4 oz	95	B
All Flavors	Nonfat	4 oz	92	A
All Flavors	Low Fat	4 oz	100	B
All Flavors	Nonfat	4 oz	80	A
All Flavors	Diet	4 oz	40	A–
Vanilla		4 oz	120	B
All Flavors	Diet	4 oz	36	A
All Flavors	Low Fat	4 oz	104	B
All Flavors	Nonfat	4 oz	97	A
All Flavors	Diet	4 oz	68	A
All Flavors	Low Fat	4 oz	108	B
All Flavors	Nonfat	4 oz	80	A
All Flavors	Nonfat	¹/₂ cup	110	A
Golden Vanilla	Regular	¹/₂ cup	130	B
Old Fashioned Vanilla	Non Fat	¹/₂ cup	110	A
Vanilla	Diet, Nonfat	¹/₂ cup	80	A
Coffee		8 oz	210	B
Lemon		8 oz	210	B
Plain		8 oz	150	B
Vanilla		8 oz	210	B
Plain		8 oz	120	A–
Berries, Mixed		8 oz	250	A
Black Cherry		8 oz	260	A
Blueberry		8 oz	250	A
Peach		8 oz	250	A
Pineapple		8 oz	250	A
Plain		8 oz	140	B
Raspberry		8 oz	250	A
Strawberry		8 oz	250	A
Strawberry & Banana		8 oz	250	A
Vanilla Bean		8 oz	230	A
French Vanilla		8 oz	215	B
Strawberry		8 oz	210	B
Plain		8 oz	110	A–
Vanilla		8 oz	160	A
All Fruit Flavors		4.4 oz	100	A
Plain		8 oz	160	D
All Fruit Flavors		8 oz	230	B

"+" indicates the food meets minimum fiber requirements; "–" indicates the food has a high sodium content.

Food	Processing Category	Brand
Yogurt	Ready to Eat	Colombo Nonfat Fruit on the Bottom
Yogurt	Ready to Eat	Crowley
Yogurt	Ready to Eat	Crowley Low Fat
Yogurt	Ready to Eat	Crowley Low Fat
Yogurt	Ready to Eat	Crowley Nonfat
Yogurt	Ready to Eat	Crowley Nonfat
Yogurt	Ready to Eat	Crowley Nonfat
Yogurt	Ready to Eat	Crowley Sundae Style
Yogurt	Ready to Eat	Crowley Swiss Style
Yogurt	Ready to Eat	Dannon Extra Smooth
Yogurt	Ready to Eat	Dannon Fresh Flavors
Yogurt	Ready to Eat	Dannon Fresh Flavors
Yogurt	Ready to Eat	Dannon Fresh Flavors
Yogurt	Ready to Eat	Dannon Fresh Flavors
Yogurt	Ready to Eat	Dannon Fruit on the Bottom
Yogurt	Ready to Eat	Dannon Fruit on the Bottom
Yogurt	Ready to Eat	Dannon Hearty Nuts & Raisins
Yogurt	Ready to Eat	Dannon Hearty Nuts & Raisins
Yogurt	Ready to Eat	Dannon Low Fat
Yogurt	Ready to Eat	Dannon Nonfat
Yogurt	Ready to Eat	Friendship Low Fat
Yogurt	Ready to Eat	Friendship Low Fat
Yogurt	Ready to Eat	Friendship Low Fat 1.5%
Yogurt	Ready to Eat	Kemp's
Yogurt	Ready to Eat	Kemp's
Yogurt	Ready to Eat	Kemp's
Yogurt	Ready to Eat	Knudsen
Yogurt	Ready to Eat	Knudsen Cal 70
Yogurt	Ready to Eat	Knudsen Cal 70
Yogurt	Ready to Eat	Knudsen Cal 70
Yogurt	Ready to Eat	Knudsen Cal 70
Yogurt	Ready to Eat	Knudsen Cal 70
Yogurt	Ready to Eat	Knudsen Cal 70
Yogurt	Ready to Eat	Knudsen Cal 70
Yogurt	Ready to Eat	Knudsen Cal 70
Yogurt	Ready to Eat	Knudsen Cal 70
Yogurt	Ready to Eat	Knudsen Low Fat
Yogurt	Ready to Eat	Knudsen Low Fat
Yogurt	Ready to Eat	Knudsen Low Fat
Yogurt	Ready to Eat	Light n' Lively
Yogurt	Ready to Eat	Light n' Lively
Yogurt	Ready to Eat	Light n' Lively
Yogurt	Ready to Eat	Light n' Lively
Yogurt	Ready to Eat	Light n' Lively
Yogurt	Ready to Eat	Light n' Lively
Yogurt	Ready to Eat	Light n' Lively
Yogurt	Ready to Eat	Light n' Lively
Yogurt	Ready to Eat	Light n' Lively
Yogurt	Ready to Eat	Light n' Lively
Yogurt	Ready to Eat	Light n' Lively
Yogurt	Ready to Eat	Light n' Lively
Yogurt	Ready to Eat	Light n' Lively 100
Yogurt	Ready to Eat	Light n' Lively 100

Major Description	Minor Description	Serving Size	Calories	Grade
All Fruit Flavors		8 oz	190	A
Plain		8 oz	160	D
Plain		8 oz	140	A–
Vanilla		8 oz	200	A
All Fruit Flavors		8 oz	100	A–
Plain		8 oz	120	A–
Strawberry		8 oz	190	A
All Fruit Flavors		8 oz	250	A
All Fruit Flavors		8 oz	240	A
All Fruit Flavors		4.4 oz	130	A
All Fruit Flavors	Except Lemon	8 oz	200	B
Coffee		8 oz	200	A
Lemon		8 oz	200	A
Vanilla		8 oz	200	A
All Fruit Flavors		8 oz	240	A
All Fruit Flavors		4.4 oz	130	A
All Fruit Flavors		8 oz	260	A
Vanilla		8 oz	270	B
Plain		8 oz	140	B
Plain		8 oz	110	A–
Coffee		8 oz	210	A
Vanilla		8 oz	210	A
Plain		8 oz	150	B–
Strawberry		6 oz	160	A
Strawberry	Nonfat	6 oz	80	A–
Vanilla		6 oz	160	A
Plain		8 oz	200	D
Black Cherry		6 oz	70	A
Blueberry		6 oz	70	A
Lemon		6 oz	70	A–
Peach		6 oz	70	A–
Pineapple		6 oz	70	A–
Raspberry		6 oz	70	A
Strawberry	Fruit Basket	6 oz	70	A
Strawberry & Banana		6 oz	70	A
Vanilla		6 oz	70	A–
All Fruit Flavors		8 oz	240	A
Plain		8 oz	160	B
Vanilla		8 oz	240	A
Black Cherry		8 oz	230	A
Blueberry		8 oz	240	A
Cherry		4.4 oz	140	A
Grape		4.4 oz	130	A
Peach		8 oz	240	A
Pineapple		8 oz	230	A
Raspberry		8 oz	230	A
Raspberry		4.4 oz	130	A
Strawberry		4.4 oz	130	A
Strawberry		8 oz	240	A
Strawberry	Fruit Cup	8 oz	240	A
Strawberry & Banana		8 oz	260	A
Black Cherry		8 oz	100	A
Blueberry		8 oz	90	A

"+" indicates the food meets minimum fiber requirements; "–" indicates the food has a high sodium content.

Food	Processing Category	Brand
Yogurt	Ready to Eat	Light n' Lively 100
Yogurt	Ready to Eat	Light n' Lively 100
Yogurt	Ready to Eat	Light n' Lively 100
Yogurt	Ready to Eat	Light n' Lively 100
Yogurt	Ready to Eat	Light n' Lively 100
Yogurt	Ready to Eat	Light n' Lively Free
Yogurt	Ready to Eat	Lite Line Lowfat 1%
Yogurt	Ready to Eat	Lite Line Swiss Style 1%
Yogurt	Ready to Eat	Lite Line Swiss Style 1%
Yogurt	Ready to Eat	Lite Line Swiss Style 1.5%
Yogurt	Ready to Eat	Meadow Gold Lowfat 1.5%
Yogurt	Ready to Eat	Meadow Gold Lowfat 2%
Yogurt	Ready to Eat	Mountain High
Yogurt	Ready to Eat	Mountain High
Yogurt	Ready to Eat	New Country
Yogurt	Ready to Eat	New Country Low Fat
Yogurt	Ready to Eat	New Country Supreme
Yogurt	Ready to Eat	Ripple 70
Yogurt	Ready to Eat	Stonyfield Farm
Yogurt	Ready to Eat	Stonyfield Farm
Yogurt	Ready to Eat	Stonyfield Farm
Yogurt	Ready to Eat	Stonyfield Farm
Yogurt	Ready to Eat	Stonyfield Farm
Yogurt	Ready to Eat	Stonyfield Farm
Yogurt	Ready to Eat	Stonyfield Farm
Yogurt	Ready to Eat	Stonyfield Farm
Yogurt	Ready to Eat	Stonyfield Farm
Yogurt	Ready to Eat	Stonyfield Farm
Yogurt	Ready to Eat	Weight Watchers Nonfat
Yogurt	Ready to Eat	Weight Watchers Ultimate 90
Yogurt	Ready to Eat	Yoplait
Yogurt	Ready to Eat	Yoplait
Yogurt	Ready to Eat	Yoplait
Yogurt	Ready to Eat	Yoplait
Yogurt	Ready to Eat	Yoplait
Yogurt	Ready to Eat	Yoplait
Yogurt	Ready to Eat	Yoplait Breakfast Yogurt
Yogurt	Ready to Eat	Yoplait Breakfast Yogurt
Yogurt	Ready to Eat	Yoplait Breakfast Yogurt
Yogurt	Ready to Eat	Yoplait Breakfast Yogurt
Yogurt	Ready to Eat	Yoplait Breakfast Yogurt
Yogurt	Ready to Eat	Yoplait Custard Style
Yogurt	Ready to Eat	Yoplait Custard Style
Yogurt	Ready to Eat	Yoplait Custard Style
Yogurt	Ready to Eat	Yoplait Custard Style
Yogurt	Ready to Eat	Yoplait Fat Free
Yogurt	Ready to Eat	Yoplait Fat Free
Yogurt	Ready to Eat	Yoplait Light
Yogurt	Ready to Eat	Yoplait Light
Yogurt	Ready to Eat	Yoplait Nonfat
Yogurt	Ready to Eat	Yoplait Nonfat

Major Description	Minor Description	Serving Size	Calories	Grade
Lemon		8 oz	100	A–
Peach		8 oz	100	A
Raspberry		8 oz	90	A
Strawberry		8 oz	90	A
Strawberry	Fruit Cup	8 oz	90	A
All Flavors		4.4 oz	50	A
Strawberry		1 cup	240	A
Cherry Vanilla		8 oz	240	A
Peach		8 oz	240	A
Plain		8 oz	140	A
Raspberry		8 oz	250	A
Plain		8 oz	160	B
Blueberry	Other Natural Flavors	8 oz	220	B
Plain		8 oz	200	D
Strawberry & Banana		6 oz	150	A
All Flavors		6 oz	150	A
All Flavors		6 oz	150	A
All Fruit Flavors		6 oz	70	A
All Flavors	Whole Milk	8 oz	210	C
Apricot & Mango		8 oz	160	A
Blueberry, Wild		8 oz	160	A
Cappuccino	Nonfat	8 oz	170	A
Lemon	Nonfat	8 oz	160	A
Most Flavors	Nonfat	8 oz	160	A
Peach		8 oz	160	A
Plain	Whole Milk	8 oz	170	D
Raspberry		8 oz	160	A
Strawberry Banana	Nonfat	8 oz	160	A
Plain		8 oz	90	A–
All Flavors		8 oz	90	A–
All Fruit Flavors		4 oz	120	A
All Fruit Flavors		6 oz	190	A
Piña Colada or Pineapple		6 oz	190	A
Plain		6 oz	130	B
Strawberry & Rhubarb		6 oz	190	A
Vanilla		6 oz	180	A
Berries, Mixed		6 oz	210	A
Cherry with Almonds		6 oz	200	A
Strawberry & Banana		6 oz	220	A
Strawberry with Almonds		6 oz	200	A
Tropical Fruit		6 oz	210	B
All Fruit Flavors	Except Cherry & Mixed Berries	6 oz	190	B
Berries, Mixed		6 oz	180	B
Cherry		6 oz	180	B
Vanilla		6 oz	180	B
All Fruit Flavors		6 oz	150	A
Vanilla		6 oz	150	A
All Fruit Flavors		4 oz	60	A
All Fruit Flavors		6 oz	90	A
Plain		8 oz	120	A–
Vanilla		8 oz	180	A

"+" indicates the food meets minimum fiber requirements; "–" indicates the food has a high sodium content.

Soups and Mixes

Mixes

This section contains all foods that are prepared from a mix. The exceptions are bread mixes, which are in the Cereal and Grains section; and pie, cake, and other snack and dessert-type foods, which are in the Frivolous Foods section.

For mixes, serving size, calories, and grade are based on the finished product prepared according to package directions. This will include milk, butter, or eggs when required by the recipe. Exceptions to this are noted in the "Minor Description." Recipe choices—such as between margarine and butter, or between milk and water—might be listed for a particular food that has different methods of preparation. These cases will also be noted in the "Minor Description."

> NOTE: *Prepared mix calorie data frequently had to be calculated from recipe ingredients and therefore is approximate.*

Advice about Preparing Mixes

Most dry mix ingredients orignally received an A rating. The downgrading is usually the result of added ingredients such as butter, eggs, whole milk. Significant
improvements in the prepared mix grade can be made by using skim or 1% milk
for whole milk, egg substitutes for whole eggs, and smaller amounts of olive oil
instead of butter or margarine.

Food	Processing Category	Brand
Bean Mix	Mix	Fantastic Foods
Bean Mix	Mix	Fantastic Foods
Bean Mix	Mix	Lipton
Bean Mix	Mix	Lipton
Beef Entree Mix	Mix	Lipton Microeasy
Bouillon	Dehydrated	Generic
Bouillon	Dehydrated	Generic
Bouillon	Dehydrated	Featherweight
Bouillon	Dehydrated	George Washington
Bouillon	Dehydrated	George Washington
Bouillon	Dehydrated	George Washington
Bouillon	Dehydrated	George Washington
Bouillon	Dehydrated	George Washington
Bouillon	Dehydrated	Lite Line Low Sodium
Bouillon	Dehydrated	Lite Line Sodium
Bouillon	Dehydrated	Steero
Bouillon	Dehydrated	Steero
Bouillon	Dehydrated	Weight Watchers Broth Mix
Bouillon	Dehydrated	Wyler's
Bouillon	Dehydrated	Wyler's
Bouillon	Dehydrated	Wyler's
Bouillon	Dehydrated	Wyler's
Burrito Dinner	Mix	Old El Paso
Burrito Dinner	Mix	Tio Sancho Dinner Kit
Burrito Filling	Mix	Del Monte
Chicken Entree	Mix	Lipton Microeasy
Chicken Entree	Mix	Lipton Microeasy
Chicken Entree	Mix	Skillet Chicken Helper
Chicken Entree	Mix	Skillet Chicken Helper
Chicken Entree	Mix	Skillet Chicken Helper
Chicken Entree	Mix	Skillet Chicken Helper
Chicken Entree	Mix	Skillet Chicken Helper
Chili Dishes	Mix	Fantastic Foods
Chili Entree	Freeze Dried	Mountain House
Chili Entree	Freeze Dried	Mountain House Chili Mac
Chow Mein, Vegetarian	Mix	Tofu Classics
Date Bar	Mix	Betty Crocker Classic
Enchilada Dinner	Mix	Old El Paso
Enchilada Dinner	Mix	Tio Sancho Dinner Kit
Hamburger Entree	Mix	Hamburger Helper

Soups

Many soups come as mixes or condensed. Serving size, calories, and grade are reported as the finished product prepared according to container directions. In the case of condensed soups, this means with added water unless otherwise noted.

Conversion: 1 cup = 8 fluid ounces

Major Description	Minor Description	Serving Size	Calories	Grade
Black Bean	Instant	$^1/_3$ cup	120	A–+
Refried	Instant	$^1/_3$ cup	120	A–+
Cajun & Sauce		$^1/_2$ cup	160	B–
Chicken & Sauce		$^1/_2$ cup	150	B–
Stew Hearty		$^1/_4$ pkg	370	D–
Beef Flavor		1 cube	6	A–
Chicken Flavor		1 cube	9	B–
Instant		1 tsp	18	D
Brown		1 tsp	6	A–
Brown	Kosher Style	1 tsp	6	A–
Golden		1 tsp	6	A–
Onion		1 tsp	12	A–
Vegetable		1 tsp	12	A–
Instant		1 tsp	12	A
Instant		1 tsp	12	A
Instant		1 tsp	8	A–
Instant		1 tsp	6	A–
Instant		1 pkt	8	A–
Instant		1 tsp	8	A–
Instant		1 tsp	6	A–
Instant	Onion Flavor	1 tsp	10	A–
Instant	Vegetable Flavor	1 tsp	6	A–
		1 burrito	299	C–
		1 burrito	390	A–
Beans		$^1/_2$ cup	110	A–
Barbecue		$^1/_4$ pkg	220	B–
Country Style		$^1/_4$ pkg	190	B–
Cheesy		6 oz	160	A–
Creamy Chicken		6 oz	170	B–
Creamy Mushroom		6 oz	170	B–
Fettuccine Alfredo		6 oz	160	B–
Stir-fried		6 oz	170	A–
Vegetarian	Pinto Beans	1 cup	400	A–+
with Beans		1 cup	390	C
with Beef		1 cup	250	B
	Mandarin Style	$^1/_2$ cup	110	C–
		.4 oz	60	B
		1 enchilada	145	D
		1 enchilada	360	A
Beef Noodle		1 cup	320	D–

"+" indicates the food meets minimum fiber requirements; "–" indicates the food has a high sodium content.

Food	Processing Category	Brand
Hamburger Entree	Mix	Hamburger Helper
Hamburger Entree	Mix	Hamburger Helper
Hamburger Entree	Mix	Hamburger Helper
Hamburger Entree	Mix	Hamburger Helper
Hamburger Entree	Mix	Hamburger Helper
Hamburger Entree	Mix	Hamburger Helper
Hamburger Entree	Mix	Hamburger Helper
Hamburger Entree	Mix	Hamburger Helper
Hamburger Entree	Mix	Hamburger Helper
Hamburger Entree	Mix	Hamburger Helper
Hamburger Entree	Mix	Hamburger Helper
Hamburger Entree	Mix	Hamburger Helper
Hamburger Entree	Mix	Hamburger Helper
Hamburger Entree	Mix	Hamburger Helper
Hamburger Entree	Mix	Hamburger Helper
Hamburger Entree	Mix	Hamburger Helper
Hamburger Entree	Mix	Hamburger Helper
Hamburger Entree	Mix	Hamburger Helper
Hamburger Entree	Mix	Hamburger Helper
Hamburger Entree	Mix	Hamburger Helper
Hamburger Entree	Mix	Hamburger Helper
Hamburger Entree	Mix	Hamburger Helper
Hamburger Entree	Mix	Hamburger Helper Pizzabake
Hamburger Entree	Mix	Hamburger Helper Sloppy Joe Bake
Hamburger Entree	Mix	Hamburger Helper Tacobake
Macaroni Dishes	Mix	Fantastic Foods
Macaroni Dishes	Mix	Fantastic Foods
Macaroni Dishes	Mix	Fantastic Foods
Macaroni Dishes	Mix	Fantastic Foods Traditional
Macaroni Dishes	Mix	Kraft Deluxe Dinner
Macaroni Dishes	Mix	Kraft Dinner
Macaroni Dishes	Mix	Kraft Dinner
Macaroni Dishes	Mix	Kraft Dinomac/Teddy
Macaroni Dishes	Mix	Kraft Family Size Dinner
Macaroni Dishes	Mix	Mexican Velveeta Touch of Mexico
Macaroni Dishes	Mix	Tofu Classics
Macaroni Dishes	Mix	Tofu Classics
Macaroni Dishes	Mix	Velveeta
Macaroni Dishes	Mix	Velveeta Bits of Bacon
Meat Extender	All Forms	Generic
Meat Loaf Entree	Mix	Lipton Microeasy
Meat Loaf Entree	Mix	Natural Touch Loaf Mix
Meat Loaf Seasoning	Mix	French's
Meat Loaf Seasoning	Mix	Lawry's Seasoning Blends
Meat Marinade	Mix	French's
Noodle Dishes	Mix	Golden Grain/Noodle Roni
Noodle Dishes	Mix	Golden Grain/Noodle Roni
Noodle Dishes	Mix	Golden Grain/Noodle Roni
Noodle Dishes	Mix	Kraft Dinner
Noodle Dishes	Mix	Kraft Dinner
Noodle Dishes	Mix	Lipton Noodles and Sauce
Noodle Dishes	Mix	Lipton Noodles and Sauce

Major Description	Minor Description	Serving Size	Calories	Grade
Beef Taco		1 cup	330	C–
Beef Teriyaki		1 cup	360	C–
Cheeseburger Macaroni		1 cup	370	D–
Chili	Beans	1 cup	280	D–
Chili	Macaroni	1 cup	330	C–
Chili	Tomato	1 cup	330	C–
Hamburger	Hash	1 cup	320	D–
Hamburger	Stew	1 cup	300	D–
Italian Style	Cheesy	1 cup	360	D–
Italian Style	Zesty	1 cup	340	C–
Lasagne		1 cup	340	C–
Meatloaf		1 cup	360	D–
Mushroom	Wild Rice	1 cup	380	C–
Nacho Cheese		1 cup	360	C–
Pizza	Dish	1 cup	360	C–
Potato	au Gratin	1 cup	320	D–
Potato	Stroganoff	1 cup	320	D–
Rice, Oriental Style		1 cup	340	C–
Romanoff		1 cup	350	D–
Spaghetti		1 cup	340	C–
Stroganoff	Creamy	1 cup	390	D–
Tamale Pie		1 cup	380	C–
Pizza		6 oz	427	C–
Sloppy Joe		6 oz	408	C–
Taco		5.75 oz	320	D–
Cheddar Cheese		2 oz	200	A–+
Parmesan Cheese		2 oz	200	A–+
Parmesan Cheese		$^1/_2$ cup	109	B–
Cheddar Cheese		$^1/_2$ cup	112	B–
Cheese		$^1/_2$ cup	172	B–
Cheese		$^1/_2$ cup	224	D–
Cheese	Spirals	$^1/_2$ cup	191	D–
Cheese		$^1/_2$ cup	206	D–
Cheese		$^1/_2$ cup	191	D–
Cheese	Shells	$^1/_2$ cup	210	C–
Shells & Curry		$^1/_2$ cup	143	D–
Shells & Curry		$^1/_2$ cup	103	B–
Cheese	Shells	$^1/_2$ cup	210	C–
Cheese	Shells with Bacon	$^1/_2$ cup	240	C–
Soybean		1 oz	88	A
Homestyle		$^1/_4$ pkg	390	D–
		4 oz	180	C
		$^1/_8$ pkg	20	A–
		$^1/_8$ pkg	44	A–
		$^1/_8$ pkg	10	A–
Garlic, Creamy		$^1/_2$ cup	300	D–
Herb & Butter		$^1/_2$ cup	160	C–
Stroganoff		$^1/_2$ cup	350	D–
		$^1/_2$ cup	224	D–
Chicken or Chicken Flavor		$^1/_2$ cup	158	C–
Alfredo	Milk & Butter	$^1/_2$ cup	220	D–
Alfredo	Skim Milk & Margarine	$^1/_2$ cup	180	C–

"+" indicates the food meets minimum fiber requirements; "–" indicates the food has a high sodium content.

Food	Processing Category	Brand
Noodle Dishes	Mix	Lipton Noodles and Sauce
Noodle Dishes	Mix	Lipton Noodles and Sauce
Noodle Dishes	Mix	Lipton Noodles and Sauce
Noodle Dishes	Mix	Lipton Noodles and Sauce
Noodle Dishes	Mix	Lipton Noodles and Sauce
Noodle Dishes	Mix	Lipton Noodles and Sauce
Noodle Dishes	Mix	Lipton Noodles and Sauce
Noodle Dishes	Mix	Lipton Noodles and Sauce
Noodle Dishes	Mix	Lipton Noodles and Sauce
Noodle Dishes	Mix	Lipton Noodles and Sauce
Noodle Dishes	Mix	Lipton Noodles and Sauce
Noodle Dishes	Mix	Lipton Noodles and Sauce
Noodle Dishes	Mix	Lipton Noodles and Sauce
Noodle Dishes	Mix	Lipton Noodles and Sauce
Noodle Dishes	Mix	Lipton Noodles and Sauce
Noodle Dishes	Mix	Lipton Noodles and Sauce
Noodle Dishes	Mix	Lipton Noodles and Sauce
Noodle Dishes	Mix	Lipton Noodles and Sauce
Noodle Dishes	Mix	Lipton Noodles and Sauce
Noodle Dishes	Mix	Lipton Noodles and Sauce
Noodle Dishes	Mix	Minute Microwave Family Size
Noodle Dishes	Mix	Minute Microwave Family Size
Noodle Dishes	Mix	Minute Microwave Family Size
Noodle Dishes	Mix	Minute Microwave Single Serve
Noodle Dishes	Mix	Minute Microwave Single Serve
Noodle Dishes	Mix	Minute Microwave Single Serve
Noodle Dishes	Mix	Mueller's Chef Series
Noodle Dishes	Mix	Mueller's Chef Series
Noodle Dishes	Mix	Mueller's Chef Series
Noodle Dishes	Mix	Mueller's Chef Series
Noodle Dishes	Mix	Mueller's Chef Series
Pasta Dishes	Mix	Country Recipe Pasta Salad
Pasta Dishes	Mix	Country Recipe Pasta Salad
Pasta Dishes	Mix	Country Recipe Pasta Salad
Pasta Dishes	Mix	Country Recipe Pasta Salad
Pasta Dishes	Mix	Country Recipe Pasta Salad
Pasta Dishes	Mix	Country Recipe Pasta Salad
Pasta Dishes	Mix	Fantastic Pasta Salad
Pasta Dishes	Mix	Fantastic Pasta Salad
Pasta Dishes	Mix	Hain
Pasta Dishes	Mix	Hain
Pasta Dishes	Mix	Hain
Pasta Dishes	Mix	Hain
Pasta Dishes	Mix	Hain
Pasta Dishes	Mix	Hain
Pasta Dishes	Mix	Hain Pasta & Sauce
Pasta Dishes	Mix	Hain Pasta & Sauce
Pasta Dishes	Mix	Hain Pasta & Sauce
Pasta Dishes	Mix	Hain Pasta & Sauce
Pasta Dishes	Mix	Hain Pasta & Sauce, Tangy

Major Description	Minor Description	Serving Size	Calories	Grade
Beef	Butter	$^1/_2$ cup	180	C–
Beef	Margarine	$^1/_2$ cup	150	B–
Butter	Butter	$^1/_2$ cup	200	D–
Butter	Margarine	$^1/_2$ cup	180	C–
Butter & Herb		$^1/_2$ cup	170	C–
Butter & Herb	Butter	$^1/_2$ cup	190	D–
Carbonara Alfredo	Milk & Butter	$^1/_2$ cup	210	D–
Carbonara Alfredo	Skim Milk & Margarine	$^1/_2$ cup	180	C–
Cheese	Butter	$^1/_2$ cup	190	C–
Cheese	Margarine	$^1/_2$ cup	170	B–
Chicken or Chicken Flavor	Broccoli with Milk & Butter	$^1/_2$ cup	200	D–
Chicken or Chicken Flavor	Broccoli with Skim Milk & Margarine	$^1/_2$ cup	160	B–
Chicken or Chicken Flavor	Butter	$^1/_2$ cup	180	C–
Chicken or Chicken Flavor	Margarine	$^1/_2$ cup	160	B–
Parmesan	Butter	$^1/_2$ cup	210	D–
Parmesan	Margarine	$^1/_2$ cup	180	C–
Sour Cream & Chives	Butter	$^1/_2$ cup	200	D–
Sour Cream & Chives	Margarine	$^1/_2$ cup	170	C–
Stroganoff	Butter	$^1/_2$ cup	200	D–
Stroganoff	Margarine	$^1/_2$ cup	170	B–
Alfredo		$^1/_2$ cup	170	C–
Chicken or Chicken Flavor		$^1/_2$ cup	160	B–
Parmesan		$^1/_2$ cup	170	C–
Alfredo		$^1/_2$ cup	160	B–
Chicken or Chicken Flavor		$^1/_2$ cup	160	B–
Parmesan		$^1/_2$ cup	160	B–
Alfredo		$^1/_2$ cup	190	D–
Chicken or Chicken Flavor		$^1/_2$ cup	160	D–
Garlic & Butter		$^1/_2$ cup	170	C–
Sour Cream & Chives		$^1/_2$ cup	190	C–
Stroganoff		$^1/_2$ cup	190	D–
Bacon Vinaigrette		$^1/_2$ cup	110	A–
Bacon Vinaigrette		$^1/_2$ cup	140	B–
Dijon Style, Creamy		$^1/_2$ cup	190	D–
Dijon Style, Creamy	without Additives	$^1/_2$ cup	110	A–
Italian Style, Creamy		$^1/_2$ cup	160	C–
Italian Style, Creamy	without Additives	$^1/_2$ cup	100	A–
Italian Style, Herb		$^1/_2$ cup	167	D
Oriental Style, Spicy		$^1/_2$ cup	175	D
Cheddar		$^1/_2$ cup	190	D–+
Dill, Creamy	Multi Bran	$^1/_2$ cup	150	C–+
Fettuccine Alfredo		$^1/_2$ cup	190	D–
Italian Style, Multibran		$^1/_2$ cup	120	D–+
Multibran Salsa		$^1/_2$ cup	130	D–+
Primavera		$^1/_2$ cup	180	D–
Cheese	Parmesan, Creamy	$^1/_4$ pkg	150	B–
Italian Style, Herb		$^1/_5$ pkg	110	B–
Primavera		$^1/_4$ pkg	140	B–
Swiss Style, Creamy		$^1/_5$ pkg	170	B–
Cheddar Cheese		$^1/_4$ pkg	180	B–

"+" indicates the food meets minimum fiber requirements; "–" indicates the food has a high sodium content.

Food	Processing Category	Brand
Pasta Dishes	Mix	Kraft Light Pasta Salad
Pasta Dishes	Mix	Kraft Light Rancher's Choice
Pasta Dishes	Mix	Kraft Pasta & Cheese
Pasta Dishes	Mix	Kraft Pasta & Cheese
Pasta Dishes	Mix	Kraft Pasta & Cheese
Pasta Dishes	Mix	Kraft Pasta & Cheese
Pasta Dishes	Mix	Kraft Pasta & Cheese
Pasta Dishes	Mix	Kraft Pasta Salad
Pasta Dishes	Mix	Kraft Pasta Salad
Pasta Dishes	Mix	Kraft Pasta Salad
Pasta Dishes	Mix	Kraft Rancher's Choice Pasta Salad
Pasta Dishes	Mix	Lipton Pasta & Sauce
Pasta Dishes	Mix	Lipton Pasta & Sauce
Pasta Dishes	Mix	Lipton Pasta & Sauce
Pasta Dishes	Mix	Lipton Pasta & Sauce
Pasta Dishes	Mix	Lipton Pasta & Sauce
Pasta Dishes	Mix	Lipton Pasta & Sauce
Pasta Dishes	Mix	Lipton Pasta & Sauce
Pasta Dishes	Mix	Lipton Pasta Salad
Pasta Dishes	Mix	McCormick/Schilling Pasta Prima
Pasta Dishes	Mix	McCormick/Schilling Pasta Prima
Pasta Dishes	Mix	McCormick/Schilling Pasta Prima
Pasta Dishes	Mix	McCormick/Schilling Pasta Prima
Pasta Dishes	Mix	McCormick/Schilling Pasta Prima
Pasta Dishes	Mix	Minute Microwave Family Size
Pasta Dishes	Mix	Mueller's Salad Bar
Pasta Dishes	Mix	Mueller's Salad Bar
Pasta Dishes	Mix	Mueller's Salad Bar
Pasta Dishes	Mix	Mueller's Salad Bar
Pasta Dishes	Mix	Mueller's Salad Bar
Pasta Salad	Mix	Fantastic Foods
Pasta Salad	Mix	Fantastic Foods
Pasta Salad	Mix	Suddenly Salad
Pasta Salad	Mix	Suddenly Salad
Pasta Salad	Mix	Suddenly Salad
Pasta Salad	Mix	Suddenly Salad
Pasta Salad	Mix	Suddenly Salad
Pizza	Mix	Chef Boyardee
Pizza	Mix	Chef Boyardee
Pizza	Mix	Chef Boyardee 2 Complete
Pizza	Mix	Chef Boyardee Complete
Pizza	Mix	Chef Boyardee Complete
Pizza Crust	Mix	Chef Boyardee Quick & Easy
Pizza Crust	Mix	Pillsbury All Ready
Pizza Crust	Mix	Robin Hood/Gold Medal Pouch Mix
Potato	Mix	Generic
Potato	Mix	Generic
Potato	Mix	Generic
Potato	Mix	Generic
Potato	Mix	Generic
Potato	Mix	Betty Crocker
Potato	Mix	Betty Crocker
Potato	Mix	Betty Crocker

Major Description	Minor Description	Serving Size	Calories	Grade
Italian Style, Creamy		$^1/_2$ cup	130	B–
		$^1/_2$ cup	170	C–
Cheddar Cheese		$^1/_2$ cup	180	C–
Cheese	3 Cheese with Vegetables	$^1/_2$ cup	180	C–
Cheese	Parmesan	$^1/_2$ cup	180	C–
Chicken with Herbs		$^1/_2$ cup	170	C–
Sour Cream & Chives		$^1/_2$ cup	180	C–
Broccoli	& Vegetable	$^1/_2$ cup	210	D–
Homestyle		$^1/_2$ cup	240	D–
Primavera Garden		$^1/_2$ cup	170	C–
		$^1/_2$ cup	250	D–
Carbonara Alfredo		$^1/_2$ cup	140	B–
Cheese	Supreme	$^1/_2$ cup	139	A–
Chicken & Broccoli		$^1/_2$ cup	129	A–
Herb Tomato	Butter	$^1/_2$ cup	180	C–
Herb Tomato	Margarine	$^1/_2$ cup	160	B–
Mushroom & Chicken Flavors		$^1/_2$ cup	124	A–
Oriental Style, with Fusilli		$^1/_2$ cup	130	A–
Broccoli, Creamy		$^1/_2$ cup	200	D
Alfredo		$^1/_2$ cup	253	D–
Herb & Garlic		$^1/_2$ cup	326	C–
Marinara		$^1/_2$ cup	329	B–
Pasta Salad		$^1/_2$ cup	390	D–
Pesto		$^1/_2$ cup	193	B–
Cheddar Cheese		$^1/_2$ cup	160	C–
Buttermilk, Country Style		$^1/_2$ cup	250	D–
Cucumber, Creamy		$^1/_2$ cup	250	D–
Homestyle		$^1/_2$ cup	250	D–
Italian Style, Creamy		$^1/_2$ cup	290	D–
Italian Style, Zesty		$^1/_2$ cup	140	C–
Italian Style, Herb		1.75 oz	170	A–
Oriental Style, Spicy		2 oz	200	A–+
Caesar		$^1/_2$ cup	170	D–
Classic		$^1/_2$ cup	160	C–
Creamy Macaroni		$^1/_2$ cup	200	D–
Primavera		$^1/_2$ cup	190	D–
Tortellini		$^1/_2$ cup	160	C–
Plain		$^1/_4$ pkg	180	A–
Sausage		$^1/_4$ pkg	270	C–
Pepperoni		$^1/_4$ pkg	420	B–
Cheese		$^1/_4$ pkg	230	B–
Pepperoni		$^1/_4$ pkg	250	C–
		$^1/_6$ pkg	150	A–
		$^1/_6$ of crust	120	A–
		$^1/_6$ pkg	110	A–
au Gratin	Milk & Margarine	$^1/_2$ cup	105	D–
Granules	Milk & Butter	$^1/_2$ cup	137	D–
Mashed Flakes	Milk & Butter	$^1/_2$ cup	118	D–
Mashed Flakes	Water Only	$^1/_2$ cup	78	A
Scalloped	Milk & Margarine	$^1/_2$ cup	105	D–
au Gratin	Prepared	$^1/_2$ cup	150	B–
Cheddar & Bacon		$^1/_2$ cup	140	C–
Hash Brown	Onions	$^1/_2$ cup	160	C

"+" indicates the food meets minimum fiber requirements; "–" indicates the food has a high sodium content.

Food	Processing Category	Brand
Potato	Mix	Betty Crocker
Potato	Mix	Betty Crocker
Potato	Mix	Betty Crocker
Potato	Mix	Betty Crocker
Potato	Mix	Betty Crocker
Potato	Mix	Betty Crocker Potato Buds
Potato	Mix	Betty Crocker Twice Baked
Potato	Mix	Betty Crocker Twice Baked
Potato	Mix	Betty Crocker Twice Baked
Potato	Mix	Betty Crocker Twice Baked
Potato	Mix	Country Store Flakes
Potato	Mix	Fantastic Foods
Potato	Mix	Fantastic Foods
Potato	Mix	Fantastic Foods
Potato	Mix	Fantastic Foods
Potato	Mix	French's
Potato	Mix	French's
Potato	Mix	French's
Potato	Mix	French's
Potato	Mix	French's
Potato	Mix	French's
Potato	Mix	French's
Potato	Mix	French's Idaho
Potato	Mix	French's Idaho Spuds
Potato	Mix	Idahoan
Potato	Mix	Idahoan
Potato	Mix	Idahoan
Potato	Mix	Idahoan
Potato	Mix	Idahoan
Potato	Mix	Idahoan
Potato	Mix	Idahoan Instamash
Potato	Mix	Idahoan Quick One-Pan
Potato	Mix	Pillsbury
Potato	Mix	Pillsbury
Potato	Mix	Pillsbury
Potato	Mix	Pillsbury Hungry Jack
Potato	Mix	Pillsbury Hungry Jack
Potato	Mix	Pillsbury Idaho
Potato	Mix	Pillsbury Idaho Spuds
Potato Dishes	Mix	Betty Crocker Potato Medleys
Potato Dishes	Mix	Betty Crocker Potato Medleys
Potato Dishes	Mix	Betty Crocker Potato Medleys
Potato Dishes	Mix	Betty Crocker Potato Medleys
Potato Dishes	Mix	Kraft Potatoes & Cheese
Potato Dishes	Mix	Kraft Potatoes & Cheese
Potato Dishes	Mix	Kraft Potatoes & Cheese
Potato Dishes	Mix	Kraft Potatoes & Cheese
Potato Dishes	Mix	Kraft Potatoes & Cheese
Potato Dishes	Mix	Kraft Potatoes & Cheese
Rice Dishes	Mix	Casbah
Rice Dishes	Mix	Casbah

Major Description	Minor Description	Serving Size	Calories	Grade
Hash Brown	Onions & Salt	¹/₂ cup	160	C–
Scalloped		¹/₂ cup	140	C–
Scalloped	Cheesy	¹/₆ pkg or ¹/₂ cup	140	C–
Scalloped	Ham	¹/₅ pkg or ¹/₂ cup	160	C–
Sour Cream & Chives		¹/₂ cup	140	C–
		¹/₂ cup	130	D–
Bacon & Cheddar		¹/₂ cup	210	D–
Butter, Herb		¹/₂ cup	220	D–
Cheddar, Mild	Onion	¹/₂ cup	190	D–
Sour Cream & Chives		¹/₂ cup	200	D–
		¹/₂ cup	105	A
au Gratin	Milk	¹/₂ cup	156	B–
au Gratin	Milk & Butter	¹/₂ cup	196	C–
Country Style		¹/₂ cup	85	A–
Country Style		¹/₂ cup	118	C–
au Gratin	Tangy	¹/₂ cup	130	C–
Cheddar & Bacon	Casserole	¹/₂ cup	130	C–
Scalloped	Cheese, Real	¹/₂ cup	140	C–
Scalloped	Crispy Top with Savory Onion	¹/₂ cup	140	C–
Scalloped	Italian Style, Creamy	¹/₂ cup	120	B–
Sour Cream & Chives		¹/₂ cup	150	D–
Stroganoff, Creamy		¹/₂ cup	130	B–
		¹/₂ cup	130	D–
		¹/₂ cup	140	D–
au Gratin	Milk & Butter	¹/₂ cup	130	C–
Cheddar	Spicy	¹/₂ cup	140	C–
Granules	Milk	¹/₂ cup	140	D–
Scalloped		¹/₂ cup	140	C–
Sour Cream & Chives		¹/₂ cup	130	C–
Western Style		¹/₂ cup	120	B–
Microwave		¹/₂ cup	80	A–
Hash Brown		¹/₂ cup	140	D–
au Gratin		¹/₂ cup	140	C–
Cheddar & Bacon	Milk & Butter	¹/₂ cup	140	C–
Sour Cream	Milk & Butter	¹/₂ cup	150	C–
Flakes		¹/₂ cup	140	D–
Mashed Potato	Natural	¹/₂ cup	150	C–
Mashed Granules		¹/₂ cup	130	D–
Mashed Potato		¹/₂ cup	150	C–
Broccoli au Gratin		¹/₂ cup	140	B–
Cheddar with Mushrooms		¹/₂ cup	140	B–
Scalloped	Broccoli	¹/₂ cup	140	C–
Scalloped	Green Beans & Mushrooms	¹/₂ cup	140	C–
Cheese, Sour Cream & Chives		¹/₂ cup	150	B–
2 Cheese		¹/₂ cup	130	B–
au Gratin	Broccoli & Cheese	¹/₂ cup	150	B–
au Gratin	Cheese	¹/₂ cup	130	C–
Scalloped	Cheese	¹/₂ cup	140	C–
Scalloped	Cheese & Ham	¹/₂ cup	150	B–
Pilaf		¹/₂ cup	90	A
Pilaf	Spanish Style	¹/₂ cup	90	A

"+" indicates the food meets minimum fiber requirements; "–" indicates the food has a high sodium content.

Food	Processing Category	Brand
Rice Dishes	Mix	Casbah
Rice Dishes	Mix	El Paso
Rice Dishes	Mix	Fantastic Foods
Rice Dishes	Mix	Fantastic Foods
Rice Dishes	Mix	Fantastic Foods
Rice Dishes	Mix	Fantastic Foods
Rice Dishes	Mix	Fantastic Foods
Rice Dishes	Mix	Fantastic Foods
Rice Dishes	Mix	Fantastic Foods
Rice Dishes	Mix	Fantastic Foods
Rice Dishes	Mix	Fantastic Foods
Rice Dishes	Mix	Goya
Rice Dishes	Mix	Goya
Rice Dishes	Mix	Hain 3-Grain Goodness
Rice Dishes	Mix	Hain 3-Grain Side Dish
Rice Dishes	Mix	Knorr Pilafs
Rice Dishes	Mix	Knorr Pilafs
Rice Dishes	Mix	Knorr Pilafs
Rice Dishes	Mix	Lipton Fast Cook
Rice Dishes	Mix	Lipton Fast Cook
Rice Dishes	Mix	Lipton Fast Cook
Rice Dishes	Mix	Lipton Fast Cook
Rice Dishes	Mix	Lipton Rice and Sauce
Rice Dishes	Mix	Lipton Rice and Sauce
Rice Dishes	Mix	Lipton Rice and Sauce
Rice Dishes	Mix	Lipton Rice and Sauce
Rice Dishes	Mix	Lipton Rice and Sauce
Rice Dishes	Mix	Lipton Rice and Sauce
Rice Dishes	Mix	Lipton Rice and Sauce
Rice Dishes	Mix	Lipton Rice and Sauce
Rice Dishes	Mix	Lipton Rice and Sauce
Rice Dishes	Mix	Lipton Rice and Sauce
Rice Dishes	Mix	Lipton Rice and Sauce
Rice Dishes	Mix	Lipton Rice and Sauce
Rice Dishes	Mix	Mahatma
Rice Dishes	Mix	Mahatma
Rice Dishes	Mix	Mahatma
Rice Dishes	Mix	Mahatma
Rice Dishes	Mix	Mahatma/Success
Rice Dishes	Mix	Minute
Rice Dishes	Mix	Minute
Rice Dishes	Mix	Minute Microwave Family Size
Rice Dishes	Mix	Near East
Rice Dishes	Mix	Near East
Rice Dishes	Mix	Near East
Rice Dishes	Mix	Near East
Rice Dishes	Mix	Near East
Rice Dishes	Mix	Near East
Rice Dishes	Mix	Near East
Rice Dishes	Mix	Pritikin
Rice Dishes	Mix	Pritikin
Rice Dishes	Mix	Quick Pilaf
Rice Dishes	Mix	Quick Pilaf

Major Description	Minor Description	Serving Size	Calories	Grade
Pilaf	with Nuts	$^1/_2$ cup	160	A
Mexican Style		$^1/_2$ cup	140	A–
3 Grain	Herbs	$^1/_2$ cup	120	A–+
Brown	Miso	$^1/_2$ cup	125	A–
Cajun Style		$^1/_2$ cup	110	A–+
Caribbean Style		$^1/_2$ cup	95	A–+
Curry	Bombay Style	$^1/_2$ cup	115	A–+
Northern Italian Style		$^1/_2$ cup	110	A–+
Spanish Style	Rice & Beans	$^1/_2$ cup	110	A+
Szechuan Style		$^1/_2$ cup	95	A–+
Tex-Mex Style		$^1/_2$ cup	115	A–+
Primavera		$^1/_2$ cup	90	A–
Yellow	Spanish Style	$^1/_2$ cup	90	A–
Oriental Style		$^1/_2$ cup	120	C–
Almondine		$^1/_2$ cup	130	C–
Basmati	Tomato & Herbs	$^1/_2$ cup	200	A–
Harvest Medley		$^1/_2$ cup	110	A–
Lemon Herb & Jasmine		$^1/_2$ cup	140	A–
Alfredo Broccoli		$^1/_2$ cup	170	B–
Cheddar & Broccoli		$^1/_2$ cup	140	B–
Chicken	Parmesan Risotto	$^1/_2$ cup	140	B–
Mushroom		$^1/_2$ cup	135	B–
Asparagus with Hollandaise	Margarine	$^1/_2$ cup	150	B–
Beef Flavor		$^1/_2$ cup	290	B–
Cajun Style	Butter	$^1/_2$ cup	150	B–
Chicken & Chicken Flavor	Butter	$^1/_2$ cup	150	B–
Herb & Butter		$^1/_2$ cup	150	B–
Long Grain & Wild	Butter	$^1/_2$ cup	150	B–
Long Grain & Wild	Mushrooms & Herbs	$^1/_2$ cup	150	B–
Mushroom	Butter	$^1/_2$ cup	150	B–
Pilaf	Butter	$^1/_2$ cup	170	C–
Pilaf	Margarine	$^1/_2$ cup	140	B–
Spanish Style	Butter	$^1/_2$ cup	140	B–
Vegetables	Margarine	$^1/_2$ cup	160	B–
Beef Flavor		$^1/_2$ cup	100	A–
Chicken & Chicken Flavor		$^1/_2$ cup	100	A–
Long Grain & Wild Rice		$^1/_2$ cup	100	A–
Spanish Style		$^1/_2$ cup	100	A–
Yellow		$^1/_2$ cup	100	A–
Fried		$^1/_2$ cup	160	B–
Long Grain & Wild		$^1/_2$ cup	150	B–
Beef Flavor		$^1/_2$ cup	160	B–
Long Grain & Wild		$^1/_2$ cup	130	B–
Pilaf		$^1/_2$ cup	140	A–
Pilaf	Beef Flavor	$^1/_2$ cup	140	B–
Pilaf	Chicken Flavor	$^1/_2$ cup	140	B–
Pilaf	Lentil	$^1/_2$ cup	170	B–
Pilaf	Wheat	$^1/_2$ cup	150	B–
Spanish Style		$^1/_2$ cup	170	B–
Mexican-style Dinner		$^1/_2$ cup	300	A+
Oriental-style Dinner		$^1/_2$ cup	285	A–+
Pilaf	Brown with Miso	$^1/_2$ cup	105	A–
Pilaf	Spanish Style, Brown	$^1/_2$ cup	98	A–

"+" indicates the food meets minimum fiber requirements; "–" indicates the food has a high sodium content.

Food	Processing Category	Brand
Rice Dishes	Mix	Rice-A-Roni
Rice Dishes	Mix	Rice-A-Roni
Rice Dishes	Mix	Rice-A-Roni
Rice Dishes	Mix	Rice-A-Roni
Rice Dishes	Mix	Rice-A-Roni
Rice Dishes	Mix	Rice-A-Roni
Rice Dishes	Mix	Rice-A-Roni
Rice Dishes	Mix	Rice-A-Roni
Rice Dishes	Mix	Rice-A-Roni
Rice Dishes	Mix	Rice-A-Roni
Rice Dishes	Mix	Rice-A-Roni
Rice Dishes	Mix	Rice-A-Roni
Rice Dishes	Mix	Rice-A-Roni
Rice Dishes	Mix	Rice-A-Roni
Rice Dishes	Mix	Rice-A-Roni
Rice Dishes	Mix	Rice-A-Roni
Rice Dishes	Mix	Rice-A-Roni
Rice Dishes	Mix	Rice-A-Roni
Rice Dishes	Mix	Rice-A-Roni
Rice Dishes	Mix	Rice-A-Roni
Rice Dishes	Mix	Rice-A-Roni
Rice Dishes	Mix	Rice-A-Roni Fast Cook
Rice Dishes	Mix	Rice-A-Roni Fast Cook
Rice Dishes	Mix	Rice-A-Roni Less Salt
Rice Dishes	Mix	Rice-A-Roni Less Salt
Rice Dishes	Mix	Rice-A-Roni Less Salt
Rice Dishes	Mix	Rice-A-Roni Original
Rice Dishes	Mix	Rice-A-Roni Savory Classics
Rice Dishes	Mix	Rice-A-Roni Savory Classics
Rice Dishes	Mix	Rice-A-Roni Savory Classics
Rice Dishes	Mix	Rice-A-Roni Savory Classics
Rice Dishes	Mix	Rice-A-Roni Savory Classics
Rice Dishes	Mix	Rice-A-Roni Savory Classics
Rice Dishes	Mix	Rice-A-Roni Savory Classics
Rice Dishes	Mix	Rice-A-Roni Savory Classics
Rice Dishes	Mix	Success
Rice Dishes	Mix	Success
Rice Dishes	Mix	Success
Rice Dishes	Mix	Success
Rice Dishes	Mix	Success
Rice Dishes	Mix	Suzi Wan
Rice Dishes	Mix	Suzi Wan
Rice Dishes	Mix	Suzi Wan
Rice Dishes	Mix	Suzi Wan
Rice Dishes	Mix	Suzi Wan
Rice Dishes	Mix	Suzi Wan Dinner Recipe
Rice Dishes	Mix	Suzi Wan Dinner Recipe
Rice Dishes	Mix	Suzi Wan Dinner Recipe
Rice Dishes	Mix	Uncle Ben's
Rice Dishes	Mix	Uncle Ben's
Rice Dishes	Mix	Uncle Ben's
Rice Dishes	Mix	Uncle Ben's Country Inn

Major Description	Minor Description	Serving Size	Calories	Grade
Beef Flavor		¹/₂ cup	170	B–
Beef Flavor	Mushroom	¹/₂ cup	150	B–
Broccoli au Gratin		¹/₂ cup	185	D–
Cajun Style with Beans		¹/₂ cup	140	B–
Cheddar Cheese & Herbs		¹/₂ cup	170	C–
Chicken & Chicken Flavor		¹/₂ cup	150	B–
Chicken & Chicken Flavor	Broccoli	¹/₂ cup	150	B–
Chicken & Chicken Flavor	Mushrooms	¹/₂ cup	180	C–
Chicken & Chicken Flavor	Vegetables	¹/₂ cup	140	B–
Fried	Almonds	¹/₂ cup	140	C–
Fried Rice		¹/₂ cup	160	C–
Herb & Butter		¹/₂ cup	130	B–
Herb & Butter		¹/₂ cup	155	B–
Long Grain & Wild		¹/₂ cup	130	B–
Oriental Style		¹/₂ cup	145	B–
Pilaf	Long Grain & Wild Rice	¹/₂ cup	155	B–
Red Beans		¹/₂ cup	140	B–+
Risotto		¹/₂ cup	200	B–
Spanish Style		¹/₂ cup	150	B–
Stroganoff		¹/₂ cup	200	C–
Yellow		¹/₂ cup	140	B–
Broccoli with Cheese		¹/₂ cup	150	C–
Oriental Style		¹/₂ cup	145	C–
Beef		¹/₂ cup	140	B–
Broccoli au Gratin		¹/₂ cup	160	C–
Chicken		¹/₂ cup	140	B–
Long Grain & Wild Rice		¹/₂ cup	130	B–
Broccoli au Gratin		¹/₂ cup	180	D–
Cauliflower au Gratin		¹/₂ cup	170	C–
Cheddar, Zesty		¹/₂ cup	180	C–
Chicken Florentine		¹/₂ cup	130	B–
Garden-style Pilaf		¹/₂ cup	140	B–
Green Bean Almondine		¹/₂ cup	210	D–
Parmesan & Herbs	Creamy	¹/₂ cup	170	C–
Spring Vegetables & Cheese		¹/₂ cup	170	C–
au Gratin, Herb		¹/₂ cup	100	A–
Broccoli	Cheese	¹/₂ cup	115	B–
Brown & Wild		¹/₂ cup	120	A–
Chicken & Chicken Flavor		¹/₂ cup	110	B–
Pilaf		¹/₂ cup	120	A–
3 Flavor		¹/₂ cup	120	A–
Chicken & Chicken Flavor	Broccoli	¹/₂ cup	120	A–
Chicken & Chicken Flavor	Vegetables	¹/₂ cup	120	A–
Sweet & Sour		¹/₂ cup	130	A–
Teriyaki		¹/₂ cup	120	A–
Broccoli Stir-fry		¹/₂ cup	120	A–
Sweet & Sour	No Butter	¹/₂ cup	130	A–
Teriyaki	No Butter	¹/₂ cup	120	A–
Brown & Wild Rice		¹/₂ cup	130	A–
Brown & Wild Rice	Mushroom Recipe	¹/₂ cup	130	A–
Long Grain & Wild Rice	Chicken Stock Sauce	¹/₂ cup	140	A–
Alfredo		¹/₂ cup	140	B–

"+" indicates the food meets minimum fiber requirements; "–" indicates the food has a high sodium content.

Food	Processing Category	Brand
Rice Dishes	Mix	Uncle Ben's Country Inn
Rice Dishes	Mix	Uncle Ben's Country Inn
Rice Dishes	Mix	Uncle Ben's Country Inn
Rice Dishes	Mix	Uncle Ben's Country Inn
Rice Dishes	Mix	Uncle Ben's Country Inn
Rice Dishes	Mix	Uncle Ben's Country Inn
Rice Dishes	Mix	Uncle Ben's Country Inn
Rice Dishes	Mix	Uncle Ben's Country Inn
Rice Dishes	Mix	Uncle Ben's Country Inn
Rice Dishes	Mix	Uncle Ben's Country Inn
Rice Dishes	Mix	Uncle Ben's Country Inn
Rice Dishes	Mix	Uncle Ben's Country Inn
Rice Dishes	Mix	Uncle Ben's Country Inn
Rice Dishes	Mix	Uncle Ben's Country Inn
Rice Dishes	Mix	Uncle Ben's Country Inn
Rice Dishes	Mix	Uncle Ben's Fast Cooking
Rice Dishes	Mix	Uncle Ben's Original
Risotto	Mix	Knorr
Risotto	Mix	Knorr
Risotto	Mix	Knorr
Risotto	Mix	Knorr
Risotto	Mix	Knorr
Roll	Mix	Dromedary
Roll	Mix	Pillsbury
Sesame Nut Mix	Mix	Planters
Soup	Base	Tone's
Soup	Canned Condensed	Generic
Soup	Canned Condensed	Generic
Soup	Canned Condensed	Generic
Soup	Canned Condensed	Generic
Soup	Canned Condensed	Generic
Soup	Canned Condensed	Generic
Soup	Canned Condensed	Generic
Soup	Canned Condensed	Generic
Soup	Canned Condensed	Generic
Soup	Canned Condensed	Generic
Soup	Canned Condensed	Generic
Soup	Canned Condensed	Generic
Soup	Canned Condensed	Generic
Soup	Canned Condensed	Generic
Soup	Canned Condensed	Generic
Soup	Canned Condensed	Generic
Soup	Canned Condensed	Generic
Soup	Canned Condensed	Generic
Soup	Canned Condensed	Generic
Soup	Canned Condensed	Generic
Soup	Canned Condensed	Generic
Soup	Canned Condensed	Generic
Soup	Canned Condensed	Generic
Soup	Canned Condensed	Generic
Soup	Canned Condensed	Generic

Major Description	Minor Description	Serving Size	Calories	Grade
Asparagus	au Gratin	$^1/_2$ cup	130	B–
au Gratin Herb		$^1/_2$ cup	140	B–
Broccoli Almondine		$^1/_2$ cup	130	A–
Broccoli au Gratin		$^1/_2$ cup	130	B–
Cauliflower au Gratin		$^1/_2$ cup	130	B–
Chicken	Vegetables	$^1/_2$ cup	130	B–
Chicken & Chicken Flavor	Homestyle	$^1/_2$ cup	140	B–
Chicken & Chicken Flavor	Mushroom Cream	$^1/_2$ cup	140	B–
Chicken & Chicken Flavor	Royale	$^1/_2$ cup	120	A–
Chicken & Chicken Flavor	Stock	$^1/_2$ cup	130	A–
Florentine Style		$^1/_2$ cup	140	B–
Mexican Style	Mushroom Cream & Wild Rice	$^1/_2$ cup	140	B–
Pilaf	Vegetable	$^1/_2$ cup	120	A–
Risotto	Chicken & Cheese	$^1/_2$ cup	120	A–
Vegetable Medley		$^1/_2$ cup	140	A–
Long Grain & Wild Rice		$^1/_2$ cup	100	A–
Long Grain & Wild Rice		$^1/_2$ cup	100	A–
Milanese		$^1/_2$ cup	150	A–
Mushroom		$^1/_2$ cup	150	A–
Onion Herb		$^1/_2$ cup	170	A–
Primavera		$^1/_2$ cup	150	A–
Tomato		$^1/_2$ cup	160	A–
Hot		1 piece	239	B–
Hot		1 piece	270	D–
Dry Roasted		1 oz	160	D–
Beef		1 tsp	11	D
Asparagus, Cream of		1 cup	87	D–
Bean Black		1 cup	116	A–
Bean with Bacon		1 cup	173	C–
Beef Noodle		1 cup	84	C–
Celery, Cream of		1 cup	90	D–
Celery, Cream of	Whole Milk	1 cup	165	D–
Cheese		1 cup	155	D–
Cheese	Whole Milk	1 cup	230	D–
Chicken & Dumplings		1 cup	97	D–
Chicken Broth		1 cup	39	C–
Chicken Gumbo		1 cup	56	B–
Chicken Noodle		1 cup	75	B–
Chicken Rice		1 cup	60	B–
Chicken Vegetable		1 cup	74	C–
Chicken, Cream of		1 cup	116	D–
Chicken, Cream of	Whole Milk	1 cup	191	D–
Chili Beef		1 cup	169	C–
Clam Chowder, Manhattan		1 cup	77	B–
Clam Chowder, New England		1 cup	95	B–
Clam Chowder, New England	Whole Milk	1 cup	163	C–
Consommé with Gelatin		1 cup	29	A–
Minestrone		1 cup	83	B–
Mushroom with Beef Stock		1 cup	85	D–
Mushroom, Cream of		1 cup	129	D–
Mushroom, Cream of		1 cup	203	D–
Onion		1 cup	57	B–

"+" indicates the food meets minimum fiber requirements; "–" indicates the food has a high sodium content.

Food	Processing Category	Brand
Soup	Canned Condensed	Generic
Soup	Canned Condensed	Generic
Soup	Canned Condensed	Generic
Soup	Canned Condensed	Generic
Soup	Canned Condensed	Generic
Soup	Canned Condensed	Generic
Soup	Canned Condensed	Generic
Soup	Canned Condensed	Generic
Soup	Canned Condensed	Generic
Soup	Canned Condensed	Generic
Soup	Canned Condensed	Generic
Soup	Canned Condensed	Generic
Soup	Canned Condensed	Generic
Soup	Canned Condensed	Generic
Soup	Canned Condensed	Generic
Soup	Canned Condensed	Generic
Soup	Canned Condensed	Generic
Soup	Canned Condensed	Campbell's
Soup	Canned Condensed	Campbell's
Soup	Canned Condensed	Campbell's
Soup	Canned Condensed	Campbell's
Soup	Canned Condensed	Campbell's
Soup	Canned Condensed	Campbell's
Soup	Canned Condensed	Campbell's
Soup	Canned Condensed	Campbell's
Soup	Canned Condensed	Campbell's
Soup	Canned Condensed	Campbell's
Soup	Canned Condensed	Campbell's
Soup	Canned Condensed	Campbell's
Soup	Canned Condensed	Campbell's
Soup	Canned Condensed	Campbell's
Soup	Canned Condensed	Campbell's
Soup	Canned Condensed	Campbell's
Soup	Canned Condensed	Campbell's
Soup	Canned Condensed	Campbell's
Soup	Canned Condensed	Campbell's
Soup	Canned Condensed	Campbell's
Soup	Canned Condensed	Campbell's
Soup	Canned Condensed	Campbell's
Soup	Canned Condensed	Campbell's
Soup	Canned Condensed	Campbell's
Soup	Canned Condensed	Campbell's
Soup	Canned Condensed	Campbell's
Soup	Canned Condensed	Campbell's
Soup	Canned Condensed	Campbell's
Soup	Canned Condensed	Campbell's
Soup	Canned Condensed	Campbell's

Major Description	Minor Description	Serving Size	Calories	Grade
Oyster Stew		1 cup	59	D–
Pea Green		1 cup	164	B–
Pea, Split with Ham		1 cup	189	B–
Pepper Pot		1 cup	103	D–
Potato, Cream of		1 cup	73	B–
Scotch Broth		1 cup	80	B–
Shrimp, Cream of		1 cup	90	D–
Shrimp, Cream of	Whole Milk	1 cup	165	D–
Stockpot		1 cup	100	C–
Tomato		1 cup	86	B–
Tomato Beef with Noodle		1 cup	140	B–
Tomato Bisque		1 cup	123	B–
Tomato Rice		1 cup	120	B–
Turkey Noodle		1 cup	69	B–
Turkey Vegetable		1 cup	74	C–
Vegetable Beef		1 cup	79	B–
Vegetable with Beef Broth		1 cup	81	B–
Vegetable, Vegetarian		1 cup	72	B–
Asparagus, Cream of		1 cup	80	D–
Bean with Bacon		1 cup	140	B–
Bean with Frankfurters		1 cup	187	C–
Beef		1 cup	80	B–
Beef Broth or Bouillon		1 cup	16	A–
Beef Noodle		1 cup	70	C–
Broccoli, Cream of		1 cup	80	D–
Broccoli, Cream of		1 cup	140	D–
Celery, Cream of		1 cup	100	D–
Cheese, Cheddar		1 cup	110	D–
Cheese, Nacho		1 cup	110	D–
Chicken & Star		1 cup	60	B–
Chicken Alphabet		1 cup	80	C–
Chicken Barley		1 cup	70	B–
Chicken Broth		1 cup	30	D–
Chicken Broth	Noodles	1 cup	45	B–
Chicken Gumbo		1 cup	60	B–
Chicken Mushroom		1 cup	120	D–
Chicken Noodle		1 cup	60	B–
Chicken Rice		1 cup	60	D–
Chicken Vegetable		1 cup	70	C–
Chicken, Cream of		1 cup	110	D–
Chili Beef		1 cup	140	C–
Clam Chowder, Manhattan		1 cup	70	B–
Clam Chowder, New England		1 cup	80	C–
Consommé with Gelatin	Beef	1 cup	25	A–
French Onion		1 cup	60	B–
Italian Tomato	Basil & Oregano	1 cup	90	A–
Minestrone		1 cup	80	B–
Mushroom, Beefy		1 cup	60	D–
Mushroom, Cream of		1 cup	100	D–
Mushroom, Golden		1 cup	70	C–
Noodle	Curly, with Chicken	1 cup	80	C–
Noodle	Ground Beef	1 cup	90	C–
Onion, Cream of		1 cup	100	D–

"+" indicates the food meets minimum fiber requirements; "–" indicates the food has a high sodium content.

Food	Processing Category	Brand
Soup	Canned Condensed	Campbell's
Soup	Canned Condensed	Campbell's
Soup	Canned Condensed	Campbell's
Soup	Canned Condensed	Campbell's
Soup	Canned Condensed	Campbell's
Soup	Canned Condensed	Campbell's
Soup	Canned Condensed	Campbell's
Soup	Canned Condensed	Campbell's
Soup	Canned Condensed	Campbell's
Soup	Canned Condensed	Campbell's
Soup	Canned Condensed	Campbell's
Soup	Canned Condensed	Campbell's
Soup	Canned Condensed	Campbell's
Soup	Canned Condensed	Campbell's
Soup	Canned Condensed	Campbell's
Soup	Canned Condensed	Campbell's
Soup	Canned Condensed	Campbell's
Soup	Canned Condensed	Campbell's
Soup	Canned Condensed	Campbell's
Soup	Canned Condensed	Campbell's Chicken 'n
Soup	Canned Condensed	Campbell's Healthy Request
Soup	Canned Condensed	Campbell's Healthy Request
Soup	Canned Condensed	Campbell's Healthy Request
Soup	Canned Condensed	Campbell's Healthy Request
Soup	Canned Condensed	Campbell's Healthy Request
Soup	Canned Condensed	Campbell's Healthy Request
Soup	Canned Condensed	Campbell's Healthy Request
Soup	Canned Condensed	Campbell's Healthy Request
Soup	Canned Condensed	Campbell's Healthy Request
Soup	Canned Condensed	Campbell's Healthy Request
Soup	Canned Condensed	Campbell's Healthy Request
Soup	Canned Condensed	Campbell's Healthy Request
Soup	Canned Condensed	Campbell's Healthy Request
Soup	Canned Condensed	Campbell's Healthy Request
Soup	Canned Condensed	Campbell's Healthy Request
Soup	Canned Condensed	Campbell's Healthy Request
Soup	Canned Condensed	Campbell's Homestyle
Soup	Canned Condensed	Campbell's Homestyle
Soup	Canned Condensed	Campbell's Homestyle
Soup	Canned Condensed	Campbell's Homestyle
Soup	Canned Condensed	Campbell's Homestyle
Soup	Canned Condensed	Campbell's Noodle-O's
Soup	Canned Condensed	Campbell's Old Fashioned
Soup	Canned Condensed	Campbell's Old Fashioned
Soup	Canned Condensed	Campbell's Special Request $1/3$ Less Salt
Soup	Canned Condensed	Campbell's Special Request $1/3$ Less Salt
Soup	Canned Condensed	Campbell's Special Request $1/3$ Less Salt
Soup	Canned Condensed	Campbell's Special Request $1/3$ Less Salt

Major Description	Minor Description	Serving Size	Calories	Grade
Oyster Stew		1 cup	70	D–
Oyster Stew		1 cup	80	D–
Oyster Stew	Whole Milk	1 cup	130	D–
Pea, Green		1 cup	160	B–
Pea, Split	Ham & Bacon	1 cup	160	B–
Pepper Pot		1 cup	90	C–
Potato, Cream of		1 cup	80	C–
Scotch Broth		1 cup	80	C–
Shrimp, Cream of		1 cup	90	D–
Teddy Bear		1 cup	60	A–
Tomato		1 cup	90	B–
Tomato	Zesty	1 cup	100	B–
Tomato Bisque		1 cup	120	B–
Turkey Noodle		1 cup	70	B–
Turkey Vegetable		1 cup	70	C–
Vegetable		1 cup	90	B–
Vegetable Beef		1 cup	70	B–
Vegetable Vegetarian		1 cup	80	B–
Won Ton		1 cup	40	B–
Chicken & Dumplings		1 cup	80	C–
Bean	Bacon	1 cup	150	B–+
Chicken	Noodle	1 cup	60	B–
Chicken	Rice	1 cup	60	D–
Chicken & Rice	Hearty	1 cup	110	B–
Chicken Broth		1 cup	10	A–
Chicken Noodle	Hearty	1 cup	80	B–
Chicken Vegetable	Hearty	1 cup	120	B–
Chicken, Cream of		1 cup	70	B–
Clam Chowder, New England		1 cup	100	B–
Minestrone	Hearty	1 cup	90	B–
Mushroom, Cream of		1 cup	60	B–
Tomato		1 cup	90	B–
Tomato	Low Fat Milk	1 cup	140	B–
Vegetable		1 cup	90	B–
Vegetable	Hearty	1 cup	90	B–
Vegetable Beef		1 cup	90	B–
Vegetable Beef	Hearty	1 cup	120	A–
Bean		1 cup	130	A–
Beef Noodle		1 cup	80	D–
Chicken Noodle		1 cup	70	C–
Tomato, Cream of		1 cup	110	B–
Vegetable		1 cup	60	B–
Chicken Noodle		1 cup	70	B–
Tomato Rice		1 cup	110	B–
Vegetable		1 cup	60	B–
Bean with Bacon		1 cup	140	B–
Chicken Noodle		1 cup	60	B–
Chicken Rice		1 cup	60	D–
Chicken, Cream of		1 cup	110	D–

"+" indicates the food meets minimum fiber requirements; "–" indicates the food has a high sodium content.

Food	Processing Category	Brand
Soup	Canned Condensed	Campbell's Special Request $^1/_3$ Less Salt
Soup	Canned Condensed	Campbell's Special Request $^1/_3$ Less Salt
Soup	Canned Condensed	Campbell's Special Request $^1/_3$ Less Salt
Soup	Canned Condensed	Campbell's Special Request $^1/_3$ Less Salt
Soup	Canned Condensed	Doxsee
Soup	Canned Condensed	Gorton's
Soup	Canned Condensed	Rokeach
Soup	Canned Condensed	Rokeach
Soup	Canned Condensed	Snow's
Soup	Canned Condensed	Snow's
Soup	Canned Condensed	Snow's
Soup	Canned Condensed	Snow's
Soup	Canned Condensed	Snow's
Soup	Canned Ready to Serve	Generic
Soup	Canned Ready to Serve	Generic
Soup	Canned Ready to Serve	Generic
Soup	Canned Ready to Serve	Generic
Soup	Canned Ready to Serve	Generic
Soup	Canned Ready to Serve	Generic
Soup	Canned Ready to Serve	Generic
Soup	Canned Ready to Serve	Generic
Soup	Canned Ready to Serve	Generic
Soup	Canned Ready to Serve	Generic
Soup	Canned Ready to Serve	Generic
Soup	Canned Ready to Serve	Generic
Soup	Canned Ready to Serve	Generic
Soup	Canned Ready to Serve	Generic
Soup	Canned Ready to Serve	Generic
Soup	Canned Ready to Serve	Generic
Soup	Canned Ready to Serve	Campbell's Chunky
Soup	Canned Ready to Serve	Campbell's Chunky
Soup	Canned Ready to Serve	Campbell's Chunky
Soup	Canned Ready to Serve	Campbell's Chunky
Soup	Canned Ready to Serve	Campbell's Chunky
Soup	Canned Ready to Serve	Campbell's Chunky
Soup	Canned Ready to Serve	Campbell's Chunky
Soup	Canned Ready to Serve	Campbell's Chunky
Soup	Canned Ready to Serve	Campbell's Chunky
Soup	Canned Ready to Serve	Campbell's Chunky
Soup	Canned Ready to Serve	Campbell's Chunky
Soup	Canned Ready to Serve	Campbell's Chunky
Soup	Canned Ready to Serve	Campbell's Chunky
Soup	Canned Ready to Serve	Campbell's Chunky
Soup	Canned Ready to Serve	Campbell's Chunky
Soup	Canned Ready to Serve	Campbell's Chunky
Soup	Canned Ready to Serve	Campbell's Chunky
Soup	Canned Ready to Serve	Campbell's Chunky
Soup	Canned Ready to Serve	Campbell's Chunky

Major Description	Minor Description	Serving Size	Calories	Grade
Mushroom, Cream of		1 cup	100	D–
Tomato		1 cup	90	B–
Vegetable	Beef Stock	1 cup	90	B–
Vegetable Beef		1 cup	70	B–
Clam Chowder, Manhattan		1 cup	70	B–
Clam Chowder, New England		1/4 can	140	C–
Barley & Mushroom		1 cup	85	A–
Pea, Split with Egg Barley		1 cup	132	A–
Clam Chowder, Manhattan		1 cup	70	B–
Clam Chowder, New England		1 cup	140	C–
Corn Chowder		1 cup	150	C–
Fish Chowder		1 cup	130	D–
Seafood Chowder		1 cup	140	C–
Bean with Ham	Chunky	8 oz	231	C–
Beef	Chunky	8 oz	160	B–
Beef	Chunky	8 oz	171	B–
Beef Broth	or Bouillon	8 oz	16	B–
Chicken	Chunky	8 oz	160	C–
Chicken Noodle	Meatballs	8 oz	91	C–
Chicken Vegetable	Chunky	8 oz	157	B–
Clam Chowder, Manhattan	Chunky	8 oz	125	B–
Crab		8 oz	70	B–
Escarole		8 oz	25	D–+
Gazpacho		8 oz	55	C–
Lentil with Ham		8 oz	197	B–
Minestrone	Chunky	8 oz	120	B–
Vegetable	Chunky	8 oz	122	B–
Vegetable	Chunky	8 oz	115	B–
Beef	Chunky	8 oz	148	B–
Beef Stroganoff Style		8 oz	236	D–
Chicken Corn Chowder		8 oz	258	D–
Chicken Mushroom		8 oz	205	D–
Chicken Noodle		8 oz	148	C–
Chicken Nuggets	Vegetables & Noodles	8 oz	141	B–
Chicken Vegetable	Chunky	8 oz	143	C–
Chicken with Rice		8 oz	118	B–
Chili Beef		8 oz	210	B–
Clam Chowder, Manhattan	Chunky	8 oz	119	B–
Clam Chowder, New England		8 oz	216	D–
Creole Style		8 oz	180	B–
Ham & Butter Bean		8 oz	207	C–
Minestrone		8 oz	135	B–
Pea, Split with Ham		8 oz	170	B–
Pepper Steak		8 oz	80	A–
Sirloin Burger		8 oz	162	C–
Steak & Potato		8 oz	148	B–
Turkey Vegetable		8 oz	126	C–
Vegetable	Chunky	8 oz	115	B–
Vegetable	Mediterranean Style	8 oz	143	C–

"+" indicates the food meets minimum fiber requirements; "–" indicates the food has a high sodium content.

Food	Processing Category	Brand
Soup	Canned Ready to Serve	Campbell's Chunky Low Sodium
Soup	Canned Ready to Serve	Campbell's Chunky Old Fashioned
Soup	Canned Ready to Serve	Campbell's Chunky Old Fashioned
Soup	Canned Ready to Serve	Campbell's Chunky Old Fashioned
Soup	Canned Ready to Serve	Campbell's Chunky Old Fashioned
Soup	Canned Ready to Serve	Campbell's Home Cookin'
Soup	Canned Ready to Serve	Campbell's Home Cookin'
Soup	Canned Ready to Serve	Campbell's Home Cookin'
Soup	Canned Ready to Serve	Campbell's Home Cookin'
Soup	Canned Ready to Serve	Campbell's Home Cookin'
Soup	Canned Ready to Serve	Campbell's Home Cookin'
Soup	Canned Ready to Serve	Campbell's Home Cookin'
Soup	Canned Ready to Serve	Campbell's Home Cookin'
Soup	Canned Ready to Serve	Campbell's Home Cookin'
Soup	Canned Ready to Serve	Campbell's Home Cookin'
Soup	Canned Ready to Serve	Campbell's Home Cookin'
Soup	Canned Ready to Serve	Campbell's Home Cookin'
Soup	Canned Ready to Serve	Campbell's Low Sodium
Soup	Canned Ready to Serve	Campbell's Low Sodium
Soup	Canned Ready to Serve	Campbell's Low Sodium
Soup	Canned Ready to Serve	Campbell's Low Sodium
Soup	Canned Ready to Serve	Campbell's Low Sodium
Soup	Canned Ready to Serve	Campbell's Microwave
Soup	Canned Ready to Serve	Campbell's Microwave
Soup	Canned Ready to Serve	Chunky Weight Watchers
Soup	Canned Ready to Serve	College Inn
Soup	Canned Ready to Serve	College Inn
Soup	Canned Ready to Serve	Gold's
Soup	Canned Ready to Serve	Gold's
Soup	Canned Ready to Serve	Gold's
Soup	Canned Ready to Serve	Grandma Brown's
Soup	Canned Ready to Serve	Grandma Brown's
Soup	Canned Ready to Serve	Great Impressions
Soup	Canned Ready to Serve	Great Impressions
Soup	Canned Ready to Serve	Great Impressions
Soup	Canned Ready to Serve	Great Impressions
Soup	Canned Ready to Serve	Hain
Soup	Canned Ready to Serve	Hain
Soup	Canned Ready to Serve	Hain
Soup	Canned Ready to Serve	Hain
Soup	Canned Ready to Serve	Hain
Soup	Canned Ready to Serve	Hain
Soup	Canned Ready to Serve	Hain
Soup	Canned Ready to Serve	Hain
Soup	Canned Ready to Serve	Hain
Soup	Canned Ready to Serve	Hain
Soup	Canned Ready to Serve	Hain
Soup	Canned Ready to Serve	Hain
Soup	Canned Ready to Serve	Hain
Soup	Canned Ready to Serve	Hain
Soup	Canned Ready to Serve	Hain

Major Description	Minor Description	Serving Size	Calories	Grade
Vegetable Beef		8 oz	133	B
Bean with Ham	Chunky	8 oz	212	B–
Chicken	Chunky	8 oz	133	B–
Chicken	Chunky	8 oz	126	B–
Vegetable Beef		8 oz	140	B–
Bean with Ham		8 oz	155	B–
Beef with Vegetables		8 oz	104	A–
Chicken Gumbo with Sausage		8 oz	104	B–
Chicken Minestrone		8 oz	133	B–
Chicken with Noodles		8 oz	104	B–
Chicken Rice		8 oz	110	C–
Lentil	Hearty	8 oz	125	A–
Minestrone		8 oz	103	B–
Pea, Split with Ham		8 oz	170	A–
Tomato	Garden Style	8 oz	110	B–
Vegetable	Country Style	8 oz	88	A–
Vegetable Beef		8 oz	103	B–
Chicken Broth		8 oz	22	B–
Chicken with Noodles		8 oz	125	B
Mushroom, Cream of		8 oz	155	D
Pea, Split		8 oz	170	B
Tomato	Tomato Pieces	8 oz	140	B
Bean with Bacon & Ham		8 oz	245	B–
Vegetable Beef		8 oz	107	B–
Vegetable, Vegetarian		8 oz	74	B–
Beef Broth		8 oz	18	A–
Chicken Broth		8 oz	35	D–
Borscht		8 oz	100	A–
Borscht	Low Calorie	8 oz	20	A–
Schav		8 oz	25	A–
Bean		8 oz	190	B–+
Pea, Split		8 oz	208	B–+
Cherry Fruit		8 oz	160	A
Berry Fruit, Three		8 oz	139	A
Blueberry Fruit		8 oz	124	A
Lemon Fruit		8 oz	117	A
Chicken Broth		8 oz	70	D–
Chicken Broth	No Salt Added	8 oz	60	D–
Chicken Noodle		8 oz	100	B–
Chicken Noodle Soup	No Salt Added	8 oz	100	C
Chicken Vegetable Soup	No Salt Added	8 oz	100	B
Clam Chowder, New England		8 oz	155	B–
Lentil, Vegetarian		8 oz	134	B–
Minestrone		8 oz	143	A–
Minestrone	No Salt Added	8 oz	135	B
Mushroom Barley		8 oz	84	B–
Mushroom, Creamy		8 oz	95	C–
Pea, Split		8 oz	143	A–
Vegetarian Split Pea		8 oz	142	A–
Turkey Rice		8 oz	84	B–
Turkey Rice Soup	No Salt Added	8 oz	100	B
Veg Vegetable Soup	No Salt Added	8 oz	126	B
Vegetable Broth		8 oz	38	A–

"+" indicates the food meets minimum fiber requirements; "–" indicates the food has a high sodium content.

Food	Processing Category	Brand
Soup	Canned Ready to Serve	Hain
Soup	Canned Ready to Serve	Hain
Soup	Canned Ready to Serve	Hain
Soup	Canned Ready to Serve	Hain 99% Fat Free
Soup	Canned Ready to Serve	Hain 99% Fat Free
Soup	Canned Ready to Serve	Hain 99% Fat Free
Soup	Canned Ready to Serve	Hain 99% Fat Free
Soup	Canned Ready to Serve	Hain 99% Fat Free
Soup	Canned Ready to Serve	Hain 99% Fat Free
Soup	Canned Ready to Serve	Hain 99% Fat Free
Soup	Canned Ready to Serve	Hain 99% Fat Free
Soup	Canned Ready to Serve	Hain Low Sodium
Soup	Canned Ready to Serve	Hain Low Sodium
Soup	Canned Ready to Serve	Hain No Salt Added
Soup	Canned Ready to Serve	Hain No Salt Added
Soup	Canned Ready to Serve	Hain No Salt Added
Soup	Canned Ready to Serve	Hain No Salt Added
Soup	Canned Ready to Serve	Hain No Salt Added
Soup	Canned Ready to Serve	Hain No Salt Added
Soup	Canned Ready to Serve	Hain No Salt Added
Soup	Canned Ready to Serve	Hain No Salt Added
Soup	Canned Ready to Serve	Hain No Salt Added
Soup	Canned Ready to Serve	Health Valley
Soup	Canned Ready to Serve	Health Valley
Soup	Canned Ready to Serve	Health Valley
Soup	Canned Ready to Serve	Health Valley
Soup	Canned Ready to Serve	Health Valley
Soup	Canned Ready to Serve	Health Valley
Soup	Canned Ready to Serve	Health Valley
Soup	Canned Ready to Serve	Health Valley
Soup	Canned Ready to Serve	Health Valley
Soup	Canned Ready to Serve	Health Valley
Soup	Canned Ready to Serve	Health Valley
Soup	Canned Ready to Serve	Health Valley
Soup	Canned Ready to Serve	Health Valley
Soup	Canned Ready to Serve	Health Valley Fat Free
Soup	Canned Ready to Serve	Health Valley Fat Free
Soup	Canned Ready to Serve	Health Valley Fat Free
Soup	Canned Ready to Serve	Health Valley Fat Free
Soup	Canned Ready to Serve	Health Valley Fat Free
Soup	Canned Ready to Serve	Health Valley Fat Free
Soup	Canned Ready to Serve	Health Valley Fat Free
Soup	Canned Ready to Serve	Health Valley Fat Free
Soup	Canned Ready to Serve	Health Valley Fat Free
Soup	Canned Ready to Serve	Health Valley Fat Free
Soup	Canned Ready to Serve	Health Valley Fat Free
Soup	Canned Ready to Serve	Health Valley Fat Free
Soup	Canned Ready to Serve	Health Valley No Salt Added
Soup	Canned Ready to Serve	Health Valley No Salt Added
Soup	Canned Ready to Serve	Health Valley No Salt Added
Soup	Canned Ready to Serve	Health Valley No Salt Added
Soup	Canned Ready to Serve	Health Valley No Salt Added
Soup	Canned Ready to Serve	Health Valley No Salt Added

Major Description	Minor Description	Serving Size	Calories	Grade
Vegetable Chicken		8 oz	100	B–
Vegetable Pasta, Italian Style		8 oz	134	B–
Vegetable, Vegetarian		8 oz	118	B–
Black Bean		8 oz	107	A–+
Mushroom Barley		8 oz	75	B–
Vegetarian Lentil		8 oz	122	A–+
Vegetarian Lentil	No Salt Added	8 oz	115	A+
Vegetarian Split Pea		8 oz	137	A–+
Vegetarian Split Pea	No Salt Added	8 oz	130	A+
Vegetarian Vegetable Broth	No Salt Added	8 oz	38	A–
Wild Rice		8 oz	70	A–
Vegetable Broth		8 oz	34	B–
Vegetable Pasta, Italian Style		8 oz	118	C
Chicken Broth		8 oz	55	D–
Chicken Noodle		8 oz	100	B
Lentil, Vegetarian		8 oz	134	B
Minestrone		8 oz	134	B
Pea, Split		8 oz	143	A
Vegetarian Split Pea		8 oz	143	A
Turkey Rice		8 oz	100	B
Vegetable Chicken		8 oz	109	B
Vegetable, Vegetarian		8 oz	126	B
Beef Broth		8 oz	18	D–
Black Bean		8 oz	170	B–+
Chicken Broth		8 oz	37	D–
Chicken Vegetable	Chunky	8 oz	133	A–+
Clam Chowder, Manhattan		8 oz	117	B–+
Lentil		8 oz	180	A–+
Minestrone		8 oz	136	B–+
Mushroom Barley		8 oz	106	B–+
Pea, Split	Green	8 oz	100	A–+
Potato Leek		8 oz	138	A–+
Tomato		8 oz	11	D–+
Vegetable		8 oz	117	A–+
Vegetable	5 Bean, Chunky	8 oz	117	B–+
14 Garden Vegetables		8 oz	53	A–+
Beef Broth		8 oz	11	A–
Beef Broth	No Salt Added	8 oz	11	A
Black Bean	Vegetable	8 oz	74	A–+
Chicken Broth		8 oz	22	A–
Country-style Corn	Vegetable	8 oz	74	A–+
Five Bean	Vegetable	8 oz	106	A–+
Lentil	Carrots	8 oz	95	A–+
Minestrone	Italian Style	8 oz	85	A–+
Pea, Split	Carrots	8 oz	85	A–+
Tomato	Vegetable	8 oz	53	A–+
Vegetable Barley		8 oz	62	A–+
Beef Broth		8 oz	18	D
Black Bean		8 oz	166	B+
Chicken Broth		8 oz	37	D
Chicken Vegetable	Chunky	8 oz	133	A+
Clam Chowder, Manhattan		8 oz	117	B+
Lentil		8 oz	180	A+

"+" indicates the food meets minimum fiber requirements; "–" indicates the food has a high sodium content.

Food	Processing Category	Brand
Soup	Canned Ready to Serve	Health Valley No Salt Added
Soup	Canned Ready to Serve	Health Valley No Salt Added
Soup	Canned Ready to Serve	Health Valley No Salt Added
Soup	Canned Ready to Serve	Health Valley No Salt Added
Soup	Canned Ready to Serve	Health Valley No Salt Added
Soup	Canned Ready to Serve	Health Valley No Salt Added
Soup	Canned Ready to Serve	Health Valley No Salt Added
Soup	Canned Ready to Serve	Healthy Choice
Soup	Canned Ready to Serve	Healthy Choice
Soup	Canned Ready to Serve	Healthy Choice
Soup	Canned Ready to Serve	Healthy Choice
Soup	Canned Ready to Serve	Healthy Choice
Soup	Canned Ready to Serve	Healthy Choice
Soup	Canned Ready to Serve	Healthy Choice
Soup	Canned Ready to Serve	Healthy Choice
Soup	Canned Ready to Serve	Healthy Choice
Soup	Canned Ready to Serve	Healthy Choice
Soup	Canned Ready to Serve	Healthy Choice
Soup	Canned Ready to Serve	Healthy Choice
Soup	Canned Ready to Serve	Healthy Choice
Soup	Canned Ready to Serve	Healthy Choice
Soup	Canned Ready to Serve	Healthy Choice
Soup	Canned Ready to Serve	Healthy Choice
Soup	Canned Ready to Serve	Healthy Choice
Soup	Canned Ready to Serve	Hormel Micro Cup Hearty Soups
Soup	Canned Ready to Serve	Hormel Micro-Cup Hearty Soups
Soup	Canned Ready to Serve	Hormel Micro-Cup Hearty Soups
Soup	Canned Ready to Serve	Hormel Micro-Cup Hearty Soups
Soup	Canned Ready to Serve	Hormel Micro-Cup Hearty Soups
Soup	Canned Ready to Serve	Hormel Micro-Cup Hearty Soups
Soup	Canned Ready to Serve	Hormel Micro-Cup Hearty Soups
Soup	Canned Ready to Serve	Lipton Hearty Ones
Soup	Canned Ready to Serve	Lipton Hearty Ones
Soup	Canned Ready to Serve	Lipton Hearty Ones Homestyle
Soup	Canned Ready to Serve	Manischewitz
Soup	Canned Ready to Serve	Manischewitz
Soup	Canned Ready to Serve	Old El Paso
Soup	Canned Ready to Serve	Old El Paso
Soup	Canned Ready to Serve	Old El Paso
Soup	Canned Ready to Serve	Old El Paso
Soup	Canned Ready to Serve	Old El Paso
Soup	Canned Ready to Serve	Old El Paso
Soup	Canned Ready to Serve	Pritikin
Soup	Canned Ready to Serve	Pritikin
Soup	Canned Ready to Serve	Pritikin
Soup	Canned Ready to Serve	Pritikin
Soup	Canned Ready to Serve	Pritikin
Soup	Canned Ready to Serve	Pritikin
Soup	Canned Ready to Serve	Pritikin
Soup	Canned Ready to Serve	Pritikin
Soup	Canned Ready to Serve	Pritikin
Soup	Canned Ready to Serve	Pritikin
Soup	Canned Ready to Serve	Pritikin

Major Description	Minor Description	Serving Size	Calories	Grade
Minestrone		8 oz	138	B+
Mushroom Barley		8 oz	106	B+
Pea, Split	Green	8 oz	200	A+
Potato Leek		8 oz	138	A+
Tomato		8 oz	106	B
Vegetable		8 oz	117	A+
Vegetable	5 Bean, Chunky	8 oz	117	B+
Bean & Ham		8 oz	233	B–
Beef	Hearty	8 oz	127	A–
Beef & Potato		8 oz	117	A–
Chicken	Hearty	8 oz	117	B–
Chicken	Rice	8 oz	95	A–
Chicken Noodle	Old Fashioned	8 oz	95	B–
Chicken Pasta		8 oz	106	B–
Chili Beef		8 oz	159	A–
Garden-style Vegetable		8 oz	106	A–
Lentil		8 oz	148	A–
Minestrone		8 oz	166	A–
Pea, Split with Ham		8 oz	180	B–
Tomato, Garden Style		8 oz	138	B–
Turkey	Vegetables	8 oz	117	B–
Turkey	White & Wild Rice	8 oz	106	B–
Vegetable	Country Style	8 oz	127	A–
Vegetable Beef		8 oz	138	A–
Bean with Ham	Chowder	8 oz.	191	A–
Beef Vegetable		8 oz.	71	A–
Chicken Noodle		8 oz.	108	B–
Chicken Vegetable	Rice	8 oz.	114	B–
Clam Chowder, New England		8 oz.	118	C–
Minestrone		8 oz.	104	B–
Vegetable	Country Style	8 oz.	89	B–
Beef Vegetable		8 oz	165	A–
Minestrone		8 oz	137	B–
Chicken Noodle		8 oz	163	B–
Borscht	Beets	8 oz	80	A–
Borscht	Low Calorie	8 oz	20	A–
Beef	Hearty	8 oz	120	B–
Black Bean	Bacon	8 oz	160	A–+
Chicken	Hearty	8 oz	110	B–
Chicken	Rice	8 oz	90	B–
Chicken	Vegetable	8 oz	110	B–
Vegetable	Garden Style	8 oz	110	B–
Chicken	Broth	1 cup	15	A–
Chicken	Pasta	1 cup	100	A–
Chicken	Rice	1 cup	80	A–+
Chili	3 Bean	1 cup	180	A–+
Lentil		1 cup	130	A–+
Minestrone		1 cup	90	A–+
Pea, Split		1 cup	140	A–+
Three Bean		1 cup	180	A–+
Vegetable	Broth	1 cup	20	A–
Vegetable	Hearty	1 cup	90	A–+
Vegetable	Vegetarian	1 cup	100	A–+

"+" indicates the food meets minimum fiber requirements; "–" indicates the food has a high sodium content.

Food	Processing Category	Brand
Soup	Canned Ready to Serve	Progresso
Soup	Canned Ready to Serve	Progresso
Soup	Canned Ready to Serve	Progresso
Soup	Canned Ready to Serve	Progresso
Soup	Canned Ready to Serve	Progresso
Soup	Canned Ready to Serve	Progresso
Soup	Canned Ready to Serve	Progresso
Soup	Canned Ready to Serve	Progresso
Soup	Canned Ready to Serve	Progresso
Soup	Canned Ready to Serve	Progresso
Soup	Canned Ready to Serve	Progresso
Soup	Canned Ready to Serve	Progresso
Soup	Canned Ready to Serve	Progresso
Soup	Canned Ready to Serve	Progresso
Soup	Canned Ready to Serve	Progresso
Soup	Canned Ready to Serve	Progresso
Soup	Canned Ready to Serve	Progresso
Soup	Canned Ready to Serve	Progresso
Soup	Canned Ready to Serve	Progresso
Soup	Canned Ready to Serve	Progresso
Soup	Canned Ready to Serve	Progresso
Soup	Canned Ready to Serve	Progresso
Soup	Canned Ready to Serve	Progresso
Soup	Canned Ready to Serve	Progresso
Soup	Canned Ready to Serve	Progresso
Soup	Canned Ready to Serve	Progresso
Soup	Canned Ready to Serve	Progresso
Soup	Canned Ready to Serve	Progresso
Soup	Canned Ready to Serve	Progresso
Soup	Canned Ready to Serve	Progresso
Soup	Canned Ready to Serve	Progresso
Soup	Canned Ready to Serve	Progresso
Soup	Canned Ready to Serve	Progresso
Soup	Canned Ready to Serve	Progresso
Soup	Canned Ready to Serve	Progresso
Soup	Canned Ready to Serve	Progresso
Soup	Canned Ready to Serve	Progresso
Soup	Canned Ready to Serve	Progresso
Soup	Canned Ready to Serve	Progresso
Soup	Canned Ready to Serve	Progresso
Soup	Canned Ready to Serve	Progresso
Soup	Canned Ready to Serve	Progresso
Soup	Canned Ready to Serve	Progresso
Soup	Canned Ready to Serve	Progresso
Soup	Canned Ready to Serve	Progresso Healthy Classics
Soup	Canned Ready to Serve	Progresso Healthy Classics
Soup	Canned Ready to Serve	Progresso Healthy Classics
Soup	Canned Ready to Serve	Progresso Healthy Classics
Soup	Canned Ready to Serve	Progresso Healthy Classics
Soup	Canned Ready to Serve	Progresso Healthy Classics
Soup	Canned Ready to Serve	Progresso Healthy Classics
Soup	Canned Ready to Serve	Progresso Homestyle

Major Description	Minor Description	Serving Size	Calories	Grade
Beef		8 oz	138	B–
Beef	Hearty	8 oz	134	B–
Beef Barley		8 oz	118	B–+
Beef Barley		8 oz	114	B–+
Beef Broth	Seasoned	8 oz	20	A–
Beef Minestrone		8 oz	138	B–
Beef Noodle		8 oz	144	B–
Beef Vegetable		8 oz	129	B–
Beef Vegetable	Pasta	8 oz	106	B–+
Black Bean	Hearty	8 oz	118	A–+
Chickarina		8 oz	109	C–
Chicken	Hearty	8 oz	99	B–
Chicken	Pasta, Hearty	8 oz	109	B–
Chicken Barley		8 oz	85	B–+
Chicken Broth		8 oz	16	A–
Chicken Minestrone		8 oz	106	B–
Chicken Noodle		8 oz	91	B–
Chicken Rice		8 oz	91	B–
Chicken Vegetable		8 oz	118	B–
Chicken, Cream of		8 oz	160	D–
Clam Chowder, Manhattan		8 oz	100	A–
Clam Chowder, New England		8 oz	167	D–
Corn Chowder		8 oz	170	D–
Escarole	In Chicken Broth	8 oz	26	B–
Ham & Bean		8 oz	119	A–+
Lentil		8 oz	106	A–+
Lentil	Sausage	8 oz	143	C–+
Lentil & Shells		8 oz	126	A–
Lentil with Sausage		8 oz	143	D–+
Macaroni & Bean		8 oz	114	B–+
Minestrone		8 oz	91	B–+
Minestrone	Hearty	8 oz	126	B–+
Minestrone & Shells	Hearty	8 oz	76	B–
Mushroom, Cream of		8 oz	136	D–
Penne in Chicken	Hearty	8 oz	67	A–
Pea, Split	Green	8 oz	152	A–
Pea, Split with Ham		8 oz	122	B–+
Tomato		8 oz	101	B–
Tomato	Tortellini	8 oz	111	C–
Tomato & Rotini	Hearty	8 oz	84	A–
Tomato Beef with Rotini		8 oz	144	C–
Tortellini		8 oz	76	B–
Tortellini, Creamy		8 oz	204	D–
Vegetable		8 oz	67	B–+
Vegetable & Rotini	Hearty	8 oz	84	A–+
Beef Barley		8 oz	140	B–
Chicken Noodle		8 oz	80	B–
Chicken Rice	Vegetables	8 oz	80	B–
Clam Chowder, New England		8 oz	110	B–
Lentil		8 oz	120	A–
Minestrone		8 oz	120	A–
Vegetable		8 oz	80	A–
Chicken		8 oz	92	B–

"+" indicates the food meets minimum fiber requirements; "–" indicates the food has a high sodium content.

Food	Processing Category	Brand
Soup	Canned Ready to Serve	Rokeach
Soup	Canned Ready to Serve	Rokeach, Diet
Soup	Canned Ready to Serve	Rokeach, Unsalted
Soup	Canned Ready to Serve	Swanson
Soup	Canned Ready to Serve	Swanson
Soup	Canned Ready to Serve	Swanson Natural Goodness
Soup	Canned Ready to Serve	Weight Watchers
Soup	Canned Ready to Serve	Weight Watchers
Soup	Canned Ready to Serve	Weight Watchers
Soup	Canned Ready to Serve	Weight Watchers
Soup	Canned Ready to Serve	Weight Watchers
Soup	Canned Ready to Serve	Weight Watchers
Soup	Canned Ready to Serve	Weight Watchers
Soup	Frozen	Kettle Ready
Soup	Frozen	Kettle Ready
Soup	Frozen	Kettle Ready
Soup	Frozen	Kettle Ready
Soup	Frozen	Kettle Ready
Soup	Frozen	Kettle Ready
Soup	Frozen	Kettle Ready
Soup	Frozen	Kettle Ready
Soup	Frozen	Kettle Ready
Soup	Frozen	Kettle Ready
Soup	Frozen	Kettle Ready
Soup	Frozen	Kettle Ready
Soup	Frozen	Kettle Ready
Soup	Frozen	Kettle Ready
Soup	Frozen	Kettle Ready
Soup	Frozen	Kettle Ready
Soup	Frozen	Kettle Ready
Soup	Frozen	Kettle Ready
Soup	Frozen	Kettle Ready
Soup	Frozen	Kettle Ready
Soup	Frozen	Kettle Ready
Soup	Frozen	Kettle Ready
Soup	Frozen	Myer's
Soup	Frozen	Myer's
Soup	Frozen	Myer's
Soup	Frozen	Myer's
Soup	Frozen	Myer's
Soup	Frozen	Myer's
Soup	Frozen	Myer's
Soup	Frozen	Myer's
Soup	Frozen	Stouffer's
Soup	Frozen	Stouffer's
Soup	Frozen	Tabatchnick
Soup	Frozen	Tabatchnick
Soup	Frozen	Tabatchnick
Soup	Frozen	Tabatchnick
Soup	Frozen	Tabatchnick
Soup	Frozen	Tabatchnick
Soup	Frozen	Tabatchnick

Major Description	Minor Description	Serving Size	Calories	Grade
Borscht		8 oz	96	A–
Borscht		8 oz	29	A–+
Borscht		8 oz	103	A
Beef Broth		8 oz	20	D–
Chicken Broth		8 oz	33	D–
Chicken Broth		8 oz	22	D–
Chicken Noodle		8 oz	61	B–
Chunky Beef Stew		7.5 oz	120	A–+
Clam Chowder, New England		7.5 oz	90	A–+
Mushroom, Cream of		8 oz	68	B–
Turkey Vegetable		8 oz	53	B–
Vegetable	Beef Stock	8 oz	68	B–
Vegetable Beef		7.5 oz	80	A–
Asparagus, Cream of		6 oz	62	D–
Bean	Black, with Ham	6 oz	154	C–
Bean	Savory, with Ham	6 oz	113	B–
Beef, Hearty Vegetable		6 oz	85	C–
Broccoli, Cream of		6 oz	94	D–
Cauliflower, Cream of		6 oz	93	D–
Cheddar Cheese	Broccoli, Cream of	6 oz	137	D–
Cheddar Cheese, Cream of		6 oz	158	D–
Chicken Gumbo		6 oz	94	C–
Chicken Noodle		6 oz	94	B–
Chicken, Cream of		6 oz	98	D–
Chili, Jalapeño		6 oz	173	D–
Chili, Traditional		6 oz	161	C–
Clam Chowder, Boston		6 oz	131	D–
Clam Chowder, Manhattan		6 oz	69	C–
Clam Chowder, New England		6 oz	116	D–
Corn & Broccoli Chowder		6 oz	102	D–
French Onion		6 oz	42	D–
Minestrone, Hearty		6 oz	104	C–
Mushroom, Cream of		6 oz	85	D–
Pea	Tortellini in Tomato Sauce	6 oz	122	C–
Pea, Split with Ham		6 oz	155	B–
Vegetable Garden		6 oz	85	C–
Asparagus, Cream of		8 oz	125	D–
Broccoli, Cream of		8 oz	143	D–
Cheese & Broccoli		8 oz	266	D–
Chicken	Noodle	8 oz	71	D–
Clam Chowder, New England		8 oz	125	B–
Seafood Bisque		8 oz	134	D–
Spinach, Cream of		8 oz	142	D–
Vegetable Beef		8 oz	100	D–
Clam Chowder, New England		8 oz	180	D–
Spinach, Cream of		8 oz	210	D–
Barley & Bean		8 oz	138	A–
Bean	Northern Style	8 oz	175	A–
Broccoli, Cream of		8 oz	96	C–
Cabbage		8 oz	117	B–
Chicken		8 oz	69	B–
Lentil		8 oz	181	A–
Minestrone		8 oz	146	A–

"+" indicates the food meets minimum fiber requirements; "–" indicates the food has a high sodium content.

Food	Processing Category	Brand
Soup	Frozen	Tabatchnick
Soup	Frozen	Tabatchnick
Soup	Frozen	Tabatchnick
Soup	Frozen	Tabatchnick
Soup	Frozen	Tabatchnick
Soup	Frozen	Tabatchnick
Soup	Frozen	Tabatchnick
Soup	Frozen	Tabatchnick
Soup	Frozen	Tabatchnick No Salt
Soup	Frozen	Tabatchnick No Salt
Soup	Frozen	Tabatchnick No Salt
Soup	Mix	Generic
Soup	Mix	Generic
Soup	Mix	Generic
Soup	Mix	Generic
Soup	Mix	Generic
Soup	Mix	Generic
Soup	Mix	Generic
Soup	Mix	Generic
Soup	Mix	Generic
Soup	Mix	Generic
Soup	Mix	Generic
Soup	Mix	Generic
Soup	Mix	Generic
Soup	Mix	Generic
Soup	Mix	Generic
Soup	Mix	Generic
Soup	Mix	Generic
Soup	Mix	Generic
Soup	Mix	Generic
Soup	Mix	Generic
Soup	Mix	Generic
Soup	Mix	Campbell's Cup 2 Minute Soup
Soup	Mix	Campbell's Cup 2 Minute Soup
Soup	Mix	Campbell's Cup 2 Minute Soup
Soup	Mix	Campbell's Cup Microwave
Soup	Mix	Campbell's Cup Microwave
Soup	Mix	Campbell's Cup Microwave
Soup	Mix	Campbell's Cup Microwave
Soup	Mix	Campbell's Cup-A-Ramen
Soup	Mix	Campbell's Cup-A-Ramen
Soup	Mix	Campbell's Cup-A-Ramen
Soup	Mix	Campbell's Cup-A-Ramen Low Fat
Soup	Mix	Campbell's Cup-A-Ramen Low Fat
Soup	Mix	Campbell's Cup-A-Ramen Low Fat
Soup	Mix	Campbell's Quality Recipe
Soup	Mix	Campbell's Quality Recipe
Soup	Mix	Campbell's Quality Recipe
Soup	Mix	Campbell's Quality Recipe
Soup	Mix	Campbell's Quality Recipe

Major Description	Minor Description	Serving Size	Calories	Grade
Mushroom Barley		8 oz	98	B–
Mushroom, Cream of		8 oz	100	B–
New England Chowder		8 oz	104	B–
Pea		8 oz	187	A–
Spinach, Cream of		8 oz	90	B–
Tomato Rice		8 oz	98	A–
Vegetable		8 oz	103	A–
Zucchini		8 oz	106	B–
Mushroom Barley		8 oz	103	A
Pea		8 oz	187	A
Vegetable		8 oz	98	B
Asparagus, Cream of		1 cup	59	B–
Bean with Bacon		1 cup	105	B–
Beef or Beef Flavor	Broth or Bouillon	1 cup	19	C–
Beef or Beef Flavor	Noodle	1 cup	41	B–
Cauliflower		1 cup	68	B–
Celery, Cream of		1 cup	63	B–
Chicken or Chicken Flavor	Broth or Bouillon	1 cup	21	D–
Chicken or Chicken Flavor	Cream of	1 cup	107	D–
Chicken or Chicken Flavor	Noodle	1 cup	53	B–
Chicken or Chicken Flavor	Rice	1 cup	60	B–
Chicken or Chicken Flavor	Vegetable	1 cup	49	A–
Consommé with Gelatin		1 cup	17	A–
Pea, Green or Split		1 cup	133	A–
Leek		1 cup	71	B–
Minestrone		1 cup	79	B–
Mushroom		1 cup	96	D–
Onion		1 cup	28	B–
Oxtail		1 cup	71	C–
Tomato		1 cup	102	B–
Tomato	Vegetable	1 cup	55	A–
Vegetable Beef		1 cup	53	B–
Vegetable, Cream of		1 cup	105	D–
Chicken or Chicken Flavor	Creamy with White Meat	1 cup	110	C–
Chicken or Chicken Flavor	Noodle with White Meat	1 cup	110	B–
Noodle	with Chicken Broth	1 cup	110	B–
Beef or Beef Flavor		1 container	130	A–
Chicken or Chicken Flavor	Noodle	1 container	140	B–
Hearty Vegetable	with Noodles	1 container	180	A–
Noodle	with Chicken Broth	1 container	130	A–
Beef or Beef Flavor	Vegetables	1 cup	270	C–
Chicken or Chicken Flavor	Noodle with Vegetables	1 cup	270	C–
Shrimp Flavor	Vegetables	1 cup	280	C–
Beef or Beef Flavor	Vegetables	1 cup	220	A–
Chicken or Chicken Flavor	Noodle with Vegetables	1 cup	220	A–
Shrimp Flavor	Vegetables	1 cup	230	A–
Chicken or Chicken Flavor	Noodle	1 cup	100	B–
Hearty Noodle		1 cup	90	A–
Noodle		1 cup	110	B–
Onion		1 cup	30	A–
Vegetable		1 cup	40	A–

"+" indicates the food meets minimum fiber requirements; "–" indicates the food has a high sodium content.

Food	Processing Category	Brand
Soup	Mix	Campbell's Ramen Noodle
Soup	Mix	Campbell's Ramen Noodle
Soup	Mix	Campbell's Ramen Noodle
Soup	Mix	Campbell's Ramen Noodle
Soup	Mix	Campbell's Ramen Noodle Low Fat
Soup	Mix	Campbell's Ramen Noodle Low Fat
Soup	Mix	Campbell's Ramen Noodle Low Fat
Soup	Mix	Campbell's Ramen Noodle Low Fat
Soup	Mix	Country Cup O'Noodles Hearty
Soup	Mix	Cup O'Noodles
Soup	Mix	Cup O'Noodles
Soup	Mix	Cup O'Noodles
Soup	Mix	Cup O'Noodles Hearty
Soup	Mix	Cup O'Noodles Hearty
Soup	Mix	Cup O'Noodles Hearty
Soup	Mix	Estee
Soup	Mix	Estee
Soup	Mix	Estee Instant
Soup	Mix	Estee Instant
Soup	Mix	Estee Instant
Soup	Mix	Fantastic Foods
Soup	Mix	Fantastic Foods
Soup	Mix	Fantastic Foods
Soup	Mix	Fantastic Foods
Soup	Mix	Fantastic Foods
Soup	Mix	Fantastic Foods
Soup	Mix	Fantastic Foods
Soup	Mix	Fantastic Foods
Soup	Mix	Fantastic Foods
Soup	Mix	Fantastic Foods
Soup	Mix	Fantastic Foods
Soup	Mix	Fantastic Foods
Soup	Mix	Fantastic Foods
Soup	Mix	Fantastic Foods
Soup	Mix	Fantastic Foods
Soup	Mix	Fantastic Foods
Soup	Mix	Fantastic Foods
Soup	Mix	Fantastic Foods
Soup	Mix	Golden Dipt
Soup	Mix	Golden Dipt
Soup	Mix	Golden Dipt
Soup	Mix	Golden Dipt
Soup	Mix	Golden Dipt
Soup	Mix	Hain Savory Soup & Recipe Mix
Soup	Mix	Hain Savory Soup & Recipe Mix
Soup	Mix	Hain Savory Soup & Recipe Mix No Salt
Soup	Mix	Hain Savory Soup & Sauce Mix
Soup	Mix	Hain Savory Soup Dip & Recipe Mix
Soup	Mix	Hain Savory Soup Dip & Recipe Mix
Soup	Mix	Hain Savory Soup Mix

Major Description	Minor Description	Serving Size	Calories	Grade
Beef or Beef Flavor		1 cup	190	C–
Chicken or Chicken Flavor	Noodle	1 cup	190	C–
Oriental Style		1 cup	190	C–
Pork Flavor		1 cup	200	C–
Beef or Beef Flavor		1 cup	160	A–
Chicken or Chicken Flavor		1 cup	160	A–
Oriental Style		1 cup	150	A–
Pork Flavor		1 cup	150	A–
Chicken or Chicken Flavor		1 cup	300	D–
Beef		1 cup	290	D–
Chicken or Chicken Flavor		1 cup	300	D–
Shrimp		1 cup	300	D–
Seafood, Savory		1 cup	300	D–
Vegetable Beef		1 cup	290	D–
Vegetable, Old Fashioned		1 cup	290	D–
Beef or Beef Flavor		1 cup	27	D–
Onion		1 cup	33	C–
Chicken or Chicken Flavor	Noodle	1 cup	33	C–
Mushroom		1 cup	53	D–
Tomato		1 cup	53	B–
Black Bean		1 cup	170	A–+
Broccoli & Cheddar		1 cup	150	A–+
Cheddar, Creamy	with Noodles	1 cup	178	D–
Chicken Free	with Noodles	1 cup	140	A–+
Chili		1 cup	200	A–+
Corn & Potato Chowder		1 cup	160	A–
Couscous	Lentils	1 cup	220	A–+
Five Bean		1 cup	200	A–+
Lentil	Country	1 cup	200	A–+
Minestrone		1 cup	130	A–+
Mushroom		1 cup	130	A–+
Pea, Split		1 cup	160	A–
Tomato Rice	Parmesan	1 cup	190	A–
Vegetable Barley		1 cup	140	A–+
Vegetable, Curry	with Noodles	1 cup	140	A–+
Vegetable, Curry	with Noodles	1 cup	150	D–
Vegetable, Miso	with Noodles	1 cup	152	C–
Vegetable, Miso	with Noodles	1 cup	130	A–+
Vegetable, Tomato	with Noodles	1 cup	150	A–+
Vegetable, Tomato	with Noodles	1 cup	158	D–
Clam Chowder, Manhattan		1/4 pkg	80	B–
Clam Chowder, New England		1/4 pkg	70	B–
Lobster Bisque		1/4 pkg	30	B–
Seafood Chowder		1/4 pkg	70	B–
Shrimp Bisque		1/4 pkg	30	B–
Mushroom		6 oz	210	D–
Tomato		6 oz	220	D–
Mushroom		6 oz	250	D
Cheese		6 oz	250	D–
Onion		6 oz	50	C–
Onion		6 oz	50	B–
Lentil		6 oz	130	A–

"+" indicates the food meets minimum fiber requirements; "–" indicates the food has a high sodium content.

Food	Processing Category	Brand
Soup	Mix	Hain Savory Soup Mix
Soup	Mix	Hain Savory Soup Mix
Soup	Mix	Hain Savory Soup Mix
Soup	Mix	Hain Savory Soup Mix
Soup	Mix	Hain Savory Soup Mix No Salt Added
Soup	Mix	Hain Soup & Recipe Mix
Soup	Mix	Hearty Lipton
Soup	Mix	Hearty Lipton Lots-a-Noodles
Soup	Mix	Hearty Lipton Lots-a-Noodles
Soup	Mix	Knorr
Soup	Mix	Knorr
Soup	Mix	Knorr
Soup	Mix	Knorr
Soup	Mix	Knorr
Soup	Mix	Knorr
Soup	Mix	Knorr
Soup	Mix	Knorr
Soup	Mix	Knorr
Soup	Mix	Knorr
Soup	Mix	Knorr
Soup	Mix	Knorr Cup-a-Soup
Soup	Mix	Knorr Cup-a-Soup
Soup	Mix	Knorr Cup-a-Soup
Soup	Mix	Knorr Cup-a-Soup
Soup	Mix	Knorr Cup-a-Soup
Soup	Mix	Knorr Cup-a-Soup
Soup	Mix	Lipton
Soup	Mix	Lipton
Soup	Mix	Lipton
Soup	Mix	Lipton
Soup	Mix	Lipton
Soup	Mix	Lipton
Soup	Mix	Lipton
Soup	Mix	Lipton
Soup	Mix	Lipton
Soup	Mix	Lipton
Soup	Mix	Lipton
Soup	Mix	Lipton
Soup	Mix	Lipton
Soup	Mix	Lipton Cup-a-Soup
Soup	Mix	Lipton Cup-a-Soup
Soup	Mix	Lipton Cup-a-Soup
Soup	Mix	Lipton Cup-a-Soup
Soup	Mix	Lipton Cup-a-Soup
Soup	Mix	Lipton Cup-a-Soup
Soup	Mix	Lipton Cup-a-Soup
Soup	Mix	Lipton Cup-a-Soup
Soup	Mix	Lipton Cup-a-Soup
Soup	Mix	Lipton Cup-a-Soup
Soup	Mix	Lipton Cup-a-Soup

Major Description	Minor Description	Serving Size	Calories	Grade
Minestrone		6 oz	110	A–
Potato Leek		6 oz	260	D–
Pea, Split		6 oz	310	B–
Vegetable		6 oz	80	A–
Vegetable		6 oz	80	A–
Cheese & Broccoli		6 oz	310	D–
Chicken or Chicken Flavor	Noodle	1 cup	83	A–
Chicken or Chicken Flavor	Noodle	1 cup	125	A–
Chicken or Chicken Flavor	Noodle	1 cup	135	A–
Bouillabaisse		1 cup	28	C–
Clam Chowder, New England		1 cup	100	C–
Fine Herb	in Water	1 cup	110	D–
Leek	in Water	1 cup	70	B–
Oriental Style Hot & Sour	in Water	1 cup	50	B–
Oxtail Hearty Beef	in Water	1 cup	70	B–
Shrimp Bisque		1 cup	70	D–
Snow Pea, Cream of		1 cup	80	B–
Spring Vegetable & Herbs	in Water	1 cup	30	A–
Tomato Basil	in Water	1 cup	90	B–
Vegetable	in Water	1 cup	35	B–
Black Bean		1¼ cup	160	A–+
Lentil		1¼ cup	176	A–+
Minestrone	Hearty	1¼ cup	120	A–
Navy Bean		1¼ cup	112	A–+
Potato Leek		1¼ cup	96	A–
Vegetable	Chicken Flavor	1¼ cup	80	A–
Beef Flavor	Mushroom	1 cup	38	A–
Beef Noodle	with Vegetables	1 cup	75	B–
Beef or Beef Flavor	Hearty & Noodles	1 cup	107	A–
Chicken or Chicken Flavor	Noodle	1 cup	81	B–
Chicken or Chicken Flavor	Noodle with Vegetables	1 cup	75	B–
Chicken or Chicken Flavor	Noodle with White Meat	1 cup	81	B–
Hearty Noodle	Beef with Vegetables	1 cup	85	A–
Onion		1 cup	20	A–
Onion	Beef	1 cup	29	C–
Onion	Golden with Chicken Broth	1 cup	62	B–
Onion	Mushroom	1 cup	41	B–
Vegetable		1 cup	39	A–
Vegetable	Country Style	1 cup	80	A–
Beef or Beef Flavor		6 oz	44	A–
Broccoli	Cheese	6 oz	70	D–
Broccoli	Creamy	6 oz	62	C–
Chicken or Chicken Flavor	Broth	6 oz	20	B–
Chicken or Chicken Flavor	Cream of	6 oz	84	D–
Chicken or Chicken Flavor	Creamy, with Vegetables	6 oz	93	B–
Chicken or Chicken Flavor	Hearty Supreme	6 oz	107	D–
Chicken or Chicken Flavor	Noodle	6 oz	48	B–
Chicken or Chicken Flavor	Noodle with Meat	6 oz	46	B–
Chicken or Chicken Flavor	Rice	6 oz	47	B–
Chicken or Chicken Flavor	Vegetable	6 oz	47	A–

"+" indicates the food meets minimum fiber requirements; "–" indicates the food has a high sodium content.

Food	Processing Category	Brand
Soup	Mix	Lipton Cup-a-Soup
Soup	Mix	Lipton Cup-a-Soup
Soup	Mix	Lipton Cup-a-Soup
Soup	Mix	Lipton Cup-a-Soup
Soup	Mix	Lipton Cup-a-Soup
Soup	Mix	Lipton Cup-a-Soup
Soup	Mix	Lipton Cup-a-Soup Country Style
Soup	Mix	Lipton Cup-a-Soup Country Style
Soup	Mix	Lipton Cup-a-Soup Country Style
Soup	Mix	Lipton Cup-a-Soup Country Style
Soup	Mix	Lipton Cup-a-Soup Country Style
Soup	Mix	Lipton Cup-a-Soup Country Style
Soup	Mix	Lipton Cup-a-Soup Country Style
Soup	Mix	Lipton Cup-a-Soup Country Style
Soup	Mix	Lipton Cup-a-Soup Food Service
Soup	Mix	Lipton Cup-a-Soup Food Service
Soup	Mix	Lipton Cup-a-Soup Food Service
Soup	Mix	Lipton Cup-a-Soup Food Service
Soup	Mix	Lipton Cup-a-Soup Lite
Soup	Mix	Lipton Cup-a-Soup Lite
Soup	Mix	Lipton Cup-a-Soup Lite
Soup	Mix	Lipton Cup-a-Soup Lite
Soup	Mix	Lipton Cup-a-Soup Lite
Soup	Mix	Lipton Cup-a-Soup Ring Noodle
Soup	Mix	Lipton Giggle Noodle
Soup	Mix	Lipton Lots-a-Noodles Cup-a-Soup
Soup	Mix	Lipton Lots-a-Noodles Cup-a-Soup
Soup	Mix	Lipton Ring-O-Noodle
Soup	Mix	Manischewitz
Soup	Mix	Manischewitz
Soup	Mix	Manischewitz
Soup	Mix	Mrs. Grass Chickeny Rich
Soup	Mix	Mrs. Grass Soup & Dip Mix
Soup	Mix	Nile Spice Soups in a Cup
Soup	Mix	Nile Spice Soups in a Cup
Soup	Mix	Nile Spice Soups in a Cup
Soup	Mix	Nile Spice Soups in a Cup
Soup	Mix	Nile Spice Soups in a Cup
Soup	Mix	Nile Spice Soups in a Cup
Soup	Mix	Nile Spice Soups in a Cup
Soup	Mix	Nile Spice Soups in a Cup
Soup	Mix	Nile Spice Soups in a Cup
Soup	Mix	Nile Spice Soups in a Cup
Soup	Mix	Nile Spice Soups in a Cup
Soup	Mix	Nile Spice Soups in a Cup
Soup	Mix	Nile Spice Soups in a Cup
Soup	Mix	Nile Spice Soups in a Cup
Soup	Mix	Nile Spice Soups in a Cup
Soup	Mix	Nile Spice Soups in a Cup
Soup	Mix	Nile Spice Soups in a Cup
Soup	Mix	Nile Spice Soups in a Cup

Major Description	Minor Description	Serving Size	Calories	Grade
Mushroom, Cream of		6 oz	71	D–
Onion		6 oz	27	B–
Onion, Creamy		6 oz	70	C–
Pea, Green		6 oz	113	C–
Tomato		6 oz	103	A–
Vegetable	Spring Style	6 oz	33	B–
Chicken or Chicken Flavor		6 oz	107	D–
Chicken or Chicken Flavor	Hearty	6 oz	69	A–
Chicken or Chicken Flavor	with Sweet Corn	6 oz	133	C–
Pea	Virginia Style	6 oz	113	C–
Pea	Virginia Style	6 oz	148	C–
Vegetable	Harvest Style	6 oz	91	A–
Vegetable	Harvest Style	6 oz	95	A–
Vegetable	Noodle with Meatballs	6 oz	95	B–
Broccoli, Creamy		6 oz	62	C–
Chicken or Chicken Flavor, Cream of		6 oz	84	D–
Pea, Green		6 oz	115	C–
Tomato		6 oz	100	A–
Broccoli, Golden		6 oz	42	B–
Chicken or Chicken Flavor	Florentine Style	6 oz	42	A–
Chicken or Chicken Flavor	Lemon	6 oz	48	A–
Oriental		6 oz	45	C–
Tomato	Creamy Herb	6 oz	66	A–
		6 oz	47	A–
		1 cup	77	B–
Chicken or Chicken Flavor	Hearty Noodle, Creamy	7 oz	179	D–
Vegetable	Garden Style	7 oz	123	A–
		1 cup	71	B–
Minestrone		6 oz	50	B–
Pea, Split		6 oz	45	B–
Vegetable		6 oz	50	B–
Chicken or Chicken Flavor	Noodle	1/4 pkg	70	B–
Onion		1/4 pkg	35	B–
Almondine		1 container	200	A–
Black Bean		1 container	190	A–
Chicken Vegetable		1 container	120	A–
Chili	Original	1 container	150	A–+
Chili	Spicy	1 container	150	A–+
Garbanzo		1 container	220	A–
Italian Tomato		1 container	140	B–
Lentil		1 container	180	A–+
Lentil Curry		1 container	200	A–+
Minestrone		1 container	160	A–+
Pasta	Mediterranean Style	1 container	210	B–
Pasta	Parmesan Cheese	1 container	200	A–
Pasta	Primavera	1 container	200	B–
Potato Leek		1 container	150	C–
Potato Romano		1 container	140	C–+
Red Bean	Rice	1 container	190	A–+
Pea, Split		1 container	200	A–+
Sweet Corn Chowder		1 container	120	B–
Tomato Minestrone		1 container	180	A–

"+" indicates the food meets minimum fiber requirements; "–" indicates the food has a high sodium content.

Food	Processing Category	Brand
Soup	Mix	Nile Spice Soups in a Cup
Soup	Mix	Oodles of Noodles/Top Ramen
Soup	Mix	Oodles of Noodles/Top Ramen
Soup	Mix	Oodles of Noodles/Top Ramen
Soup	Mix	Oodles of Noodles/Top Ramen
Spaghetti Dishes	Mix	Chef Boyardee Dinner
Spaghetti Dishes	Mix	Chef Boyardee Dinner
Spaghetti Dishes	Mix	Chef Boyardee Dinner
Spaghetti Dishes	Mix	Kraft Dinner
Spaghetti Dishes	Mix	Kraft Italian Style Dinner
Spaghetti Dishes	Mix	Kraft Mild American Dinner
Tabbouleh	Mix	Casbah
Tabbouleh	Mix	Fantastic Foods
Tabbouleh	Mix	Fantastic Foods
Tabbouleh	Mix	Near East
Taco	Mix	Natural Touch
Taco	Mix	Old El Paso
Taco	Mix	Tio Sancho
Taco	Mix	Tio Sancho
Taco	Mix	Tio Sancho
Tahini Mix	*See also* Sesame Butter	All Brands
Tempura Batter	Mix	Golden Dipt
Tofu Dishes	Mix	Fantastic Foods
Tofu Dishes	Mix	Fantastic Foods
Tofu Dishes	Mix	Fantastic Foods
Tofu Dishes	Mix	Fantastic Foods
Tofu Dishes	Mix	Fantastic Foods
Tuna Entree	Mix	Tuna Helper
Tuna Entree	Mix	Tuna Helper
Tuna Entree	Mix	Tuna Helper
Tuna Entree	Mix	Tuna Helper
Tuna Entree	Mix	Tuna Helper
Tuna Entree	Mix	Tuna Helper
Tuna Entree	Mix	Tuna Helper
Tuna Entree	Mix	Tuna Helper
Tuna Entree	Mix	Tuna Helper
Tuna Entree	Mix	Tuna Helper
Tuna Entree	Mix	Tuna Helper
Tuna Entree	Mix	Tuna Helper

Major Description	Minor Description	Serving Size	Calories	Grade
Vegetable Parmesan		1 container	200	A–
Beef Flavor	Noodle	1 cup	390	D–
Chicken or Chicken Flavor	Noodle	1 cup	400	D–
Noodle	Oriental Style	1 cup	390	D–
Pork Flavor	Noodle	1 cup	390	D–
in Condensed Meat Sauce		3.25 oz	250	B–
in Meat Sauce		7.9 oz	240	A–
in Mushroom Sauce		7.9 oz	210	A–
in Meat Sauce		1 cup	360	C–
Tangy		1 cup	310	B–
		1 cup	300	B–
Salad		1 oz dry	126	A
in Oil		1/2 cup	160	D–
Salad	No Oil	1/2 cup	80	A–+
in Oil		1/2 cup	170	D–
Vegetarian		2 Tbsp	90	B
		1 taco	67	D–
Taco Sauce		2 oz	62	A–
Taco Seasoning		1.25 oz	104	A–+
Taco Shell		1 piece	64	D
		1 oz dry	25	D
		1 oz	100	A–
Burger		1 cup	540	B–+
Chow Mein	Mandarin Style	1 cup	330	A–+
Scrambler		3 tsp	72	A–+
Shells & Curry		1 cup	440	A–+
Stroganoff, Creamy		1 cup	430	B–
au Gratin		6 oz	280	C–
Buttery Rice		6 oz	160	A–
Cheesy Noodle		7.75 oz	250	C–
Creamy Noodle		8 oz	300	D–
Fettuccine Alfredo		7 oz	300	C–
Mushroom, Creamy		6 oz	140	A–
Mushroom, Creamy		7 oz	220	B–
Pot Pie		5.1 oz	420	D–
Rice, Buttery		6 oz	280	C–
Romanoff		6 oz	210	A–
Salad		5.5 oz	420	D–
Tetrazzini		6 oz	240	B–

"+" indicates the food meets minimum fiber requirements; "–" indicates the food has a high sodium content.

Frivolous Foods

Stop!

Before entering this section, you must pass a test. If you fail, you cannot indulge in any of the foods in this section. Many nutritionists try to be all things for all people. They try to teach you it's okay to have a small portion or a snack of this or that horribly unhealthful food. The fact that even after three decades of nutritional education by a multi-billion dollar diet industry Americans are fatter then ever is testament to the fantasy of the "occasional snack" and "just a small portion" approach to nutrition. So ask yourself these questions:

- Are you overweight—even a little?
- Do you have heart disease?
- Do you have diabetes?
- Do you have a cholesterol problem?
- Do you exercise less than every other day?

If you answered yes to *any* of these questions, you simply can't even think of eating any of the thousands of foods listed in this section; for you, they are, in a sense, poison. The idea that you can have just one cookie or a small scoop of ice cream is a deception. These foods are very alluring; you can't stop eating them. In this context, the A and B ratings represent the "best of the worst."

Food	Processing Category	Brand
Brownie	Frozen	Nestlé Toll House
Brownie	Frozen	Pepperidge Farm Newport
Brownie	Frozen	Weight Watchers
Brownie	Frozen	Weight Watchers
Brownie	Frozen	Weight Watchers
Brownie	Frozen	Weight Watchers
Brownie	Mix	Betty Crocker
Brownie	Mix	Betty Crocker
Brownie	Mix	Betty Crocker
Brownie	Mix	Betty Crocker
Brownie	Mix	Betty Crocker
Brownie	Mix	Betty Crocker
Brownie	Mix	Betty Crocker Family Size
Brownie	Mix	Betty Crocker Micro Rave
Brownie	Mix	Betty Crocker Micro Rave
Brownie	Mix	Betty Crocker Micro Rave
Brownie	Mix	Betty Crocker Supreme
Brownie	Mix	Duncan Hines
Brownie	Mix	Duncan Hines
Brownie	Mix	Duncan Hines
Brownie	Mix	Duncan Hines
Brownie	Mix	Duncan Hines
Brownie	Mix	Duncan Hines Gourmet
Brownie	Mix	Duncan Hines Gourmet
Brownie	Mix	Estee
Brownie	Mix	Finast Ultra Moist
Brownie	Mix	Finast Ultra Moist
Brownie	Mix	Great Additions
Brownie	Mix	Great Additions
Brownie	Mix	Great Additions
Brownie	Mix	Pillsbury
Brownie	Mix	Pillsbury
Brownie	Mix	Pillsbury
Brownie	Mix	Pillsbury
Brownie	Mix	Pillsbury
Brownie	Mix	Pillsbury
Brownie	Mix	Pillsbury Family Size
Brownie	Mix	Pillsbury Microwave
Brownie	Mix	Robin Hood/Gold
Brownie	Packaged	Awrey's Cake
Brownie	Packaged	Awrey's Sheet Cake
Brownie	Packaged	Freihofer
Brownie	Packaged	Little Debbie
Brownie	Packaged	Tastycake
Bun, Sweet	Fresh Baked	Aunt Fanny's Honey Bun
Bun, Sweet	Fresh Baked	Aunt Fanny's Honey Bun

On the other hand, the A- and B-rated foods in this section are excellent calorie sources to be taken before, during, and after exercise. They provide exactly what the muscles crave, readily available carbohydrate.

Major Description	Minor Description	Serving Size	Calories	Grade
Double Chocolate Chip		1.4 oz piece	150	D
Hot Fudge		1 ramekin	400	D
Chocolate		1/3 pkg	100	B–
Mint Frosted		1.2 oz piece	100	B–+
Peanut Butter Fudge		1.2 oz piece	100	B–+
Swiss Mocha Fudge		1.2 oz piece	90	B–+
Caramel Swirl		1 oz piece	120	B
Chocolate Chip		1 oz piece	140	C
Frosted		1 oz piece	160	C
Fudge		1 oz piece	150	B
German Chocolate		1 oz piece	130	B
Walnut		1 oz piece	140	D
Fudge		1 oz piece	140	C
Frosted		1.3 oz piece	180	C
Fudge		1 oz piece	150	C
Walnut		1 oz piece	160	C
Fudge		1 oz piece	120	B
Milk Chocolate		1 piece	160	C
Fudge		1 piece	160	C
Fudge	Chewy	1 piece	130	C
Fudge	Peanut Butter	1 piece	150	D
Vienna White		1 piece	240	D
		1 piece	280	D
		1 piece	240	C
		2" square	50	C
Fudge		1/16 pkg	130	C
Walnut		1/16 pkg	130	D
Double Chocolate		1 oz piece	140	C
Funfetti		1 oz piece	160	C
Walnut		1 oz piece	140	D
Caramel Fudge Chunk		2" square	170	C
Double Fudge		2" square	160	C
Fudge	Deluxe	2" square	150	C
Fudge	Deluxe with Walnuts	2" square	150	D
Rocky Road Fudge		2" square	170	D
Triple Chunky Fudge		2" square	170	C
Fudge	Deluxe	2" square	150	D
Fudge		1 piece	190	D
Fudge		1/16 pkg	100	C
Dutch Chocolate		1/16 cake	340	D
Fudge	Nut	2.5 oz piece	300	D
Fudge	Fat Free	1/10 package	110	A–
Fudge		2 oz piece	240	B
Fudge	Walnut	3 oz piece	335	C+
Apple Bear		1 bun	440	D+
Birdie	Jelly Filled	1 bun	460	D+

"+" indicates the food meets minimum fiber requirements; "–" indicates the food has a high sodium content.

Food	Processing Category	Brand
Bun, Sweet	Fresh Baked	Aunt Fanny's Honey Bun
Bun, Sweet	Fresh Baked	Aunt Fanny's Honey Bun
Bun, Sweet	Fresh Baked	Aunt Fanny's Honey Bun
Bun, Sweet	Fresh Baked	Aunt Fanny's Honey Bun
Bun, Sweet	Fresh Baked	Hostess Breakfast
Bun, Sweet	Fresh Baked	Hostess Breakfast
Bun, Sweet	Fresh Baked	Tastykake
Bun, Sweet	Fresh Baked	Tastykake
Bun, Sweet	Frozen	Rich's Ever Fresh
Bun, Sweet	Frozen	Rich's Ever Fresh
Buns	Fresh Baked	Entenmann's
Buns	Fresh Baked	Entenmann's
Buns	Fresh Baked	Entenmann's
Buns	Fresh Baked	Entenmann's
Buns	Fresh Baked	Entenmann's
Buns	Fresh Baked	Freihofer
Buns	Fresh Baked	Freihofer
Buns	Fresh Baked	Freihofer
Buns	Fresh Baked	Freihofer
Buns	Fresh Baked	Freihofer
Butterscotch Chips, Baking	Packaged	Nestlé Toll House Morsels
Butterscotch Topping	All Forms	Kraft
Butterscotch Topping	All Forms	Smucker's
Butterscotch Topping	All Forms	Smucker's Special Recipe
Cake	Fresh Baked	Generic [1]
Cake	Fresh Baked	Generic
Cake	Fresh Baked	Generic
Cake	Fresh Baked	Generic
Cake	Fresh Baked	Generic
Cake	Fresh Baked	Generic
Cake	Fresh Baked	Generic
Cake	Fresh Baked	Generic
Cake	Fresh Baked	Generic
Cake	Fresh Baked	Generic
Cake	Fresh Baked	Generic
Cake	Fresh Baked	Generic
Cake	Fresh Baked	Generic
Cake	Fresh Baked	Generic
Cake	Fresh Baked	Generic
Cake	Fresh Baked	Generic
Cake	Fresh Baked	Generic
Cake	Processing	Generic
Cake	Fresh Baked	Generic
Cake	Fresh Baked	Generic
Cake	Fresh Baked	Generic
Cake	Fresh Baked	Generic
Cake	Fresh Baked	Generic
Cake	Fresh Baked	Generic
Cake	Fresh Baked	Generic
Cake	Fresh Baked	Generic

[1] Generic cake recipes based on standard USDA formulas.

Major Description	Minor Description	Serving Size	Calories	Grade
Bogie	Cream Filled	1 bun	460	D+
Lemon Bear		1 bun	440	D+
Regular		1 bun	390	D
Snow Bear		1 bun	430	D
Glazed		1 bun	360	D
Iced		1 bun	430	D
Glazed		1 bun	362	D
Iced		1 bun	348	C
Cinnamon		1 bun	293	D
Honey, Mini		1 bun	133	D
Apple	Fat Free	1 bun	140	A
Cheese		1 bun	240	D
Cinnamon		1 bun	230	C
Pineapple Cheese	Fat Free	1 oz bun	120	A
Raspberry Cheese	Fat Free	1 bun	160	A
Apple	Fat Free	1 bun	150	A
Blueberry Cheese	Fat Free	1 bun	140	A
Cinnamon Raisin	Fat Free	1 bun	160	A
Pineapple Cheese	Fat Free	1 bun	140	A
Raspberry Cheese	Fat Free	1 bun	160	A
		1 oz	150	D
		2 Tbsp	120	A
		2 Tbsp	140	A
Caramel Flavor		2 Tbsp	160	B
Angel Food		1 oz piece	73	A–
Angel Food	Prepared with Water	1 oz piece	72	A–
Boston Cream		1 oz piece	89	C
Boston Cream	Prepared With Shortening	1 oz piece	72	B
Carrot	Cream Cheese Frosting	1 oz piece	125	D
Carrot	No Frosting	1 oz piece	96	D
Cheesecake		1 oz piece	91	D
Cherry Fudge	Chocolate Frosting	1 oz piece	75	D
Chocolate	Chocolate Frosting	1 oz piece	104	D
Chocolate	Diet, Low Sodium	1 oz piece	109	B
Chocolate Fudge	with Water & Eggs	1 oz piece	88	C–
Coffee Cake	Cheese	1 oz piece	96	D
Coffee Cake	Cinnamon Crumb	1 oz piece	119	D
Coffee Cake	Fruit	1 oz piece	88	B
Devil's Food	Microwave	1 oz piece	98	D–
Fruitcake		1 oz piece	92	B
German Chocolate	Coconut Nut Frosting	1 oz piece	103	D
Gingerbread	Traditional Recipe	1 oz piece	101	D
Gingerbread	Water & Eggs	1 oz piece	88	B–
Marble	Water & Eggs	1 oz piece	100	D
Pineapple	Upside-Down	1 oz piece	90	C
Pound	Old Fashioned, Butter	1 oz piece	123	D
Pound	Reduced Butter Content	1 oz piece	110	D
Pound	Sour Cream	1 oz piece	110	D
Pound	with Margarine	1 oz piece	108	C
Shortcake		1 oz piece	98	C–
Snack Cake	Chocolate, Cream Filled	1 oz piece	107	C
Sponge		1 oz piece	82	A

"+" indicates the food meets minimum fiber requirements; "–" indicates the food has a high sodium content.

Food	Processing Category	Brand
Cake	Fresh Baked	Generic
Cake	Fresh Baked	Generic
Cake	Fresh Baked	Generic
Cake	Fresh Baked	Generic
Cake	Fresh Baked	Generic
Cake	Fresh Baked	Generic
Cake	Fresh Baked	Generic
Cake	Fresh Baked	Aunt Fanny's
Cake	Fresh Baked	Aunt Fanny's
Cake	Fresh Baked	Aunt Fanny's
Cake	Fresh Baked	Awrey's
Cake	Fresh Baked	Awrey's
Cake	Fresh Baked	Awrey's
Cake	Fresh Baked	Awrey's
Cake	Fresh Baked	Awrey's
Cake	Fresh Baked	Awrey's
Cake	Fresh Baked	Awrey's
Cake	Fresh Baked	Awrey's
Cake	Fresh Baked	Awrey's
Cake	Fresh Baked	Awrey's
Cake	Fresh Baked	Awrey's
Cake	Fresh Baked	Awrey's
Cake	Fresh Baked	Awrey's
Cake	Fresh Baked	Awrey's
Cake	Fresh Baked	Awrey's
Cake	Fresh Baked	Awrey's
Cake	Fresh Baked	Awrey's
Cake	Fresh Baked	Awrey's
Cake	Fresh Baked	Awrey's
Cake	Fresh Baked	Awrey's
Cake	Fresh Baked	Awrey's
Cake	Fresh Baked	Awrey's
Cake	Fresh Baked	Awrey's
Cake	Fresh Baked	Awrey's
Cake	Fresh Baked	Awrey's
Cake	Fresh Baked	Awrey's
Cake	Fresh Baked	Awrey's
Cake	Fresh Baked	Awrey's
Cake	Fresh Baked	Awrey's
Cake	Fresh Baked	Awrey's
Cake	Fresh Baked	Awrey's
Cake	Fresh Baked	Awrey's Best Wishes
Cake	Fresh Baked	Awrey's Four in One Occasion
Cake	Fresh Baked	Drake's
Cake	Fresh Baked	Entenmann's
Cake	Fresh Baked	Entenmann's
Cake	Fresh Baked	Entenmann's

Major Description	Minor Description	Serving Size	Calories	Grade
White	Coconut Frosting	1 oz piece	101	B
White	No Frosting, Pudding Type	1 oz piece	98	C–
White	No Frosting, Regular	1 oz piece	76	B–
Yellow	Chocolate Frosting	1 oz piece	107	D–
Yellow	No Frosting, Pudding Type	1 oz piece	103	D
Yellow	No Frosting, Regular	1 oz piece	90	B–
Yellow	Vanilla Frosting	1 oz piece	106	C
Applesauce		1 oz piece	100	C
Chocolate Fudge		1 oz piece	80	B–
Pound		1 oz piece	88	C–
Apple Streusel		2" × 2" piece	160	D
Banana, Iced		2" × 2" piece	140	D
Black Forest Torte		$1/_{14}$ cake	350	D
Carrot Supreme, Iced		2" square	210	D
Carrot, Cream Cheese Iced	Three Layer	$1/_{12}$ cake	390	D
Chocolate		.8 oz piece	70	C–
Chocolate		1.4 oz piece	150	D
Chocolate	Double, Iced	2" square	130	D
Chocolate	Double, Three Layer	$1/_{12}$ cake	310	D
Chocolate	Double, Torte	$1/_{14}$ cake	340	C
Chocolate	Double, Two Layer	$1/_{12}$ cake	250	C
Chocolate	White Iced, Two Layer	$1/_{12}$ cake	270	D
Chocolate	Yellow Iced, Two Layer	$1/_{12}$ cake	290	D
Coconut	Three Layer	$1/_{12}$ cake	350	D
Coconut Butter Cream		2" square	160	D
Coffee Cake	Caramel Nut	$1/_{12}$ cake	140	D
Coffee Cake	Long John	$1/_{12}$ cake	160	D
Devil's Food	White Iced	2" square	150	D
German Chocolate	Iced	2" square	160	D
German Chocolate	Three Layer	$1/_{12}$ cake	350	D
Lemon	Three Layer	$1/_{12}$ cake	320	D
Lemon	Two Layer	$1/_{12}$ cake	290	D
Neapolitan Torte		$1/_{14}$ cake	380	D
Orange	Frosty Iced	2" square	150	D
Orange	Three Layer	$1/_{12}$ cake	320	D
Peanut Butter Torte		$1/_{14}$ cake	380	D
Pistachio Torte		$1/_{14}$ cake	370	D
Pound, Golden		$1/_{14}$ loaf	130	C
Raisin Spice	Iced	2" square	160	D
Raspberry Nut		$1/_{16}$ cake	310	D
Sponge		2" square	80	C–
Strawberry Supreme Torte		$1/_{14}$ cake	270	C
Walnut Torte		$1/_{14}$ cake	320	D
Yellow		.9 oz piece	80	C–
Yellow	White Iced	2" square	150	D
		3 oz piece	320	D
		1.3 oz piece	150	D
Pound		1 oz piece	110	D
Apple Puff		1 piece	280	D
Apple Sauce	Fat Free	1 oz piece	80	A
Apple Strudel	Old Fashioned	1 oz piece	80	C

"+" indicates the food meets minimum fiber requirements; "–" indicates the food has a high sodium content.

Food	Processing Category	Brand
Cake	Fresh Baked	Entenmann's
Cake	Fresh Baked	Entenmann's
Cake	Fresh Baked	Entenmann's
Cake	Fresh Baked	Entenmann's
Cake	Fresh Baked	Entenmann's
Cake	Fresh Baked	Entenmann's
Cake	Fresh Baked	Entenmann's
Cake	Fresh Baked	Entenmann's
Cake	Fresh Baked	Entenmann's
Cake	Fresh Baked	Entenmann's
Cake	Fresh Baked	Entenmann's
Cake	Fresh Baked	Entenmann's
Cake	Fresh Baked	Entenmann's
Cake	Fresh Baked	Entenmann's
Cake	Fresh Baked	Entenmann's
Cake	Fresh Baked	Entenmann's
Cake	Fresh Baked	Entenmann's
Cake	Fresh Baked	Entenmann's
Cake	Fresh Baked	Entenmann's
Cake	Fresh Baked	Entenmann's
Cake	Fresh Baked	Entenmann's
Cake	Fresh Baked	Entenmann's
Cake	Fresh Baked	Entenmann's
Cake	Fresh Baked	Entenmann's
Cake	Fresh Baked	Entenmann's
Cake	Fresh Baked	Entenmann's
Cake	Fresh Baked	Entenmann's
Cake	Fresh Baked	Entenmann's
Cake	Fresh Baked	Entenmann's
Cake	Fresh Baked	Entenmann's
Cake	Fresh Baked	Freihofer
Cake	Fresh Baked	Freihofer
Cake	Fresh Baked	Freihofer
Cake	Fresh Baked	Freihofer
Cake	Fresh Baked	Freihofer
Cake	Fresh Baked	Freihofer
Cake	Fresh Baked	Freihofer
Cake	Fresh Baked	Freihofer
Cake	Fresh Baked	Freihofer
Cake	Fresh Baked	Freihofer
Cake	Fresh Baked	Freihofer
Cake	Fresh Baked	Freihofer
Cake	Fresh Baked	Freihofer
Cake	Fresh Baked	Freihofer
Cake	Fresh Baked	Freihofer
Cake	Fresh Baked	Freihofer
Cake	Fresh Baked	Freihofer
Cake	Fresh Baked	Freihofer
Cake	Frozen	Pepperidge Farm
Cake	Frozen	Pepperidge Farm
Cake	Frozen	Pepperidge Farm
Cake	Frozen	Pepperidge Farm

Major Description	Minor Description	Serving Size	Calories	Grade
Banana Crunch	Fat Free	1 oz piece	80	A–
Banana Loaf	Fat Free	1.3 oz piece	90	A–
Black Forest	Fat Free	1 oz piece	69	A
Blueberry Crunch	Fat Free	1 oz piece	70	A–
Carrot	Fat Free	1 oz piece	71	A–
Cheese & Crumb Coffee Cake		1 oz piece	93	D
Cheese Coffee Cake		1 oz piece	94	D
Chocolate Crunch	Fat Free	1 oz piece	70	A–
Chocolate Loaf	Fat Free	1 oz piece	70	A–
Cinnamon Apple Coffee Cake	Fat Free	1 oz piece	69	A
Cinnamon Filbert Ring		1 oz piece	127	D
Crumb Coffee Cake		1 oz piece	123	C
Cupcakes	Fat Free	1 cupcake	190	A
Devil's Food	Fudge Iced	1 oz piece	108	C
French Crumb	All Butter	1 oz piece	113	C
Fudge Iced, Golden	Fat Free	1 oz piece	69	A
Golden Chocolatey Chip Loaf	Fat Free	1 oz piece	80	A
Golden French Crumb	Fat Free	1 oz piece	80	A
Golden Loaf	Fat Free	1 oz piece	70	A–
Golden Thick Fudge		1 oz piece	108	C
Lemon Twist	Fat Free	1 oz piece	80	A
Louisiana Crunch		1 oz piece	106	C
Louisiana Crunch	Fat Free	1 oz piece	80	A–
Marble Loaf	Fat Free	1 oz piece	70	A–
Orange	Fat Free	1 oz piece	70	A–
Pineapple Crunch		1 oz piece	70	A
Pineapple Crunch	Fat Free	1 oz piece	70	A–
Pound	All Butter	1 oz piece	110	C–
Pound	Sour Cream	1 oz piece	120	D
Raisin Loaf	Fat Free	1 oz piece	80	A
Applesauce	Fat Free	$1/6$ cake	167	A+
Banana Crunch	Fat Free	$1/6$ cake	183	A
Banana Loaf	Fat Free	$1/6$ cake	190	A–
Blueberry Crunch	Fat Free	$1/6$ cake	180	A–
Carrot	Fat Free	$1/6$ cake	227	A–
Chocolate Crunch	Fat Free	$1/6$ cake	175	A–
Chocolate Loaf	Fat Free	$1/6$ cake	175	A–
Cinnamon Apple Twist	Fat Free	2 oz piece	150	A
Fudge	Iced Chocolate, Fat Free	$1/6$ cake	210	A–
Fudge	Iced Golden, Fat Free	$1/6$ cake	220	A
Golden Chocolatey Chip Loaf	Fat Free	$1/6$ cake	183	A–
Golden French Crumb	Fat Free	$1/6$ cake	192	A
Golden Loaf	Fat Free	2 oz piece	147	A–
Lemon Twist	Fat Free	2 oz piece	130	A–
Louisiana Crunch	Fat Free	$1/6$ cake	220	A
Marble Loaf	Fat Free	2 oz piece	133	A–
Pineapple Crunch	Fat Free	$1/6$ cake	190	A–
Raisin Loaf	Fat Free	2 oz piece	150	A–
Raspberry Twist	Fat Free	2 oz piece	140	A
Carrot	Cream Cheese Iced	1 oz piece	100	D
Chocolate	Fudge Layer	1 oz piece	113	D
Chocolate	Fudge Stripe Layer	1 oz piece	106	D
Chocolate	German Layer	1 oz piece	113	D

"+" indicates the food meets minimum fiber requirements; "–" indicates the food has a high sodium content.

Food	Processing Category	Brand
Cake	Frozen	Pepperidge Farm
Cake	Frozen	Pepperidge Farm
Cake	Frozen	Pepperidge Farm
Cake	Frozen	Pepperidge Farm
Cake	Frozen	Pepperidge Farm
Cake	Frozen	Pepperidge Farm
Cake	Frozen	Pepperidge Farm Supreme
Cake	Frozen	Pepperidge Farm Supreme
Cake	Frozen	Pepperidge Farm Supreme
Cake	Frozen	Pepperidge Farm Supreme
Cake	Frozen	Pepperidge Farm Supreme
Cake	Frozen	Pepperidge Farm Supreme
Cake	Frozen	Sara Lee
Cake	Frozen	Sara Lee
Cake	Frozen	Sara Lee
Cake	Frozen	Sara Lee
Cake	Frozen	Sara Lee
Cake	Frozen	Sara Lee
Cake	Frozen	Sara Lee
Cake	Frozen	Sara Lee
Cake	Frozen	Sara Lee
Cake	Frozen	Sara Lee
Cake	Frozen	Sara Lee
Cake	Frozen	Sara Lee
Cake	Frozen	Sara Lee Classics
Cake	Frozen	Sara Lee Classics
Cake	Frozen	Sara Lee Family Size
Cake	Frozen	Sara Lee Free & Light
Cake	Frozen	Sara Lee Free & Light
Cake	Frozen	Sara Lee Original
Cake	Frozen	Tofutti Better Than Cheesecake
Cake	Frozen	Weight Watchers
Cake	Frozen	Weight Watchers
Cake	Frozen	Weight Watchers
Cake	Frozen	Weight Watchers
Cake	Frozen	Weight Watchers
Cake	Frozen	Weight Watchers
Cake	Frozen	Weight Watchers
Cake	Frozen	Weight Watchers
Cake	Frozen	Weight Watchers
Cake	Frozen	Weight Watchers
Cake	Mix [2]	Aunt Jemima Easy
Cake	Mix	Betty Crocker
Cake	Mix	Betty Crocker
Cake	Mix	Betty Crocker Classic
Cake	Mix	Betty Crocker Classic
Cake	Mix	Betty Crocker Classic
Cake	Mix	Betty Crocker Classic
Cake	Mix	Betty Crocker Classic
Cake	Mix	Betty Crocker Classic

[2] Use of cholesterol-free egg product as a substitute when cake mix recipe calls for eggs generally raises rating one letter grade.

Major Description	Minor Description	Serving Size	Calories	Grade
Coconut	Layer	1 oz piece	113	C
Devil's Food	Layer	1 oz piece	113	D
Golden	Layer	1 oz piece	113	D
Pound		1 oz piece	110	D
Strawberry Stripe	Layer	1 oz piece	107	D
Vanilla	Layer	1 oz piece	120	C
Boston Cream		1 oz piece	100	D
Chocolate		1 oz piece	200	D
Lemon Coconut		1 oz piece	93	D
Lemon Cream		1 oz piece	106	D
Pineapple Cream		1 oz piece	95	C
Strawberry Cream		1 oz piece	95	C
Banana	Layer	$^1/_8$ cake	170	C
Black Forest	Two Layer	$^1/_8$ cake	190	C
Carrot	Layer, Iced	$^1/_8$ cake	250	D
Cheesecake, Cherry Cream		$^1/_8$ cake	243	B
Cheesecake, French Strawberry		$^1/_8$ cake	240	D
Cheesecake, Plain Cream		$^1/_8$ cake	230	D
Cheesecake, Strawberry Cream		$^1/_8$ cake	222	C
Chocolate	Double, Three Layer	$^1/_8$ cake	220	D
Coffee Cake, Cheese	All Butter	$^1/_8$ cake	210	D
Coffee Cake, Pecan	All Butter	$^1/_8$ cake	160	D
Coffee Streusel	All Butter	$^1/_8$ cake	160	C
Strawberry Shortcake		$^1/_8$ cake	190	C
Cheesecake	French Style	$^1/_8$ cake	250	D
Chocolate Mousse		$^1/_8$ cake	260	D
Pound	All Butter	$^1/_8$ cake	250	D
Chocolate		$^1/_8$ cake	110	A–
Pound		$^1/_8$ cake	56	A–
Pound	All Butter	$^1/_8$ cake	104	D
Cheesecake	Nondairy, All Flavors	1 oz piece	80	D
Boston Cream Pie		1 oz piece	53	B–
Carrot		1 oz piece	57	B–
Cheesecake		1 oz piece	54	B
Cheesecake, Brownie		1 oz piece	57	B–
Cheesecake, Strawberry		1 oz piece	46	B
Cherries & Cream		1 oz piece	63	B
Chocolate		1 oz piece	72	B–
Chocolate	Double Fudge	1 oz piece	73	B
Chocolate Irish Creme		1 oz piece	57	B–+
German Chocolate		1 oz piece	80	C
Toasted Almond Amaretto		1 oz piece	57	B+
Coffee Cake		$^1/_{12}$ cake	156	B–
Angel Food	Chocolate Confetti Lemon	$^1/_{12}$ cake	150	A–
Angel Food	Strawberry	$^1/_{12}$ cake	150	A–
Boston Cream		$^1/_{12}$ cake	180	B–
Chocolate	Pudding	$^1/_{12}$ cake	165	B
Lemon	Chiffon	$^1/_{12}$ cake	200	B
Lemon	Pudding	$^1/_{12}$ cake	165	B
Pineapple	Upside-down	$^1/_{12}$ cake	188	C
Pound	Golden	$^1/_{12}$ cake	200	D

"+" indicates the food meets minimum fiber requirements; "–" indicates the food has a high sodium content.

Food	Processing Category	Brand
Cake	Mix	Betty Crocker Microrave
Cake	Mix	Betty Crocker Microrave
Cake	Mix	Betty Crocker Microrave
Cake	Mix	Betty Crocker Microrave
Cake	Mix	Betty Crocker Microrave
Cake	Mix	Betty Crocker Microrave
Cake	Mix	Betty Crocker Microrave
Cake	Mix	Betty Crocker Microrave
Cake	Mix	Betty Crocker Super Moist
Cake	Mix	Betty Crocker Super Moist
Cake	Mix	Betty Crocker Super Moist
Cake	Mix	Betty Crocker Super Moist
Cake	Mix	Betty Crocker Super Moist
Cake	Mix	Betty Crocker Super Moist
Cake	Mix	Betty Crocker Super Moist
Cake	Mix	Betty Crocker Super Moist
Cake	Mix	Betty Crocker Super Moist
Cake	Mix	Betty Crocker Super Moist
Cake	Mix	Betty Crocker Super Moist
Cake	Mix	Betty Crocker Super Moist
Cake	Mix	Betty Crocker Super Moist
Cake	Mix	Betty Crocker Super Moist
Cake	Mix	Betty Crocker Super Moist
Cake	Mix	Betty Crocker Super Moist
Cake	Mix	Betty Crocker Super Moist
Cake	Mix	Betty Crocker Super Moist
Cake	Mix	Betty Crocker Super Moist
Cake	Mix	Betty Crocker Super Moist
Cake	Mix	Betty Crocker Super Moist
Cake	Mix	Betty Crocker Super Moist
Cake	Mix	Betty Crocker Traditional
Cake	Mix	Dromedary
Cake	Mix	Dromedary
Cake	Mix	Dromedary
Cake	Mix	Duncan Hines
Cake	Mix	Duncan Hines
Cake	Mix	Duncan Hines
Cake	Mix	Duncan Hines
Cake	Mix	Duncan Hines
Cake	Mix	Duncan Hines
Cake	Mix	Duncan Hines
Cake	Mix	Duncan Hines
Cake	Mix	Duncan Hines
Cake	Mix	Duncan Hines
Cake	Mix	Duncan Hines Butter Recipe
Cake	Mix	Duncan Hines Supreme
Cake	Mix	Duncan Hines Supreme
Cake	Mix	Duncan Hines Supreme
Cake	Mix	Duncan Hines Tiarra
Cake	Mix	Duncan Hines Tiarra
Cake	Mix	Duncan Hines Tiarra
Cake	Mix	Duncan Hines Tiarra

Major Description	Minor Description	Serving Size	Calories	Grade
Apple Streusel		$^1/_{12}$ cake	120	D
Chocolate	Fudge, Vanilla Frosting	$^1/_{12}$ cake	155	D
Cinnamon	Pecan	$^1/_{12}$ cake	145	D
Devil's Food	Chocolate Frosting	$^1/_{12}$ cake	155	D
German Chocolate	Coconut Pecan Frosting	$^1/_{12}$ cake	160	D
Lemon	Lemon Frosting	$^1/_{12}$ cake	150	D
Vanilla	Rainbow Chip Frosting	$^1/_{12}$ cake	160	D
Yellow	Chocolate Frosting	$^1/_{12}$ cake	150	D
Apple	Cinnamon	$^1/_{12}$ cake	250	C
Brickle	Butter	$^1/_{12}$ cake	250	C
Carrot		$^1/_{12}$ cake	250	C
Cherry Chip		$^1/_{12}$ cake	190	A–
Chocolate	Butter	$^1/_{12}$ cake	270	D–
Chocolate Chip		$^1/_{12}$ cake	280	D
Chocolate, Chocolate Chip		$^1/_{12}$ cake	260	D–
Devil's Food		$^1/_{12}$ cake	260	D–
German Chocolate		$^1/_{12}$ cake	220	C–
German Chocolate		$^1/_{12}$ cake	260	D–
Lemon		$^1/_{12}$ cake	260	C
Marble	Fudge	$^1/_{12}$ cake	250	C
Milk Chocolate		$^1/_{12}$ cake	260	D–
Pecan	Butter	$^1/_{12}$ cake	250	C–
Rainbow Chip		$^1/_{12}$ cake	250	C–
Sour Cream	Chocolate	$^1/_{12}$ cake	260	D–
Sour Cream	White	$^1/_{12}$ cake	180	A–
Spice		$^1/_{12}$ cake	260	C
Vanilla	Golden	$^1/_{12}$ cake	280	D
White		$^1/_{12}$ cake	180	A–
Yellow		$^1/_{12}$ cake	260	C
Yellow	Butter	$^1/_{12}$ cake	260	C–
Chocolate	Fudge	$^1/_{12}$ cake	250	D–
Angel Food		$^1/_{12}$ cake	130	A–
Carrot		$^1/_{12}$ cake	232	D–
Gingerbread		2" square	100	B–
Pound		$^1/_2$" slice	150	C
Angel Food		$^1/_{12}$ cake	140	A
Butter	Golden	$^1/_{12}$ cake	270	D
Chocolate	Fudge Marble	$^1/_{12}$ cake	260	C
Chocolate	Fudge, Dark Dutch	$^1/_{12}$ cake	280	D–
Chocolate	Swiss	$^1/_{12}$ cake	280	D–
Devil's Food		$^1/_{12}$ cake	280	D–
French Vanilla		$^1/_{12}$ cake	260	C
Spice		$^1/_{12}$ cake	260	C
White		$^1/_{12}$ cake	250	C
Yellow		$^1/_{12}$ cake	260	C
Chocolate	Fudge	$^1/_{12}$ cake	270	D–
Lemon		$^1/_{12}$ cake	260	C
Pineapple		$^1/_{12}$ cake	260	C
Strawberry		$^1/_{12}$ cake	260	C
Black Forest Mousse		$^1/_{12}$ cake	260	D
Cherries & Cream		$^1/_{12}$ cake	250	C
Chocolate Mousse		$^1/_{12}$ cake	270	D
Chocolate Mousse	Amaretto	$^1/_{12}$ cake	270	D

"+" indicates the food meets minimum fiber requirements; "–" indicates the food has a high sodium content.

Food	Processing Category	Brand
Cake	Mix	Estee
Cake	Mix	Estee
Cake	Mix	Estee
Cake	Mix	Estee
Cake	Mix	Estee
Cake	Mix	Finast Ultra Moist
Cake	Mix	Finast Ultra Moist
Cake	Mix	Jell-O No Bake
Cake	Mix	Jell-O No Bake
Cake	Mix	Jell-O No Bake
Cake	Mix	Martha White
Cake	Mix	Pillsbury
Cake	Mix	Pillsbury
Cake	Mix	Pillsbury Bundt
Cake	Mix	Pillsbury Bundt
Cake	Mix	Pillsbury Bundt
Cake	Mix	Pillsbury Bundt
Cake	Mix	Pillsbury Bundt Brand
Cake	Mix	Pillsbury Bundt Brand
Cake	Mix	Pillsbury Bundt Brand
Cake	Mix	Pillsbury Bundt Brand
Cake	Mix	Pillsbury Bundt Brand
Cake	Mix	Pillsbury Microwave
Cake	Mix	Pillsbury Microwave
Cake	Mix	Pillsbury Microwave
Cake	Mix	Pillsbury Microwave
Cake	Mix	Pillsbury Microwave
Cake	Mix	Pillsbury Microwave
Cake	Mix	Pillsbury Microwave
Cake	Mix	Pillsbury Microwave
Cake	Mix	Pillsbury Microwave
Cake	Mix	Pillsbury Plus
Cake	Mix	Pillsbury Plus
Cake	Mix	Pillsbury Plus
Cake	Mix	Pillsbury Plus
Cake	Mix	Pillsbury Plus
Cake	Mix	Pillsbury Plus
Cake	Mix	Pillsbury Plus
Cake	Mix	Pillsbury Plus
Cake	Mix	Pillsbury Plus
Cake	Mix	Pillsbury Plus
Cake	Mix	Pillsbury Plus
Cake	Mix	Pillsbury Plus
Cake	Mix	Pillsbury Streusel Swirl
Cake	Mix	Pillsbury Streusel Swirl
Cake	Mix	Pillsbury Streusel Swirl
Cake	Mix	Pillsbury Streusel Swirl Microwave
Cake	Mix	Robin Hood/Gold
Cake	Mix	Robin Hood/Gold
Cake	Mix	Robin Hood/Gold
Cake	Mix	Robin Hood/Gold
Cake	Mix	Royal No Bake
Cake	Mix	Royal No Bake

Major Description	Minor Description	Serving Size	Calories	Grade
Carrot		$^1/_{12}$ cake	83	B
Chocolate		$^1/_{12}$ cake	83	B
Lemon		$^1/_{12}$ cake	83	B
Pound		$^1/_{12}$ cake	83	B
White		$^1/_{12}$ cake	83	B
Devil's Food		$^1/_{12}$ cake	250	C–
Yellow		$^1/_{12}$ cake	240	C
Cheesecake		$^1/_{12}$ cake	187	D–
Cheesecake	New York Style	$^1/_{12}$ cake	187	C–
Cheesecake, Lemon		$^1/_{12}$ cake	185	D–
Pound		$^1/_{12}$ cake	100	B
Coffee Cake	Apple Cinnamon	$^1/_{12}$ cake	160	B
Gingerbread		3" square	190	B–
Black Forest Cherry		$^1/_{12}$ cake	320	B–
Boston Cream		$^1/_{12}$ cake	360	C
Chocolate Macaroon		$^1/_{12}$ cake	320	C–
Pineapple	Cream	$^1/_{12}$ cake	347	C
Black Forest Cherry		$^1/_{16}$ cake	240	C–
Chocolate Macaroon		$^1/_{12}$ cake	320	B–
Fudge, Tunnel of		$^1/_{12}$ cake	346	D–
Lemon, Tunnel of		$^1/_{12}$ cake	360	C–
Pineapple Cream		$^1/_{12}$ cake	346	C–
Chocolate		$^1/_{12}$ cake	140	D
Chocolate	Chocolate Frosting	$^1/_{12}$ cake	200	D
Chocolate	Double Supreme	$^1/_{12}$ cake	220	D
Chocolate	Vanilla Frosting	$^1/_{12}$ cake	200	D
Lemon		$^1/_{12}$ cake	147	D
Lemon	Double Supreme	$^1/_{12}$ cake	266	D
Lemon	Lemon Frosting	$^1/_{12}$ cake	200	D
Yellow		$^1/_{12}$ cake	147	D
Yellow	Chocolate Frosting	$^1/_{12}$ cake	200	D
Banana		$^1/_{12}$ cake	250	C
Butter		$^1/_{12}$ cake	260	D–
Carrot	& Spice	$^1/_{12}$ cake	260	C–
Chocolate	Dark	$^1/_{12}$ cake	250	D–
Chocolate	Fudge Marble	$^1/_{12}$ cake	270	C
Chocolate Chip		$^1/_{12}$ cake	270	D
Devil's Food		$^1/_{12}$ cake	270	D–
German Chocolate		$^1/_{12}$ cake	250	C–
Lemon		$^1/_{12}$ cake	250	C
Strawberry		$^1/_{12}$ cake	260	C
White		$^1/_{12}$ cake	240	C
Yellow		$^1/_{12}$ cake	260	D
Blueberry		$^1/_{12}$ cake	350	C
Cinnamon		$^1/_{12}$ cake	346	C
Lemon		$^1/_{12}$ cake	360	C–
Cinnamon		$^1/_{12}$ cake	160	D
Applesauce	with Raisins	$^1/_{12}$ cake	140	B
Banana Walnut		$^1/_{12}$ cake	150	B–
Chocolate Chip Fudge		$^1/_{12}$ cake	150	B–
Golden Chocolate Chip		$^1/_{12}$ cake	140	B–
Cheesecake		$^1/_{12}$ cake	187	B–
Cheesecake	Light	$^1/_{12}$ cake	140	D–

"+" indicates the food meets minimum fiber requirements; "–" indicates the food has a high sodium content.

Food	Processing Category	Brand
Cake	Refrigerated	Pillsbury
Cake	Refrigerated	Pillsbury
Cake, Snack	Frozen	Pepperidge Farm
Cake, Snack	Frozen	Pepperidge Farm Classic
Cake, Snack	Frozen	Pepperidge Farm Classic
Cake, Snack	Frozen	Pepperidge Farm Classic
Cake, Snack	Frozen	Pepperidge Farm Classic
Cake, Snack	Frozen	Pepperidge Farm Classic
Cake, Snack	Frozen	Pepperidge Farm Dessert
Cake, Snack	Frozen	Pepperidge Farm Dessert
Cake, Snack	Frozen	Pepperidge Farm Dessert
Cake, Snack	Frozen	Pepperidge Farm Dessert
Cake, Snack	Frozen	Pepperidge Farm Dessert
Cake, Snack	Frozen	Pepperidge Farm Dessert
Cake, Snack	Frozen	Pepperidge Farm Hyannis
Cake, Snack	Frozen	Sara Lee
Cake, Snack	Frozen	Sara Lee
Cake, Snack	Frozen	Sara Lee
Cake, Snack	Frozen	Sara Lee
Cake, Snack	Frozen	Sara Lee Deluxe
Cake, Snack	Frozen	Sara Lee Individually
Cake, Snack	Frozen	Sara Lee Individually
Cake, Snack	Frozen	Sara Lee Individually
Cake, Snack	Frozen	Sara Lee Lights
Cake, Snack	Frozen	Sara Lee Lights
Cake, Snack	Frozen	Sara Lee Lights
Cake, Snack	Frozen	Sara Lee Lights
Cake, Snack	Frozen	Sara Lee Lights
Cake, Snack	Frozen	Sara Lee Lights
Cake, Snack	Frozen	Sara Lee Lights
Cake, Snack	Frozen	Sara Lee Lights
Cake, Snack	Frozen	Weight Watchers
Cake, Snack	Packaged	Drake's
Cake, Snack	Packaged	Drake's
Cake, Snack	Packaged	Drake's Devil Dog
Cake, Snack	Packaged	Drake's Funny Bone
Cake, Snack	Packaged	Drake's Jr.
Cake, Snack	Packaged	Drake's Ring-Ding
Cake, Snack	Packaged	Drake's Ring-Ding
Cake, Snack	Packaged	Drake's Ring-Ding
Cake, Snack	Packaged	Drake's Small
Cake, Snack	Packaged	Drake's Sunny Doodle
Cake, Snack	Packaged	Drake's Yodel
Cake, Snack	Packaged	Drake's Zoinks
Cake, Snack	Packaged	Hostess
Cake, Snack	Packaged	Hostess
Cake, Snack	Packaged	Hostess
Cake, Snack	Packaged	Hostess
Cake, Snack	Packaged	Hostess
Cake, Snack	Packaged	Hostess
Cake, Snack	Packaged	Hostess Choco Bliss
Cake, Snack	Packaged	Hostess Chocodiles
Cake, Snack	Packaged	Hostess Ding Dongs

Major Description	Minor Description	Serving Size	Calories	Grade
Cinnamon Swirl		$^1/_{12}$ cake	120	D
Pecan Streusel		$^1/_{12}$ cake	120	D
Cheesecake	Strawberry	1 ramekin	300	B
Carrot		1 piece	260	D
Chocolate	Double	1 piece	250	D
Coconut		1 piece	230	D
German Chocolate		1 piece	250	D
Vanilla Fudge Swirl		1 piece	250	C
Apple & Spice Bake		1 piece	170	A
Cherries Supreme		1 piece	170	A
Chocolate Mousse		1 piece	190	D–
Lemon Supreme		1 piece	170	B
Raspberry Vanilla Swirl		1 piece	160	B
Shortcake, Strawberry		1 piece	170	B
Boston Cream Pie		1 ramekin	230	C
Cheesecake	Classic	1 piece	200	D
Chocolate	Fudge	1 piece	190	D
Chocolate Mousse		1 piece	180	D
Pound	All Butter	1 piece	200	D
Carrot		1 piece	180	C
Coffee Cake, Apple Cinnamon		1 piece	290	D
Coffee Cake, Butter Streusel		1 piece	230	D
Coffee Cake, Pecan		1 piece	280	D
Apple Crisp		1 piece	150	A
Black Forest		1 piece	170	B
Carrot		1 piece	170	B
Cheesecake	French Strawberry	1 piece	150	A
Cheesecake	French Style	1 piece	150	B
Chocolate	Double	1 piece	150	B
Chocolate Mousse		1 piece	170	D
Lemon Cream		1 piece	180	B
Coffee	Cinnamon Streusel	1 piece	190	C–
Chocolate Roll, Swiss	Cream Filled	1 piece	170	D
Coffee Cake	Cinnamon Crumb	1 piece	150	C
Chocolate	Cream Filled	1 piece	160	C
Donut		1 piece	150	D
Coffee Cake		1 piece	140	C
Chocolate	Cream Filled	1 piece	180	D
Chocolate Mint	Cream Filled	1 piece	190	D
Cupcake, Chocolate	Cream Filled	1 piece	100	C
Coffee Cake		1 piece	220	C
Cupcake, Golden	Cream Filled	1 piece	100	B
Chocolate Roll	Cream Filled	1 piece	150	D
Donut		1 piece	130	C
Banana		1 piece	240	C
Coffee Crumb Cake		1 piece	120	C
Cupcake, Chocolate		1 piece	180	B–
Cupcake, Orange		1 piece	160	B
Dessert Cup		1 piece	90	B–
Pudding Cakes		1 piece	170	B
Chocolate		1 piece	200	D
Chocolate		1 piece	240	D
Chocolate		1 piece	170	D

"+" indicates the food meets minimum fiber requirements; "–" indicates the food has a high sodium content.

Food	Processing Category	Brand
Cake, Snack	Packaged	Hostess Fruit Loaf
Cake, Snack	Packaged	Hostess Ho-Hos
Cake, Snack	Packaged	Hostess Light
Cake, Snack	Packaged	Hostess Light
Cake, Snack	Packaged	Hostess Light
Cake, Snack	Packaged	Hostess Light
Cake, Snack	Packaged	Hostess Lil Angels
Cake, Snack	Packaged	Hostess Sno Balls
Cake, Snack	Packaged	Hostess Suzy-Qs
Cake, Snack	Packaged	Hostess Tiger Tail
Cake, Snack	Packaged	Hostess Twinkies
Cake, Snack	Packaged	Hostess Twinkies
Cake, Snack	Packaged	Hostess Twinkies Fruit
Cake, Snack	Packaged	Hostess Twinkies Fruit
Cake, Snack	Packaged	Hostess Twinkies Light
Cake, Snack	Packaged	Little Debbie
Cake, Snack	Packaged	Little Debbie
Cake, Snack	Packaged	Little Debbie
Cake, Snack	Packaged	Little Debbie
Cake, Snack	Packaged	Little Debbie
Cake, Snack	Packaged	Little Debbie
Cake, Snack	Packaged	Little Debbie
Cake, Snack	Packaged	Little Debbie
Cake, Snack	Packaged	Little Debbie
Cake, Snack	Packaged	Little Debbie
Cake, Snack	Packaged	Little Debbie
Cake, Snack	Packaged	Little Debbie
Cake, Snack	Packaged	Little Debbie
Cake, Snack	Packaged	Little Debbie
Cake, Snack	Packaged	Little Debbie
Cake, Snack	Packaged	Little Debbie
Cake, Snack	Packaged	Little Debbie
Cake, Snack	Packaged	Little Debbie
Cake, Snack	Packaged	Little Debbie
Cake, Snack	Packaged	Little Debbie
Cake, Snack	Packaged	Little Debbie
Cake, Snack	Packaged	Little Debbie
Cake, Snack	Packaged	Little Debbie
Cake, Snack	Packaged	Little Debbie Be My Valentine
Cake, Snack	Packaged	Little Debbie Caravella
Cake, Snack	Packaged	Little Debbie Choco-Cake
Cake, Snack	Packaged	Little Debbie Choco-Jel
Cake, Snack	Packaged	Little Debbie Christmas Tree
Cake, Snack	Packaged	Little Debbie Devil Cremes
Cake, Snack	Packaged	Little Debbie Devil Squares
Cake, Snack	Packaged	Little Debbie Doodle Dandies
Cake, Snack	Packaged	Little Debbie Easter Bunny
Cake, Snack	Packaged	Little Debbie Figaroos
Cake, Snack	Packaged	Little Debbie Holiday Cake
Cake, Snack	Packaged	Little Debbie Holiday Cake
Cake, Snack	Packaged	Little Debbie Mint Sprints

Major Description	Minor Description	Serving Size	Calories	Grade
Fruit		1 piece	400	B–
Chocolate		1 piece	120	D
Apple		1 piece	130	A
Chocolate	Vanilla Pudding Filled	1 piece	130	A–
Coffee Crumb Cake		1 piece	80	A
Cupcake, Chocolate	Cream Filled	1 piece	130	A–
Golden	Cream Filled	1 piece	90	B
Chocolate	Coconut Frosted	1 piece	150	B
Chocolate		1 piece	250	C
Golden	Cream Filled	1 piece	240	B
Banana		1 piece	150	B–
Golden	Cream Filled	1 piece	150	B–
Strawberry		1 piece	160	B–
Strawberry		1 piece	140	B–
Golden	Cream Filled	1 piece	110	B–
Apple Delights		1 pkg	140	B
Apple Spice		1 pkg	270	C
Banana	Slices	1 pkg	340	C
Banana	Twins	1 pkg	250	C
Cherry Cordial		1 pkg	170	D
Chocolate		1 pkg	320	C
Chocolate	Fudge, Crispy	1 pkg	260	B
Chocolate	Slices	1 pkg	320	B
Chocolate	Twins	1 pkg	240	B
Chocolate Chip		1 pkg	320	D
Coconut	Round	1 pkg	150	D
Coconut Crunch		1 pkg	320	D
Coffee Cake		1 pkg	250	C
Dessert Cup		1 pkg	80	A–
Fancy Cakes		1 pkg	340	D
Golden	Cream Filled	1 pkg	270	C
Jelly Roll		1 pkg	250	C
Lemon Stix		1 pkg	220	D
Marshmallow Supreme		1 pkg	150	B
Peanut Butter	Bar	1 pkg	370	D
Peanut Butter & Jelly Sandwich		1 pkg	150	C
Pecan Twins		1 pkg	220	D
Pumpkin Delights		1 pkg	140	C
Swiss Roll		1 pkg	280	C
Vanilla		1 pkg	390	D
		1 pkg	330	D
		1 pkg	200	D
Chocolate		1 pkg	270	D
Chocolate		1 pkg	150	D
		1 pkg	220	D
Devil's Food		1 pkg	300	C
Devil's Food		1 pkg	270	C
		1 pkg	320	D
		1 pkg	320	D
Fig		1 pkg	160	B
Chocolate		1 pkg	310	D
Vanilla		1 pkg	320	D
Mint Wafer	Chocolate Coated	1 pkg	200	D

"+" indicates the food meets minimum fiber requirements; "–" indicates the food has a high sodium content.

Food	Processing Category	Brand
Cake, Snack	Packaged	Little Debbie Nutty Bar
Cake, Snack	Packaged	Little Debbie Peanut Butter
Cake, Snack	Packaged	Little Debbie Peanut Cluster
Cake, Snack	Packaged	Little Debbie Star Crunch
Cake, Snack	Packaged	Sunbelt
Cake, Snack	Packaged	Tastykake
Cake, Snack	Packaged	Tastykake
Cake, Snack	Packaged	Tastykake
Cake, Snack	Packaged	Tastykake Creamie
Cake, Snack	Packaged	Tastykake Creamie
Cake, Snack	Packaged	Tastykake Creamie
Cake, Snack	Packaged	Tastykake Juniors
Cake, Snack	Packaged	Tastykake Juniors
Cake, Snack	Packaged	Tastykake Juniors
Cake, Snack	Packaged	Tastykake Juniors
Cake, Snack	Packaged	Tastykake Kandy Kakes
Cake, Snack	Packaged	Tastykake Kandy Kakes
Cake, Snack	Packaged	Tastykake Koffee Kake
Cake, Snack	Packaged	Tastykake Koffee Kake
Cake, Snack	Packaged	Tastykake Kreme Kup
Cake, Snack	Packaged	Tastykake Krimpets
Cake, Snack	Packaged	Tastykake Krimpets
Cake, Snack	Packaged	Tastykake Krimpets
Cake, Snack	Packaged	Tastykake Krimpets
Cake, Snack	Packaged	Tastykake Tasty Twist
Cake, Snack	Packaged	Tastykake Tastylite
Cake, Snack	Packaged	Tastykake Tastylite
Candy	All Forms	Barat
Candy	All Forms	Barat Bar
Candy	All Forms	Barat Bar
Candy	All Forms	Barat Bar
Candy	All Forms	Barat Bits
Candy	All Forms	Barat Bits
Candy	All Forms	Barat Bits
Candy	All Forms	Barat Bits
Candy	All Forms	Barat Passionettes
Candy	All Forms	Bearitos Little Bear
Candy	All Forms	Beich's Laffy Taffy
Candy	All Forms	Beich's Laffy Taffy
Candy	All Forms	Beich's Laffy Taffy
Candy	All Forms	Beich's Laffy Taffy
Candy	All Forms	Beich's Laffy Taffy
Candy	All Forms	Beich's Laffy Taffy
Candy	All Forms	Beich's Laffy Taffy
Candy	All Forms	Bit-O-Honey
Candy	All Forms	Bits-O-Heath
Candy	All Forms	Bonkers Chews
Candy	All Forms	Boyer
Candy	All Forms	Boyer Mallow Cup
Candy	All Forms	Boyer Smoothie
Candy	All Forms	Brach's
Candy	All Forms	Brach's

Major Description	Minor Description	Serving Size	Calories	Grade
Peanut Butter Wafer	Chocolate Coated	1 pkg	310	D
Wafer	Peanut Butter Filled	1 pkg	170	D
Chocolate	Caramel & Peanut Filled	1 pkg	230	D
		1 pkg	150	C
Apple Bar	Baked	1.31 oz pkg	130	A
Cupcake	Butter Cream Filled	1.1 oz	118	C
Cupcake	Chocolate	1.1 oz	100	B
Pecan Twirls		1 oz	109	D
Banana		1.5 oz	185	C
Chocolate		1.5 oz	168	D
Vanilla		1.5 oz	184	D
Chocolate		3.3 oz	341	C
Coconut		3.3 oz	296	B
Lemon		3.3 oz	306	A
Orange		3.3 oz	337	B
Chocolate		.7 oz	78	C
Peanut Butter		.7 oz	87	D
Coffee		2.5 oz	261	B
Coffee	Cream Filled	1 oz	110	C
Cupcake	Cream Filled	.9 oz	86	B–
Butterscotch		1 oz	103	B
Chocolate	Cream Filled	1 piece	124	C
Jelly		1 oz	85	A
Vanilla	Cream Filled	1.1 oz	116	C
Swiss Roll		1 piece	18	B
Cupcake	Chocolate, Cream Filled	1.1 oz	118	C
Cupcake	Vanilla, Cream Filled	1 piece	100	A
Chocolate Tofu	After Dinner Mints	1 piece	40	D
Chocolate Tofu	Almonds	1 oz	170	D
Chocolate Tofu	Almonds & Raisins	1 oz	160	D
Chocolate Tofu	Truffle with Praline	1 oz	170	D
Chocolate Tofu	Mints	1 oz	160	D
Chocolate Tofu	Pastilles	1 oz	160	D
Chocolate Tofu	Peanuts, Dipped	1 oz	120	D
Chocolate Tofu	Raisins	1 oz	120	D
Chocolate Tofu		1 piece	70	D
Popcorn	Caramel Coated	1 oz	110	B
Apple-flavored Chews		1 oz	110	A
Banana-flavored Chews		1 oz	120	A
Cherry-flavored Chews, Sweet & Sour		1 oz	110	A
Grape-flavored Chews		1 oz	110	A
Punch-flavored Chews		1 oz	120	A
Strawberry-flavored Chews		1 oz	110	A
Watermelon-flavored Chews		1 oz	110	A
Honey		1.7 oz piece	200	B
English Toffee		3.5 oz	520	D
All Flavors		1 piece	20	A
Peanut Butter Cup		.5 oz piece	75	D
Marshmallow		1 piece	36	D
		1 piece	125	D
Autumn, Leaves		1 oz	100	A
Bridge Mix		1 oz	130	D

"+" indicates the food meets minimum fiber requirements; "–" indicates the food has a high sodium content.

Food	Processing Category	Brand
Candy	All Forms	Brach's
Candy	All Forms	Brach's
Candy	All Forms	Brach's
Candy	All Forms	Brach's
Candy	All Forms	Brach's
Candy	All Forms	Brach's
Candy	All Forms	Brach's
Candy	All Forms	Brach's
Candy	All Forms	Brach's
Candy	All Forms	Brach's
Candy	All Forms	Brach's
Candy	All Forms	Brach's
Candy	All Forms	Brach's
Candy	All Forms	Brach's
Candy	All Forms	Brach's
Candy	All Forms	Brach's
Candy	All Forms	Brach's
Candy	All Forms	Brach's
Candy	All Forms	Brach's
Candy	All Forms	Brach's
Candy	All Forms	Brach's
Candy	All Forms	Brach's
Candy	All Forms	Brach's
Candy	All Forms	Brach's
Candy	All Forms	Brach's
Candy	All Forms	Brach's
Candy	All Forms	Brach's
Candy	All Forms	Brach's
Candy	All Forms	Brach's
Candy	All Forms	Brach's
Candy	All Forms	Brach's
Candy	All Forms	Brach's
Candy	All Forms	Brach's
Candy	All Forms	Brach's
Candy	All Forms	Brach's
Candy	All Forms	Brach's
Candy	All Forms	Brach's
Candy	All Forms	Brach's
Candy	All Forms	Brach's
Candy	All Forms	Brach's
Candy	All Forms	Brach's
Candy	All Forms	Brach's
Candy	All Forms	Brach's
Candy	All Forms	Brach's
Candy	All Forms	Brach's
Candy	All Forms	Brach's
Candy	All Forms	Brach's
Candy	All Forms	Brach's
Candy	All Forms	Brach's
Candy	All Forms	Brach's
Candy	All Forms	Brach's
Candy	All Forms	Brach's
Candy	All Forms	Brach's
Candy	All Forms	Brach's

Major Description	Minor Description	Serving Size	Calories	Grade
Cherry	Chocolate Cream	1 oz	110	B
Cherry	Dark Chocolate Coated	1 oz	110	B
Cherry	Milk Chocolate Coated	1 oz	110	B
Chocolate	Assorted	1 oz	110	B
Chocolate	Assorted, Wrapped	1 oz	110	B
Christmas Bell	Chocolate in Foil	1 oz	150	D
Christmas, Candy Cane		1 oz	110	A
Christmas, Jellies		1 oz	100	A
Christmas, Jellies	Snowbase	1 oz	100	A
Christmas, Nougat		1 oz	110	B
Christmas, Ornaments		1 oz	150	D
Christmas, Santa	Chocolate in Foil	1 oz	140	D
Christmas, Santa	Marshmallow	1 oz	120	B
Coconut	Neapolitan	1 oz	120	A
Coffee Flavor		1 oz	120	A
Easter, Corn		1 oz	100	A
Easter, Eggs	Chocolate Buttercream	1 oz	120	B
Easter, Eggs	Chocolate in Foil	1 oz	150	D
Easter, Eggs	Chocolate Malted Milk	1 oz	130	C
Easter, Eggs	Chocolate-Coated Cherries	1 oz	110	B
Easter, Eggs	Coconut	1 oz	110	B
Easter, Eggs	Maple	1 oz	110	B
Easter, Eggs	Marshmallow	1 oz	100	A
Easter, Eggs	Vanilla	1 oz	110	B
Easter, Eggs, Fruit & Nut		1 oz	110	B
Easter, Eggs, Jelly		1 oz	100	A
Easter, Eggs, Jelly	Speckled	1 oz	110	A
Easter, Eggs, Jelly	Spiced	1 oz	90	A
Easter, Nougats		1 oz	100	A
Filled, Assorted		1 oz	110	A
Halloween, Corn	Three Color	1 oz	100	A
Halloween, Holiday Mints		1 oz	110	A
Halloween, Holiday Mix		1 oz	110	A
Halloween, Indian Corn		1 oz	100	A
Halloween, Jelly Beans		1 oz	100	A
Halloween, Pumpkins		1 oz	100	A
Halloween, Witches Teeth		1 oz	100	A
Jellied & Gummed	Beans	1 oz	100	A
Jellied & Gummed	Mints, Assorted	1 oz	100	A
Jellied & Gummed	Spearmint Leaves	1 oz	100	A
Lemon Drops		1 oz	110	A
Malted Milk Balls	Milk Chocolate Coated	1 oz	130	C
Mint	Parfait	1 oz	150	D
Mint	Regular, Creme or Thin	1 oz	110	B
Nonpareils Dark Chocolate		1 oz	140	C
Nougat	Jelly	1 oz	100	A
Orange Sticks	Chocolate Coated	1 oz	110	B
Peanut	Filled	1 oz	110	A
Peanut	French Burnt	1 oz	130	C
Peanut	Milk Chocolate	1 oz	150	D
Peanut Butter	Kisses	1 oz	110	B
Peanut Caramel Cluster		1 oz	150	D

"+" indicates the food meets minimum fiber requirements; "–" indicates the food has a high sodium content.

Food	Processing Category	Brand
Candy	All Forms	Brach's
Candy	All Forms	Brach's
Candy	All Forms	Brach's
Candy	All Forms	Brach's
Candy	All Forms	Brach's
Candy	All Forms	Brach's
Candy	All Forms	Brach's
Candy	All Forms	Brach's
Candy	All Forms	Brach's
Candy	All Forms	Brach's
Candy	All Forms	Brach's
Candy	All Forms	Brach's
Candy	All Forms	Brach's
Candy	All Forms	Brach's
Candy	All Forms	Brach's Chicks & Rabbits
Candy	All Forms	Brach's Cinnamon Bears
Candy	All Forms	Brach's Conversation, Large
Candy	All Forms	Brach's Conversation, Small
Candy	All Forms	Brach's Coolers, Starlight
Candy	All Forms	Brach's Crème De Menthe
Candy	All Forms	Brach's Cut Rock
Candy	All Forms	Brach's Dessert Mints
Candy	All Forms	Brach's Disks
Candy	All Forms	Brach's Disks
Candy	All Forms	Brach's Easter Fun
Candy	All Forms	Brach's Fiesta
Candy	All Forms	Brach's Fruit Bunch
Candy	All Forms	Brach's Gummi Bears/Worms
Candy	All Forms	Brach's Heart Box, Lb.
Candy	All Forms	Brach's Hide N Seek
Candy	All Forms	Brach's I Luv U
Candy	All Forms	Brach's Imperial
Candy	All Forms	Brach's Jels
Candy	All Forms	Brach's Jordan Almonds
Candy	All Forms	Brach's Jots
Candy	All Forms	Brach's Jots
Candy	All Forms	Brach's Jots
Candy	All Forms	Brach's Jots/Pearls
Candy	All Forms	Brach's Jube
Candy	All Forms	Brach's Jube
Candy	All Forms	Brach's Jube
Candy	All Forms	Brach's Kentucky Mints
Candy	All Forms	Brach's Love
Candy	All Forms	Brach's Mellowcremes
Candy	All Forms	Brach's Mellowcremes
Candy	All Forms	Brach's Milk Maid
Candy	All Forms	Brach's Milk Maid
Candy	All Forms	Brach's Nut Goodies
Candy	All Forms	Brach's Orangettes
Candy	All Forms	Brach's Peanut Clusters
Candy	All Forms	Brach's Peanuts
Candy	All Forms	Brach's Pearls

Major Description	Minor Description	Serving Size	Calories	Grade
Peanut Parfait		1 oz	160	D
Peeps Rabbits	Marshmallow	1 piece	120	B
Peppermint Kisses		1 oz	100	A
Raisins, Chocolate Coated		1 oz	130	C
Raspberry Filled		1 oz	110	A
Ribbon Crimp		1 oz	110	A
Seasonal & Specialty	Christmas, Assorted Chocolate	1 oz	110	B
Sour Balls		1 oz	110	A
Straws	Mint Filled	1 oz	110	A
Toffee		1 oz	110	B
Valentine's Day, Hearts		1 oz	110	B
Valentine's Day, Hearts	Fruity	1 oz	100	A
Valentine's Day, Hearts	Red Jelly	1 oz	100	A
Valentine's Day, Kisses	Nougat	1 oz	110	B
Easter Assorted		1 oz	100	A
Jellied & Gummed	Cinnamon	1 oz	80	A
Valentine's Day, Hearts		1 oz	110	A
Valentine's Day, Hearts		1 oz	110	A
Mint		1 oz	110	A
Mint		1 oz	150	D
Rock		1 oz	110	A
Mint	Assorted	1 oz	110	A
Butterscotch		1 oz	110	A–
Cinnamon		1 oz	110	A
Easter, Assorted Flavors		1 oz	100	A
Easter, Eggs, Pastel		1 oz	120	B
Fruit Flavored	All Flavors	1 oz	90	A
Jellied & Gummed		1 oz	100	A
Valentine's Day		1 oz	110	B
Easter, Eggs		1 oz	110	A
Valentine's Day, Chocolate		1 oz	150	D
Valentine's Day, Hearts	Cinnamon	1 oz	110	A
Jellied & Gummed	Cherry, Sour	1 oz	100	A
Almond	Candy Coated	1 oz	120	A
Chocolate		1 oz	130	C
Christmas		1 oz	130	C
Peanut		1 oz	140	C
Mint		1 oz	120	A
Easter, Peeps Jelly Rabbits		1 oz	100	A
Jellied & Gummed		1 oz	100	A
Valentine's Day, Hearts	Cherry Jelly	1 oz	100	A
Mint		1 oz	110	A
Valentine's Day		1 oz	150	D
Halloween		1 oz	100	A
Valentine's Day		1 oz	100	A
Caramel		1 oz	110	B
Caramel	Chocolate	1 oz	110	B
Nut		1 oz	130	B
Orange		1 oz	100	A
Chocolate		1 oz	150	D
Chocolate Coated		1 oz	140	D
Christmas, Mints		1 oz	110	A

"+" indicates the food meets minimum fiber requirements; "–" indicates the food has a high sodium content.

Food	Processing Category	Brand
Candy	All Forms	Brach's Perkys
Candy	All Forms	Brach's Perkys Circus Peanuts
Candy	All Forms	Brach's Picture Pops
Candy	All Forms	Brach's Pops
Candy	All Forms	Brach's Rainbow Bears
Candy	All Forms	Brach's Red Laces/Twin Twists
Candy	All Forms	Brach's Robin Eggs
Candy	All Forms	Brach's Saltwater Taffy
Candy	All Forms	Brach's Sassy Hearts
Candy	All Forms	Brach's Scary Cats
Candy	All Forms	Brach's Spicettes
Candy	All Forms	Brach's Starlight
Candy	All Forms	Brach's Starlight
Candy	All Forms	Brach's Stars
Candy	All Forms	Brach's Tiny
Candy	All Forms	Brach's Trick or Treat Party Pack
Candy	All Forms	Brach's Twists
Candy	All Forms	Brach's Valentine Heart Box
Candy	All Forms	Breath Savers
Candy	All Forms	Butterfinger
Candy	All Forms	Cadbury
Candy	All Forms	Cadbury
Candy	All Forms	Cadbury
Candy	All Forms	Cadbury
Candy	All Forms	Cadbury Dairy Milk
Candy	All Forms	Callard & Bowser
Candy	All Forms	Callard & Bowser
Candy	All Forms	Callard & Bowser
Candy	All Forms	Callard & Bowser
Candy	All Forms	Campfire
Candy	All Forms	Caramello
Candy	All Forms	Caroby
Candy	All Forms	Certs Sugar Free
Candy	All Forms	Certs Sugar Free
Candy	All Forms	Charleston Chew
Candy	All Forms	Chunky
Candy	All Forms	Clorets
Candy	All Forms	Clorets
Candy	All Forms	Cracker Jack
Candy	All Forms	Cracker Jack
Candy	All Forms	Demet's Turtles
Candy	All Forms	Estee
Candy	All Forms	Estee
Candy	All Forms	Estee
Candy	All Forms	Estee
Candy	All Forms	Estee
Candy	All Forms	Estee
Candy	All Forms	Estee
Candy	All Forms	Estee
Candy	All Forms	Estee
Candy	All Forms	Estee
Candy	All Forms	Estee
Candy	All Forms	Estee

Major Description	Minor Description	Serving Size	Calories	Grade
Christmas		1 oz	90	A
Marshmallow		1 oz	100	A
Halloween, Lollipops		1 oz	110	A
Lollipop	All Flavors	1 oz	110	A
Jellied & Gummed	Rainbow	1 oz	100	A
Licorice		1 oz	100	A
Easter, Eggs		1 oz	140	C
Taffy, All Flavors		1 oz	100	A
Valentine's Day, Hearts		1 oz	100	A
Halloween, Cats		1 oz	100	A
Spice		1 oz	100	A
Christmas, Mints		1 oz	110	A
Easter, Mints		1 oz	110	A
Milk Chocolate		1 oz	150	D
Easter, Eggs, Jelly		1 piece	100	A
Halloween		1 piece	110	A
Licorice		1 oz	100	A
Chocolates		1 oz	110	B
Mints	All Flavors	1 piece	8	A
		1 bar	100	D
Chocolate	Almonds, Roasted	1 oz	150	D
Chocolate	with Fruit & Nuts	1 oz	150	D
Chocolate	with Krisps & Honey	1 oz	150	D
Easter, Eggs	Cream	1 egg	190	C
Milk Chocolate		1 oz	150	D
Butterscotch		1 oz	115	A
Chocolate	Cream	1 oz	120	B
Jellied & Gummed	Juicy	1 oz	90	A
Toffee		1 oz	135	D
Marshmallow		1 piece	20	A
Chocolate	Caramel	1 piece	220	D
Carob Milk Bar		1 section	38	D
Mint	Mini	1 piece	1	A
Mint	Regular	1 piece	6	A
Nougat, Chocolate Coated	All Flavors	1 oz	120	B
Chocolate	Fruit & Nuts	1 piece	210	D
Mint	Clear	1 piece	8	A
Mint	Pressed	1 piece	6	A
Popcorn	Toffee & Butter	1 oz	130	C
Popcorn, Caramel Coated	Peanuts	1 oz	120	B
Chocolate	Pecan & Caramel	1 oz	15	D
Caramel	Chocolate Vanilla	1 piece	20	D
Chocolate	Almond	2 squares	60	D
Chocolate	Coconut	2 squares	60	D
Chocolate	Crunch	2 squares	45	D
Chocolate	Dark, Deluxe	2 squares	60	D
Chocolate	Fruit & Nuts	2 squares	60	D
Chocolate	Milk	2 squares	60	D
Chocolate	Mint	2 squares	60	D
Chocolate	Peanut	2 squares	60	D
Gum Drops		1 piece	6	A
Gummy Bears		1 piece	5	A
Hard		1 piece	25	A

"+" indicates the food meets minimum fiber requirements; "−" indicates the food has a high sodium content.

Food	Processing Category	Brand
Candy	All Forms	Estee
Candy	All Forms	Estee
Candy	All Forms	Estee
Candy	All Forms	Estee
Candy	All Forms	Estee
Candy	All Forms	Estee Estee-ets
Candy	All Forms	Featherweight
Candy	All Forms	Featherweight
Candy	All Forms	Featherweight
Candy	All Forms	Featherweight
Candy	All Forms	Featherweight
Candy	All Forms	Featherweight
Candy	All Forms	Featherweight
Candy	All Forms	Featherweight Cool Blue
Candy	All Forms	Featherweights
Candy	All Forms	Flavor House
Candy	All Forms	Franklin
Candy	All Forms	Franklin
Candy	All Forms	Funmallows
Candy	All Forms	Funmallows
Candy	All Forms	Good & Fruity
Candy	All Forms	Good & Plenty
Candy	All Forms	Greenfield Healthy Foods
Candy	All Forms	Heath Bar
Candy	All Forms	Heath Bits-O-Brickle
Candy	All Forms	Heath Soft N Crunch Bar
Candy	All Forms	Hershey's
Candy	All Forms	Hershey's
Candy	All Forms	Hershey's Almond Joy
Candy	All Forms	Hershey's Golden Almond
Candy	All Forms	Hershey's Kisses
Candy	All Forms	Hershey's Kisses
Candy	All Forms	Hershey's Mounds
Candy	All Forms	Hershey's Mr. Goodbar
Candy	All Forms	Hershey's Reese's
Candy	All Forms	Hershey's Reese's Pieces
Candy	All Forms	Hershey's Rolos
Candy	All Forms	Hershey's Skor
Candy	All Forms	Hershey's Solitaires
Candy	All Forms	Hershey's Special Dark
Candy	All Forms	Hershey's Symphony
Candy	All Forms	Hershey's Symphony
Candy	All Forms	Holidays
Candy	All Forms	Hot Tamales
Candy	All Forms	Jolly Joes
Candy	All Forms	Jujyfruits
Candy	All Forms	Junior Mints
Candy	All Forms	Just Born
Candy	All Forms	Just Born
Candy	All Forms	Just Born
Candy	All Forms	Just Born

Major Description	Minor Description	Serving Size	Calories	Grade
Lollipop	All Flavors	1 piece	25	A
Peanut Brittle		.25 oz	35	B
Peanut Butter	Cup	1 piece	40	D
Popcorn, Caramel Coated		1 oz	140	B
Raisins, Chocolate Coated		10 raisins	30	B
Cream Center, Chocolate Coated		5 pieces	35	D
Butterscotch		1 piece	25	A
Caramel		1 piece	30	B
Chocolate	Almond	1 section	90	D
Chocolate	Crunch	1 section	80	D
Chocolate	Milk	1 section	80	D
Fruit Flavor	Berry Patch Orchard or Tropical Blend	1 piece	12	A
Fruit Flavored Drops	All Flavors	1 oz	90	A
Mint		1 piece	25	A
Peppermint Swirls		1 piece	20	A
Peanut	Butter Toffee	1 oz	150	D
Popcorn	Maple & Walnut	1 oz	140	B
Popcorn	Toffee & Peanuts	1 oz	140	B
Marshmallow		1 piece	30	A
Marshmallow	Miniature	1 piece	2	A
Licorice	Candy Coated	1 oz	106	A
Licorice	Candy Coated	1 oz	106	A
Popcorn	Caramel Coated	1 oz	120	A
English Toffee		1 oz	151	D
English Toffee		1 oz	150	D
English Toffee		1 oz	160	D
Chocolate		1 bar	240	D
Chocolate	Almonds	1 bar	230	D
Coconut	Almonds	1 bar	250	D
Chocolate		1 bar	260	D
Chocolate		1 piece	25	D
Chocolate	Almonds	1 piece	26	D
Coconut	Chocolate Coated	1 bar	260	D
Chocolate	with Peanuts	1 bar	290	D
Peanut Butter Cups	Chocolate Coated	1 piece	42	D
Peanut Butter	Candy Coated	1 piece	4	C
Caramel	Chocolate Coated	1 pkg	270	C
Toffee		1 bar	220	D
Chocolate	Almonds	1 bar	260	D
Chocolate	Dark, Sweet	1 bar	220	D
Chocolate	Creamy	1 bar	270	D
Chocolate	Creamy with Almonds & Toffee Chips	1 bar	280	D
Chocolate	Candy Coated	1 oz	140	C
		1 piece	9	A
Jellied & Gummed		1 piece	9	A
Jellied & Gummed		1 piece	100	A
Mint	Chocolate Coated	1 oz	120	B
Easter, Peeps	Marshmallow	1 piece	27	A
Easter, Peeps or Rabbits	Marshmallow	1 large	111	A
Halloween, Cats	Marshmallow	1 piece	28	A
Halloween, Pumpkins	Marshmallow	1 piece	111	A

"+" indicates the food meets minimum fiber requirements; "−" indicates the food has a high sodium content.

Food	Processing Category	Brand
Candy	All Forms	Just Born
Candy	All Forms	Just Born
Candy	All Forms	Just Born
Candy	All Forms	Just Born, Petite
Candy	All Forms	Just Born, Teenee Beanee Gourmet
Candy	All Forms	Kit Kat
Candy	All Forms	Kraft
Candy	All Forms	Kraft
Candy	All Forms	Kraft
Candy	All Forms	Kraft
Candy	All Forms	Kraft Fudgies
Candy	All Forms	Kraft Jet-puffed
Candy	All Forms	Krrackel
Candy	All Forms	Life Savers
Candy	All Forms	Life Savers
Candy	All Forms	Life Savers
Candy	All Forms	Life Savers
Candy	All Forms	Life Savers
Candy	All Forms	Life Savers
Candy	All Forms	Life Savers
Candy	All Forms	Life Savers
Candy	All Forms	Mars Bar
Candy	All Forms	Mars Bounty
Candy	All Forms	Mars M&M's
Candy	All Forms	Mars M&M's
Candy	All Forms	Mars M&M's
Candy	All Forms	Mars M&M's
Candy	All Forms	Mars Munch
Candy	All Forms	Mars Skittles
Candy	All Forms	Mars Snickers
Candy	All Forms	Mars Starburst
Candy	All Forms	Mars Twix
Candy	All Forms	Mars Twix
Candy	All Forms	Mars, 3 Musketeers
Candy	All Forms	Milky Way
Candy	All Forms	Milky Way Mini
Candy	All Forms	Milky Way, Dark
Candy	All Forms	Mint Meltaway
Candy	All Forms	Nabisco
Candy	All Forms	Nabisco
Candy	All Forms	Nabisco Stars
Candy	All Forms	Necco
Candy	All Forms	Necco
Candy	All Forms	Necco Sky Bar
Candy	All Forms	Nestlé
Candy	All Forms	Nestlé
Candy	All Forms	Nestlé 100 Grand
Candy	All Forms	Nestlé Alpine
Candy	All Forms	Nestlé Baby Ruth
Candy	All Forms	Nestlé Crunch

Major Description	Minor Description	Serving Size	Calories	Grade
Marshmallow	Coconut Toasted	1 piece	30	B+
Snowmen or Trees	Marshmallow	1 large	111	A
Snowmen or Trees	Marshmallow	1 small	37	A
Jellied & Gummed	Eggs	1 piece	4	A
Jellied & Gummed	Beans	1 piece	4	A
Wafer Bar	Chocolate Coated	1 bar	250	D
Butter or Party Mint		1 piece	8	A
Caramel		1 piece	30	B
Marshmallow	Mini	10 pieces	18	A
Peanut Brittle		1 oz	130	C
Fudge		1 piece	35	B
Marshmallow		1 piece	25	A
Chocolate	Crisps	1 piece	230	D
All Fruit Flavors		1 piece	8	A
All Mint Flavors except Butter Cream		1 piece	8	A
Butter Cream Mint		1 piece	8	A
Butter Rum		1 piece	8	A–
Butterscotch		1 piece	8	A–
Cinnamon		1 piece	8	A
Lollipop	All Flavors	1 piece	45	A
Root Beer		1 piece	8	A
		1 bar	240	D
Coconut	Dark or Milk Chocolate	1 bar	150	D
Chocolate	Almond	1/4 cup	230	D
Chocolate	Peanut Butter	1/4 cup	220	D
Chocolate	Peanuts	1/4 cup	220	D
Chocolate	Plain	1/4 cup	210	D
		1 bar	220	D
Fruit Flavor	All Flavors	2.3 oz pkg	265	A
		1 bar	280	D
Fruit Flavor	All Flavors, Chews	1 oz	120	B
Caramel	Chocolate Coated, with Cookies	1 piece	140	D
Peanut Butter	Chocolate Coated, with Cookies	1 piece	130	D
Chocolate		1 bar	260	B
Milk Chocolate		1 bar	280	C
Milk Chocolate		1 bar	40	C
Dark Chocolate		1 bar	220	C
		1 piece	50	D
Peanuts	Chocolate Coated	1 oz	160	D
Raisins	Chocolate Coated	1 oz	130	C
Chocolate	Milk	1 oz	160	D
Wafer	Assorted	1 piece	225	A
Wafer	Chocolate	1 piece	226	A
		1 piece	196	C
Chocolate		1 bar	220	D
Chocolate	Almonds	1 bar	230	D
Chocolate	Crisps & Peanuts	1 bar	200	C
Chocolate	White, with Almonds	1 bar	210	D
Chocolate with Peanuts	Full Size	1 bar	277	D
Chocolate	Crisps	1 bar	210	D

"+" indicates the food meets minimum fiber requirements; "–" indicates the food has a high sodium content.

Food	Processing Category	Brand
Candy	All Forms	Nestlé Goobers
Candy	All Forms	Nestlé Oh-Henry
Candy	All Forms	Nestlé Raisinets
Candy	All Forms	Nestlé Sno-Caps
Candy	All Forms	Orville Redenbacher
Candy	All Forms	PB Max
Candy	All Forms	Pearson's Licorice Nip
Candy	All Forms	Pom Poms
Candy	All Forms	Rascals
Candy	All Forms	Rodda
Candy	All Forms	Rowntree, After Eight
Candy	All Forms	Spangler
Candy	All Forms	Spangler Bittersweets
Candy	All Forms	Spangler Blo Bubble
Candy	All Forms	Spangler Circus Peanuts
Candy	All Forms	Spangler Dum Dums
Candy	All Forms	Spangler Opera Creme Chocolate Drop
Candy	All Forms	Spangler Peanut Cluster
Candy	All Forms	Spangler Peanut Cluster
Candy	All Forms	Spangler Peanut Cluster
Candy	All Forms	Spangler Peanut Cluster
Candy	All Forms	Spangler Peanut Cluster
Candy	All Forms	Spangler Pecan Cluster
Candy	All Forms	Spangler Saf-T-Tops
Candy	All Forms	Sugar Babies
Candy	All Forms	Sugar Daddy
Candy	All Forms	Sunbelt Macaroo
Candy	All Forms	Tootsie Roll
Candy	All Forms	Tootsie Roll Pop
Candy	All Forms	Tootsie Roll Pop
Candy	All Forms	Weight Watchers
Candy	All Forms	Weight Watchers Smart Snackers
Candy	All Forms	Woody's
Candy	All Forms	Woodys
Candy	All Forms	Y & S Bites
Candy	All Forms	Y & S Nibs
Candy	All Forms	Y & S Twizzlers
Candy	All Forms	York Peppermint Patties
Caramel Topping	Jar	Kraft
Caramel Topping	Jar	Smucker's
Caramel Topping	Jar	Smucker's
Cobbler	Fresh Baked	Awrey's
Cobbler	Fresh Baked	Awrey's
Cobbler	Frozen	Marie Callender's

Major Description	Minor Description	Serving Size	Calories	Grade
Peanut	Chocolate Coated	10 pieces	51	D
Caramel	Peanut, Chocolate Coated	1 bar	280	D
Raisins	Chocolate Coated	10 pieces	41	B
Nonpareils		1 oz	140	C
Popcorn	Caramel Coated	3 cups	288	D
Peanut Butter		1 piece	240	D
Licorice		1 oz	120	B
Caramel	Chocolate Coated	1 oz	100	B
Fruit Flavor	All Flavors, Chews	1 piece	4	A
Jellied & Gummed	Eggs	1 piece	7	A
Mint	Dark Chocolate	1 piece	35	B
Candy Cane		1 piece	60	A
Cream Center, Chocolate Coated	Mint, Dark Chocolate Coated	1 piece	80	B
Lollipop	Bubble Gum Center	1 pop	57	A
Marshmallow		1 piece	28	A
Lollipop	All Flavors	1 pop	25	A
Cream Center, Chocolate Coated		1 piece	80	B
Cream Center, Chocolate Coated	Caramel with Nuts	1 piece	100	D
Cream Center, Chocolate Coated	Cherry Cream with Nuts	1 piece	110	D
Cream Center, Chocolate Coated	Fudge with Nuts	1 piece	140	C
Cream Center, Chocolate Coated	Maple Cream with Nuts	1 piece	110	D
Cream Center, Chocolate Coated	Vanilla Cream with Nuts	1 piece	110	D
Cream Center, Chocolate Coated	Fudge with Nuts	1 piece	140	D
Lollipop	All Flavors	1 pop	45	A
Regular/Tidbits	Caramel	1 pkg	180	A
Caramel		1 pop	150	A
Coconut	Chocolate Coated	2 oz	288	D
Tootsie Roll		1 piece	112	B
Lollipop	All Flavors Except Chocolate	1 pop	60	A
Lollipop	Chocolate	1 pop	60	A
Popcorn	Toffee & Butter	1 oz	140	B
Popcorn	Caramel Coated	1 oz	110	A
Fudge	Chocolate or Mint with Walnuts	1 oz	120	B
Fudge	Maple Walnut	1 oz	120	B
Licorice	Cherry	1 oz	100	A
Licorice	Cherry	1 oz	100	A
Licorice	Strawberry	1 oz	100	A
Mint	Chocolate Coated, Large	1 patty	180	B
		2 Tbsp	120	A
		2 Tbsp	150	B
Flavored		2 Tbsp	140	A
Apple, Deep-dish		1/8 pie	320	C
Blueberry, Deep-dish		1/8 pie	310	C
Apple		4.5 oz	350	D

"+" indicates the food meets minimum fiber requirements; "–" indicates the food has a high sodium content.

Food	Processing Category	Brand
Cobbler	Frozen	Marie Callender's
Cobbler	Frozen	Marie Callender's
Cobbler	Frozen	Marie Callender's
Cobbler	Frozen	Marie Callender's
Cobbler	Frozen	Pet Ritz
Cobbler	Frozen	Pet Ritz
Cobbler	Frozen	Pet Ritz
Cobbler	Frozen	Pet Ritz
Cobbler	Frozen	Pet Ritz
Cobbler	Frozen	Pet Ritz
Cobbler	Frozen	Stillwell
Cobbler	Frozen	Stillwell
Cobbler	Frozen	Stillwell
Cobbler	Frozen	Stillwell
Cocoa Powder	Canned	Bensdorp
Cocoa Powder	Canned	Hershey's
Cocoa Powder	Canned	Hershey's European
Cocoa Powder	Canned	Nestlé
Cookies	Fresh Baked	Generic
Cookies	Fresh Baked	Generic
Cookies	Fresh Baked	Generic
Cookies	Fresh Baked	Almost Home
Cookies	Fresh Baked	Almost Home
Cookies	Fresh Baked	Almost Home Old Fashioned
Cookies	Fresh Baked	Almost Home Real
Cookies	Fresh Baked	Archway
Cookies	Fresh Baked	Archway
Cookies	Fresh Baked	Archway
Cookies	Fresh Baked	Archway
Cookies	Fresh Baked	Archway
Cookies	Fresh Baked	Archway
Cookies	Fresh Baked	Archway
Cookies	Fresh Baked	Archway
Cookies	Fresh Baked	Archway
Cookies	Fresh Baked	Archway
Cookies	Fresh Baked	Archway
Cookies	Fresh Baked	Archway
Cookies	Fresh Baked	Archway 54/Pkg
Cookies	Fresh Baked	Archway 80/Pkg
Cookies	Fresh Baked	Archway Homestyle
Cookies	Fresh Baked	Archway Homestyle
Cookies	Fresh Baked	Archway Homestyle
Cookies	Fresh Baked	Archway Homestyle
Cookies	Fresh Baked	Archway Homestyle
Cookies	Fresh Baked	Archway Homestyle
Cookies	Fresh Baked	Archway Homestyle
Cookies	Fresh Baked	Archway Homestyle

Major Description	Minor Description	Serving Size	Calories	Grade
Berry		4.5 oz	350	D
Blueberry		4.5 oz	340	D
Cherry		4.5 oz	390	D
Peach		4.5 oz	340	D
Apple		4.33 oz	290	B
Blackberry		4.33 oz	250	C
Blueberry		4.33 oz	370	B
Cherry		4.33 oz	280	C
Peach		4.33 oz	260	C
Strawberry		4.33 oz	290	B
Apple		4 oz	200	B
Blackberry		4 oz	280	B
Cherry		4 oz	250	B
Peach		4 oz	270	B
		1 Tbsp	37	D
		1 Tbsp	34	B
		1 Tbsp	25	B
		1 Tbsp	34	B
Apple	Fruit Filled	.5 oz cookie	50	A
Oatmeal Raisin		.5 oz cookie	60	A
Vanilla Sandwich		.5 oz cookie	70	B
Chocolate Chip	Fudge	1 cookie	70	C
Oatmeal	Raisin	1 cookie	70	C
Sugar		1 cookie	70	C
Chocolate Chip		1 cookie	60	D
Apple & Raisin		1 cookie	120	B–
Chocolate Chip		1 cookie	50	D
Molasses		1 cookie	100	B–+
Oatmeal		1 cookie	110	B
Oatmeal	Apple Filled	1 cookie	90	A–
Oatmeal	Date Filled	1 cookie	100	B
Oatmeal	Iced	1 cookie	140	C
Oatmeal	Raisin	1 cookie	100	B
Oatmeal	Raisin Bran	1 cookie	100	B
Pecan Crunch		1 cookie	60	D
Raisin Oatmeal		1 cookie	50	C
Vanilla	Wafer	1 cookie	30	B
Gingersnaps		1 cookie	35	B
Gingersnaps		1 cookie	25	C
Apple-filled Oatmeal	No Cholesterol, Low Sodium	1 cookie	90	B
Applesauce Drop	Low Cholesterol	1 cookie	80	B
Aunt Mary's Sugar Cookie	Low Cholesterol, No Palm Oil	1 cookie	140	B
Brownie Bars	No Cholesterol	1 cookie	100	C
Carrot Cake Cookie	Low Cholesterol, Low Sodium	1 cookie	140	C
Chocolate Chip Drop	Low Cholesterol, Low Sodium	1 cookie	100	B
Cinnamon Honey Gems	Fat Free, Cholesterol Free	1 cookie	33	A
Date-filled Oatmeal	Low Cholesterol, Low Sodium	1 cookie	110	B

"+" indicates the food meets minimum fiber requirements; "–" indicates the food has a high sodium content.

Food	Processing Category	Brand
Cookies	Fresh Baked	Archway Homestyle
Cookies	Fresh Baked	Archway Homestyle
Cookies	Fresh Baked	Archway Homestyle
Cookies	Fresh Baked	Archway Homestyle
Cookies	Fresh Baked	Archway Homestyle
Cookies	Fresh Baked	Archway Homestyle
Cookies	Fresh Baked	Archway Homestyle
Cookies	Fresh Baked	Archway Homestyle
Cookies	Fresh Baked	Archway Homestyle
Cookies	Fresh Baked	Archway Homestyle
Cookies	Fresh Baked	Archway Homestyle
Cookies	Fresh Baked	Archway Homestyle
Cookies	Fresh Baked	Archway Homestyle
Cookies	Fresh Baked	Archway Homestyle
Cookies	Fresh Baked	Archway Homestyle
Cookies	Fresh Baked	Archway Homestyle
Cookies	Fresh Baked	Archway Homestyle
Cookies	Fresh Baked	Archway Homestyle
Cookies	Fresh Baked	Archway Homestyle
Cookies	Fresh Baked	Archway Ruth Golden
Cookies	Fresh Baked	Archway Select
Cookies	Fresh Baked	Baker's Bonus
Cookies	Fresh Baked	Barnum's
Cookies	Fresh Baked	Bisco's
Cookies	Fresh Baked	Bisco's
Cookies	Fresh Baked	Bugs Bunny
Cookies	Fresh Baked	Cameo
Cookies	Fresh Baked	Carr's Hob Nobs
Cookies	Fresh Baked	Carr's Home Wheat Graham
Cookies	Fresh Baked	Carr's Muesli
Cookies	Fresh Baked	Chips Ahoy Selection
Cookies	Fresh Baked	Drake's
Cookies	Fresh Baked	Drake's
Cookies	Fresh Baked	Drake's
Cookies	Fresh Baked	Drake's
Cookies	Fresh Baked	Duncan Hines
Cookies	Fresh Baked	Duncan Hines
Cookies	Fresh Baked	Entenmann's
Cookies	Fresh Baked	Entenmann's
Cookies	Fresh Baked	Entenmann's
Cookies	Fresh Baked	Entenmann's
Cookies	Fresh Baked	Entenmann's

Major Description	Minor Description	Serving Size	Calories	Grade
Dutch Cocoa	No Cholesterol, Low Sodium	1 cookie	100	B
Frosty Lemon	No Cholesterol, Low Sodium	1 cookie	120	C
Iced Spice	No Cholesterol, No Palm Oil	1 cookie	120	B–
Oatmeal Apple Bran	Low Cholesterol, No Palm Oil	1 cookie	110	B–
Oatmeal Raisin	Fat Free, Cholesterol Free	1 cookie	100	A–
Oatmeal Raisin Bran	Low Cholesterol, Low Sodium	1 cookie	100	B
Ol Dutch Apple	Low Cholesterol	1 cookie	110	B
Old Fashioned Molasses	No Cholesterol, No Palm Oil	1 cookie	130	B–
Pecan Oatmeal	No Cholesterol	1 cookie	110	C
Raisin Bar	No Cholesterol, Low Sodium	1 cookie	60	A–
Strawberry Filled	No Cholesterol	1 cookie	90	B
Sugared Molasses	No Cholesterol	1 cookie	110	B–
Chocolate Chip	Low Cholesterol	1 cookie	120	D
Coconut Macaroon	Low Cholesterol, Low Sodium	1 cookie	129	D
Fruit Bar	Fat Free, Cholesterol Free	1 cookie	90	A
Iced Gingerbread	No Cholesterol	1 cookie	50	B
Oatmeal	No Cholesterol	1 cookie	100	C
Peanut Butter	Low Cholesterol	1 cookie	150	D
Raspberry Filled	Low Cholesterol, Low Sodium	1 cookie	120	B
Oatmeal		1 cookie	120	B
Assorted		1 cookie	50	C
Oatmeal		1 cookie	80	C
Animal Crackers		1 cookie	12	B
Sugar	Wafer	1 cookie	18	C
Wafer	Waffle Creams	1 cookie	35	D
Graham Cracker		1 cookie	12	B
Vanilla	Cream Sandwich	1 cookie	70	C
		1 cookie	72	C
Graham Cracker	Wheat	1 cookie	74	D
		1 cookie	84	D
Chocolate Chip	Chocolate	1 cookie	95	D
Chocolate Chip		1 cookie	70	C
Chocolate Chip	Chocolate	1 cookie	65	C
Coconut		1 cookie	65	C
Oatmeal		1 cookie	60	B
Chocolate Chip		1 cookie	55	D
Oatmeal	Raisin	1 cookie	55	D
Chocolate Brownie	Fat Free	1 cookie	40	A
Chocolate Chip		1 cookie	47	D
Oatmeal	Raisin	1 cookie	40	A–
Oatmeal Chocolate Chip	Fat Free	1 cookie	40	A–
Oatmeal Raisin	Fat Free	1 cookie	40	A–

"+" indicates the food meets minimum fiber requirements; "–" indicates the food has a high sodium content.

Food	Processing Category	Brand
Cookies	Fresh Baked	Estee
Cookies	Fresh Baked	Estee
Cookies	Fresh Baked	Estee
Cookies	Fresh Baked	Estee
Cookies	Fresh Baked	Estee
Cookies	Fresh Baked	Estee
Cookies	Fresh Baked	Estee
Cookies	Fresh Baked	Estee
Cookies	Fresh Baked	Estee
Cookies	Fresh Baked	Featherweight
Cookies	Fresh Baked	Featherweight
Cookies	Fresh Baked	Featherweight
Cookies	Fresh Baked	Featherweight
Cookies	Fresh Baked	Featherweight
Cookies	Fresh Baked	Featherweight
Cookies	Fresh Baked	Featherweight
Cookies	Fresh Baked	Featherweight
Cookies	Fresh Baked	Featherweight
Cookies	Fresh Baked	Featherweight
Cookies	Fresh Baked	FFV
Cookies	Fresh Baked	FFV
Cookies	Fresh Baked	FFV
Cookies	Fresh Baked	FFV
Cookies	Fresh Baked	FFV
Cookies	Fresh Baked	FFV
Cookies	Fresh Baked	FFV
Cookies	Fresh Baked	FFV
Cookies	Fresh Baked	FFV
Cookies	Fresh Baked	FFV
Cookies	Fresh Baked	FFV
Cookies	Fresh Baked	FFV
Cookies	Fresh Baked	FFV
Cookies	Fresh Baked	FFV
Cookies	Fresh Baked	FFV
Cookies	Fresh Baked	FFV Kreem Pilot Bread
Cookies	Fresh Baked	FFV Royal Dainty
Cookies	Fresh Baked	FFV Tango
Cookies	Fresh Baked	FFV TC Rounds
Cookies	Fresh Baked	FFV Trolley Cakes
Cookies	Fresh Baked	Fig Newtons
Cookies	Fresh Baked	Freihofer
Cookies	Fresh Baked	Freihofer
Cookies	Fresh Baked	Frookies
Cookies	Fresh Baked	Frookies
Cookies	Fresh Baked	Frookies
Cookies	Fresh Baked	Frookies
Cookies	Fresh Baked	Frookies
Cookies	Fresh Baked	Frookies
Cookies	Fresh Baked	Frookies
Cookies	Fresh Baked	Frookies
Cookies	Fresh Baked	Frookies
Cookies	Fresh Baked	Frookies Fat Free

Major Description	Minor Description	Serving Size	Calories	Grade
Chocolate Sandwich		1 cookie	50	C
Fudge		1 cookie	30	B
Oriental Sandwich		1 cookie	45	C
Raisin		1 cookie	30	C
Sandwich	Peanut Butter	1 cookie	50	D
Snack Crisp	Chocolate Strawberry	1 cookie	80	B
Wafer	Cream Filled Assorted	1 cookie	30	D
Wafer	Cream Filled Chocolate	1 cookie	20	D
Wafer	Snack, Chocolate Coated	1 cookie	130	D
Chocolate	Cream Wafer	1 cookie	20	D
Chocolate Chip		1 cookie	45	C
Chocolate Chip	Double	1 cookie	45	C
Lemon		1 cookie	45	C
Oatmeal	Raisin	1 cookie	45	C
Peanut Butter		1 cookie	40	D
Peanut Butter	Cream Wafer	1 cookie	25	C
Strawberry	Cream Wafer	1 cookie	20	D
Vanilla		1 cookie	45	C
Vanilla	Cream Wafer	1 cookie	20	D
Animal Crackers		1 pkg	160	C
Caramel Patties		1 cookie	25	D
Fig Bar	Vanilla	1 cookie	70	A
Fig Bar	Whole Wheat	1 cookie	70	B
Ginger Boys		1 pkg	150	B–
Gingersnaps		1 cookie	26	B
Jelly Tarts		1 cookie	60	B
Mint Sandwich		1 cookie	80	C
Oatmeal		1 cookie	26	B
Peach Apricot Bar	Vanilla	1 cookie	70	A
Peach Apricot Bar	Whole Wheat	1 cookie	70	B
Peanut Butter	Sandwich	1 cookie	85	D
Praline, Pecan		1 cookie	40	D
Shortbread	Country Style	1 cookie	70	D
Vanilla	Wafer	1 cookie	16	C
		1 cookie	60	B
		1 cookie	60	D
		1 cookie	80	B
		1 cookie	160	D
Devil's Food		1 cookie	120	A
Fig Bar		1 cookie	60	A
Chocolate Brownie	Fat Free	1 cookie	40	A
Oatmeal Raisin	Fat Free	1 cookie	40	A–
Animal Crackers	Chocolate	1 cookie	60	B
Animal Crackers	Cinnamon	1 cookie	60	B
Apple Cinnamon	Oat Bran	1 cookie	45	C+
Chocolate Chip		1 cookie	45	C+
Chocolate Chip	Mint	1 cookie	45	C+
Ginger Spice		1 cookie	45	C+
Oatbran Muffin		1 cookie	45	C+
Oatmeal	7 Grain	1 cookie	45	C+
Oatmeal Raisin		1 cookie	45	C+
Apple Spice		1 cookie	50	A–+

"+" indicates the food meets minimum fiber requirements; "–" indicates the food has a high sodium content.

Food	Processing Category	Brand
Cookies	Fresh Baked	Frookies Fat Free
Cookies	Fresh Baked	Frookies Fat Free
Cookies	Fresh Baked	Frookies Fat Free
Cookies	Fresh Baked	Frookies Frookwich
Cookies	Fresh Baked	Frookies Frookwich
Cookies	Fresh Baked	Frookies Frookwich
Cookies	Fresh Baked	Frookies Frookwich
Cookies	Fresh Baked	Frookies Frookwich
Cookies	Fresh Baked	Frookies Fruitins
Cookies	Fresh Baked	Frookies Fruitins
Cookies	Fresh Baked	Frookies Fruitins Fat Free
Cookies	Fresh Baked	Frookies Fruitins Fat Free
Cookies	Fresh Baked	Frookies Funky Monkey
Cookies	Fresh Baked	Frookies Funky Monkey
Cookies	Fresh Baked	Grandma's Big Cookies
Cookies	Fresh Baked	Grandma's Big Cookies
Cookies	Fresh Baked	Grandma's Big Cookies
Cookies	Fresh Baked	Grandma's Big Cookies
Cookies	Fresh Baked	Grandma's Old Time Big
Cookies	Fresh Baked	Granma's Big Cookies
Cookies	Fresh Baked	Health Valley
Cookies	Fresh Baked	Health Valley
Cookies	Fresh Baked	Health Valley
Cookies	Fresh Baked	Health Valley
Cookies	Fresh Baked	Health Valley
Cookies	Fresh Baked	Health Valley
Cookies	Fresh Baked	Health Valley
Cookies	Fresh Baked	Health Valley
Cookies	Fresh Baked	Health Valley
Cookies	Fresh Baked	Health Valley
Cookies	Fresh Baked	Health Valley
Cookies	Fresh Baked	Health Valley Amaranth
Cookies	Fresh Baked	Health Valley Fancy Fruit
Cookies	Fresh Baked	Health Valley Fruit Centers
Cookies	Fresh Baked	Health Valley Fruit Centers
Cookies	Fresh Baked	Health Valley Fruit Centers
Cookies	Fresh Baked	Health Valley Fruit Centers
Cookies	Fresh Baked	Health Valley Fruit Centers
Cookies	Fresh Baked	Health Valley Fruit Centers
Cookies	Fresh Baked	Health Valley Fruit Centers
Cookies	Fresh Baked	Health Valley Fruit Centers
Cookies	Fresh Baked	Health Valley Fruit Chunks
Cookies	Fresh Baked	Health Valley Fruit Chunks
Cookies	Fresh Baked	Health Valley Fruit Chunks
Cookies	Fresh Baked	Health Valley Fruit Jumbos
Cookies	Fresh Baked	Health Valley
Cookies	Fresh Baked	Heyday
Cookies	Fresh Baked	Honey Maid
Cookies	Fresh Baked	Honey Maid
Cookies	Fresh Baked	Honey Maid Graham Bites
Cookies	Fresh Baked	Honey Maid Graham Bites
Cookies	Fresh Baked	Honey Maid Graham Bites
Cookies	Fresh Baked	Ideal

Major Description	Minor Description	Serving Size	Calories	Grade
Banana		1 cookie	45	A–+
Cranberry Orange		1 cookie	45	A–+
Oatmeal Raisin		1 cookie	50	A–+
Chocolate		1 cookie	50	C
Chocolate & Vanilla	Duplex	1 cookie	50	C
Lemon		1 cookie	50	C
Peanut Butter		1 cookie	50	C
Vanilla		1 cookie	50	C
Apple		1 cookie	60	A
Fig		1 cookie	60	A
Fig		1 cookie	45	A
Raspberry		1 cookie	45	A
Chocolate		1 cookie	60	B
Vanilla		1 cookie	60	B
Chocolate Chip		1 cookie	185	D
Oatmeal	Apple Spice	1 cookie	165	C–
Peanut Butter		1 cookie	205	D
Raisin	Soft	1 cookie	160	B
Molasses		1 cookie	160	B–
Chocolate Chip	Fudge	1 cookie	175	C
Apple Spice		1 cookie	27	A+
Apricot		1 cookie	27	A+
Apricot Apple		1 cookie	27	A+
Date		1 cookie	27	A+
Hawaiian Fruit		1 cookie	27	A+
Jumbos	Apple Raisin	1 cookie	80	A+
Jumbos	Raisin-Raisin	1 cookie	80	A+
Mini Fruit Centers	Apple Cinnamon	1 cookie	45	A+
Mini Fruit Centers	Raspberry Apple	1 cookie	25	A+
Mini Fruit Centers	Strawberry	1 cookie	25	A+
Raisin Oatmeal		1 cookie	27	A+
	Amaranth	1 cookie	90	B+
	Apricot Almond	1 cookie	45	C+
Apple Fruit		1 cookie	80	A+
Apricot		1 cookie	80	A+
Date Fruit		1 cookie	80	A+
Orange Pineapple		1 cookie	45	A+
Peach Apricot		1 cookie	45	A+
Raisin Apple		1 cookie	70	A+
Raspberry Fruit		1 cookie	80	A+
Tropical Fruit		1 cookie	80	A+
Apple Raisin		1 cookie	28	A+
Banana Spice		1 cookie	28	A+
Oatmeal Raisin Cinnamon		1 cookie	28	A+
	Almond Date	1 cookie	70	C+
Wafer	Wheat Free	1 cookie	33	B+
Fudge Bar	Caramel & Peanut	1 cookie	110	D
Graham Cracker	Cinnamon	1 cookie	30	A–
Graham Cracker	Honey	1 cookie	30	A–
Graham Cracker	Apple Cinnamon	1 cookie	6	B–
Graham Cracker	Brown Sugar & Spice	1 cookie	6	B–
Graham Cracker	Honey & Oat Bran	1 cookie	6	B
Chocolate Peanut Butter		1 cookie	90	D

"+" indicates the food meets minimum fiber requirements; "–" indicates the food has a high sodium content.

Food	Processing Category	Brand
Cookies	Fresh Baked	Keebler
Cookies	Fresh Baked	Keebler
Cookies	Fresh Baked	Keebler
Cookies	Fresh Baked	Keebler
Cookies	Fresh Baked	Keebler
Cookies	Fresh Baked	Keebler Apple Grahams
Cookies	Fresh Baked	Keebler Baby Bear
Cookies	Fresh Baked	Keebler Chocolate
Cookies	Fresh Baked	Keebler Cinnamon Crisp
Cookies	Fresh Baked	Keebler Deluxe
Cookies	Fresh Baked	Keebler El Fudge
Cookies	Fresh Baked	Keebler El Fudge
Cookies	Fresh Baked	Keebler El Fudge
Cookies	Fresh Baked	Keebler El Fudge
Cookies	Fresh Baked	Keebler Elfin Delights
Cookies	Fresh Baked	Keebler Elfin Delights
Cookies	Fresh Baked	Keebler Elfin Delights
Cookies	Fresh Baked	Keebler Elfin Delights
Cookies	Fresh Baked	Keebler Elfin Delights
Cookies	Fresh Baked	Keebler French Vanilla
Cookies	Fresh Baked	Keebler Fudge Sticks
Cookies	Fresh Baked	Keebler Fudge Stripes
Cookies	Fresh Baked	Keebler Grasshopper
Cookies	Fresh Baked	Keebler Honey Grahams
Cookies	Fresh Baked	Keebler Magic Middles
Cookies	Fresh Baked	Keebler Magic Middles
Cookies	Fresh Baked	Keebler Magic Middles
Cookies	Fresh Baked	Keebler Old Fashioned
Cookies	Fresh Baked	Keebler Rainbow Chips
Cookies	Fresh Baked	Keebler Reduced Fat
Cookies	Fresh Baked	Keebler Reduced Fat
Cookies	Fresh Baked	Keebler Reduced Fat
Cookies	Fresh Baked	Keebler Soft Batch
Cookies	Fresh Baked	Keebler Soft Batch
Cookies	Fresh Baked	Keebler Soft Batch
Cookies	Fresh Baked	Keebler Soft Batch
Cookies	Fresh Baked	Keebler Soft Batch
Cookies	Fresh Baked	Keebler Soft Batch
Cookies	Fresh Baked	Keebler Thin Bites
Cookies	Fresh Baked	Keebler Thin Bites
Cookies	Fresh Baked	Little Debbie
Cookies	Fresh Baked	Little Debbie
Cookies	Fresh Baked	Lorna Doone
Cookies	Fresh Baked	Mallomars
Cookies	Fresh Baked	Mystic Mint
Cookies	Fresh Baked	Nabisco
Cookies	Fresh Baked	Nabisco
Cookies	Fresh Baked	Nabisco
Cookies	Fresh Baked	Nabisco
Cookies	Fresh Baked	Nabisco
Cookies	Fresh Baked	Nabisco

Major Description	Minor Description	Serving Size	Calories	Grade
Animal Crackers		1 cookie	14	B
Fig Bar		1 cookie	60	B
Graham Cracker		1 cookie	5	B
Iced Bar	Raisin	1 cookie	80	D
Wafer	Golden Vanilla	1 cookie	20	C
Graham Cracker	Cinnamon	1 cookie	12	B
Butter Flavor	Chocolate Coated	1 cookie	23	B
Chocolate Sandwich	Fudge Cream Filled	1 cookie	80	D
Graham Cracker	Cinnamon	1 cookie	5	B
Graham Cracker	Fudge Covered	1 cookie	45	C
Butter Flavor	Chocolate Coated	1 cookie	40	D
Chocolate Sandwich	Fudge with Fudge Cream Filling	1 cookie	70	C
Chocolate Sandwich	Fudge with Peanut Butter Cream	1 cookie	50	D
Chocolate-filled Sandwich	Fudge Cream	1 cookie	60	D
Chocolate Sandwich	Fudge Cream	1 cookie	50	B
Chocolate Sandwich	Vanilla Cream	1 cookie	50	B
Cream Sandwich		1 cookie	50	B
Devil's Food		1 cookie	70	A
Oatmeal	Caramel Apple	1 cookie	70	B
Vanilla	Cream Sandwich	1 cookie	80	D
Wafer	Cream Fudge Covered	1 cookie	50	D
Shortbread	Fudge Striped	1 cookie	50	D
Fudge	Mint	1 cookie	35	C
Graham Cracker	Honey	1 cookie	18	B
Chocolate Chip	Chocolate Middle	1 cookie	80	D
Oatmeal	Chocolate Middle	1 cookie	80	D
Shortbread	Chocolate Cream Center	1 cookie	80	D
Oatmeal		1 cookie	80	C–
Chocolate Chip	Candy-coated Chocolate	1 cookie	80	C
Chips Deluxe		1 cookie	70	C
Pecan Sandies		1 cookie	70	C
Vanilla Wafers		1 cookie	15	B
Chocolate Chip		1 cookie	80	D
Chocolate Chip	Mint	1 cookie	80	D
Chocolate Chip	Walnut	1 cookie	80	D
Oatmeal	Raisin	1 cookie	70	C
Peanut Butter	Chocolate Chip	1 cookie	80	D
Peanut Butter	Nut	1 cookie	80	D
Graham Cracker	Chocolate	1 cookie	6	C
Graham Cracker	Cinnamon	1 cookie	6	C
Chocolate Sandwich		1 pkg	250	D
Oatmeal		1 pkg	340	C–
Shortbread		1 cookie	23	D
Marshmallow & Chocolate Cake		1 cookie	60	D
Mint Sandwich		1 cookie	90	D
Apple Newton		1 cookie	50	A
Apple Newton	Fat Free	1 cookie	70	A
Cranberry Newton	Fat Free	1 cookie	50	A
Devil's Food Cakes		1 cookie	70	A
Fig Newton		1 cookie	60	A
Fig Newton	Fat Free	1 cookie	70	A

"+" indicates the food meets minimum fiber requirements; "–" indicates the food has a high sodium content.

Food	Processing Category	Brand
Cookies	Fresh Baked	Nabisco
Cookies	Fresh Baked	Nabisco
Cookies	Fresh Baked	Nabisco
Cookies	Fresh Baked	Nabisco
Cookies	Fresh Baked	Nabisco
Cookies	Fresh Baked	Nabisco
Cookies	Fresh Baked	Nabisco
Cookies	Fresh Baked	Nabisco Chips Ahoy
Cookies	Fresh Baked	Nabisco Chips Ahoy
Cookies	Fresh Baked	Nabisco Chips Ahoy
Cookies	Fresh Baked	Nabisco Chips Ahoy
Cookies	Fresh Baked	Nabisco Chips Ahoy
Cookies	Fresh Baked	Nabisco Chips Ahoy Pure
Cookies	Fresh Baked	Nabisco Chips Ahoy Selections
Cookies	Fresh Baked	Nabisco Chips Ahoy Selections
Cookies	Fresh Baked	Nabisco Chunky Chips Ahoy
Cookies	Fresh Baked	Nabisco Cookie Break
Cookies	Fresh Baked	Nabisco Cookies N Fudge
Cookies	Fresh Baked	Nabisco Cookies N Fudge
Cookies	Fresh Baked	Nabisco Famous Wafers
Cookies	Fresh Baked	Nabisco Giggles
Cookies	Fresh Baked	Nabisco Nilla Wafers
Cookies	Fresh Baked	Nabisco Nilla Wafers
Cookies	Fresh Baked	Nabisco Nutter Butter
Cookies	Fresh Baked	Nabisco Old Fashioned
Cookies	Fresh Baked	Nabisco Pantry
Cookies	Fresh Baked	Nabisco Pecan Chips Ahoy
Cookies	Fresh Baked	Nabisco Pecan Supremes
Cookies	Fresh Baked	Nabisco Puffs
Cookies	Fresh Baked	Nabisco Snack Wells
Cookies	Fresh Baked	Nabisco Snack Wells
Cookies	Fresh Baked	Nabisco Snack Wells
Cookies	Fresh Baked	Nabisco Snack Wells
Cookies	Fresh Baked	Nabisco Snack Wells
Cookies	Fresh Baked	Nabisco Snack Wells
Cookies	Fresh Baked	Nabisco Snack Wells
Cookies	Fresh Baked	Nabisco Snaps
Cookies	Fresh Baked	Nabisco Teddy Grahams
Cookies	Fresh Baked	Nabisco Teddy Grahams Bearwiches
Cookies	Fresh Baked	Nabisco Twirls
Cookies	Fresh Baked	Nabiscos Cookies N Fudge
Cookies	Fresh Baked	National
Cookies	Fresh Baked	Nestlé Mini Chips Ahoy
Cookies	Fresh Baked	Nutter Butter
Cookies	Fresh Baked	Nutter Butter
Cookies	Fresh Baked	Oreo
Cookies	Fresh Baked	Oreo
Cookies	Fresh Baked	Oreo
Cookies	Fresh Baked	Oreo Big Stuff
Cookies	Fresh Baked	Oreo Double Stuff
Cookies	Fresh Baked	Pepperidge Farm
Cookies	Fresh Baked	Pepperidge Farm
Cookies	Fresh Baked	Pepperidge Farm

Major Description	Minor Description	Serving Size	Calories	Grade
Graham Cracker		1 cookie	30	A–
Middles		1 cookie	80	D
Raspberry Newtons		1 cookie	50	A
Shortbread	Pecan	1 cookie	80	D
Snaps		1 cookie	18	B
Strawberry Newtons		1 cookie	50	A
Wafer	Brown Edged	1 cookie	27	C
Chocolate Chip	Chewy	1 cookie	60	D
Chocolate Chip	Rockers	1 cookie	60	D
Chocolate Chip	Sprinkled	1 cookie	50	C
Chocolate Chip	Striped	1 cookie	90	D
Chocolate Chip	White Fudge Chunk	1 cookie	90	D
Chocolate Chip		1 cookie	50	C
Chocolate Chip	Chocolate	1 cookie	90	D
Oatmeal	Chocolate Chunk	1 cookie	95	D
Chocolate Chip	Chunk	1 cookie	90	D
Vanilla	Cream Sandwich	1 cookie	50	C
Graham Cracker	Fudge Coated	1 cookie	45	C
Wafer	Fudge Striped	1 cookie	70	D
Wafer		1 cookie	70	B–
Vanilla	Cream Sandwich	1 cookie	60	D
Vanilla Wafer		1 cookie	60	B
Vanilla Wafer	Cinnamon	1 cookie	60	B
Peanut Butter Sandwich		1 cookie	70	C
Gingersnaps		1 cookie	30	B–
Molasses		1 cookie	80	C
Chocolate Chip	Chunks	1 cookie	100	D
Pecan		1 cookie	80	D
Marshmallow & Fudge Cake		1 cookie	90	C
Chocolate	Sandwich	1 cookie	50	D–
Chocolate Chip		1 cookie	50	A
Cinnamon Grahams		1 cookie	50	A
Cream Sandwich		1 cookie	50	B
Devil's Food	Cookie Cake	1 cookie	50	A
Double Fudge		1 cookie	50	A–
Oatmeal Raisin		1 cookie	55	B
Chocolate Chip		1 cookie	23	B
Graham Cracker	All Varieties	1 cookie	60	B–
Graham Sandwich	All Varieties	1 cookie	70	C
Marshmallow & Fudge Cake		1 cookie	140	C
Shortbread	Fudge Striped	1 cookie	60	D
Arrowroot Biscuit		1 cookie	20	D
Chocolate Chip	Mini	1 cookie	12	C
Peanut Butter	Sandwich	1 cookie	70	C
Peanut Cream Patties		1 cookie	40	D
Chocolate Sandwich		1 cookie	50	C–
Chocolate Sandwich	Fudge Covered	1 cookie	110	D
Chocolate Sandwich	White Fudge Covered	1 cookie	110	D
Chocolate Sandwich		1 cookie	250	D
Chocolate Sandwich		1 cookie	70	D
Carrot Walnut		1 cookie	60	A
Chocolate Chip	Chunk	1 cookie	120	D
Chocolate Chip	with Macadamia Nut	1 cookie	120	D

"+" indicates the food meets minimum fiber requirements; "–" indicates the food has a high sodium content.

Food	Processing Category	Brand
Cookies	Fresh Baked	Pepperidge Farm
Cookies	Fresh Baked	Pepperidge Farm
Cookies	Fresh Baked	Pepperidge Farm
Cookies	Fresh Baked	Pepperidge Farm Bordeaux
Cookies	Fresh Baked	Pepperidge Farm Brussels
Cookies	Fresh Baked	Pepperidge Farm Brussels
Cookies	Fresh Baked	Pepperidge Farm Cappuccino
Cookies	Fresh Baked	Pepperidge Farm Capri
Cookies	Fresh Baked	Pepperidge Farm Chantilly
Cookies	Fresh Baked	Pepperidge Farm Chantilly
Cookies	Fresh Baked	Pepperidge Farm Chessmen
Cookies	Fresh Baked	Pepperidge Farm Cheyenne
Cookies	Fresh Baked	Pepperidge Farm Dakota
Cookies	Fresh Baked	Pepperidge Farm Fruit Cookies
Cookies	Fresh Baked	Pepperidge Farm Fruit Cookies
Cookies	Fresh Baked	Pepperidge Farm Geneva
Cookies	Fresh Baked	Pepperidge Farm Kitchen
Cookies	Fresh Baked	Pepperidge Farm Kitchen
Cookies	Fresh Baked	Pepperidge Farm Lido
Cookies	Fresh Baked	Pepperidge Farm Linzer
Cookies	Fresh Baked	Pepperidge Farm Milano
Cookies	Fresh Baked	Pepperidge Farm Mint
Cookies	Fresh Baked	Pepperidge Farm Nassau
Cookies	Fresh Baked	Pepperidge Farm Old Fashioned
Cookies	Fresh Baked	Pepperidge Farm Old Fashioned
Cookies	Fresh Baked	Pepperidge Farm Old Fashioned
Cookies	Fresh Baked	Pepperidge Farm Old Fashioned
Cookies	Fresh Baked	Pepperidge Farm Old Fashioned
Cookies	Fresh Baked	Pepperidge Farm Old Fashioned
Cookies	Fresh Baked	Pepperidge Farm Old Fashioned
Cookies	Fresh Baked	Pepperidge Farm Old Fashioned
Cookies	Fresh Baked	Pepperidge Farm Old Fashioned
Cookies	Fresh Baked	Pepperidge Farm Old Fashioned
Cookies	Fresh Baked	Pepperidge Farm Old Fashioned
Cookies	Fresh Baked	Pepperidge Farm Orange
Cookies	Fresh Baked	Pepperidge Farm Orleans
Cookies	Fresh Baked	Pepperidge Farm Orleans
Cookies	Fresh Baked	Pepperidge Farm Pecan
Cookies	Fresh Baked	Pepperidge Farm Santa Fe
Cookies	Fresh Baked	Pepperidge Farm Tahiti
Cookies	Fresh Baked	Pepperidge Farm Zurich
Cookies	Fresh Baked	Pinwheels
Cookies	Fresh Baked	Pitter Patter
Cookies	Fresh Baked	Regal
Cookies	Fresh Baked	Rokeach
Cookies	Fresh Baked	Social Tea
Cookies	Fresh Baked	Stella D'oro
Cookies	Fresh Baked	Stella D'oro
Cookies	Fresh Baked	Stella D'oro
Cookies	Fresh Baked	Stella D'oro
Cookies	Fresh Baked	Stella D'oro
Cookies	Fresh Baked	Stella D'oro
Cookies	Fresh Baked	Stella D'oro
Cookies	Fresh Baked	Stella D'oro

Major Description	Minor Description	Serving Size	Calories	Grade
Chocolate Chip	Walnuts	1 cookie	120	D
Ginger		1 cookie	35	C
Vanilla		1 cookie	35	D
Vanilla	Chocolate Laced	1 cookie	35	C
Chocolate-filled Sandwich		1 cookie	55	D
Chocolate-filled Sandwich	Mint	1 cookie	65	D
Coffee Chocolate Praline Filled		1 cookie	50	D
Brownie	Cream Sandwich	1 cookie	80	D
Raspberry Filled		1 cookie	80	B
Raspberry Filled	Chocolate	1 cookie	90	B
Butter Flavored		1 cookie	45	C
Peanut Butter	Chocolate Chip Chunks	1 cookie	110	D
Oatmeal	Chocolate Chip Chunks	1 cookie	110	D
Apricot Raspberry		1 cookie	50	C
Strawberry		1 cookie	50	D
Vanilla	Chocolate Nut Coated	1 cookie	65	D
Date Pecan		1 cookie	55	D
Raisin Bran		1 cookie	55	D
Chocolate-filled Sandwich		1 cookie	90	D
Raspberry Filled		1 cookie	120	B
Chocolate-filled Sandwich		1 cookie	60	D
Chocolate-filled Sandwich	Mint	1 cookie	75	D
Peanut Butter	Chocolate Filled	1 cookie	80	D
Brownie	Chocolate Nut	1 cookie	55	D
Chocolate Chip		1 cookie	50	D
Chocolate Chip	Toffee	1 cookie	50	D
Hazelnut		1 cookie	55	D
Lemon Nut Crunch		1 cookie	55	D
Molasses	Crisps	1 cookie	35	C
Oatmeal	Irish Style	1 cookie	45	D
Oatmeal	Raisin	1 cookie	55	D
Shortbread		1 cookie	75	D
Shortbread	Pecan	1 cookie	70	D
Sugar		1 cookie	50	D
Chocolate-filled Sandwich	Orange	1 cookie	75	D
Chocolate-filled Sandwich		1 cookie	60	D
Vanilla	Chocolate Coated	1 cookie	30	D
Chocolate Chip	Chunk	1 cookie	120	D
Oatmeal	Raisin	1 cookie	100	C
Coconut	Chocolate Filled	1 cookie	90	D
Apricot Raspberry		1 cookie	60	B
Marshmallow	Chocolate Cake	1 cookie	130	C
Peanut Butter	Cream Filled	1 cookie	90	C–
Graham Cracker		1 cookie	70	D
Graham Cracker		1 cookie	15	B
Tea Biscuit		1 cookie	20	D
Apple Bar	Dutch	1 cookie	112	B
Apple Pastry	Diet	1 cookie	86	C
Coconut	Diet	1 cookie	52	D
Coconut	Macaroon	1 cookie	60	D
Egg Biscuit	Diet	1 cookie	43	B
Egg Biscuit	Roman	1 cookie	137	C
Egg Biscuit	Sugared	1 cookie	75	B

"+" indicates the food meets minimum fiber requirements; "–" indicates the food has a high sodium content.

Food	Processing Category	Brand
Cookies	Fresh Baked	Stella D'oro
Cookies	Fresh Baked	Stella D'oro
Cookies	Fresh Baked	Stella D'oro
Cookies	Fresh Baked	Stella D'oro
Cookies	Fresh Baked	Stella D'oro
Cookies	Fresh Baked	Stella D'oro
Cookies	Fresh Baked	Stella D'oro
Cookies	Fresh Baked	Stella D'oro Angel Bars
Cookies	Fresh Baked	Stella D'oro Angel Wings
Cookies	Fresh Baked	Stella D'oro Angelica
Cookies	Fresh Baked	Stella D'oro Anginetti
Cookies	Fresh Baked	Stella D'oro Anisette
Cookies	Fresh Baked	Stella D'oro Anisette Toast
Cookies	Fresh Baked	Stella D'oro Anisette Toast
Cookies	Fresh Baked	Stella D'oro Breakfast
Cookies	Fresh Baked	Stella D'oro Castelets
Cookies	Fresh Baked	Stella D'oro Castelets
Cookies	Fresh Baked	Stella D'oro Chimese
Cookies	Fresh Baked	Stella D'oro Como Delight
Cookies	Fresh Baked	Stella D'oro Golden Bars
Cookies	Fresh Baked	Stella D'oro Holiday
Cookies	Fresh Baked	Stella D'oro Hostess
Cookies	Fresh Baked	Stella D'oro Jumbo
Cookies	Fresh Baked	Stella D'oro Kitchel
Cookies	Fresh Baked	Stella D'oro Lady Stella
Cookies	Fresh Baked	Stella D'oro Love Cookies
Cookies	Fresh Baked	Stella D'oro Mandel
Cookies	Fresh Baked	Stella D'oro Margherite
Cookies	Fresh Baked	Stella D'oro Margherite
Cookies	Fresh Baked	Stella D'oro Pfefefusse
Cookies	Fresh Baked	Stella D'oro Regina
Cookies	Fresh Baked	Stella D'oro Regina
Cookies	Fresh Baked	Stella D'oro Royal Nuggets
Cookies	Fresh Baked	Stella D'oro Swiss Fudge
Cookies	Fresh Baked	Suddenly Smores
Cookies	Fresh Baked	Sunshine
Cookies	Fresh Baked	Sunshine
Cookies	Fresh Baked	Sunshine
Cookies	Fresh Baked	Sunshine
Cookies	Fresh Baked	Sunshine
Cookies	Fresh Baked	Sunshine Golden Fruit
Cookies	Fresh Baked	Sunshine Golden Fruit
Cookies	Fresh Baked	Sunshine Golden Fruit
Cookies	Fresh Baked	Sunshine Grahamy Bears
Cookies	Fresh Baked	Sunshine Oh Berry
Cookies	Fresh Baked	Tastykake
Cookies	Fresh Baked	Tastykake
Cookies	Fresh Baked	Tastykake
Cookies	Fresh Baked	Tastykake
Cookies	Fresh Baked	Tastykake
Cookies	Fresh Baked	Tastykake Soft and Chewy
Cookies	Fresh Baked	Tastykake Soft and Chewy
Cookies	Fresh Baked	Tastykake Soft and Chewy

Major Description	Minor Description	Serving Size	Calories	Grade
Fig Pastry	Diet	1 cookie	89	C
Fruit	Slices	1 cookie	60	C
Fruit Delight	Fat Free	1 cookie	70	A
Fruit Slices	Fat Free	1 cookie	50	A+
Peach Apricot Pastry		1 cookie	93	C
Peach Apricot Pastry	Diet	1 cookie	87	C
Prune Pastry	Diet	1 cookie	95	C
		1 cookie	76	D
		1 cookie	74	D
		1 cookie	106	C
Egg Biscuit		1 cookie	31	B
Anise		1 cookie	51	A
Anise		1 cookie	46	A
Anise		1 cookie	109	A
Almond		1 cookie	101	C
Chocolate		1 cookie	64	C
Vanilla		1 cookie	72	C
Almond		1 cookie	169	D
		1 cookie	145	D
Raisin		1 cookie	109	C
		1 cookie	38	D
Assorted		1 cookie	42	D
Egg Biscuit		1 cookie	47	A
Egg Biscuit	Diet	1 cookie	8	D–
Assorted		1 cookie	42	D
		1 cookie	106	D
Almond	Toast	1 cookie	58	B
Chocolate		1 cookie	72	C
Vanilla		1 cookie	72	C
Spice Drops		1 cookie	35	B
Sesame		1 cookie	48	D
Sesame	Diet	1 cookie	41	D
		1 cookie	2	D
		1 cookie	68	D
		1 cookie	100	C
Animal Crackers		1 cookie	13	B
Gingersnaps		1 cookie	20	B
Graham Cracker	Cinnamon	1 cookie	70	C–
Graham Cracker	Honey	1 cookie	60	B–
Oatmeal	Raisin	1 cookie	55	D
Fruit	Apple	1 cookie	70	A
Fruit	Cranberry	1 cookie	70	A
Fruit	Raisin	1 cookie	80	B
Graham Cracker		1 cookie	15	C
Wafer	Strawberry, Fat Free	1 cookie	13	A
Bar	Chocolate Chip	1 cookie	193	C
Bar	Fudge	1 cookie	205	B
Bar	Oatmeal Raisin	1 cookie	212	C
Shortbread	Vanilla	1 cookie	55	D
Sugar	Wafer, Vanilla	1 cookie	3	D
Chocolate Chip		1 cookie	174	C
Chocolate Chip	Chocolate	1 cookie	171	C
Oatmeal	Raisins	1 cookie	161	C

"+" indicates the food meets minimum fiber requirements; "–" indicates the food has a high sodium content.

Food	Processing Category	Brand
Cookies	Fresh Baked	Teddy Grahams
Cookies	Fresh Baked	Teddy Grahams
Cookies	Fresh Baked	Teddy Grahams
Cookies	Fresh Baked	Teddy Grahams
Cookies	Fresh Baked	Teddy Grahams Bearwichs
Cookies	Fresh Baked	Teddy Grahams Bearwichs
Cookies	Fresh Baked	Weight Watchers
Cookies	Fresh Baked	Weight Watchers
Cookies	Fresh Baked	Weight Watchers
Cookies	Fresh Baked	Weight Watchers
Cookies	Fresh Baked	Weight Watchers
Cookies	Fresh Baked	Weight Watchers
Cookies	Fresh Baked	Weight Watchers
Cookies	Fresh Baked	Weight Watchers
Cookies	Frozen	Nestlé Toll House
Cookies	Frozen	Nestlé Toll House
Cookies	Frozen	Nestlé Toll House
Cookies	Frozen	Nestlé Toll House
Cookies	Mix	Betty Crocker Big Batch
Cookies	Mix	Duncan Hines
Cookies	Mix	Duncan Hines
Cookies	Mix	Duncan Hines
Cookies	Mix	Duncan Hines
Cookies	Mix	Finast
Cookies	Refrigerated	Pillsbury
Cookies	Refrigerated	Pillsbury
Cookies	Refrigerated	Pillsbury
Cookies	Refrigerated	Pillsbury
Cream Topping, Nondairy	Frozen	Generic
Cream Topping, Nondairy	Frozen	Birds Eye Cool Whip
Cream Topping, Nondairy	Frozen	Birds Eye Cool Whip Dairy
Cream Topping, Nondairy	Frozen	Birds Eye Cool Whip Lite
Cream Topping, Nondairy	Frozen	Estee
Cream Topping, Nondairy	Frozen	Kraft Whipped Topping
Cream Topping, Nondairy	Frozen	La Creme
Cream Topping, Nondairy	Frozen	La Creme
Cream Topping, Nondairy	Frozen	Pet Whip
Cream Topping, Nondairy	Frozen	Rich's Richwhip
Cream Topping, Nondairy	Frozen	Rich's Richwhip
Cream Topping, Nondairy	Mix	D-zerta
Cream Topping, Nondairy	Mix	Dream Whip
Cream Topping, Nondairy	Mix	Featherweight
Cream Topping, Nondairy	Pressurized	Generic
Cream Topping, Nondairy	Pressurized	Rich's Richwhip
Danish Pastry	Fresh Baked	Awrey's
Danish Pastry	Fresh Baked	Awrey's
Danish Pastry	Fresh Baked	Awrey's
Danish Pastry	Fresh Baked	Awrey's
Danish Pastry	Fresh Baked	Awrey's
Danish Pastry	Fresh Baked	Awrey's Round

Major Description	Minor Description	Serving Size	Calories	Grade
Graham Cracker	Cinnamon	1 cookie	6	B–
Graham Cracker	Honey	1 cookie	6	B–
Graham Cracker	Vanilla	1 cookie	6	B–
Graham Cracker	Vanilla, Chocolate Cream	1 cookie	18	C
Graham Cracker	Chocolate, Vanilla Cream	1 cookie	18	C
Graham Cracker	Cinnamon, Vanilla Cream	1 cookie	18	C
Apple & Raisin Bar		1 cookie	100	B
Chocolate		1 cookie	27	C
Chocolate Chip		1 cookie	140	C
Chocolate Sandwich		1 cookie	140	B
Fig Bar	Fruit Filled	1 cookie	70	A
Oatmeal	Spice	1 cookie	27	B
Raspberry	Fruit Filled	1 cookie	70	A
Shortbread		1 cookie	27	B
Chocolate Chip		1 cookie	150	D
Chocolate Chip	Double	1 cookie	150	D
Chocolate Chip	Nuts	1 cookie	160	D
Oatmeal Raisin		1 cookie	130	C
Chocolate Chip		1 cookie	60	D
Chocolate Chip		1 cookie	65	C
Oatmeal Raisin		1 cookie	65	D
Peanut Butter		1 cookie	70	D
Sugar Golden		1 cookie	65	D
Chocolate Chip		1 cookie	55	D–
Chocolate Chip		1 cookie	70	C
Oatmeal Raisin		1 cookie	60	D
Peanut Butter		1 cookie	70	C
Sugar		1 cookie	70	C
Semisolid		1 Tbsp	13	D
Semisolid		1 Tbsp	12	D
Semisolid	Extra Creamy	1 Tbsp	14	D
Semisolid		1 Tbsp	8	A
Prewhipped		1 Tbsp	4	A
Semisolid		1 Tbsp	9	D
Light		1 Tbsp	8	A
Whipped		1 Tbsp	16	D
Semisolid		1 Tbsp	14	D
Prewhipped		1 Tbsp	12	D
Unwhipped		.25 oz	20	D
		1 Tbsp	8	D
		1 Tbsp	10	A
		1 Tbsp	4	A–
		.25 oz	19	D
		.25 oz	20	D
Apple Filled	Mini	1 piece	160	D
Cheese Filled	Mini	1 piece	170	D+
Cinnamon Raisin Filled	Mini	1 piece	160	D
Pineapple Filled	Mini	1 piece	157	D
Strawberry Filled	Mini	1 piece	160	D
Apple Filled		1 piece	390	D

"+" indicates the food meets minimum fiber requirements; "–" indicates the food has a high sodium content.

Food	Processing Category	Brand
Danish Pastry	Fresh Baked	Awrey's Round
Danish Pastry	Fresh Baked	Awrey's Round
Danish Pastry	Fresh Baked	Awrey's Round
Danish Pastry	Fresh Baked	Awrey's Square
Danish Pastry	Fresh Baked	Awrey's Square
Danish Pastry	Fresh Baked	Awrey's Square
Danish Pastry	Fresh Baked	Awrey's Square
Danish Pastry	Fresh Baked	Hostess Breakfast Bake Shop
Danish Pastry	Fresh Baked	Hostess Breakfast Bake Shop
Danish Pastry	Frozen	Pepperidge Farm
Danish Pastry	Frozen	Pepperidge Farm
Danish Pastry	Frozen	Pepperidge Farm
Danish Pastry	Frozen	Pepperidge Farm
Danish Pastry	Frozen	Sara Lee
Danish Pastry	Frozen	Sara Lee
Danish Pastry	Frozen	Sara Lee
Danish Pastry	Frozen	Sara Lee Free & Light
Danish Pastry	Frozen	Sara Lee Individual
Danish Pastry	Frozen	Sara Lee Individual
Danish Pastry	Frozen	Sara Lee Individual
Danish Pastry	Refrigerated	Pillsbury
Danish Pastry	Refrigerated	Pillsbury
Danish Pastry	Refrigerated	Pillsbury
Donut	Fresh Baked	Awrey's
Donut	Fresh Baked	Awrey's
Donut	Fresh Baked	Awrey's
Donut	Fresh Baked	Entenmann's
Donut	Fresh Baked	Entenmann's
Donut	Fresh Baked	Entenmann's
Donut	Fresh Baked	Hostess Breakfast Bake Shop
Donut	Fresh Baked	Hostess Breakfast Bake Shop
Donut	Fresh Baked	Hostess Breakfast Bake Shop
Donut	Fresh Baked	Hostess Breakfast Bake Shop
Donut	Fresh Baked	Hostess Breakfast Bake Shop Donette Gems
Donut	Fresh Baked	Hostess Breakfast Bake Shop Donette Gems
Donut	Fresh Baked	Hostess Breakfast Bake Shop Donette Gems
Donut	Fresh Baked	Hostess Breakfast Bake Shop Donette Gems
Donut	Fresh Baked	Hostess Breakfast Bake Shop Donette Gems
Donut	Fresh Baked	Hostess Breakfast Bake Shop Donette Gems
Donut	Fresh Baked	Hostess Breakfast Bake Shop Donette Gems
Donut	Fresh Baked	Hostess Breakfast Bake Shop Donette Gems
Donut	Fresh Baked	Hostess Breakfast Bake Shop Family Pack
Donut	Fresh Baked	Hostess Breakfast Bake Shop Family Pack

Major Description	Minor Description	Serving Size	Calories	Grade
Cheese Filled		1 piece	420	D–
Cinnamon-walnut		1 piece	300	D
Strawberry Filled		1 piece	400	D
Apple Filled		1 piece	220	C
Cheese Filled		1 piece	210	D–
Cinnamon Raisin Filled		1 piece	290	C
Raspberry Filled		1 piece	260	B
Apple Filled		1 piece	400	D
Raspberry Filled		1 piece	390	D
Apple		1 piece	220	C
Cheese		1 piece	240	D
Cinnamon Raisin		1 piece	250	C
Raspberry		1 piece	220	C
Apple Twist		1 piece	190	D
Cheese Twist		1 piece	200	D–
Raspberry Twist		1 piece	200	D
Apple		1 piece	130	A
Apple		1 piece	120	D
Cheese		1 piece	130	D
Cinnamon Raisin		1 piece	150	D
Caramel	with Nuts	1 piece	160	D–
Cinnamon Raisin	Iced	1 piece	150	D–
Orange	Iced	1 piece	150	D–
Crunch		1 piece	600	D
Plain		1 piece	490	D–
Powdered Sugar		1 piece	610	D
Crumb Topped		1 piece	260	D
Devil's Food Crumb		1 piece	250	D
Frosted Rich		1 piece	280	D
Crumb		1 piece	160	D
Frosted		1 piece	190	D
Glazed Whirl		1 piece	190	C
Honey Wheat		1 piece	250	D
Cinnamon	Apple Filled, Mini	1 piece	70	C
Cinnamon	Mini	1 piece	60	D
Crumb	Mini	1 piece	80	D
Frosted	Mini	1 piece	80	D
Frosted	Strawberry Filled, Mini	1 piece	80	D
Plain	Mini	1 piece	60	D–
Powdered Sugar	Mini	1 piece	60	D
Powdered Sugar	Mini Strawberry Filled	1 piece	70	C
Cinnamon		1 piece	120	D
Plain		1 piece	120	D–

"+" indicates the food meets minimum fiber requirements; "–" indicates the food has a high sodium content.

Food	Processing Category	Brand
Donut	Fresh Baked	Hostess Breakfast Bake Shop Family Pack
Donut	Fresh Baked	Hostess Breakfast Bake Shop Old Fashioned
Donut	Fresh Baked	Hostess Breakfast Bake Shop Old Fashioned
Donut	Fresh Baked	Hostess Breakfast Bake Shop Pantry
Donut	Fresh Baked	Hostess Breakfast Bake Shop Pantry
Donut	Fresh Baked	Hostess Breakfast Bake Shop Pantry
Donut	Fresh Baked	Hostess Krunch
Donut	Fresh Baked	Hostess Os
Donut	Fresh Baked	Hostess Os
Donut	Fresh Baked	Little Debbie
Donut	Fresh Baked	Tastykake
Donut	Fresh Baked	Tastykake
Donut	Fresh Baked	Tastykake
Donut	Fresh Baked	Tastykake
Donut	Fresh Baked	Tastykake
Donut	Fresh Baked	Tastykake
Donut	Fresh Baked	Tastykake
Donut	Fresh Baked	Tastykake, Assorted
Donut	Fresh Baked	Tastykake, Assorted
Donut	Fresh Baked	Tastykake, Assorted
Eclair	Frozen	Weight Watchers Sweet Celebrations
Frosting	Mix	Betty Crocker Creamy
Frosting	Mix	Betty Crocker Creamy
Frosting	Mix	Betty Crocker Creamy
Frosting	Mix	Betty Crocker Creamy
Frosting	Mix	Betty Crocker Creamy
Frosting	Mix	Betty Crocker Creamy
Frosting	Mix	Betty Crocker Creamy
Frosting	Mix	Betty Crocker Creamy
Frosting	Mix	Betty Crocker Fluffy
Frosting	Mix	Estee
Frosting	Ready to Use	Betty Crocker Creamy Deluxe
Frosting	Ready to Use	Betty Crocker Creamy Deluxe
Frosting	Ready to Use	Betty Crocker Creamy Deluxe
Frosting	Ready to Use	Betty Crocker Creamy Deluxe
Frosting	Ready to Use	Betty Crocker Creamy Deluxe
Frosting	Ready to Use	Betty Crocker Creamy Deluxe
Frosting	Ready to Use	Betty Crocker Creamy Deluxe
Frosting	Ready to Use	Betty Crocker Creamy Deluxe
Frosting	Ready to Use	Betty Crocker Creamy Deluxe
Frosting	Ready to Use	Betty Crocker Creamy Deluxe
Frosting	Ready to Use	Betty Crocker Creamy Deluxe
Frosting	Ready to Use	Betty Crocker Creamy Deluxe
Frosting	Ready to Use	Betty Crocker Creamy Deluxe
Frosting	Ready to Use	Betty Crocker Creamy Deluxe
Frosting	Ready to Use	Betty Crocker Creamy Deluxe
Frosting	Ready to Use	Betty Crocker Creamy Deluxe
Frosting	Ready to Use	Betty Crocker Creamy Deluxe
Frosting	Ready to Use	Betty Crocker Creamy Deluxe Party
Frosting	Ready to Use	Betty Crocker Creamy Deluxe Party

Major Description	Minor Description	Serving Size	Calories	Grade
Powdered Sugar		1 piece	120	D
Glazed		1 piece	250	D
Honey Wheat		1 piece	200	D–
Cinnamon		1 piece	190	D–
Plain		1 piece	190	D–
Powdered Sugar		1 piece	190	D
Crunch		1 piece	110	C
Frosted		1 piece	260	D
Honey Wheat		1 piece	230	C
Powdered Sugar	Stick	1 piece	230	D
Cinnamon	Mini	1 piece	48	D
Frosted		1 piece	258	D
Frosted	Mini	1 piece	61	D
Honey Wheat		1 piece	209	C
Honey Wheat	Mini	1 piece	40	B
Orange Glazed		1 piece	219	C
Powdered Sugar	Mini	1 piece	42	B–
Cinnamon		1 piece	179	D
Plain		1 piece	185	D
Powdered Sugar		1 piece	188	D
Chocolate		1 piece	150	B
Cherry		$^1/_{12}$ pkg	180	B
Chocolate	Fudge	$^1/_{12}$ pkg	180	B
Chocolate	Milk	$^1/_{12}$ pkg	170	B
Coconut Pecan		$^1/_{12}$ pkg	150	D
Rainbow Chip		$^1/_{12}$ pkg	190	C
Sour Cream	Fudge	$^1/_{12}$ pkg	180	B
Sour Cream	White	$^1/_{12}$ pkg	170	B
Vanilla		$^1/_{12}$ pkg	170	B
White		$^1/_{12}$ pkg	70	A
		$1^1/_2$ Tbsp	50	B
Amaretto Almond		$^1/_{12}$ tub	160	C
Butter Pecan		$^1/_{12}$ tub	170	C
Cherry		$^1/_{12}$ tub	160	C
Chocolate		$^1/_{12}$ tub	160	C
Chocolate	Light	$^1/_{12}$ tub	130	A
Chocolate	Fudge, Dark Dutch	$^1/_{12}$ tub	160	C
Chocolate Chip		$^1/_{12}$ tub	170	C
Chocolate Chip	Double	$^1/_{12}$ tub	170	D
Chocolate Coconut Almond		$^1/_{12}$ tub	160	D
Coconut Pecan		$^1/_{12}$ tub	160	D
Cream Cheese		$^1/_{12}$ tub	160	C
Lemon		$^1/_{12}$ tub	170	C
Rainbow Chip		$^1/_{12}$ tub	170	C
Rocky Road		$^1/_{12}$ tub	150	D
Sour Cream	Chocolate	$^1/_{12}$ tub	160	C
Sour Cream	White	$^1/_{12}$ tub	160	C
Vanilla		$^1/_{12}$ tub	160	C
Chocolate	Dinosaurs	$^1/_{12}$ tub	160	C
Chocolate Chip	Candy Coated	$^1/_{12}$ tub	160	C

"+" indicates the food meets minimum fiber requirements; "–" indicates the food has a high sodium content.

Food	Processing Category	Brand
Frosting	Ready to Use	Betty Crocker Creamy Deluxe Party
Frosting	Ready to Use	Duncan Hines
Frosting	Ready to Use	Duncan Hines
Frosting	Ready to Use	Duncan Hines
Frosting	Ready to Use	Pillsbury
Frosting	Ready to Use	Pillsbury
Frosting	Ready to Use	Pillsbury
Frosting	Ready to Use	Pillsbury
Frosting	Ready to Use	Pillsbury
Frosting	Ready to Use	Pillsbury Frost it Hot
Frosting	Ready to Use	Pillsbury Frost it Hot
Frosting	Ready to Use	Pillsbury Frosting Supreme
Frosting	Ready to Use	Pillsbury Frosting Supreme
Frosting	Ready to Use	Pillsbury Frosting Supreme
Frosting	Ready to Use	Pillsbury Frosting Supreme
Frosting	Ready to Use	Pillsbury Frosting Supreme
Frosting	Ready to Use	Pillsbury Frosting Supreme
Frosting	Ready to Use	Pillsbury Frosting Supreme
Frosting	Ready to Use	Pillsbury Frosting Supreme
Frosting	Ready to Use	Pillsbury Frosting Supreme
Frosting	Ready to Use	Pillsbury Frosting Supreme
Frosting	Ready to Use	Pillsbury Frosting Supreme
Frosting	Ready to Use	Pillsbury Frosting Supreme
Frosting	Ready to Use	Pillsbury Frosting Supreme
Frosting	Ready to Use	Pillsbury Frosting Supreme
Frosting	Ready to Use	Pillsbury Funfetti
Frosting	Ready to Use	Pillsbury Funfetti Pink and White
Frosting	Ready to Use	Pillsbury Lovin' Lites
Frosting	Ready to Use	Pillsbury Lovin' Lites
Frosting	Ready to Use	Pillsbury Lovin' Lites
Fruit Bar	Frozen	Dole Fresh Lites
Fruit Bar	Frozen	Dole Fresh Lites
Fruit Bar	Frozen	Dole Fresh Lites
Fruit Bar	Frozen	Dole Fresh Lites
Fruit Bar	Frozen	Dole Fruit & Cream
Fruit Bar	Frozen	Dole Fruit & Cream
Fruit Bar	Frozen	Dole Fruit & Cream
Fruit Bar	Frozen	Dole Fruit & Cream
Fruit Bar	Frozen	Dole Fruit & Cream
Fruit Bar	Frozen	Dole Fruit & Cream
Fruit Bar	Frozen	Dole Fruit & Yogurt
Fruit Bar	Frozen	Dole Fruit & Yogurt
Fruit Bar	Frozen	Dole Fruit & Yogurt
Fruit Bar	Frozen	Dole Fruit 'N Juice
Fruit Bar	Frozen	Dole Fruit 'N Juice
Fruit Bar	Frozen	Dole Fruit 'N Juice
Fruit Bar	Frozen	Dole Fruit 'N Juice
Fruit Bar	Frozen	Dole Suntops
Fruit Bar	Frozen	Dole Suntops
Fruit Bar	Frozen	Dole Suntops
Fruit Bar	Frozen	Dole Suntops
Fruit Bar	Frozen	Minute Maid Fruit Juice
Fruit Bar	Frozen	Sunkist

Major Description	Minor Description	Serving Size	Calories	Grade
Vanilla	Teddy Bears	$^1/_{12}$ tub	160	C
Chocolate		$^1/_{12}$ tub	160	C
Chocolate	Fudge, Dark Dutch	$^1/_{12}$ tub	160	C
Vanilla		$^1/_{12}$ tub	160	C
Chocolate	Fudge	$^1/_{12}$ tub	73	D
Coconut Almond		$^1/_{12}$ tub	160	D
Coconut Pecan		$^1/_{12}$ tub	150	D
Vanilla		$^1/_{12}$ tub	80	C
White	Fluffy	$^1/_{12}$ tub	60	A
Chocolate		$^1/_{12}$ tub	34	A
White	Fluffy	$^1/_{12}$ tub	34	A
Caramel Pecan		$^1/_{12}$ tub	160	D
Chocolate Chip		$^1/_{12}$ tub	150	B
Chocolate, Double Dutch		$^1/_{12}$ tub	140	C
Chocolate, Fudge		$^1/_{12}$ tub	150	C
Chocolate, Mint		$^1/_{12}$ tub	150	D
Chocolate, Mocha		$^1/_{12}$ tub	150	C
Coconut Almond		$^1/_{12}$ tub	150	D
Coconut Pecan		$^1/_{12}$ tub	160	D
Cream Cheese		$^1/_{12}$ tub	160	C
Lemon		$^1/_{12}$ tub	160	C
Milk Chocolate		$^1/_{12}$ tub	150	C
Sour Cream	Vanilla	$^1/_{12}$ tub	160	C
Strawberry		$^1/_{12}$ tub	160	C
Vanilla		$^1/_{12}$ tub	160	C
Chocolate Fudge		$^1/_{12}$ tub	140	C
Vanilla		$^1/_{12}$ tub	150	C
Chocolate Fudge		$^1/_{12}$ tub	130	A
Milk Chocolate		$^1/_{12}$ tub	130	A
Vanilla		$^1/_{12}$ tub	130	A
Cherry		1 bar	25	A
Lemon		1 bar	25	A
Pineapple Orange		1 bar	25	A
Raspberry		1 bar	25	A
Blueberry		1 bar	90	A
Chocolate & Banana		1 bar	175	D
Chocolate & Strawberry		1 bar	140	D
Peach		1 bar	90	A
Raspberry		1 bar	90	A
Strawberry		1 bar	90	A
Cherry		1 bar	80	A
Raspberry		1 bar	70	A
Strawberry		1 bar	70	A
Piña Colada		1 bar	90	B
Pineapple		1 bar	70	A
Raspberry		1 bar	70	A
Strawberry		1 bar	70	A
Grape		1 bar	40	A
Lemonade		1 bar	40	A
Orange Tropical		1 bar	40	A
Punch		1 bar	40	A
All Flavors		1 bar	60	A
Coconut		4 fl oz	170	D

"+" indicates the food meets minimum fiber requirements; "–" indicates the food has a high sodium content.

Food	Processing Category	Brand
Fruit Bar	Frozen	Sunkist
Fruit Bar	Frozen	Sunkist
Fruit Bar	Frozen	Sunkist
Fruit Bar	Frozen	Sunkist Juice Bar
Fruit Snack	All Forms	Berry Bears
Fruit Snack	All Forms	Flavor Tree
Fruit Snack	All Forms	Flavor Tree Fruit Circus/Fruit Bears
Fruit Snack	All Forms	Fruit Corners/Fruit Roll Ups, Peelouts
Fruit Snack	All Forms	Fruit Wrinkles
Fruit Snack	All Forms	Garfield & Friends
Fruit Snack	All Forms	Garfield & Friends 1-2 Punch
Fruit Snack	All Forms	Garfield & Friends Fruity Party
Fruit Snack	All Forms	Garfield & Friends Wild Blue
Fruit Snack	All Forms	Shark Bites
Fruit Snack	All Forms	Squeezit
Fruit Snack	All Forms	Sunkist Fun Fruits
Fruit Snack	All Forms	Sunkist Fun Fruits Berry Bunch
Fruit Snack	All Forms	Sunkist Fun Fruits Creme Supremes
Fruit Snack	All Forms	Sunkist Fun Fruits Fantastic Fruit
Fruit Snack	All Forms	Thunder Jets
Fruit Snack	All Forms	Weight Watchers
Fudge Bar	Frozen	Borden
Fudge Bar	Frozen	Good Humor
Fudge Bar	Frozen	Good Humor
Fudge Bar	Frozen	Good Humor
Fudge Bar	Frozen	Good Humor
Fudge Bar	Frozen	Trix Fudge N Fruity
Fudge Bar	Frozen	Weight Watchers
Gelatin	Unflavored	Knox
Gelatin Bar	Frozen	Jell-O Gelatin Pops
Gelatin Dessert	Mix	D-zerta
Gelatin Dessert	Mix	Featherweight
Gelatin Dessert	Mix	Jell-O
Gelatin Dessert	Mix	Royal
Gelatin Dessert	Mix	Royal Sugar Free
Hush Puppy	Frozen	Seapak Regular
Hush Puppy	Mix	Golden Dipt
Hush Puppy	Mix	Golden Dipt
Hush Puppy	Mix	Golden Dipt
Ice	Frozen	Baskin-Robbins
Ice	Frozen	Ben & Jerry's
Ice	Frozen	Ben & Jerry's
Ice	Frozen	Ben & Jerry's
Ice	Frozen	Ben & Jerry's
Ice	Frozen	Ben & Jerry's
Ice	Frozen	Good Humor
Ice Bar	Frozen	Gold Bond Twin Pop
Ice Bar	Frozen	Good Humor Calippo
Ice Bar	Frozen	Good Humor Calippo
Ice Bar	Frozen	Good Humor Calippo
Ice Bar	Frozen	Good Humor Ice Stripes
Ice Bar	Frozen	Popsicle All Natural

Major Description	Minor Description	Serving Size	Calories	Grade
Lemonade		4 fl oz	90	A
Strawberry	& Cream	4 fl oz	90	A
Wildberry		4 fl oz	140	A
Orange		4 fl oz	100	A
All Flavors		1 pouch	100	A
All Flavors		1 piece	75	A
Assorted		1 piece	117	A
All Flavors		1 roll	50	A
All Flavors		1 pouch	100	A
Strawberry		1 pouch	90	A
Fruit Punch		1 pouch	100	B
Fruit		1 roll	50	A
Blueberry		1 roll	50	A
All Flavors		1 pouch	100	A
All Flavors		1 pouch	110	A
All Flavors		1 pouch	100	A
Berry		1 pouch	100	A
Strawberry	Yogurt Coated	1 pouch	114	B
Fruit Punch		1 pouch	100	A
All Flavors		1 pouch	100	A
All Flavors		1 pouch	50	A–
All Flavors	Fudge Bar	3 oz	130	A
	Fudge Bar	2.5 oz	90	A
	Fudgesicle Pop	1.75 oz	60	A
	Sugar-free Fudgesicle	1.75 oz	35	B–
Banana	Fudge Pop	1.76 oz	60	A
All Flavors		1.75 oz	80	A
Chocolate	Chocolate Treat	2.75 oz	100	A–
		1 pkt	25	A
All Flavors		1 bar	35	A
All Flavors		1/2 cup	8	A
All Flavors		1/2 cup	10	A
All Flavors		1/2 cup	80	A
All Flavors		1/2 cup	80	A–
All Flavors		1/2 cup	6	A–
		4 oz	330	B–
Deluxe		1.25 oz	120	A–
Jalapeño		1.25 oz	120	A–
with Onion		1.25 oz	120	A–
Daiquiri		1 regular scoop	140	A
Grapefruit		1/2 cup	130	A
Lemon Daiquri		1/2 cup	120	A
Mandarin		1/2 cup	130	A
Marguerita Lime		1/2 cup	120	A
Raspberry		1/2 cup	120	A
Cherry Italian		6 fl oz	138	A
All Flavors		1 pop	60	A
Cherry		1 bar	138	A
Lemon		1 bar	112	A
Orange		1 bar	111	A
All Flavors		1 bar	35	A
All Flavors		1 bar	60	A

"+" indicates the food meets minimum fiber requirements; "–" indicates the food has a high sodium content.

Food	Processing Category	Brand
Ice Bar	Frozen	Popsicle Water Ice
Ice Bar	Frozen	Popsicle Water Ice
Ice Bar	Frozen	Popsicle Water Ice
Ice Cream	Frozen	Generic
Ice Cream	Frozen	Generic
Ice Cream	Frozen	Generic
Ice Cream	Frozen	Baskin-Robbins
Ice Cream	Frozen	Baskin-Robbins
Ice Cream	Frozen	Baskin-Robbins
Ice Cream	Frozen	Baskin-Robbins
Ice Cream	Frozen	Baskin-Robbins
Ice Cream	Frozen	Baskin-Robbins
Ice Cream	Frozen	Baskin-Robbins International Creams
Ice Cream	Frozen	Baskin-Robbins Jamoca
Ice Cream	Frozen	Baskin-Robbins Very Berry
Ice Cream	Frozen	Baskin-Robbins World Class
Ice Cream	Frozen	Ben & Jerry's
Ice Cream	Frozen	Ben & Jerry's
Ice Cream	Frozen	Ben & Jerry's
Ice Cream	Frozen	Ben & Jerry's
Ice Cream	Frozen	Ben & Jerry's
Ice Cream	Frozen	Ben & Jerry's
Ice Cream	Frozen	Ben & Jerry's
Ice Cream	Frozen	Ben & Jerry's
Ice Cream	Frozen	Ben & Jerry's
Ice Cream	Frozen	Ben & Jerry's
Ice Cream	Frozen	Ben & Jerry's
Ice Cream	Frozen	Ben & Jerry's
Ice Cream	Frozen	Ben & Jerry's
Ice Cream	Frozen	Ben & Jerry's
Ice Cream	Frozen	Ben & Jerry's
Ice Cream	Frozen	Ben & Jerry's
Ice Cream	Frozen	Ben & Jerry's
Ice Cream	Frozen	Ben & Jerry's
Ice Cream	Frozen	Ben & Jerry's
Ice Cream	Frozen	Ben & Jerry's
Ice Cream	Frozen	Ben & Jerry's
Ice Cream	Frozen	Ben & Jerry's
Ice Cream	Frozen	Ben & Jerry's
Ice Cream	Frozen	Ben & Jerry's
Ice Cream	Frozen	Borden
Ice Cream	Frozen	Borden Olde Fashioned Recipe
Ice Cream	Frozen	Borden Olde Fashioned Recipe
Ice Cream	Frozen	Breyers
Ice Cream	Frozen	Breyers
Ice Cream	Frozen	Breyers

[3] *One scoop is approximately 3 oz.*

Major Description	Minor Description	Serving Size	Calories	Grade
All Flavors		1 bar	50	A
Cherry		1 bar	70	A
Wildberry		1 bar	40	A
Vanilla	Regular 10% Fat	1 oz	134	D
Vanilla	Rich 16% Fat	$^1/_2$ cup	175	D
Vanilla	Soft-serve	$^1/_2$ cup	189	D
Chocolate		1 regular scoop [3]	270	D
Chocolate Chip		1 regular scoop	260	D
French Vanilla		1 regular scoop	280	D
Pralines & Cream		1 regular scoop	280	D
Rocky Road		1 regular scoop	300	D
Vanilla		1 regular scoop	240	D
Chocolate Raspberry Truffle		1 regular scoop	310	D
Almond Fudge		1 regular scoop	270	D
Strawberry		1 regular scoop	220	D
Chocolate		1 regular scoop	280	D
Aztec Harvest Coffee	Smooth Line	$^1/_2$ cup	230	D
Banana Walnut	Metro Line	$^1/_2$ cup	290	D
Butter Pecan		$^1/_2$ cup	310	D
Cherry Garcia	Cherry with Chocolate Chunks, Cherries	$^1/_2$ cup	240	D
Cherry Vanilla	Metro Line	$^1/_2$ cup	240	D
Chocolate Chip Cookie Dough		$^1/_2$ cup	270	D
Chocolate Fudge Brownie		$^1/_2$ cup	250	D
Chocolate Peanut Butter Cookie Dough		$^1/_2$ cup	300	D
Chunky Monkey	Vanilla with Chocolate Chunks, Walnuts	$^1/_2$ cup	280	D
Coconut Almond	Metro Line	$^1/_2$ cup	260	D
Coconut Almond Fudge Chip		$^1/_2$ cup	320	D
Coffee Almond Fudge		$^1/_2$ cup	290	D
Coffee Toffee Crunch		$^1/_2$ cup	280	D
Deep Dark Chocolate	Smooth Line	$^1/_2$ cup	260	D
Double Chocolate Fudge	Smooth Line	$^1/_2$ cup	280	D
English Toffee Crunch		$^1/_2$ cup	310	D
Mint with Chocolate Cookie		$^1/_2$ cup	260	D
Mocha Fudge	Smooth Line	$^1/_2$ cup	270	D
New York Super Fudge Chunk		$^1/_2$ cup	290	D
Peanut Butter Cup		$^1/_2$ cup	370	D
Rainforest Crunch		$^1/_2$ cup	300	D
Vanilla		$^1/_2$ cup	230	D
Vanilla	Smooth Line	$^1/_2$ cup	230	D
Vanilla Bean	Smooth Line	$^1/_2$ cup	230	D
Vanilla Caramel Fudge	Smooth Line	$^1/_2$ cup	280	D
Wavy Gravy		$^1/_2$ cup	330	D
White Russian	Smooth Line	$^1/_2$ cup	240	D
All Flavors		$^1/_2$ cup	130	D
Strawberry Cream		$^1/_2$ cup	130	C
Vanilla		$^1/_2$ cup	130	D
Butter Almond		$^1/_2$ cup	170	D
Butter Pecan		$^1/_2$ cup	180	D
Cherry Vanilla		$^1/_2$ cup	150	D

"+" indicates the food meets minimum fiber requirements; *"–"* indicates the food has a high sodium content.

Food	Processing Category	Brand
Ice Cream	Frozen	Breyers
Ice Cream	Frozen	Breyers
Ice Cream	Frozen	Breyers
Ice Cream	Frozen	Breyers
Ice Cream	Frozen	Breyers
Ice Cream	Frozen	Breyers
Ice Cream	Frozen	Breyers
Ice Cream	Frozen	Breyers
Ice Cream	Frozen	Breyers
Ice Cream	Frozen	Breyers
Ice Cream	Frozen	Carnation Bon Bons
Ice Cream	Frozen	Darigold Classic
Ice Cream	Frozen	Darigold Classic
Ice Cream	Frozen	Darigold/Darigold Alpine
Ice Cream	Frozen	Darigold/Darigold Alpine
Ice Cream	Frozen	Dreyer's
Ice Cream	Frozen	Dreyer's
Ice Cream	Frozen	Dreyer's
Ice Cream	Frozen	Dreyer's
Ice Cream	Frozen	Dreyer's
Ice Cream	Frozen	Eagle Brand Homestyle
Ice Cream	Frozen	Frusen Glädjé
Ice Cream	Frozen	Frusen Glädjé
Ice Cream	Frozen	Frusen Glädjé
Ice Cream	Frozen	Frusen Glädjé
Ice Cream	Frozen	Frusen Glädjé
Ice Cream	Frozen	Frusen Glädjé
Ice Cream	Frozen	Frusen Glädjé
Ice Cream	Frozen	Frusen Glädjé
Ice Cream	Frozen	Good Humor Cup
Ice Cream	Frozen	Gorden Ole Fashioned Recipe
Ice Cream	Frozen	Häagen-Dazs
Ice Cream	Frozen	Häagen-Dazs
Ice Cream	Frozen	Häagen-Dazs
Ice Cream	Frozen	Häagen-Dazs
Ice Cream	Frozen	Häagen-Dazs
Ice Cream	Frozen	Häagen-Dazs
Ice Cream	Frozen	Häagen-Dazs
Ice Cream	Frozen	Häagen-Dazs
Ice Cream	Frozen	Häagen-Dazs
Ice Cream	Frozen	Häagen-Dazs
Ice Cream	Frozen	Häagen-Dazs
Ice Cream	Frozen	Häagen-Dazs
Ice Cream	Frozen	Häagen-Dazs
Ice Cream	Frozen	Häagen-Dazs
Ice Cream	Frozen	Häagen-Dazs
Ice Cream	Frozen	Häagen-Dazs
Ice Cream	Frozen	Häagen-Dazs
Ice Cream	Frozen	Häagen-Dazs
Ice Cream	Frozen	Häagen-Dazs
Ice Cream	Frozen	Häagen-Dazs

Major Description	Minor Description	Serving Size	Calories	Grade
Chocolate		$^1/_2$ cup	160	D
Chocolate Mint		$^1/_2$ cup	170	D
Coffee		$^1/_2$ cup	150	D
Cookies & Cream		$^1/_2$ cup	170	D
Peach Natural		$^1/_2$ cup	130	D
Strawberry		$^1/_2$ cup	130	D
Vanilla		$^1/_2$ cup	150	D
Vanilla Chocolate		$^1/_2$ cup	160	D
Vanilla Chocolate Strawberry		$^1/_2$ cup	150	D
Vanilla Fudge Twirl		$^1/_2$ cup	160	D
Vanilla	Nuggets, Dark Chocolate Coated	5 pieces	170	D
Chocolate		$^1/_2$ cup	180	D
Vanilla		$^1/_2$ cup	180	D
Chocolate		$^1/_2$ cup	140	D
Vanilla		$^1/_2$ cup	130	D
Chocolate Chip		$^1/_2$ cup	150	D
Cookies & Cream		$^1/_2$ cup	160	D
Fudge Marble		$^1/_2$ cup	150	D
Rocky Road		$^1/_2$ cup	170	D
Vanilla		$^1/_2$ cup	160	D
Vanilla		$^1/_2$ cup	150	D
Butter Pecan		$^1/_2$ cup	280	D
Chocolate		$^1/_2$ cup	240	D
Chocolate Chip		$^1/_2$ cup	270	D
Chocolate Swiss Almond		$^1/_2$ cup	270	D
Strawberry		$^1/_2$ cup	230	D
Vanilla		$^1/_2$ cup	230	D
Vanilla Swiss Almond		$^1/_2$ cup	270	D
Vanilla Toffee Chunk		$^1/_2$ cup	270	D
Vanilla		3 oz	98	D
Dutch Chocolate		$^1/_2$ cup	130	D
Belgian Chocolate		$^1/_2$ cup	330	D
Brandied Cherry		$^1/_2$ cup	250	D
Butter Pecan		$^1/_2$ cup	390	D
Cappuccino		$^1/_2$ cup	340	D
Caramel Cone		$^1/_2$ cup	330	D
Caramel Nut Sundae		$^1/_2$ cup	310	D
Carrot Cake		$^1/_2$ cup	310	D
Chocolate		$^1/_2$ cup	270	D
Chocolate Chip		$^1/_2$ cup	290	D
Chocolate Mint		$^1/_2$ cup	300	D
Chocolate Peanut Butter, Deep		$^1/_2$ cup	330	D
Chocolate Swiss Almond		$^1/_2$ cup	300	D
Chocolate, Deep		$^1/_2$ cup	290	D
Chocolate, Fudge, Deep		$^1/_2$ cup	290	D
Coffee		$^1/_2$ cup	270	D
Coffee Chip		$^1/_2$ cup	300	D
Coffee Toffee Crunch		$^1/_2$ cup	300	D
Cookie Dough		$^1/_2$ cup	300	D
Cookies & Cream		$^1/_2$ cup	280	D
Macadamia Brittle		$^1/_2$ cup	280	D
Macademia Nut		$^1/_2$ cup	330	D

"+" indicates the food meets minimum fiber requirements; "–" indicates the food has a high sodium content.

Food	Processing Category	Brand
Ice Cream	Frozen	Häagen-Dazs
Ice Cream	Frozen	Häagen-Dazs
Ice Cream	Frozen	Häagen-Dazs
Ice Cream	Frozen	Häagen-Dazs
Ice Cream	Frozen	Häagen-Dazs
Ice Cream	Frozen	Häagen-Dazs
Ice Cream	Frozen	Häagen-Dazs
Ice Cream	Frozen	Häagen-Dazs
Ice Cream	Frozen	Häagen-Dazs
Ice Cream	Frozen	Häagen-Dazs
Ice Cream	Frozen	Häagen-Dazs
Ice Cream	Frozen	Häagen-Dazs
Ice Cream	Frozen	Lady Borden
Ice Cream	Frozen	Sealtest
Ice Cream	Frozen	Sealtest
Ice Cream	Frozen	Sealtest
Ice Cream	Frozen	Sealtest
Ice Cream	Frozen	Sealtest
Ice Cream	Frozen	Sealtest
Ice Cream	Frozen	Sealtest
Ice Cream	Frozen	Sealtest
Ice Cream	Frozen	Sealtest
Ice Cream	Frozen	Sealtest
Ice Cream	Frozen	Sealtest
Ice Cream	Frozen	Sealtest
Ice Cream	Frozen	Sealtest
Ice Cream	Frozen	Sealtest
Ice Cream	Frozen	Sealtest Cubic Scoops
Ice Cream	Frozen	Sealtest Cubic Scoops
Ice Cream	Frozen	Seatlest Cubic Scoops
Ice Cream	Frozen	Weight Watchers
Ice Cream	Frozen	Weight Watchers
Ice Cream	Frozen	Weight Watchers
Ice Cream	Frozen	Weight Watchers
Ice Cream	Frozen	Weight Watchers
Ice Cream	Frozen	Weight Watchers
Ice Cream	Frozen	Weight Watchers
Ice Cream	Frozen	Weight Watchers
Ice Cream	Frozen	Weight Watchers
Ice Cream	Frozen	Weight Watchers
Ice Cream	Frozen	Weight Watchers
Ice Cream	Mix	Salada
Ice Cream	Mix	Salada
Ice Cream, Bar	Frozen	Baker's Fudgetastic
Ice Cream, Bar	Frozen	Baker's Fudgetastic
Ice Cream, Bar	Frozen	Good Humor
Ice Cream, Bar	Frozen	Good Humor
Ice Cream, Bar	Frozen	Good Humor
Ice Cream, Bar	Frozen	Good Humor
Ice Cream, Bar	Frozen	Good Humor
Ice Cream, Bar	Frozen	Good Humor
Ice Cream, Bar	Frozen	Good Humor Fat Frog
Ice Cream, Bar	Frozen	Good Humor Halo Bar

Major Description	Minor Description	Serving Size	Calories	Grade
Maple Walnut		$^1/_2$ cup	330	D
Peanut Butter		$^1/_2$ cup	340	D
Pralines & Cream		$^1/_2$ cup	290	D
Rum Raisin		$^1/_2$ cup	250	D
Strawberry		$^1/_2$ cup	250	D
Triple Brownie		$^1/_2$ cup	330	D
Vanilla		$^1/_2$ cup	260	D
Vanilla Chip		$^1/_2$ cup	300	D
Vanilla Fudge		$^1/_2$ cup	270	D
Vanilla Honey		$^1/_2$ cup	250	D
Vanilla Peanut Butter Swirl		$^1/_2$ cup	280	D
Vanilla Swiss Almond		$^1/_2$ cup	290	D
Butter Pecan		$^1/_2$ cup	180	D
Butter Crunch		$^1/_2$ cup	150	D
Butter Pecan		$^1/_2$ cup	160	D
Chocolate		$^1/_2$ cup	140	C
Chocolate	Triple Stripes	$^1/_2$ cup	140	D
Chocolate Chip		$^1/_2$ cup	150	D
Chocolate Marshmallow Sundae		$^1/_2$ cup	150	C
Coffee		$^1/_2$ cup	140	D
Fudge		$^1/_2$ cup	140	D
Heavenly Hash		$^1/_2$ cup	150	D
Maple Walnut		$^1/_2$ cup	160	D
Peanut Fudge Sundae		$^1/_2$ cup	140	D
Strawberry		$^1/_2$ cup	130	C
Vanilla		$^1/_2$ cup	140	D
Vanilla Chocolate Strawberry		$^1/_2$ cup	140	C
Vanilla Chocolate Strawberry		$^1/_2$ cup	130	D
Vanilla Orange		$^1/_2$ cup	130	B
Vanilla Raspberry		$^1/_2$ cup	130	B
Artic D Lites	Low Fat	2.5 oz	130	D
Berries & Cream Mousse	Low Fat	3.5 oz	70	B
Caramel Fudge Sundae		4.5 oz	160	B
Chocolate Fudge Sundae		4.5 oz	160	B
Cookie Dough	Light	$^1/_2$ cup	140	B
Double Fudge Brownie Parfait		5.3 oz	190	A
Praline Crunch	Light	$^1/_2$ cup	140	B
Praline Toffee Crunch Parfait		5.1 oz	190	A
Rocky Road	Light	$^1/_2$ cup	140	B
Triple Chocolate	Light	$^1/_2$ cup	150	B
Vanilla	Light	$^1/_2$ cup	120	B
Dutch Chocolate	Prepared	1 cup	310	D
Peach Vanilla or Wild Strawberry	Prepared	1 cup	310	D
Chocolate Fudge Sundae		1 bar	220	D
Chocolate Fudge Sundae, Crunchy		1 bar	230	D
Almond	Toasted	1 bar	212	D
Chip Candy Crunch		1 bar	255	D
Chocolate Eclair		1 bar	188	D
Chocolate Fudge Cake		1 bar	214	D
Strawberry Shortcake		1 bar	176	D
Vanilla	Chocolate Coated	1 bar	198	D
		1 bar	154	D
		1 bar	230	D

"+" indicates the food meets minimum fiber requirements; "−" indicates the food has a high sodium content.

Food	Processing Category	Brand
Ice Cream, Bar	Frozen	Good Humor Whammy
Ice Cream, Bar	Frozen	Häagen-Daz Crunch Bar
Ice Cream, Bar	Frozen	Häagen-Dazs
Ice Cream, Bar	Frozen	Häagen-Dazs
Ice Cream, Bar	Frozen	Häagen-Dazs
Ice Cream, Bar	Frozen	Häagen-Dazs
Ice Cream, Bar	Frozen	Häagen-Dazs
Ice Cream, Bar	Frozen	Häagen-Dazs
Ice Cream, Bar	Frozen	Häagen-Dazs
Ice Cream, Bar	Frozen	Häagen-Dazs
Ice Cream, Bar	Frozen	Häagen-Dazs
Ice Cream, Bar	Frozen	Häagen-Dazs Crunch Bar
Ice Cream, Bar	Frozen	Häagen-Dazs Crunch Bar
Ice Cream, Bar	Frozen	Heath
Ice Cream, Bar	Frozen	Klondike
Ice Cream, Bar	Frozen	Klondike
Ice Cream, Bar	Frozen	Klondike Krispy
Ice Cream, Bar	Frozen	Klondike Lite
Ice Cream, Bar	Frozen	Nestlé Alpine Premium
Ice Cream, Bar	Frozen	Nestlé Crunch
Ice Cream, Bar	Frozen	Nestlé Premium
Ice Cream, Bar	Frozen	Nestlé Quick
Ice Cream, Bar	Frozen	Oh-Henry
Ice Cream, Sandwich [4]	Frozen	Good Humor
Ice Cream, Sandwich	Frozen	Good Humor
Ice Cream, Sandwich	Frozen	Good Humor
Ice Cream, Sandwich	Frozen	Good Humor
Ice Cream, Sandwich	Frozen	Klondike
Ice Milk	Frozen	Generic
Ice Milk	Frozen	Generic
Ice Milk	Frozen	Borden
Ice Milk	Frozen	Borden
Ice Milk	Frozen	Borden
Ice Milk	Frozen	Breyers Light
Ice Milk	Frozen	Breyers Light
Ice Milk	Frozen	Breyers Light
Ice Milk	Frozen	Breyers Light
Ice Milk	Frozen	Breyers Light
Ice Milk	Frozen	Breyers Light
Ice Milk	Frozen	Breyers Light
Ice Milk	Frozen	Bryers Light
Ice Milk	Frozen	Bryers Light
Ice Milk	Frozen	Darigold
Ice Milk	Frozen	Darigold Lite
Ice Milk	Frozen	Kemp's
Ice Milk	Frozen	Light n' Lively
Ice Milk	Frozen	Light n' Lively

[4] For all ice cream sandwich products, serving size indicates 1 item.

Major Description	Minor Description	Serving Size	Calories	Grade
Assorted		1 bar	95	D
Peanut Butter		1 bar	270	D
Chocolate	Dark Chocolate Coated	1 bar	390	D
Coffee	Almonds Crunch	1 bar	360	D
Peanut Butter	Chocolate	1 bar	390	D
Vanilla	Almonds	1 bar	370	D
Vanilla	Caramel	1 bar	370	D
Vanilla	Chocolate Almond Coated	1 bar	370	D
Vanilla	Chocolate Brittle Coated	1 bar	370	D
Vanilla	Chocolate Coated	1 bar	360	D
Vanilla	Dark Chocolate Coated	1 bar	390	D
Caramel Almond		1 bar	240	D
Vanilla		1 bar	220	D
		1 bar	170	D
		1 bar	280	D
Chocolate		1 bar	270	D
		1 bar	290	D
		1 bar	140	D
with White Chocolate Coating		1 bar	350	D
Vanilla	Chocolate Coated & Crisps	1 bar	180	D
Chocolate	with Almonds & Chocolate Coated	1 bar	350	D
Chocolate	Chocolate Coated	1 bar	210	D
Vanilla	Caramel Peanut Center & Chocolate Coated	1 bar	320	D
Chocolate Chip Cookie		2.7 oz	204	C
Chocolate Chip Cookie		4 oz	246	C
Vanilla		2.5 oz	165	B
Vanilla		3 oz	191	B
Vanilla		5 oz	230	C
Vanilla	Hard	1/2 cup	92	B
Vanilla	Soft	1/2 cup	112	B
Chocolate		1/2 cup	100	B
Strawberry		1/2 cup	90	B
Vanilla		1/2 cup	90	B
Fudge Twirl		1/2 cup	130	B
Heavenly Hash		1/2 cup	150	B
Praline Almond		1/2 cup	130	C
Strawberry		1/2 cup	110	B
Vanilla		1/2 cup	120	B
Vanilla Chocolate Strawberry		1/2 cup	120	B
Vanilla Raspberry Parfait		1/2 cup	130	B
Chocolate		1/2 cup	120	B
Toffee Fudge Parfait		1/2 cup	140	C
Vanilla		1/2 cup	110	B
Chocolate		1/2 cup	110	B
Vanilla	Light	1/2 cup	100	B
Caramel Nut		1/2 cup	120	B
Chocolate Chip		1/2 cup	120	B

"+" indicates the food meets minimum fiber requirements; "–" indicates the food has a high sodium content.

Food	Processing Category	Brand
Ice Milk	Frozen	Light n' Lively
Ice Milk	Frozen	Light n' Lively
Ice Milk	Frozen	Light n' Lively
Ice Milk	Frozen	Light n' Lively
Ice Milk	Frozen	Light n' Lively
Ice Milk	Frozen	Light n' Lively
Ice Milk	Frozen	Light n' Lively
Ice Milk	Frozen	Light n' Lively
Ice Milk	Frozen	Weight Watchers
Ice Milk	Frozen	Weight Watchers Grand Collection
Ice Milk	Frozen	Weight Watchers Grand Collection
Ice Milk	Frozen	Weight Watchers Grand Collection
Ice Milk	Frozen	Weight Watchers Grand Collection
Ice Milk	Frozen	Weight Watchers Grand Collection
Ice Milk	Frozen	Weight Watchers Grand Collection
Mousse	Frozen	Weight Watchers
Mousse	Frozen	Weight Watchers
Mousse	Frozen	Weight Watchers
Mousse	Frozen	Weight Watchers Sweet Celebration
Mousse	Frozen	Weight Watchers Sweet Celebration
Mousse	Mix	Jell-O Rich & Luscious
Mousse	Mix	Jell-O Rich & Luscious
Mousse	Mix	Knorr
Mousse	Mix	Knorr
Mousse	Mix	Knorr
Mousse	Mix	Weight Watchers
Mousse	Mix	Weight Watchers
Mousse	Mix	Weight Watchers
Mousse	Mix	Weight Watchers
Pie	Fresh Baked	Generic or Homemade [5]
Pie	Fresh Baked	Generic or Homemade
Pie	Fresh Baked	Generic or Homemade
Pie	Fresh Baked	Generic or Homemade
Pie	Fresh Baked	Generic or Homemade
Pie	Fresh Baked	Generic or Homemade
Pie	Fresh Baked	Generic or Homemade
Pie	Fresh Baked	Generic or Homemade
Pie	Fresh Baked	Generic or Homemade
Pie	Fresh Baked	Generic or Homemade
Pie	Fresh Baked	Generic or Homemade
Pie	Fresh Baked	Generic or Homemade
Pie	Fresh Baked	Generic or Homemade
Pie	Fresh Baked	Generic or Homemade
Pie	Fresh Baked	Generic or Homemade
Pie	Fresh Baked	Generic or Homemade
Pie	Fresh Baked	Generic or Homemade
Pie	Fresh Baked	Generic or Homemade
Pie	Fresh Baked	Generic or Homemade
Pie	Fresh Baked	Generic or Homemade
Pie	Fresh Baked	Generic or Homemade
Pie	Fresh Baked	Generic or Homemade
Pie	Fresh Baked	Generic or Homemade
Pie	Fresh Baked	Generic or Homemade

[5] Generic or homemade pie recipes based on USDA formulas for 9-inch pie.

Major Description	Minor Description	Serving Size	Calories	Grade
Coffee		$^1/_2$ cup	100	B
Cookies & Cream		$^1/_2$ cup	110	B
Heavenly Hash		$^1/_2$ cup	120	B
Vanilla		$^1/_2$ cup	100	B
Vanilla Chocolate Almond		$^1/_2$ cup	120	B
Vanilla Chocolate Strawberry		$^1/_2$ cup	100	B
Vanilla Fudge Twirl		$^1/_2$ cup	110	B
Vanilla Raspberry Swirl		$^1/_2$ cup	110	B
Pecan Pralines & Cream Bars		2.1 oz	120	D
Chocolate		$^1/_2$ cup	110	B
Chocolate Chip		$^1/_2$ cup	120	B
Chocolate Swirl		$^1/_2$ cup	120	B
Neapolitan		$^1/_2$ cup	110	B
Pecan Pralines & Cream		$^1/_2$ cup	120	B
Vanilla		$^1/_2$ cup	100	B
Berries & Creme		3.5 oz	70	B
Chocolate		2.5 oz	170	C
Pecan Praline		2.71 oz	190	C
Chocolate		2.7 oz	190	B+
Triple Chocolate Caramel		2.7 oz	190	B
Chocolate		$^1/_2$ cup	150	C
Chocolate	Fudge	$^1/_2$ cup	140	C
Chocolate		$^1/_2$ cup	80	D
Dark Chocolate		$^1/_2$ cup	80	D
White Chocolate		$^1/_2$ cup	70	C
Cheesecake		$^1/_2$ cup	60	B–
Chocolate		$^1/_2$ cup	60	D
Raspberry		$^1/_2$ cup	60	D–
White Chocolate	with Almonds	$^1/_2$ cup	60	D
Apple		$^1/_8$ pie	280	C
Banana Custard		$^1/_8$ pie	252	C
Blackberry		$^1/_8$ pie	287	D
Blueberry		$^1/_8$ pie	286	C
Butterscotch		$^1/_8$ pie	304	C
Cherry		$^1/_8$ pie	308	C
Chocolate Chiffon		$^1/_8$ pie	266	D
Chocolate Cream		$^1/_8$ pie	301	D
Chocolate Mousse		$^1/_8$ pie	259	D
Coconut Cream		$^1/_8$ pie	258	D
Coconut Custard		$^1/_8$ pie	268	D
Lemon Chiffon		$^1/_8$ pie	254	C
Lemon Meringue		$^1/_8$ pie	350	C
Mincemeat		$^1/_8$ pie	320	C–
Peach		$^1/_8$ pie	301	C
Pecan		$^1/_8$ pie	431	D
Pineapple		$^1/_8$ pie	299	C
Pineapple Chiffon		$^1/_8$ pie	233	C
Pineapple Custard		$^1/_8$ pie	251	C
Pumpkin		$^1/_8$ pie	241	D
Raisin		$^1/_8$ pie	319	C
Rhubarb		$^1/_8$ pie	299	C
Strawberry		$^1/_8$ pie	184	C
Sweet Potato		$^1/_8$ pie	243	D

"+" indicates the food meets minimum fiber requirements; "–" indicates the food has a high sodium content.

Food	Processing Category	Brand
Pie	Fresh Baked	Entenmann's
Pie	Fresh Baked	Entenmann's
Pie	Fresh Baked	Entenmann's
Pie	Fresh Baked	Entenmann's
Pie	Fresh Baked	Freihofer
Pie	Fresh Baked	Freihofer
Pie	Frozen	Banquet
Pie	Frozen	Banquet
Pie	Frozen	Banquet
Pie	Frozen	Banquet
Pie	Frozen	Banquet
Pie	Frozen	Banquet Family Size [6]
Pie	Frozen	Banquet Family Size
Pie	Frozen	Banquet Family Size
Pie	Frozen	Banquet Family Size
Pie	Frozen	Banquet Family Size
Pie	Frozen	Banquet Family Size
Pie	Frozen	Banquet Family Size
Pie	Frozen	McMillin's Pies
Pie	Frozen	McMillin's Pies
Pie	Frozen	McMillin's Pies
Pie	Frozen	McMillin's Pies
Pie	Frozen	McMillin's Pies
Pie	Frozen	McMillin's Pies
Pie	Frozen	McMillin's Pies
Pie	Frozen	McMillin's Pies
Pie	Frozen	McMillin's Pies
Pie	Frozen	Mrs. Smith's [7]
Pie	Frozen	Mrs. Smith's
Pie	Frozen	Mrs. Smith's
Pie	Frozen	Mrs. Smith's
Pie	Frozen	Mrs. Smith's
Pie	Frozen	Mrs. Smith's
Pie	Frozen	Mrs. Smith's
Pie	Frozen	Pepperidge Farm
Pie	Frozen	Pet-Ritz [7]
Pie	Frozen	Pet-Ritz
Pie	Frozen	Pet-Ritz
Pie	Frozen	Pet-Ritz
Pie	Frozen	Pet-Ritz
Pie	Frozen	Pet-Ritz
Pie	Frozen	Pet-Ritz
Pie	Frozen	Pet-Ritz
Pie	Frozen	Pet-Ritz
Pie	Frozen	Pet-Ritz
Pie	Frozen	Pet-Ritz
Pie	Frozen	Pet-Ritz
Pie	Frozen	Pet-Ritz
Pie	Frozen	Sara Lee Free & Light
Pie	Frozen	Sara Lee Free & Light

[6] *Fractions of a Banquet Family Sized pie are approximately 2 to 3.5 ozs.*
[7] *Fractions of a Mrs. Smith, Pet-Ritz, or Sara Lee Homestyle pie are approximately 2 to 3.5 ozs.*

Major Description	Minor Description	Serving Size	Calories	Grade
Apple	Homestyle	2.1 oz	140	D
Apple Beehive	Fat Free	$^1/_6$ pie	270	A–
Cherry Beehive	Fat Free	$^1/_6$ pie	260	A
Coconut Custard		1.8 oz	140	D
Apple Beehive	Fat Free	$^1/_6$ pie	225	A
Cherry Beehive	Fat Free	$^1/_6$ pie	225	A
Banana Cream		$^1/_6$ pie	180	D
Chocolate Cream		$^1/_6$ pie	190	D
Coconut Cream		$^1/_6$ pie	190	D
Lemon Cream		$^1/_6$ pie	170	D
Strawberry Cream		$^1/_6$ pie	170	D
Apple		$^1/_6$ pie	250	C
Blackberry		$^1/_6$ pie	270	C–
Blueberry		$^1/_6$ pie	270	C–
Cherry		$^1/_6$ pie	250	C
Mincemeat		$^1/_6$ pie	260	C–
Peach		$^1/_6$ pie	245	D
Pumpkin		$^1/_6$ pie	200	C–
Apple		4 oz	460	D
Berry		4 oz	440	D
Boston Cream		4 oz	440	D
Cherry		4 oz	430	D
Chocolate Pudding		4 oz	450	D
Coconut Pudding		4 oz	440	D
Lemon		4 oz	430	D
Peach		4 oz	440	D
Strawberry		4 oz	420	D
Vanilla Pudding		4 oz	400	D
Apple		$^1/_8$ of pie	210	C
Blueberry		$^1/_8$ of pie	220	C
Cherry		$^1/_8$ of pie	220	C
Lemon Meringue		$^1/_8$ of pie	210	B
Peach		$^1/_8$ of pie	210	C
Pecan		$^1/_8$ of pie	330	C
Pumpkin		$^1/_8$ of pie	190	B
Mississippi Mud		1 ramekin	310	D
Apple		$^1/_6$ pie	330	C
Banana Cream		$^1/_6$ pie	170	D
Blueberry		$^1/_6$ pie	370	B
Cherry		$^1/_6$ pie	300	C
Chocolate Cream		$^1/_6$ pie	190	C
Coconut Cream		$^1/_6$ pie	190	C
Custard		$^1/_6$ pie	200	C
Lemon Cream		$^1/_6$ pie	190	D
Mincemeat		$^1/_6$ pie	280	B
Neapolitan Cream		$^1/_6$ pie	180	D
Peach		$^1/_6$ pie	320	C
Pumpkin		$^1/_6$ pie	250	C
Strawberry Cream		$^1/_6$ pie	170	D
Sweet Potato		$^1/_6$ pie	150	D
Apple	Streusel	$^1/_{10}$ pie	136	A
Cherry	Streusel	$^1/_{10}$ pie	160	A

"+" indicates the food meets minimum fiber requirements; "–" indicates the food has a high sodium content.

Food	Processing Category	Brand
Pie	Frozen	Sara Lee Homestyle [7]
Pie	Frozen	Sara Lee Homestyle
Pie	Frozen	Sara Lee Homestyle
Pie	Frozen	Sara Lee Homestyle
Pie	Frozen	Sara Lee Homestyle
Pie	Frozen	Sara Lee Homestyle
Pie	Frozen	Sara Lee Homestyle
Pie	Frozen	Sara Lee Homestyle
Pie	Frozen	Sara Lee Homestyle
Pie	Frozen	Sara Lee Homestyle High
Pie	Frozen	Weight Watchers
Pie	Frozen	Weight Watchers
Pie	Frozen	Weight Watchers Sweet Celebrations
Pie	Mix	Jell-O No Bake
Pie	Mix	Jell-O No Bake
Pie	Mix	Jell-O No Bake
Pie	Mix	Jell-O No Bake
Pie	Mix	Libby
Pie	Mix	Royal No Bake
Pie	Mix	Royal No Bake
Pie	Mix	Royal No Bake
Pie Crust	Ready to Eat	Nabisco
Pie Crust	Ready to Eat	Nabisco
Pie Crust	Ready to Eat	Nabisco
Pie Crust	Ready to Eat	Nabisco Premium
Pie Crust Shell	Frozen	Mrs. Smith's
Pie Crust Shell	Frozen	Pet-Ritz
Pie Crust Shell	Frozen	Pet-Ritz
Pie Crust Shell	Frozen	Pet-Ritz
Pie Crust Shell	Frozen	Pet-Ritz
Pie Crust Shell	Mix	Betty Crocker
Pie Crust Shell	Mix	Flako
Pie Crust Shell	Mix	Pillsbury
Pie Crust Shell	Refrigerated	Pillsbury All Ready
Pie Filling	Canned	Generic
Pie Filling	Canned	Borden None Such
Pie Filling	Canned	Borden None Such
Pie Filling	Canned	Borden None Such
Pie Filling	Canned	Comstock
Pie Filling	Canned	Comstock
Pie Filling	Canned	Comstock
Pie Filling	Canned	Comstock
Pie Filling	Canned	Comstock
Pie Filling	Canned	Comstock
Pie Filling	Canned	Comstock
Pie Filling	Canned	Comstock
Pie Filling	Canned	Comstock
Pie Filling	Canned	Comstock
Pie Filling	Canned	Comstock
Pie Filling	Canned	Comstock
Pie Filling	Canned	Comstock
Pie Filling	Canned	Comstock

[7] *Fractions of a Mrs. Smith, Pet-Ritz, or Sara Lee Homestyle pie are approximately 2 to 3.5 ozs.*

Major Description	Minor Description	Serving Size	Calories	Grade
Apple		$^1/_{10}$ of pie	280	C
Blueberry		$^1/_{10}$ of pie	300	C
Cherry		$^1/_{10}$ of pie	270	D
Dutch Apple		$^1/_{10}$ of pie	300	C
Mincemeat		$^1/_{10}$ of pie	300	C
Peach		$^1/_{10}$ of pie	280	C
Pecan		$^1/_{10}$ of pie	400	D
Pumpkin		$^1/_{10}$ of pie	240	C
Raspberry		$^1/_{10}$ of pie	280	D
Apple		$^1/_{10}$ of pie	400	D
Chocolate Mocha		$^1/_2$ pie	160	B
Apple		$^1/_2$ pie	200	B–
Chocolate Mocha		2.7 oz	160	B
Banana Cream		$^1/_8$ pie	240	D–
Chocolate Mousse		$^1/_8$ pie	260	D–
Coconut Cream		$^1/_8$ pie	260	D
Pumpkin		$^1/_8$ pie	250	D–
Pumpkin		$^1/_8$ pie	390	C
Chocolate	Mint	$^1/_8$ pie	260	D
Chocolate	Mousse	$^1/_8$ pie	230	D
Lemon Meringue		$^1/_8$ pie	310	C
Graham Cracker	Honey Maid	$^3/_4$ oz slice	110	D
Nilla		$^3/_4$ oz slice	110	D
Oreo		$^3/_4$ oz slice	110	D–
Cracker Crumbs	Fat Free	2 tbs	50	A
		$^1/_8$ of 8" shell	80	D–
		$^1/_6$ shell	110	D
All Vegetable Shortening		$^1/_6$ shell	110	D
Deep-dish		$^1/_6$ shell	130	D
Graham Cracker		$^1/_6$ chell	110	D
		$^1/_{16}$ pkg	120	D
		$^1/_6$ of pie	247	D–
		$^1/_8$ of shell	100	D–
		$^1/_8$ of double crust pie	240	D
Pumpkin		$^1/_2$ cup	141	A–
Mincemeat	Condensed	$^1/_4$ can	220	A–
Mincemeat	Ready to Use	$^1/_3$ cup	200	A–
Mincemeat	Ready to Use with Brandy & Rum	$^1/_3$ cup	220	A
Apple		3.5 oz	120	A
Apricot		3.5 oz	110	A
Banana		3.5 oz	110	B–
Blueberry		3.5 oz	110	A
Cherry		3.5 oz	110	A
Chocolate		3.5 oz	130	B–
Coconut		3.5 oz	120	B–
Lemon		3.5 oz	140	A
Mincemeat		3.5 oz	150	A
Peach		3.5 oz	110	A
Pineapple		3.5 oz	100	A
Pumpkin		3.5 oz	100	A–
Raisin		3.5 oz	120	A

"+" indicates the food meets minimum fiber requirements; "–" indicates the food has a high sodium content.

Food	Processing Category	Brand
Pie Filling	Canned	Comstock
Pie Filling	Canned	Comstock Lite
Pie Filling	Canned	Comstock Lite
Pie Filling	Canned	Comstock Lite
Pie Filling	Canned	Libby
Pie Filling	Canned	Lucky Leaf
Pie Filling	Canned	Lucky Leaf
Pie Filling	Canned	Lucky Leaf
Pie Filling	Canned	Lucky Leaf
Pie Filling	Canned	Lucky Leaf
Pie Filling	Canned	Lucky Leaf
Pie Filling	Canned	Lucky Leaf
Pie Filling	Canned	Lucky Leaf
Pie Filling	Canned	Lucky Leaf
Pie Filling	Canned	Lucky Leaf
Pie Filling	Canned	Lucky Leaf
Pie Filling	Canned	Lucky Leaf
Pie Filling	Canned	Lucky Leaf
Pie Filling	Canned	Lucky Leaf
Pie Filling	Canned	Lucky Leaf
Pie Filling	Canned	Lucky Leaf
Pie Filling	Canned	Lucky Leaf
Pie Filling	Canned	Lucky Leaf
Pie Filling	Canned	Lucky Leaf
Pie Filling	Canned	Lucky Leaf
Pie Filling	Canned	Lucky Leaf
Pie Filling	Canned	Lucky Leaf Plus
Pie Filling	Canned	Lucky Leaf Plus
Pie Filling	Canned	Lucky Leaf Plus
Pie Filling	Canned	Lucky Leaf Plus
Pie Filling	Canned	Lucky Leaf Plus
Pie Filling	Canned	Lucky Leaf Plus
Pie Filling	Canned	Pathmark No Frills
Pie Filling	Canned	Pathmark No Frills
Pie Filling	Canned	S & W Old Fashioned
Pie Filling	Canned	Stokely
Pie Filling	Canned	White House
Pie Filling	Canned	White House
Pie Filling	Canned	White House
Pie Filling	Canned	White House
Pie, Snack	Packaged	Drake's
Pie, Snack	Packaged	Drake's
Pie, Snack	Packaged	Drake's
Pie, Snack	Packaged	Hostess
Pie, Snack	Packaged	Hostess
Pie, Snack	Packaged	Hostess
Pie, Snack	Packaged	Hostess
Pie, Snack	Packaged	Hostess
Pie, Snack	Packaged	Hostess
Pie, Snack	Packaged	Hostess
Pie, Snack	Packaged	Hostess
Pie, Snack	Packaged	Hostess
Pie, Snack	Packaged	Little Debbie
Pie, Snack	Packaged	Little Debbie

Major Description	Minor Description	Serving Size	Calories	Grade
Strawberry		3.5 oz	100	A
Apple		3.5 oz	80	A
Blueberry		3.5 oz	75	A
Cherry		3.5 oz	75	A
Pumpkin		1 cup	260	A–
Apple		4 oz	120	A
Apricot		4 oz	150	A
Blackberry		4 oz	120	A
Blueberry		4 oz	120	A–
Boysenberry		4 oz	120	A
Cherry		4 oz	120	A
Gooseberry		4 oz	180	A
Lemon		4 oz	200	A
Lemon, French		4 oz	180	A
Mincemeat		4 oz	190	A
Peach		4 oz	150	A
Pineapple		4 oz	110	A
Pumpkin		4 oz	170	B
Raisin		4 oz	130	A
Raspberry, Black		4 oz	190	A
Raspberry, Red		4 oz	190	A
Strawberry		4 oz	120	A
Strawberry Rhubarb		4 oz	120	A
Turnover, Diced		4 oz	120	A
Vanilla Cream		4 oz	150	B
Apple		4 oz	121	A
Blackberry		4 oz	121	A
Blueberry		4 oz	145	A
Cherry		4 oz	108	A
Peach		4 oz	113	A
Strawberry		4 oz	138	A
Apple		4 oz	130	A
Cherry		4 oz	130	A
Mincemeat	Brandy	4 oz	234	A
Pumpkin		½ cup	170	A–
Apple		3.5 oz	121	A
Blueberry		3.5 oz	118	A
Cherry		3.5 oz	141	A
Peach		3.5 oz	117	A
Apple		1 piece	210	D
Blueberry	Apple	1 piece	210	D
Lemon		1 piece	210	D
Apple		1 piece	430	D
Apple, French		1 piece	430	D
Blackberry		1 piece	420	C
Blueberry		1 piece	420	C
Cherry		1 piece	460	C
Chocolate Pudding		1 piece	490	C
Lemon		1 piece	440	D
Peach		1 piece	420	C
Strawberry		1 piece	410	D
Apple, Dutch		1 piece	230	C
Marshmallow	Banana	1 piece	360	B

"+" indicates the food meets minimum fiber requirements; "–" indicates the food has a high sodium content.

Food	Processing Category	Brand
Pie, Snack	Packaged	Little Debbie
Pie, Snack	Packaged	Little Debbie
Pie, Snack	Packaged	Little Debbie
Pie, Snack	Packaged	Little Debbie
Pie, Snack	Packaged	Little Debbie
Pie, Snack	Packaged	Tasty Klair
Pie, Snack	Packaged	Tastykake
Pie, Snack	Packaged	Tastykake
Pie, Snack	Packaged	Tastykake
Pie, Snack	Packaged	Tastykake
Pie, Snack	Packaged	Tastykake
Pie, Snack	Packaged	Tastykake
Pie, Snack	Packaged	Tastykake
Pie, Snack	Packaged	Tastykake
Pie, Snack	Packaged	Tastykake
Pie, Snack	Packaged	Tastykake
Pie, Snack	Packaged	Tastykake
Pie, Snack	Packaged	Tastykake
Pie, Snack	Packaged	Tastykake
Popcorn	Microwave Popped	Betty Crocker Pop Secret
Popcorn	Microwave Popped	Betty Crocker Pop Secret
Popcorn	Microwave Popped	Betty Crocker Pop Secret
Popcorn	Microwave Popped	Betty Crocker Pop Secret
Popcorn	Microwave Popped	Betty Crocker Pop Secret by Request
Popcorn	Microwave Popped	Betty Crocker Pop Secret by Request
Popcorn	Microwave Popped	Betty Crocker Pop Secret, Pop Quiz
Popcorn	Microwave Popped	Jolly Time
Popcorn	Microwave Popped	Jolly Time
Popcorn	Microwave Popped	Jolly Time
Popcorn	Microwave Popped	Jolly Time Natural
Popcorn	Microwave Popped	Orville Redenbacher's
Popcorn	Microwave Popped	Orville Redenbacher's
Popcorn	Microwave Popped	Orville Redenbacher's
Popcorn	Microwave Popped	Pillsbury
Popcorn	Microwave Popped	Pillsbury Original
Popcorn	Microwave Popped	Pillsbury Original
Popcorn	Microwave Popped	Pillsbury Salt Free
Popcorn	Microwave Popped	Planters
Popcorn	Microwave Popped	Planters Natural
Popcorn	Microwave Popped	Pop Rites Natural
Popcorn	Microwave Popped	Pop Weavers
Popcorn	Microwave Popped	Pop Weavers Natural
Popcorn	Microwave Popped	Pops Rite
Popcorn	Microwave Popped	Weight Watchers
Popcorn	Popped	Generic
Popcorn	Popped	Generic
Popcorn	Popped	Bachman
Popcorn	Popped	Bachman
Popcorn	Popped	Bachman
Popcorn	Popped	Bachman Lite
Popcorn	Popped	Bearitos Organic
Popcorn	Popped	Bearitos Organic
Popcorn	Popped	Bearitos Organic Lite

Major Description	Minor Description	Serving Size	Calories	Grade
Marshmallow	Banana or Chocolate	1 piece	170	C
Marshmallow	Chocolate	1 piece	370	C
Oatmeal Cream		1 piece	160	C
Pecan		1 piece	170	A
Raisin Cream		1 piece	140	C
		1 piece	402	D
Apple		1 piece	296	C
Apple, French		1 piece	353	B
Banana Cream		1 piece	382	C
Blueberry		1 piece	308	B–
Cherry		1 piece	298	B
Chocolate Pudding		1 piece	443	C
Coconut Cream		1 piece	377	D
Lemon		1 piece	319	C
Lemon Lime		1 piece	310	B
Peach		1 piece	310	B
Pineapple Cheese		1 piece	343	C
Pumpkin		1 piece	324	C–
Strawberry		1 piece	342	C
Butter Flavor		3 cups	100	D–+
Butter Flavor, Light		3 cups	70	C–+
Cheese Flavor		3 cups	170	D–
Natural		3 cups	70	C–+
Butter Flavor		3 cups	60	A–
Natural		3 cups	60	A–
Butter Flavor or Natural		3 cups	90	D–+
Cheddar Cheese Flavor		3 cups	155	D
Natural Light		3 cups	70	B
Light Butter Flavor		3 cups	60	B
Natural		3 cups	120	D
Butter Flavor		3 cups	50	C–+
Butter, Light		3 cups	50	C–
Natural, Light		3 cups	60	B–
Butter Flavor		3 cups	210	D–
		3 cups	210	D–
Frozen		3 cups	210	D–
Frozen		3 cups	170	C
Butter Flavor		3 cups	140	D–
		3 cups	140	D–
		3 cups	90	D–
Butter Flavor		3 cups	105	D–+
		3 cups	105	D–+
Butter Flavor		3 cups	90	D–
		1 oz pkg	100	A
Air-Popped		3 cups	90	A
Oil Popped	Vegetable Oil	3 cups	165	D–
		3 cups	160	D–
Cheese & Cheese Flavor		3 cups	180	D–
Cheese & Cheese Flavor	Cheddar, White	3 cups	140	D–
		3 cups	100	B+
		3 cups	140	D+
Cheese & Cheese Flavor		3 cups	137	D
		3 cups	132	D+

"+" indicates the food meets minimum fiber requirements; "–" indicates the food has a high sodium content.

Food	Processing Category	Brand
Popcorn	Popped	Bearitos Organic Salt
Popcorn	Popped	Bonnie Lee
Popcorn	Popped	Jolly Time
Popcorn	Popped	Keebler Deluxe
Popcorn	Popped	Keebler Pop Deluxe
Popcorn	Popped	Laura Scudder's
Popcorn	Popped	Laura Scudder's
Popcorn	Popped	Orville Redenbacher's
Popcorn	Popped	Orville Redenbacher's
Popcorn	Popped	Orville Redenbacher's
Popcorn	Popped	Orville Redenbacher's
Popcorn	Popped	Orville Redenbacher's
Popcorn	Popped	Orville Redenbacher's
Popcorn	Popped	Pops Rite
Popcorn	Popped	Pops Rite
Popcorn	Popped	Pops Rite
Popcorn	Popped	Pops Rite
Popcorn	Popped	Smartfood
Popcorn	Popped	Tone's
Popcorn	Popped	Weight Watchers
Popcorn	Popped	Weight Watchers
Popcorn	Popped	Wise
Popcorn	Popped	Wise
Popcorn	Popped	Wise
Popcorn	Popped	Wise Tender Eating
Potato Chips & Crisps	All Forms	Generic
Potato Chips & Crisps	All Forms	Generic
Potato Chips & Crisps	All Forms	Generic
Potato Chips & Crisps	All Forms	American Grains Popsters
Potato Chips & Crisps	All Forms	American Grains Popsters
Potato Chips & Crisps	All Forms	American Grains Popsters
Potato Chips & Crisps	All Forms	Bachman
Potato Chips & Crisps	All Forms	Bachman Kettle Cooked
Potato Chips & Crisps	All Forms	Bachman Kettle Cooked
Potato Chips & Crisps	All Forms	Bachman Ridge/Ruffled
Potato Chips & Crisps	All Forms	Bachman Unsalted
Potato Chips & Crisps	All Forms	Barrel O Fun
Potato Chips & Crisps	All Forms	Cape Cod
Potato Chips & Crisps	All Forms	Cape Cod No Salt Added
Potato Chips & Crisps	All Forms	Cape Cod No Salt Added
Potato Chips & Crisps	All Forms	Cape Cod Waves
Potato Chips & Crisps	All Forms	Cottage Fries No Salt Added
Potato Chips & Crisps	All Forms	Eagle
Potato Chips & Crisps	All Forms	Eagle
Potato Chips & Crisps	All Forms	Eagle
Potato Chips & Crisps	All Forms	Eagle
Potato Chips & Crisps	All Forms	Eagle
Potato Chips & Crisps	All Forms	Eagle
Potato Chips & Crisps	All Forms	Eagle
Potato Chips & Crisps	All Forms	Eagle
Potato Chips & Crisps	All Forms	Eagle Extra Crunchy

Major Description	Minor Description	Serving Size	Calories	Grade
		3 cups	108	A
Popped without Oil & Salt		3 cups	82	A
White Prepared without Salt		3 cups	56	A+
Cheese & Cheese Flavor	Cheddar, White	3 cups	140	D–
Honey Caramel		3 cups	120	B–
		3 cups	160	D–
Cheese & Cheese Flavor	Cheddar White	3 cups	140	D–
		3 cups	50	B–+
Butter Flavor		3 cups	80	D–+
Butter Flavor		3 cups	80	D+
Cheese & Cheese Flavor	Cheddar	3 cups	160	D–+
Hot Air		3 cups	40	A+
Original		3 cups	80	D+
Air Popped	White, Prepared without Salt	3 cups	100	B
Oil Popped	White, Prepared without Salt	3 cups	220	D
Yellow, Prepared without Salt	Air Popped	3 cups	100	B
Yellow, Prepared without Salt	Oil Popped	3 cups	220	D
Cheese & Cheese Flavor	Cheddar, White	3 cups	160	D–
		3 cups	90	A+
		.66 oz pkg	80	D
Cheese & Cheese Flavor	Cheddar, White	.66 oz bag	100	D
Butter Flavor		3 cups	150	D–
Butter Flavor	Reduced Calorie	3 cups	130	C–
Cheese & Cheese Flavor	Cheddar, White	3 cups	240	D–
Baby Corn		3 cups	210	D–
		1 oz	148	D
No Salt Added		1 oz	148	D
Reformulated from Dried Potatoes		1 oz	164	D–
		1 oz	100	A–
Herb & Garlic		1 oz	100	A–
Salt & Vinegar		1 oz	100	A–
All Flavors		1 oz	160	D–
		1 oz	140	D
Saratoga Style		1 oz	140	D
		1 oz	160	D–
		1 oz	160	D
		1 oz	150	D
Dill & Sour Cream		1 oz	150	D
		1 oz	150	D
Dill & Sour Cream		1 oz	150	D
		1 oz	150	D
		1 oz	160	D
	Thins	1 oz	160	D
Cheddar & Sour Cream	Ripples	1 oz	160	D–
Idaho Russet	Dark & Crunchy	1 oz	140	D
Mesquite Barbeque	Ripples	1 oz	160	D
Mesquite Barbeque	Thins	1 oz	160	D
Natural	Ripples	1 oz	160	D
No Salt Added	Thins	1 oz	160	D
Sour Cream & Onion	Thins	1 oz	160	D
Barbecue		1 oz	150	D–

"+" indicates the food meets minimum fiber requirements; "–" indicates the food has a high sodium content.

Food	Processing Category	Brand
Potato Chips & Crisps	All Forms	Eagle Extra Crunchy Louisiana
Potato Chips & Crisps	All Forms	Eagle Extra Crunchy/Idaho Russet
Potato Chips & Crisps	All Forms	Eagle Ridged
Potato Chips & Crisps	All Forms	Eagle Ridged/Eagle Thins
Potato Chips & Crisps	All Forms	Eagle Thins
Potato Chips & Crisps	All Forms	Featherweight Low Salt
Potato Chips & Crisps	All Forms	Health Valley Country
Potato Chips & Crisps	All Forms	King Kold
Potato Chips & Crisps	All Forms	King Kold
Potato Chips & Crisps	All Forms	King Kold
Potato Chips & Crisps	All Forms	King Kold
Potato Chips & Crisps	All Forms	King Kold
Potato Chips & Crisps	All Forms	King Kold BBQ
Potato Chips & Crisps	All Forms	King Kold Rip-L
Potato Chips & Crisps	All Forms	Lay's
Potato Chips & Crisps	All Forms	Lay's
Potato Chips & Crisps	All Forms	Lay's
Potato Chips & Crisps	All Forms	Lay's Bar-B-Q
Potato Chips & Crisps	All Forms	Lay's Unsalted
Potato Chips & Crisps	All Forms	Louise's Fat Free
Potato Chips & Crisps	All Forms	Louise's Fat Free
Potato Chips & Crisps	All Forms	Louise's Fat Free
Potato Chips & Crisps	All Forms	Louise's Fat Free Original
Potato Chips & Crisps	All Forms	Louise's Low Fat
Potato Chips & Crisps	All Forms	Munchos
Potato Chips & Crisps	All Forms	Nabisco Mr. Phipps Tater Crisps
Potato Chips & Crisps	All Forms	Nabisco Mr. Phipps Tater Crisps
Potato Chips & Crisps	All Forms	Nabisco Mr. Phipps Tater Crisps
Potato Chips & Crisps	All Forms	O'Boisies
Potato Chips & Crisps	All Forms	O'Boisies
Potato Chips & Crisps	All Forms	Pacific Grain No Fries
Potato Chips & Crisps	All Forms	Pringles
Potato Chips & Crisps	All Forms	Pringles
Potato Chips & Crisps	All Forms	Pringles Cheez-ums
Potato Chips & Crisps	All Forms	Pringles Idaho Rippled
Potato Chips & Crisps	All Forms	Pringles Light
Potato Chips & Crisps	All Forms	Ruffles
Potato Chips & Crisps	All Forms	Ruffles
Potato Chips & Crisps	All Forms	Ruffles
Potato Chips & Crisps	All Forms	Ruffles
Potato Chips & Crisps	All Forms	Ruffles
Potato Chips & Crisps	All Forms	Ruffles
Potato Chips & Crisps	All Forms	Ruffles Light
Potato Chips & Crisps	All Forms	Ruffles Mesquite Grille
Potato Chips & Crisps	All Forms	Snack Appeal
Potato Chips & Crisps	All Forms	Snacktime Krunchers
Potato Chips & Crisps	All Forms	Snacktime Krunchers
Potato Chips & Crisps	All Forms	Snacktime Krunchers
Potato Chips & Crisps	All Forms	Tato Skins
Potato Chips & Crisps	All Forms	Wise
Potato Chips & Crisps	All Forms	Wise
Potato Chips & Crisps	All Forms	Wise
Potato Chips & Crisps	All Forms	Wise New York Deli

Major Description	Minor Description	Serving Size	Calories	Grade
Barbecue		1 oz	150	D
		1 oz	150	D
Sour Cream & Onion Flavor		1 oz	150	D–
		1 oz	150	D–
Barbecue Flavor		1 oz	150	D–
		1 oz	160	D
		1 oz	160	D
		1 oz	150	D
au Gratin		1 oz	150	D–
Dill		1 oz	150	D–
Onion & Garlic		1 oz	150	D–
Sour Cream & Onion		1 oz	150	D–
Barbecue		1 oz	140	D–
		1 oz	150	D
		1 oz	150	D–
Salt & Vinegar		1 oz	150	D–
Sour Cream & Onion		1 oz	160	D–
Barbecue		1 oz	150	D–
		1 oz	150	D
Mesquite Barbeque		1 oz	100	A–
Onion		1 oz	100	A–
Salt & Vinegar		1 oz	100	A–
		1 oz	100	A–
		1 oz	120	B–
		1 oz	150	D–
		1 oz	120	B–
Barbeque		1 oz	120	B–
Sour Cream & Onion		1 oz	120	B–
		1 oz	150	D
Sour Cream & Onion		1 oz	150	D–
		1 oz	100	A
Regular		1 oz	170	D
Sour Cream & Onion		1 oz	170	D
Cheese Flavor		1 oz	170	D
All Flavors		1 oz	170	D
All Flavors		1 oz	150	D
		1 oz	150	D–
Barbecue		1 oz	150	D–
Cajun Spice		1 oz	150	D–
Cheddar & Sour Cream		1 oz	150	D–
Ranch		1 oz	160	D–
Sour Cream & Onion		1 oz	150	D–
		1 oz	130	D–
Mesquite Barbecue		1 oz	160	D–
Crisps	All Flavors	1 oz	110	A–
		1 oz	150	D
Jalapeño Pepper		1 oz	150	D–
Mesquite Barbecue		1 oz	150	D–
All Flavors		1 oz	150	D
Barbecue		1 oz	150	D–
Hot		1 oz	160	D–
Onion & Garlic		1 oz	150	D–
		1 oz	160	D

"+" indicates the food meets minimum fiber requirements; "–" indicates the food has a high sodium content.

Food	Processing Category	Brand
Potato Chips & Crisps	All Forms	Wise Plain or Rippled
Potato Chips & Crisps	All Forms	Wise Ridgies
Potato Chips & Crisps	All Forms	Wise Ridgies
Potato Chips & Crisps	All Forms	Wise Ridgies
Potato Chips & Crisps	All Forms	Wise Ridgies Super Crispy
Potato Chips & Crisps	All Forms	Zapp's Lite
Potato Chips & Crisps	All Forms	Zapp's Lite/Original Kettle
Potato Sticks	Canned	Allen's
Potato Sticks	Canned	Allen's No Salt
Pudding	Frozen	Rich's
Pudding	Frozen	Rich's
Pudding	Frozen	Rich's
Pudding	Mix	D-zerta
Pudding	Mix	D-zerta
Pudding	Mix	D-zerta
Pudding	Mix	Featherweight
Pudding	Mix	Featherweight
Pudding	Mix	Featherweight
Pudding	Mix	Featherweight
Pudding	Mix	Featherweight Instant
Pudding	Mix	Featherweight Instant
Pudding	Mix	Featherweight Instant
Pudding	Mix	French's
Pudding	Mix	Jell-O
Pudding	Mix	Jell-O
Pudding	Mix	Jell-O
Pudding	Mix	Jell-O
Pudding	Mix	Jell-O
Pudding	Mix	Jell-O Americana
Pudding	Mix	Jell-O Americana
Pudding	Mix	Jell-O Americana
Pudding	Mix	Jell-O Cook N Serve Sugar Free
Pudding	Mix	Jell-O Cook N Serve Sugar Free
Pudding	Mix	Jell-O Instant
Pudding	Mix	Jell-O Instant
Pudding	Mix	Jell-O Instant
Pudding	Mix	Jell-O Instant
Pudding	Mix	Jell-O Instant
Pudding	Mix	Jell-O Instant
Pudding	Mix	Jell-O Instant
Pudding	Mix	Jell-O Instant
Pudding	Mix	Jell-O Instant
Pudding	Mix	Jell-O Instant Sugar Free
Pudding	Mix	Jell-O Instant Sugar Free
Pudding	Mix	Jell-O Instant Sugar Free
Pudding	Mix	Jell-O Instant Sugar Free
Pudding	Mix	Jell-O Instant Sugar Free
Pudding	Mix	Jell-O Instant Sugar Free
Pudding	Mix	Jell-O Microwave
Pudding	Mix	Jell-O Microwave
Pudding	Mix	Jell-O Microwave
Pudding	Mix	Jell-O Microwave
Pudding	Mix	Junket

Major Description	Minor Description	Serving Size	Calories	Grade
		1 oz	150	D–
		1 oz	150	D–
Barbecue		1 oz	150	D–
Sour Cream & Onion		1 oz	160	D–
		1 oz	150	D–
Sour Cream & Onion		1 oz	150	D
All Flavors		1 oz	150	D
Shoestring		1 oz	140	D–
Shoestring		1 oz	140	D
Butterscotch		3 oz	130	D
Chocolate		3 oz	140	D
Vanilla		3 oz	130	D
Butterscotch	Skim Milk	$1/2$ cup	70	A
Chocolate	Skim Milk	$1/2$ cup	60	A
Vanilla	Skim Milk	$1/2$ cup	70	A
Butterscotch		$1/2$ cup	12	A
Chocolate		$1/2$ cup	12	A–
Custard	Lemon or Vanilla	$1/2$ cup	40	A
Vanilla		$1/2$ cup	12	A
Butterscotch		$1/2$ cup	100	A–
Chocolate		$1/2$ cup	110	A–
Vanilla		$1/2$ cup	100	A–
Lemon		$1/2$ cup	110	A
Butterscotch		$1/2$ cup	170	B
Chocolate	All Varieties	$1/2$ cup	160	B
Flan		$1/2$ cup	150	B
French Vanilla		$1/2$ cup	170	B
Vanilla		$1/2$ cup	160	B–
Custard	Egg, Golden	$1/2$ cup	160	B–
Rice		$1/2$ cup	170	B
Tapioca, Vanilla		$1/2$ cup	160	B
Chocolate		$1/2$ cup	90	B–
Vanilla		$1/2$ cup	80	B–
Banana Cream		$1/2$ cup	160	B–
Butter Pecan		$1/2$ cup	170	B–
Butterscotch		$1/2$ cup	160	B–
Chocolate	All Varieties	$1/2$ cup	180	B–
Coconut Cream		$1/2$ cup	180	B–
French Vanilla		$1/2$ cup	160	B–
Lemon		$1/2$ cup	170	B–
Pistachio		$1/2$ cup	170	B–
Vanilla		$1/2$ cup	170	B–
Banana	2% Low Fat Milk	$1/2$ cup	80	B–
Butterscotch	2% Low Fat Milk	$1/2$ cup	90	B–
Chocolate	2% Low Fat Milk	$1/2$ cup	90	B–
Chocolate	Fudge	$1/2$ cup	100	B–
Pistachio		$1/2$ cup	90	B
Vanilla		$1/2$ cup	90	B–
Banana Cream		$1/2$ cup	150	B–
Butterscotch		$1/2$ cup	170	B
Chocolate		$1/2$ cup	170	B
Vanilla		$1/2$ cup	160	B
Rennet Custard All Flavors		$1/2$ cup	120	B

"+" indicates the food meets minimum fiber requirements; "–" indicates the food has a high sodium content.

Food	Processing Category	Brand
Pudding	Mix	Junket
Pudding	Mix	Knorr Maizena
Pudding	Mix	Knorr Maizena
Pudding	Mix	Knorr Maizena
Pudding	Mix	Knorr Maizena
Pudding	Mix	Knorr Maizena
Pudding	Mix	Royal
Pudding	Mix	Royal
Pudding	Mix	Royal
Pudding	Mix	Royal
Pudding	Mix	Royal
Pudding	Mix	Royal
Pudding	Mix	Royal
Pudding	Mix	Royal
Pudding	Mix	Royal
Pudding	Mix	Royal Instant
Pudding	Mix	Royal Instant
Pudding	Mix	Royal Instant
Pudding	Mix	Royal Instant
Pudding	Mix	Royal Instant
Pudding	Mix	Royal Instant
Pudding	Mix	Royal Instant
Pudding	Mix	Royal Instant
Pudding	Mix	Royal Instant
Pudding	Mix	Royal Instant
Pudding	Mix	Royal Instant
Pudding	Mix	Royal Instant Sugar Free
Pudding	Mix	Royal Instant Sugar Free
Pudding	Mix	Royal Instant Sugar Free
Pudding	Mix	Salada Danish Dessert
Pudding	Mix	Salada Danish Dessert
Pudding	Mix	Weight Watchers
Pudding	Ready to Serve	Crowley
Pudding	Ready to Serve	Crowley
Pudding	Ready to Serve	Crowley
Pudding	Ready to Serve	Crowley
Pudding	Ready to Serve	Crowley
Pudding	Ready to Serve	Del Monte Pudding Cup [8]
Pudding	Ready to Serve	Del Monte Pudding Cup
Pudding	Ready to Serve	Del Monte Pudding Cup
Pudding	Ready to Serve	Del Monte Pudding Cup
Pudding	Ready to Serve	Del Monte Pudding Cup
Pudding	Ready to Serve	Del Monte Pudding Cup
Pudding	Ready to Serve	Estee
Pudding	Ready to Serve	Estee
Pudding	Ready to Serve	Featherweight
Pudding	Ready to Serve	Featherweight
Pudding	Ready to Serve	Featherweight
Pudding	Ready to Serve	Hunt's Snack Pack [9]
Pudding	Ready to Serve	Hunt's Snack Pack
Pudding	Ready to Serve	Hunt's Snack Pack
Pudding	Ready to Serve	Hunt's Snack Pack Lite

[8] One container of Del Monte Pudding equals 5 oz.
[9] One container of Hunt's Snack Pack Pudding equals 4 or 4.5 oz.

Major Description	Minor Description	Serving Size	Calories	Grade
Rennet Custard All Flavors	Skim Milk	1/2 cup	90	A
Chocolate		1/2 cup	30	A
Coconut		1/2 cup	30	A–
Flan	Caramel	1/2 cup	60	A
Lemon		1/2 cup	30	A–
Vanilla		1/2 cup	30	A–
Banana Cream		1/2 cup	160	B–
Butterscotch		1/2 cup	160	B–
Chocolate	All Varieties	1/2 cup	180	B
Custard		1/2 cup	150	B
Flan	in Caramel Sauce	1/2 cup	150	B
Key Lime		1/2 cup	160	B
Lemon		1/2 cup	160	B
Tapioca Vanilla		1/2 cup	160	B
Vanilla		1/2 cup	160	B–
Banana Cream		1/2 cup	180	B–
Butter Almond, Toasted		1/2 cup	170	B–
Butterscotch		1/2 cup	180	B–
Chocolate		1/2 cup	190	B–
Chocolate	Chocolate Chip	1/2 cup	190	B–
Chocolate	Dark & Sweet	1/2 cup	190	B–
Chocolate Mint		1/2 cup	190	B–
Coconut, Toasted		1/2 cup	170	B–
Lemon		1/2 cup	180	B–
Pistachio	Nut	1/2 cup	170	B–
Vanilla		1/2 cup	180	B–
Butterscotch	2% Low Fat Milk	1/2 cup	100	B–
Chocolate	2% Low Fat Milk	1/2 cup	110	B–
Vanilla		1/2 cup	100	B–
Raspberry Pie & Pudding		1/2 cup	130	A
Strawberry Pie & Pudding		1/2 cup	130	A
All Flavors	Instant, Skim Milk	1/2 cup	90	A–
Butterscotch		4.5 oz	150	B–
Chocolate		4.5 oz	190	A
Rice		4.5 oz	125	A
Tapioca		4.5 oz	135	A
Vanilla		4.5 oz	140	B
Banana		1 container	180	B–
Butterscotch		1 container	180	B–
Chocolate		1 container	190	B–
Chocolate	Fudge	1 container	190	B–
Tapioca		1 container	180	B–
Vanilla		1 container	180	B–
Chocolate		1/2 cup	70	A
Vanilla		1/2 cup	70	A
Butterscotch		1/2 cup	100	A–
Chocolate		1/2 cup	100	A
Vanilla		1/2 cup	100	B–
Chocolate		1 container	160	B
Tapioca		1 container	160	B–
Vanilla		1 container	170	C
Chocolate		1 container	100	B

"+" indicates the food meets minimum fiber requirements; "–" indicates the food has a high sodium content.

Food	Processing Category	Brand
Pudding	Ready to Serve	Hunt's Snack Pack Lite
Pudding	Ready to Serve	Hunt's Snack Pack Lite
Pudding	Ready to Serve	Jell-O Light Pudding Snacks [10]
Pudding	Ready to Serve	Jell-O Light Pudding Snacks
Pudding	Ready to Serve	Jell-O Light Pudding Snacks
Pudding	Ready to Serve	Jell-O Light Pudding Snacks
Pudding	Ready to Serve	Jell-O Pudding Snacks
Pudding	Ready to Serve	Jell-O Pudding Snacks
Pudding	Ready to Serve	Jell-O Pudding Snacks
Pudding	Ready to Serve	Jell-O Pudding Snacks
Pudding	Ready to Serve	Jell-O Pudding Snacks
Pudding	Ready to Serve	Jell-O Pudding Snacks
Pudding	Ready to Serve	Jell-O Pudding Snacks
Pudding	Ready to Serve	Jell-O Pudding Snacks
Pudding	Ready to Serve	Jell-O Pudding Snacks
Pudding	Ready to Serve	Jell-O Pudding Snacks
Pudding	Ready to Serve	Lucky Leaf
Pudding	Ready to Serve	Lucky Leaf
Pudding	Ready to Serve	Lucky Leaf
Pudding	Ready to Serve	Lucky Leaf
Pudding	Ready to Serve	Lucky Leaf
Pudding	Ready to Serve	Lucky Leaf
Pudding	Ready to Serve	Lucky Leaf
Pudding	Ready to Serve	Swiss Miss
Pudding	Ready to Serve	Swiss Miss
Pudding	Ready to Serve	Swiss Miss
Pudding	Ready to Serve	Swiss Miss Lite
Pudding	Ready to Serve	Swiss Miss Lite
Pudding	Ready to Serve	Swiss Miss Lite
Pudding	Ready to Serve	White House
Pudding	Ready to Serve	White House
Pudding	Ready to Serve	White House
Pudding	Ready to Serve	White House
Pudding	Ready to Serve	White House
Pudding	Ready to Serve	White House
Puff Pastry	Frozen	Pepperidge Farm
Puff Pastry	Frozen	Pepperidge Farm
Sherbert	Frozen	Baskin-Robbins
Sherbert	Frozen	Borden
Sherbert	Frozen	Darigold
Sherbert	Frozen	Sealtest
Sherbert Bar	Frozen	Borden
Sherbert Bar	Frozen	Borden
Sherbert Bar	Frozen	Good Humor Creamsicle
Sherbert Bar	Frozen	Nestlé Flinstones Treat
Sherbert Bar	Frozen	Nestlé Flinstones Treat
Sherbert Bar	Frozen	Nestlé Flinstones Treat
Sherbert Bar	Frozen	Nestlé Flinstones Treat
Sherbert Bar	Frozen	Nestlé Flinstones Treat
Sherbert Bar	Frozen	Nestlé Flinstones Treat
Sorbet	Frozen	Baskin-Robbins

[10] One container of Jell-O Pudding equals 4 oz, except where indicated.

Major Description	Minor Description	Serving Size	Calories	Grade
Tapioca		1 container	100	B
Vanilla		1 container	100	B
Chocolate		1 container	100	B–
Chocolate	Fudge	1 container	100	A–
Chocolate Vanilla	Combo	1 container	100	B–
Vanilla		1 container	100	B–
Butterscotch Chocolate Vanilla Swirl		1 container	180	B
Chocolate		5.5 oz container	230	C
Chocolate	Fudge	1 container	170	C
Chocolate	Milk	1 container	170	C
Chocolate Caramel Swirl		1 container	170	C
Chocolate Fudge Milk Chocolate Swirl		1 container	170	C
Chocolate Vanilla Swirl		5.5 oz container	240	B
Tapioca		1 container	170	B
Vanilla		5.5 oz container	250	C
Vanilla Chocolate Swirl		1 container	180	B
Banana		4 oz	150	B
Butterscotch		4 oz	170	C
Chocolate		4 oz	180	C
Chocolate	Fudge	4 oz	180	C
Rice		4 oz	120	B
Tapioca		4 oz	140	C
Vanilla		4 oz	170	C
Chocolate		4 oz	180	B
Tapioca		4 oz	150	B–
Vanilla		4 oz	160	C–
Chocolate		4 oz	100	A
Tapioca		4 oz	100	B
Vanilla		4 oz	100	B
Butterscotch		3.5 oz	113	B–
Chocolate		3.5 oz	120	B
Lemon		3.5 oz	152	A
Rice		3.5 oz	111	B
Tapioca		3.5 oz	131	C
Vanilla		3.5 oz	111	B
Sheets		1/4 sheet	260	D
Shells, Mini		1 shell	50	D
Rainbow		1 regular scoop	160	A
All Flavors		1/2 cup	110	A
All Flavors		1/2 cup	120	A
All Flavors		1/2 cup	130	A
Orange Swirl		1 bar	110	B
Raspberry Swirl		1 bar	110	B
All Flavors		1 bar	100	B
All Flavors	Push Up	1 bar	90	B
Berry	Push Up	1 bar	90	A
Lime	Push Up	1 bar	90	A
Orange	Original Push Up	1 bar	100	B
Raspberry	Push Up	1 bar	90	A
Strawberry	Original Push Up	1 bar	100	B
Raspberry		1 regular scoop	140	A

"+" indicates the food meets minimum fiber requirements; "–" indicates the food has a high sodium content.

Food	Processing Category	Brand
Sorbet	Frozen	Dole
Sorbet	Frozen	Dole
Sorbet	Frozen	Dole
Sorbet	Frozen	Dole
Sorbet	Frozen	Dole
Sorbet	Frozen	Frusen Glädjé
Sorbet	Frozen	Häagen-Dazs
Sorbet	Frozen	Häagen-Dazs
Sorbet	Frozen	Häagen-Dazs
Sorbet	Frozen	Häagen-Dazs
Sorbet	Frozen	Häagen-Dazs
Sorbet	Frozen	Häagen-Dazs
Sorbet	Frozen	Häagen-Dazs
Sorbet	Frozen	TCBY

Major Description	Minor Description	Serving Size	Calories	Grade
Orange Mandarin		4 oz	110	A
Peach		4 oz	120	A
Pineapple		4 oz	120	A
Raspberry		4 oz	110	A
Strawberry		4 oz	110	A
Raspberry		$^1/_2$ cup	140	A
Blueberry & Vanilla		$^1/_2$ cup	190	C
Key Lime & Vanilla		$^1/_2$ cup	200	C
Lemon		4 oz	140	A
Orange		4 oz	140	A
Orange & Vanilla		$^1/_2$ cup	190	C
Raspberry		4 oz	110	A
Raspberry & Vanilla		$^1/_2$ cup	180	C
All Flavors		$^1/_2$ cup	100	A

"+" indicates the food meets minimum fiber requirements; "−" indicates the food has a high sodium content.

Fast Foods

I've always been curious about the origin of the term "fast foods." Did this originally mean you could get food quickly or very quickly get sick from the food? Regardless, anyone on a diet heavy in typical fast foods is on the fast track to major medical problems. Besides giving one very little value for one's money, these foods have a disproportionately high level of fat, sodium, and calories.

Unless you have just traveled across the desert, finished drinking the water from your car's radiator and—as you are on your last gasp of energy and hydration—look up and see a familiar fast-food franchise symbol beckoning, I can't see a place in *anyone's* diet for many of these foods! They are strictly convenience foods. Yes, there are items on most menus that are acceptable foods, but one has to resist the alluring aromas of the unhealthful fatty choices strongly contending for your attention.

Food	Processing Category	Brand
Arby's	Breakfast Items	
Arby's	Breakfast Items	
Arby's	Breakfast Items	
Arby's	Breakfast Items	
Arby's	Breakfast Items	
Arby's	Breakfast Items	
Arby's	Breakfast Items	
Arby's	Breakfast Items	
Arby's	Breakfast Items	
Arby's	Breakfast Items	
Arby's	Breakfast Items	
Arby's	Breakfast Items	
Arby's	Breakfast Items	
Arby's	Breakfast Items	
Arby's	Breakfast Items	
Arby's	Breakfast Items	
Arby's	Condiments	
Arby's	Condiments	
Arby's	Condiments	
Arby's	Desserts	
Arby's	Desserts	
Arby's	Desserts	
Arby's	Desserts	
Arby's	Desserts	
Arby's	Desserts	
Arby's	Desserts	
Arby's	Desserts	
Arby's	Desserts	
Arby's	Desserts	
Arby's	Desserts	
Arby's	Desserts	
Arby's	Dressings	
Arby's	Dressings	
Arby's	Dressings	
Arby's	Dressings	
Arby's	Dressings	
Arby's	Light Menu	
Arby's	Light Menu	
Arby's	Light Menu	
Arby's	Light Menu	
Arby's	Light Menu	
Arby's	Light Menu	
Arby's	Light Menu	
Arby's	Potatoes	
Arby's	Potatoes	
Arby's	Potatoes	
Arby's	Potatoes	
Arby's	Potatoes	
Arby's	Potatoes	
Arby's	Potatoes	
Arby's	Potatoes	

Major Description	Minor Description	Serving Size	Calories	Grade
Bacon & Egg Croissant		1 item	430	D–
Bacon Biscuit		1 item	318	D–
Bacon Platter		1 item	593	D–
Blueberry Muffin		1 item	240	B
Cinnamon Nut Danish		1 item	360	B
Egg Platter		1 item	460	D–
Ham & Cheese Croissant		1 item	345	D–
Ham Biscuit		1 item	323	D–
Ham Platter		1 item	518	D–
Mushroom & Cheese Croissant		1 item	493	D–
Plain Biscuit		1 item	280	D–
Plain Croissant		1 item	260	D
Sausage & Egg Croissant		1 item	519	D
Sausage Biscuit		1 item	460	D–
Sausage Platter		1 platter	640	D–
Toastix		1 item	420	D
Arby's Sauce		1 oz	30	A–
au Jus		1 oz	2	A–
Horsey Sauce		1 oz	110	D–
Apple Turnover		1 item	303	D
Blueberry Turnover		1 item	320	D
Butterfinger Polar Swirl		1 item	457	C
Cheese Cake		1 item	306	D
Cherry Turnover		1 item	280	D
Chocolate Chip Cookie		1 item	130	B
Chocolate Shake		1 item	451	B
Heath Polar Swirl		1 item	543	C
Jamocha Shake		1 item	368	B
Oreo Polar Swirl		1 item	482	C
Peanut Butter Cup Polar Swirl		1 item	517	D
Snickers Polar Swirl		1 item	511	C
Vanilla Shake		1 item	330	C
Blue Cheese Dressing		2.0 oz	295	D–
Buttermilk Ranch Dressing	Reduced Calorie	2.0 oz	349	A–
Honey French Dressing		2.0 oz	322	D–
Light Italian Dressing		2.0 oz	23	D–
Thousand Island Dressing		2.0 oz	298	D–
Chef Salad		1 item	205	D–
Garden Salad		1 item	117	A
Light Roast Beef Deluxe		1 item	294	B–
Light Roast Chicken Deluxe		1 item	276	A–
Light Roast Turkey Deluxe		1 item	260	B–
Roast Chicken Salad		1 item	204	C–
Side Salad		1 item	25	A
Baked Potato		1 item	463	D
Broccoli & Cheese Baked Potato		1 item	417	C
Cheddar Fries		1 serving	399	D
Curly Fries		1 serving	337	D
Deluxe Baked Potato		1 item	621	D
French Fries	Small	1 serving	246	D
Mushroom & Cheese Baked Potato		1 item	515	D–
Plain Baked Potato		1 item	240	A

"+" indicates the food meets minimum fiber requirements; "–" indicates the food has a high sodium content.

Food	Processing Category	Brand
Arby's	Potatoes	
Arby's	Sandwiches	
Arby's	Sandwiches	
Arby's	Sandwiches	
Arby's	Sandwiches	
Arby's	Sandwiches	
Arby's	Sandwiches	
Arby's	Sandwiches	
Arby's	Sandwiches	
Arby's	Sandwiches	
Arby's	Sandwiches	
Arby's	Sandwiches	
Arby's	Sandwiches	
Arby's	Sandwiches	
Arby's	Sandwiches	
Arby's	Sandwiches	
Arby's	Sandwiches	
Arby's	Sandwiches	
Arby's	Soups	
Arby's	Soups	
Arby's	Soups	
Arby's	Soups	
Arby's	Soups	
Arby's	Soups	
Arby's	Sub Shop	
Arby's	Sub Shop	
Arby's	Sub Shop	
Arby's	Sub Shop	
Boston Market	Baked Goods	
Boston Market	Baked Goods	
Boston Market	Baked Goods	
Boston Market	Baked Goods	
Boston Market	Entrees	
Boston Market	Entrees	
Boston Market	Entrees	
Boston Market	Entrees	
Boston Market	Entrees	
Boston Market	Entrees	
Boston Market	Entrees	
Boston Market	Side Dishes	
Boston Market	Side Dishes	
Boston Market	Side Dishes	
Boston Market	Side Dishes	
Boston Market	Side Dishes	
Boston Market	Side Dishes	
Boston Market	Side Dishes	
Boston Market	Side Dishes	
Boston Market	Side Dishes	

Major Description	Minor Description	Serving Size	Calories	Grade
Potato Cakes		1 serving	204	D–
Chicken	Chicken Breast Fillet	1 sandwich	575	D–
Chicken	Chicken Cordon Bleu	1 sandwich	518	D–
Chicken	Grilled Chicken Barbeque	1 sandwich	386	C–
Chicken	Grilled Chicken Deluxe	1 sandwich	430	D–
Chicken	Roasted Chicken Club	1 sandwich	503	D–
Fish Fillet		1 sandwich	526	D–
Ham & Cheese		1 sandwich	355	C–
Roast Beef	Arby Q	1 sandwich	389	C–
Roast Beef	Bacon & Cheese Deluxe	1 sandwich	512	D–
Roast Beef	Beef & Cheddar Cheese	1 sandwich	508	D–
Roast Beef	French Dip	1 sandwich	368	C–
Roast Beef	French Dip & Swiss Cheese	1 sandwich	429	C–
Roast Beef	Giant Roast Beef	1 sandwich	544	D–
Roast Beef	Junior Roast Beef	1 sandwich	233	D–
Roast Beef	Philly Beef & Swiss Cheese	1 sandwich	467	D–
Roast Beef	Regular Roast Beef	1 sandwich	383	D–
Roast Beef	Super Roast Beef	1 sandwich	552	D–
Clam Chowder, Boston		8 oz	193	D–
Cream of Broccoli		8 oz	166	C–
Lumberjack Mixed Vegetable		8 oz	89	C–
Old Fashioned Chicken Noodle		8 oz	99	B–
Potato with Bacon		8 oz	184	C–
Wisconsin Cheese		8 oz	281	D–
Italian Sub		1 sub	671	D–
Roast Beef Sub		1 sub	623	D–
Tuna Sub		1 sub	663	D–
Turkey Sub		1 sub	486	C–
Brownie		1 piece	452	D
Chocolate Chip Cookie		1 piece	369	C
Corn Bread		1 piece	253	B–
Oatmeal Raisin Cookie		1 piece	341	C
$^{1}/_{2}$ Chicken with Skin		1 item	642	D–
$^{1}/_{4}$ Dark Meat Chicken with Skin		1 item	330	D–
$^{1}/_{4}$ Dark Meat Chicken without Skin		1 item	218	D–
$^{1}/_{4}$ White Meat Chicken with Skin		1 item	332	D–
$^{1}/_{4}$ White Meat Chicken without Skin		1 item	164	B–
Chicken Pot Pie		1 item	703	D–
Chunky Chicken Salad		1 item	460	D–
Barbequed Baked Beans		1 serving	290	B–+
Buttered Corn		1 serving	181	B+
Butternut Squash		1 serving	247	C–+
Coleslaw		1 serving	289	D–
Cranberry Relish		1 serving	371	A
Creamed Spinach		1 serving	298	D–
Cucumber Salad		1 serving	79	D–
Fruit Salad, Seasonal		1 serving	49	A

"+" indicates the food meets minimum fiber requirements; "–" indicates the food has a high sodium content.

Food	Processing Category	Brand
Boston Market	Side Dishes	
Boston Market	Side Dishes	
Boston Market	Side Dishes	
Boston Market	Side Dishes	
Boston Market	Side Dishes	
Boston Market	Side Dishes	
Boston Market	Side Dishes	
Boston Market	Side Dishes	
Boston Market	Side Dishes	
Burger King	Breakfast	
Burger King	Breakfast	
Burger King	Breakfast	
Burger King	Breakfast	
Burger King	Breakfast	
Burger King	Breakfast	
Burger King	Breakfast	
Burger King	Burgers	
Burger King	Burgers	
Burger King	Burgers	
Burger King	Burgers	
Burger King	Burgers	
Burger King	Burgers	
Burger King	Burgers	
Burger King	Burgers	
Burger King	Burgers	
Burger King	Burgers	
Burger King	Burgers	
Burger King	Condiments	
Burger King	Condiments	
Burger King	Condiments	
Burger King	Condiments	
Burger King	Condiments	
Burger King	Condiments	
Burger King	Condiments	
Burger King	Condiments	
Burger King	Condiments	
Burger King	Condiments	
Burger King	Condiments	
Burger King	Condiments	
Burger King	Condiments	
Burger King	Condiments	
Burger King	Shakes	
Burger King	Shakes	
Burger King	Shakes	
Burger King	Shakes	
Burger King	Sandwiches	

Major Description	Minor Description	Serving Size	Calories	Grade
Homestyle Mashed Potatoes & Gravy		1 serving	205	D–
Macaroni & Cheese		1 serving	290	C–
Mediterranean Pasta Salad		1 serving	160	D–+
New Potatoes		1 serving	129	B+
Rice Pilaf		1 serving	188	B–
Steamed Vegetables		1 serving	32	A+
Stuffing		1 serving	282	C–
Tortellini Salad		1 serving	430	D–
Zucchini Marinara		1 serving	80	D–+
Breakfast Buddy with Sausage, Egg & Cheese		1 item	255	D–
Croissanwich with Bacon, Egg & Cheese		1 item	353	D–
Croissanwich with Ham, Egg & Cheese		1 item	351	D–
Croissanwich with Sausage, Egg & Cheese		1 item	600	D–
French Toast Sticks		1 item	500	D
Hash Browns		1 serving	213	D–
Mini Muffins, Blueberry		1 item	292	D
Bacon Double Cheeseburger		1 item	470	D–
Bacon Double Cheeseburger	Deluxe	1 item	570	D–
Cheeseburger		1 item	300	D–
Double Cheeseburger		1 item	450	D–
Double Whopper Sandwich		1 item	860	D
Double Whopper with Cheese		1 item	950	D–
Hamburger		1 item	260	C–
Whopper Jr.		1 item	330	D–
Whopper Jr. with Cheese		1 item	380	D–
Whopper Sandwich		1 item	630	D–
Whopper with Cheese		1 item	720	D–
Bacon Bits		1 serving	16	D
Bacon Bits	Croutons	1 serving	31	B–
Dipping Sauce	AM Express	1 oz serving	84	A
Dipping Sauce	Barbecue	1 oz serving	36	A–
Dipping Sauce	Honey	1 oz serving	91	A
Dipping Sauce	Ranch	1 oz serving	171	D
Dipping Sauce	Sweet & Sour	1 oz serving	45	A
Salad Dressing	Bleu Cheese	1 oz serving	150	D–
Salad Dressing	French	1 oz serving	145	D–
Salad Dressing	Light Italian	1 oz serving	15	D–
Salad Dressing	Ranch	1 oz serving	175	D
Salad Dressing	Thousand Island	1 oz serving	145	D–
Sandwich Condiments/Toppings	Broiler Sauce	.4 oz serving	37	D–
Sandwich Condiments/Toppings	Cocktail Sauce	.75 oz serving	20	A–
Chocolate Shake, Medium		1 shake	320	B
Chocolate Shake, Medium, Syrup Added		1 shake	400	B
Strawberry Shake, Medium, Syrup Added		1 shake	370	A
Vanilla Shake, Medium		1 shake	310	B
Big Fish		1 item	710	D–

"+" indicates the food meets minimum fiber requirements; "–" indicates the food has a high sodium content.

Food	Processing Category	Brand
Burger King	Sandwiches	
Burger King	Sandwiches	
Burger King	Side Orders	
Burger King	Side Orders	
Burger King	Side Orders	
Burger King	Side Orders	
Burger King	Side Orders	
Burger King	Side Orders	
Burger King	Side Orders	
Burger King	Side Orders	
Burger King	Side Orders	
Burger King	Side Orders	
Burger King	Side Orders	
Burger King	Side Orders	
Church's Fried Chicken	Dessert	
Church's Fried Chicken	Entree	
Church's Fried Chicken	Entree	
Church's Fried Chicken	Entree	
Church's Fried Chicken	Entree	
Church's Fried Chicken	Side Dishes	
Church's Fried Chicken	Side Dishes	
Church's Fried Chicken	Side Dishes	
Church's Fried Chicken	Side Dishes	
Church's Fried Chicken	Side Dishes	
Church's Fried Chicken	Side Dishes	
Church's Fried Chicken	Side Dishes	
Domino's Pizza	Deep-Dish	
Domino's Pizza	Deep-Dish	
Domino's Pizza	Deep-Dish	
Domino's Pizza	Deep-Dish	
Domino's Pizza	Deep-Dish	
Domino's Pizza	Deep-Dish	
Domino's Pizza	Hand-tossed	
Domino's Pizza	Hand-tossed	
Domino's Pizza	Hand-tossed	
Domino's Pizza	Hand-tossed	
Domino's Pizza	Hand-tossed	
Domino's Pizza	Hand-tossed	
Domino's Pizza	Thin Crust	
Domino's Pizza	Thin Crust	
Domino's Pizza	Thin Crust	
Domino's Pizza	Thin Crust	
Domino's Pizza	Thin Crust	
Domino's Pizza	Thin Crust	
Dunkin' Donuts	Bagels	
Dunkin' Donuts	Bagels	
Dunkin' Donuts	Bagels	
Dunkin' Donuts	Bagels	
Dunkin' Donuts	Cookies	
Dunkin' Donuts	Cookies	
Dunkin' Donuts	Cookies	
Dunkin' Donuts	Croissants	

Major Description	Minor Description	Serving Size	Calories	Grade
BK Broiler Chicken		1 item	379	D–
Chicken	Regular	1 item	700	D–
Baked Potato		1 item	210	A
Chef Salad		1 item	178	D–
Chicken Tenders		1 serving or 6 pieces	236	D–
Chunky Chicken Salad		1 serving	142	B–
Dinner Roll		1 item	80	B–
Dinner Salad or Side Salad		1 item	20	A
Dutch Apple Pie		1 piece	308	D
French Fries, Salted	Medium	1 serving	372	D
Garden Salad		1 item	95	D–
Onion Rings		1 serving	339	D–
Popcorn		1 oz serving	130	D–
Snickers Ice Cream Bar		1 bar	220	D
Apple Pie		1 piece	280	C
Breast		1 piece	200	D–
Leg		1 piece	140	D
Thigh		1 piece	230	D–
Wing		1 piece	250	D–
Biscuits		1 piece	250	D–
Cajun Rice		1 serving	130	D–
Cole Slaw		1 serving	92	D–
Corn on the Cob		1 serving	190	B
French Fries		1 serving	210	D
Okra		1 serving	210	D–
Potatoes & Gravy		1 serving	90	C–
Cheese	12" Pie	2 slices	560	C–
Extra Cheese & Pepperoni	12" Pie	2 slices	670	D–
Ham	12" Pie	2 slices	577	C–
Italian Sausage & Mushroom	12" Pie	2 slices	618	D–
Pepperoni	12" Pie	2 slices	622	D–
Veggie	12" Pie	2 slices	576	C–
Cheese	12" Pie	2 slices	344	B–
Extra Cheese & Pepperoni	12" Pie	2 slices	455	C–
Ham	12" Pie	2 slices	361	B–
Italian Sausage & Mushroom	12" Pie	2 slices	402	C–
Pepperoni	12" Pie	2 slices	406	C–
Veggie	12" Pie	2 slices	360	A–
Cheese	12" Pie	2 slices	364	C–
Extra Cheese & Pepperoni	12" Pie	2 slices	512	D–
Ham	12" Pie	2 slices	387	C–
Italian Sausage & Mushroom	12" Pie	2 slices	442	D–
Pepperoni	12" Pie	2 slices	447	D–
Veggie	12" Pie	2 slices	385	C–
Cinnamon & Raisin		1 item	250	A–
Egg		1 item	250	A–
Onion		1 item	250	A–
Plain		1 item	250	A–
Chocolate Chunk		1 item	200	D
Chocolate Chunk with Nuts		1 item	210	D
Oatmeal Pecan Raisin		1 item	200	D
Almond		1 item	420	D

"+" indicates the food meets minimum fiber requirements; *"–"* indicates the food has a high sodium content.

Food	Processing Category	Brand
Dunkin' Donuts	Croissants	
Dunkin' Donuts	Croissants	
Dunkin' Donuts	Donuts	
Dunkin' Donuts	Donuts	
Dunkin' Donuts	Donuts	
Dunkin' Donuts	Donuts	
Dunkin' Donuts	Donuts	
Dunkin' Donuts	Donuts	
Dunkin' Donuts	Donuts	
Dunkin' Donuts	Donuts	
Dunkin' Donuts	Muffins	
Dunkin' Donuts	Muffins	
Dunkin' Donuts	Muffins	
Dunkin' Donuts	Muffins	
Dunkin' Donuts	Muffins	
Dunkin' Donuts	Muffins	
Dunkin' Donuts	Rings	
Dunkin' Donuts	Rings	
Dunkin' Donuts	Rings	
Dunkin' Donuts	Rings	
Dunkin' Donuts	Rings	
Dunkin' Donuts	Rings	
Dunkin' Donuts	Rolls	
Hardee's	Breakfast	
Hardee's	Breakfast	
Hardee's	Breakfast	
Hardee's	Breakfast	
Hardee's	Breakfast	
Hardee's	Breakfast	
Hardee's	Breakfast	
Hardee's	Breakfast	
Hardee's	Breakfast	
Hardee's	Breakfast	
Hardee's	Breakfast	
Hardee's	Breakfast	
Hardee's	Breakfast	
Hardee's	Breakfast	
Hardee's	Breakfast	
Hardee's	Breakfast	
Hardee's	Breakfast	
Hardee's	Breakfast	
Hardee's	Breakfast	
Hardee's	Breakfast	
Hardee's	Fried Chicken Side Orders	
Hardee's	Fried Chicken Side Orders	
Hardee's	Fried Chicken Side Orders	
Hardee's	Fried Chicken Side Orders	
Hardee's	Fried Chicken Side Orders	
Hardee's	Fried Chicken Side Orders	
Hardee's	Salads/Fries	
Hardee's	Salads/Fries	

Major Description	Minor Description	Serving Size	Calories	Grade
Chocolate		1 item	440	D
Plain		1 item	310	D
Apple Cinnamon		1 item	190	D
Bavarian Filled with Chocolate Frosting		1 item	240	D
Blueberry		1 item	210	C
Boston Cream		1 item	240	D
Honey-dipped Yeast		1 item	200	D
Jelly Filled		1 item	220	C–
Lemon Filled		1 item	260	D
Plain Cake		1 item	262	D–
Apple & Spice		1 item	300	B
Banana Nut		1 item	310	B
Blueberry		1 item	280	B
Bran & Raisin		1 item	310	B–
Corn		1 item	340	C–
Cranberry Nut		1 item	290	B
Chocolate-Frosted Yeast		1 item	200	D
Glazed Buttermilk		1 item	290	D–
Glazed Chocolate		1 item	324	D
Glazed Whole Wheat		1 item	330	D
Glazed Yeast		1 item	200	D
Powdered Cake		1 item	270	D–
Glazed Coffee		1 item	280	C
3 Pancakes		1 serving	280	A–
3 Pancakes with 1 Sausage Patty		1 serving	430	C–
3 Pancakes with 2 Bacon Strips		1 serving	350	B–
Bacon & Egg Biscuit		1 item	490	D–
Bacon, Egg & Cheese Biscuit		1 item	530	D–
Big Country Breakfast Bacon		1 item	740	D–
Big Country Breakfast Sausage		1 item	930	D–
Biscuit & Gravy		1 item	510	D–
Blueberry Muffin		1 item	400	C
Canadian Rise & Shine Biscuit		1 item	570	D–
Chicken Fillet Biscuit		1 item	510	D–
Cinnamon & Raisin Biscuit		1 item	370	D
Country Ham Biscuit		1 item	430	D–
Frisco Breakfast Sandwich, Ham		1 item	460	D–
Ham Biscuit		1 item	400	D–
Ham, Egg & Cheese Biscuit		1 item	500	D–
Regular Hash Rounds		1 serving	230	D–
Rise & Shine Biscuit		1 item	390	D–
Sausage & Egg Biscuit		1 item	560	D–
Sausage Biscuit		1 item	510	D–
Steak Biscuit		1 item	580	D–
Breast		1 item	370	C–
Gravy		1 serving	20	A–
Leg		1 item	170	C–
Mashed Potatoes		1 serving	70	A–
Thigh		1 item	330	D–
Wing		1 item	200	C–
Chef Salad		1 serving	200	D–
Crispy Curls		1 serving	300	D–

"+" indicates the food meets minimum fiber requirements; "–" indicates the food has a high sodium content.

Food	Processing Category	Brand
Hardee's	Salads/Fries	
Hardee's	Salads/Fries	
Hardee's	Salads/Fries	
Hardee's	Salads/Fries	
Hardee's	Salads/Fries	
Hardee's	Sandwiches	
Hardee's	Sandwiches	
Hardee's	Sandwiches	
Hardee's	Sandwiches	
Hardee's	Sandwiches	
Hardee's	Sandwiches	
Hardee's	Sandwiches	
Hardee's	Sandwiches	
Hardee's	Sandwiches	
Hardee's	Sandwiches	
Hardee's	Sandwiches	
Hardee's	Sandwiches	
Hardee's	Sandwiches	
Hardee's	Sandwiches	
Hardee's	Shakes/Desserts	
Hardee's	Shakes/Desserts	
Hardee's	Shakes/Desserts	
Hardee's	Shakes/Desserts	
Hardee's	Shakes/Desserts	
Hardee's	Shakes/Desserts	
Hardee's	Shakes/Desserts	
Hardee's	Shakes/Desserts	
Hardee's	Shakes/Desserts	
Hardee's	Shakes/Desserts	
Long John Silver's	Long John's Meals	
Long John Silver's	Long John's Meals	
Long John Silver's	Long John's Meals	
Long John Silver's	Long John's Meals	
Long John Silver's	Long John's Meals	
Long John Silver's	Long John's Meals	
Long John Silver's	Long John's Meals	
Long John Silver's	Long John's Meals	
Long John Silver's	Long John's Meals	
Long John Silver's	Long John's Meals	
Long John Silver's	Long John's Meals	
Long John Silver's	Long John's Meals	
Long John Silver's	Long John's Meals	
Long John Silver's	Long John's Meals	
Long John Silver's	Long John's Meals	
Long John Silver's	Long John's Meals	

Major Description	Minor Description	Serving Size	Calories	Grade
French Fries, Large		1 serving	430	C
French Fries, Small		1 serving	240	C
Garden Salad		1 serving	190	D–
Grilled Chicken Salad		1 serving	120	B–
Side Salad		1 item	20	A
Bacon Cheeseburger		1 item	600	D–
Big Deluxe Burger		1 item	530	D–
Big Roast Beef		1 item	370	C–
Cheeseburger		1 item	300	C–
Chicken Fillet		1 item	400	C–
Fisherman's Fillet		1 item	500	C–
Frisco Burger		1 item	760	D–
Frisco Grilled Chicken		1 item	620	D–
Hamburger		1 item	260	C–
Hot Dog		1 item	450	C–
Hot Ham & Cheese		1 item	530	D–
Mushroom & Swiss Burger		1 item	520	D–
Quarterpound Cheeseburger		1 item	490	D–
Regular Roast Beef		1 item	270	C–
Big Cookie		1 item	280	C
Cool Twist Cone, Chocolate		1 serving	180	B
Cool Twist Cone, Chocolate & Vanilla		1 serving	170	B
Cool Twist Cone, Vanilla		1 serving	180	B
Cool Twist Hot Fudge Sundae		1 serving	320	B
Cool Twist Strawberry Sundae		1 serving	260	B
Shake, Chocolate		1 item	390	B
Shake, Peach		1 item	530	B
Shake, Strawberry		1 item	390	B
Shake, Vanilla		1 item	370	B
Baked Chicken	with Rice Pilaf	1 meal	630	B–
Baked Fish with Lemon Crumb	Rice, Green Beans, Coleslaw & Breadstick	1 meal	640	B–
Baked Fish with Paprika Fries	2 Hush Puppies	1 meal	610	B–
Baked Fish with Scampi Sauce	Rice, Green Beans & Coleslaw	1 meal	660	B–
Baked Shrimp Scampi	with Rice Pilaf	1 meal	610	B–
Chicken Planks Dinner	3 Planks Fries	1 meal	860	C–
Chicken Planks Dinner	4 Planks Fries	1 meal	990	C–
Fish & More	2 Fish, Fries	1 meal	860	D–
Fish & More (3 Fish)	Fries	1 meal	1070	D–
Fish (1 Piece) & Chicken (2 Pieces)	Fries	1 meal	930	D–
Fish (2 Pieces)	& Fries with 2 Hush Puppies	1 meal	720	D–
Fish (3 Pieces)	& Fries	1 meal	930	D–
Fish Sandwich, Batter Dipped	with Tartar Sauce, Fries, Salad, Apple Pie	1 meal	965	C–
Homestyle Shrimp Dinner	6 Pieces with Fries	1 meal	740	D
Homestyle Shrimp Dinner	9 Shrimp with Fries	1 meal	880	D
Light Portion Baked Fish with Lemon Crumb Rice		1 meal	320	A–

"+" indicates the food meets minimum fiber requirements; "–" indicates the food has a high sodium content.

Food	Processing Category	Brand
Long John Silver's	Long John's Meals	
Long John Silver's	Long John's Meals	
Long John Silver's	Long John's Meals	
Long John Silver's	Long John's Meals	
Long John Silver's	Long John's Meals	
Long John Silver's	Long John's Meals	
Long John Silver's	Single Items	
Long John Silver's	Single Items	
Long John Silver's	Single Items	
Long John Silver's	Single Items	
Long John Silver's	Single Items	
Long John Silver's	Single Items	
Long John Silver's	Single Items	
Long John Silver's	Single Items	
Long John Silver's	Single Items	
Long John Silver's	Single Items	
Long John Silver's	Single Items	
Long John Silver's	Single Items	
Long John Silver's	Single Items	
Long John Silver's	Single Items	
Long John Silver's	Single Items	
Long John Silver's	Single Items	
Long John Silver's	Single Items	
Long John Silver's	Single Items	
Long John Silver's	Single Items	
Long John Silver's	Single Items	
Long John Silver's	Single Items	
Long John Silver's	Single Items	
Long John Silver's	Single Items	
Long John Silver's	Single Items	
McDonald's	Breakfast	
McDonald's	Breakfast	
McDonald's	Breakfast	
McDonald's	Breakfast	
McDonald's	Breakfast	
McDonald's	Breakfast	
McDonald's	Breakfast	
McDonald's	Breakfast	
McDonald's	Breakfast	
McDonald's	Breakfast	
McDonald's	Breakfast	
McDonald's	Breakfast	
McDonald's	Breakfast	
McDonald's	Breakfast	
McDonald's	Chicken	
McDonald's	Chicken	
McDonald's	Chicken	
McDonald's	Desserts/Shakes	

Major Description	Minor Description	Serving Size	Calories	Grade
Light Portion Baked Fish with Paprika Rice		1 meal	300	A–
Long John's Homestyle Fish	3 Pieces with Fries	1 meal	830	D
Long John's Homestyle Fish	4 Pieces with Fries & 2 Hush Puppies	1 meal	960	D
Ocean Chef Salad with Dressing Gumbo		1 meal	395	D–
Shrimp Dinner, Batter Dipped	6 Shrimp with Fries	1 meal	800	D–
Shrimp, Batter Dipped	9 Shrimp with Fries	1 meal	970	D–
Chicken Plank		1 item	130	D–
Chicken Sandwich, Baked	without Sauce	1 item	320	B–
Chicken Sandwich, Batter Dipped	without Sauce	1 item	440	C–
Chowder, Seafood with Cod		1 serving	140	C–
Clams, Breaded		1 serving	240	D–
Corn Cobbette		1 item	140	D
Dijon Herb Sauce		1 oz serving	90	D–
Fish Sandwich, Batter Dipped	without Sauce	1 item	380	C–
Fish, Battered		1 item	210	D–
Fish, Homestyle		1 item	125	D–
Fries		1 serving	170	C
Pie	Apple	1 slice	320	C–
Pie	Cherry	1 slice	360	C
Pie	Lemon	1 slice	340	B
Rice	Pilaf	1 serving	210	A–
Salad	Ocean, Chef	1 item	150	B–
Salad	Seafood	1 item	230	B–
Salad	Side Order	1 item	25	A
Salad Dressing	Lite Italian	1 oz	12	A–
Salad Dressing	Ranch	1 oz	90	B–
Salad Dressing	Sea Salad	1 oz	90	C–
Seafood Gumbo with Cod		1 serving	120	D–
Seafood Sauce		1 oz	35	A–
Shrimp, Battered		1 piece	60	D–
Shrimp, Homestyle		1 piece	45	D–
Bacon, Egg & Cheese Biscuit		1 item	440	D–
Biscuit		1 item	260	D–
Breakfast Burrito		1 item	290	D–
Egg McMuffin		1 item	280	C–
English Muffin		1 item	170	B–
Hash Browns		1 serving	130	D–
Hotcakes Plain		1 serving	250	A–
Hotcakes with Syrup & Margarine 2 Pats		1 serving	410	B–
Sausage		1 piece	160	D–
Sausage Biscuit		1 item	420	D–
Sausage Biscuit with Egg		1 item	520	D–
Sausage McMuffin		1 item	350	D–
Sausage McMuffin with Egg		1 item	430	D–
Scrambled Eggs (2)		1 serving	140	D–
Chicken McNuggets 4 Piece		1 serving	180	D–
Chicken McNuggets 6 Piece		1 serving	270	D–
Chicken McNuggets 9 Piece		1 serving	400	D–
Baked Apple Pie		1 slice	280	D

"+" indicates the food meets minimum fiber requirements; "–" indicates the food has a high sodium content.

Food	Processing Category	Brand
McDonald's	Desserts/Shakes	
McDonald's	Desserts/Shakes	
McDonald's	Desserts/Shakes	
McDonald's	Desserts/Shakes	
McDonald's	Desserts/Shakes	
McDonald's	Desserts/Shakes	
McDonald's	Desserts/Shakes	
McDonald's	Desserts/Shakes	
McDonald's	Desserts/Shakes	
McDonald's	Desserts/Shakes	
McDonald's	French Fries	
McDonald's	Muffins/Danish	
McDonald's	Muffins/Danish	
McDonald's	Muffins/Danish	
McDonald's	Muffins/Danish	
McDonald's	Muffins/Danish	
McDonald's	Salad Dressings	
McDonald's	Salad Dressings	
McDonald's	Salads	
McDonald's	Salads	
McDonald's	Salads	
McDonald's	Salads	
McDonald's	Salads	
McDonald's	Sandwiches	
McDonald's	Sandwiches	
McDonald's	Sandwiches	
McDonald's	Sandwiches	
McDonald's	Sandwiches	
McDonald's	Sandwiches	
McDonald's	Sandwiches	
McDonald's	Sandwiches	
McDonald's	Sandwiches	
McDonald's	Sandwiches	
McDonald's	Sandwiches	
Pizza Hut	Pizza	
Pizza Hut	Pizza	
Pizza Hut	Pizza	
Pizza Hut	Pizza	
Pizza Hut	Pizza	
Pizza Hut	Pizza	
Pizza Hut	Pizza	
Pizza Hut	Pizza	
Pizza Hut	Pizza	
Pizza Hut	Pizza	
Pizza Hut	Pizza	
Pizza Hut	Pizza	
Pizza Hut	Pizza	
Pizza Hut	Pizza	
Pizza Hut	Pizza	
Pizza Hut	Pizza	
Pizza Hut	Pizza	
Pizza Hut	Pizza	

Major Description	Minor Description	Serving Size	Calories	Grade
Chocolate Shake		1 shake	350	B
Chocolaty Chip Cookies		1 pkg	330	D
Hot Caramel, Lowfat Frozen Yogurt		1 serving	270	A
Hot Fudge, Lowfat Frozen Yogurt		1 serving	240	A
McDonaldland Cookies		1 pkg	290	B
Nuts Sundaes		1 serving	40	D
Strawberry Lowfat	Frozen	1 serving	210	A
Strawberry Shake	Small	1 shake	340	A
Vanilla Shake	Small	1 shake	310	A
Vanilla, Lowfat, Frozen Yogurt Cone		1 item	110	A
Large French Fries		1 serving	400	D
Apple Bran Muffin		1 item	180	A
Apple Danish		1 item	360	C
Cheese Danish		1 item	400	D
Cinnamon Raisin Danish		1 item	430	D
Raspberry Danish		1 item	390	C
Lite Vinaigrette		1 pkg	50	C−
Red French, Reduced Calorie		1 pkg	160	D−
Bacon Bits		1 pkg	15	D−
Chef Salad		1 item	170	D−
Chunky Garden Salad		1 item	150	B−
Garden Salad		1 item	50	C−+
Side Salad		1 item	30	B+
Big Mac		1 item	490	D−
Cheeseburger		1 item	300	C−
Chicken Fajita		1 item	190	C−
Filet-o-Fish		1 item	370	D−
Hamburger		1 item	250	C−
McChicken Sandwich		1 item	490	D−
McGrilled Chicken Sandwich		1 item	260	A−
McLean Deluxe		1 item	320	B−
McLean Deluxe with Cheese		1 item	370	C−
Quarter Pounder		1 item	400	D−
Quarter Pounder with Cheese		1 item	490	D−
Beef	Hand Tossed	1 slice	261	C−
Beef	Pan	1 slice	288	D−
Beef	Thin N Crispy	1 slice	231	D−
Bigfoot	Cheese	1 slice	179	B−
Bigfoot	Pepperoni	1 slice	195	C−
Bigfoot	Pepperoni & Mushroom	1 slice	213	C−
Cheese	Hand Tossed	1 slice	235	B−
Cheese	Pan	1 slice	260	D−
Cheese	Thin N Crispy	1 slice	205	C−
Chunky Combo	Hand Tossed	1 slice	280	C−
Chunky Combo	Pan	1 slice	306	D−
Chunky Combo	Thin N Crispy	1 slice	250	D−
Chunky Meat	Hand Tossed	1 slice	325	D−
Chunky Meat	Pan	1 slice	352	D−
Chunky Meat	Thin N Crispy	1 slice	295	D−
Chunky Veggie	Hand Tossed	1 slice	224	B−
Chunky Veggie	Pan	1 slice	251	C−

"+" indicates the food meets minimum fiber requirements; "−" indicates the food has a high sodium content.

Food	Processing Category	Brand
Pizza Hut	Pizza	
Pizza Hut	Pizza	
Pizza Hut	Pizza	
Pizza Hut	Pizza	
Pizza Hut	Pizza	
Pizza Hut	Pizza	
Pizza Hut	Pizza	
Pizza Hut	Pizza	
Pizza Hut	Pizza	
Pizza Hut	Pizza	
Pizza Hut	Pizza	
Pizza Hut	Pizza	
Pizza Hut	Pizza	
Pizza Hut	Pizza	
Pizza Hut	Pizza	
Pizza Hut	Pizza	
Pizza Hut	Pizza	
Pizza Hut	Pizza	
Pizza Hut	Pizza	
Pizza Hut	Pizza	
Pizza Hut	Pizza	
Pizza Hut	Pizza	
Pizza Hut	Pizza	
Pizza Hut	Pizza	
Pizza Hut	Pizza	
Pizza Hut	Pizza	
Pizza Hut	Pizza	
Subway	Salad	
Subway	Salad	
Subway	Sandwich	
Subway	Sandwich	
Subway	Sandwich	
Subway	Sandwich	
Subway	Sandwich	
Subway	Sandwich	
Subway	Sandwich	
Subway	Sandwich	
Subway	Sandwich	
Subway	Sandwich	
Subway	Sandwich	
Subway	Sandwich	
Subway	Sandwich	
Subway	Sandwich	
Subway	Sandwich	
Taco Bell	Burritos	
Taco Bell	Burritos	
Taco Bell	Burritos	
Taco Bell	Burritos	
Taco Bell	Burritos	
Taco Bell	Specialties	
Taco Bell	Specialties	
Taco Bell	Specialties	
Taco Bell	Specialties	
Taco Bell	Specialties	
Taco Bell	Specialties	

Major Description	Minor Description	Serving Size	Calories	Grade
Chunky Veggie	Thin N Crispy	1 slice	193	C–
Italian Sausage	Hand Tossed	1 slice	267	C–
Italian Sausage	Pan	1 slice	293	D–
Italian Sausage	Thin N Crispy	1 slice	236	D–
Meat Lovers	Hand Tossed	1 slice	314	C–
Meat Lovers	Pan	1 slice	347	D–
Meat Lovers	Thin N Crispy	1 slice	288	D–
Pepperoni	Hand Tossed	1 slice	240	C–
Pepperoni	Pan	1 slice	265	D–
Pepperoni	Thin N Crispy	1 slice	230	D–
Pepperoni Lovers	Thin N Crispy	1 slice	290	D–
Pepperoni Lovers	Hand Tossed	1 slice	306	D–
Pepperoni Lovers	Pan	1 slice	332	D–
Personal Pan Pizza	Pepperoni	1 slice	640	C–
Personal Pan Pizza	Supreme	1 slice	720	D–
Pork	Hand Tossed	1 slice	270	C–
Pork	Pan	1 slice	296	D–
Pork	Thin N Crispy	1 slice	240	D–
Super Supreme	Hand Tossed	1 slice	295	C–
Super Supreme	Pan	1 slice	320	D–
Super Supreme	Thin N Crispy	1 slice	253	D–
Supreme	Hand Tossed	1 slice	289	C–
Supreme	Pan	1 slice	315	D–
Supreme	Thin N Crispy	1 slice	260	D–
Veggie Lovers	Hand Tossed	1 slice	222	B–
Veggie Lovers	Pan	1 slice	249	C–
Veggie Lovers	Thin N Crispy	1 slice	192	C–+
Chef	Small	1 item	189	D–
Garden	Large	1 item	46	A–
Ham	Jumbo	1 item	260	B–
Ham	Junior	1 item	210	B–
Meatball	6"	1 item	429	C–
Roast Beef	Jumbo	1 item	350	B–
Roast Beef	Junior	1 item	250	B–
Seafood & Crab	Jumbo	1 item	470	D–
Seafood & Crab	Junior	1 item	280	D–
Steak	6"	1 item	423	B–
Subway Club	6"	1 item	300	B–
Tuna	6"	1 item	522	D–
Tuna	Junior	1 item	330	D–
Turkey	6"	1 item	275	A–
Turkey	Junior	1 item	220	B–
Bean Burrito		1 item	381	C–
Beef Burrito		1 item	431	C–
Burrito Supreme		1 item	440	C–
Chicken Burrito		1 item	334	C–
Combo Burrito		1 item	407	C–
Beef Meximelt		1 item	266	D–
Chicken Meximelt		1 item	257	D–
Chilito		1 item	383	D–
Cinnamon Twists		1 item	171	D–
Mexican Pizza		1 item	575	D–
Nachos		1 item	346	D

"+" indicates the food meets minimum fiber requirements; "–" indicates the food has a high sodium content.

Food	Processing Category	Brand
Taco Bell	Specialties	
Taco Bell	Specialties	
Taco Bell	Specialties	
Taco Bell	Specialties	
Taco Bell	Specialties	
Taco Bell	Tacos & Tostadas	
Taco Bell	Tacos & Tostadas	
Taco Bell	Tacos & Tostadas	
Taco Bell	Tacos & Tostadas	
Taco Bell	Tacos & Tostadas	
Taco Bell	Tacos & Tostadas	
Wendy's	Baked Potato	
Wendy's	Baked Potato	
Wendy's	Baked Potato	
Wendy's	Baked Potato	
Wendy's	Baked Potato	
Wendy's	Baked Potato	
Wendy's	Chicken	
Wendy's	Chili	
Wendy's	Desserts	
Wendy's	Desserts	
Wendy's	French Fries	
Wendy's	Fresh Salads to Go	
Wendy's	Fresh Salads to Go	
Wendy's	Fresh Salads to Go	
Wendy's	Fresh Salads to Go	
Wendy's	Fresh Salads to Go	
Wendy's	Fresh Salads to Go	
Wendy's	Garden Spot Salad Bar	
Wendy's	Garden Spot Salad Bar	
Wendy's	Garden Spot Salad Bar	
Wendy's	Garden Spot Salad Bar	
Wendy's	Garden Spot Salad Bar	
Wendy's	Salad Dressing	
Wendy's	Salad Dressing	
Wendy's	Salad Dressing	
Wendy's	Salad Dressing	
Wendy's	Salad Dressing	
Wendy's	Salad Dressing	
Wendy's	Salad Dressing	
Wendy's	Salad Dressing	
Wendy's	Salad Dressing	
Wendy's	Salad Dressing	
Wendy's	Salad Dressing	
Wendy's	Sandwich Components	
Wendy's	Sandwich Components	
Wendy's	Sandwich Components	
Wendy's	Sandwich Components	
Wendy's	Sandwich Components	
Wendy's	Sandwich Components	
Wendy's	Sandwich Components	
Wendy's	Sandwiches	
Wendy's	Sandwiches	

Major Description	Minor Description	Serving Size	Calories	Grade
Nachos Bellgrande		1 item	649	D–
Nachos Supreme		1 item	367	D–
Pintos N Cheese		1 item	190	D–
Taco Salad		1 item	905	D
Taco Salad without Shell		1 item	484	D–
Chicken Soft Taco		1 item	213	D–
Soft Taco		1 item	225	D–
Soft Taco Supreme		1 item	272	D–
Taco		1 item	183	D–
Taco Supreme		1 item	230	D
Tostada		1 item	243	D–
Bacon & Cheese		1 item	530	C–
Broccoli & Cheese		1 item	460	B+
Cheese		1 item	560	C
Chili & Cheese		1 item	610	C
Plain		1 item	310	A+
Sour Cream & Chives		1 item	380	A+
Chicken Nuggets	6 Pieces	1 serving	280	D–
Large		1 serving	290	B–+
Chocolate Chip Cookie		1 piece	280	D
Frosty Dairy Dessert		12 oz	340	B
Biggie		1 serving	420	D
Caesar Side Salad	without Dressing	1 item	110	D–+
Deluxe Garden Salad	without Dressing	1 item	110	D–+
Grilled Chicken Salad	without Dressing	1 item	200	C–+
Side Salad	without Dressing	1 item	60	D–+
Soft Breadstick	without Dressing	1 item	130	B–
Taco Salad	without Dressing	1 item	580	D–+
Chicken Salad		2 Tbsp	70	D–
Potato Salad		2 Tbsp	80	D–
Pudding	Chocolate or Vanilla	$^{1}/_{4}$ cup	70	C
Seafood Salad		$^{1}/_{4}$ cup	70	D–
Turkey Ham Diced		2 Tbsp	50	D–
Bleu Cheese		2 Tbsp	180	D
Celery Seed		2 Tbsp	100	D–
French		2 Tbsp	120	D–
French, Fat Free		2 Tbsp	35	A–
French, Sweet Red		2 Tbsp	130	D–
Hidden Valley Ranch		2 Tbsp	90	D–
Hidden Valley Ranch	Reduced Fat	2 Tbsp	60	D–
Italian Caesar		2 Tbsp	150	D–
Italian Golden		2 Tbsp	90	D–
Italian Red	Reduced Fat	2 Tbsp	40	D–
Thousand Island		2 Tbsp	130	D
$^{1}/_{4}$ lb Hamburger Patty		1 item	190	D
American Cheese		1 item	70	D–
American Cheese Jr.		1 item	45	D–
Bacon		1 item	30	D–
Breaded Chicken Fillet		1 item	220	D–
Grilled Chicken Fillet		1 item	100	B–
Jr. Hamburger Patty		1 item	90	D
Big Bacon Classic		1 item	640	D–
Breaded Chicken Sandwich		1 item	450	C–

"+" indicates the food meets minimum fiber requirements; "–" indicates the food has a high sodium content.

Food	Processing Category	Brand
Wendy's	Sandwiches	
Wendy's	Sandwiches	
Wendy's	Sandwiches	
Wendy's	Sandwiches	
Wendy's	Sandwiches	
Wendy's	Sandwiches	
Wendy's	Sandwiches	
Wendy's	Sandwiches	
Wendy's	Sandwiches	
Wendy's	Sandwiches	
Wendy's	Superbar	
Wendy's	Superbar	
Wendy's	Superbar	
Wendy's	Superbar	
Wendy's	Superbar	
Wendy's	Superbar	
Wendy's	Superbar	
Wendy's	Superbar	
Wendy's	Superbar	
Wendy's	Superbar	
Wendy's	Superbar	
Wendy's	Superbar	
Wendy's	Superbar	
Wendy's	Superbar	
Wendy's	Superbar	

Major Description	Minor Description	Serving Size	Calories	Grade
Cheeseburger Kids Meal		1 item	310	C–
Chicken Club Sandwich		1 item	520	D–
Grilled Chicken Sandwich		1 item	290	B–
Hamburger Kids Meal		1 item	270	B–
Jr. Bacon Cheeseburger		1 item	440	D–
Jr. Cheeseburger		1 item	320	C–
Jr. Cheeseburger Deluxe		1 item	390	D–
Jr. Hamburger		1 item	270	B–
Plain Single		1 item	350	C–
Single with Everything		1 item	440	D–
Alfredo Sauce		$^1/_4$ cup	30	D–
Macaroni & Cheese		$^1/_2$ cup	130	D–
Parmesan Cheese, Grated		2 Tbsp	70	D–
Picante Sauce		2 Tbsp	10	A–
Refried Beans		$^1/_4$ cup	80	C–+
Rotini		$^1/_2$ cup	90	B
Sour Topping		2 Tbsp	60	D
Spaghetti Meat Sauce		$^1/_4$ cup	45	B–+
Spaghetti Sauce		$^1/_4$ cup	30	A–
Spanish Rice		$^1/_4$ cup	60	A–+
Taco Chips		8 pieces	120	D+
Taco Meat		2 Tbsp	80	D–
Taco Sauce		2 Tbsp	10	A–
Taco Shells		1 piece	60	D+
Tortilla, Flour		1 piece	110	B–

"+" indicates the food meets minimum fiber requirements; "–" indicates the food has a high sodium content.

Appendix

Food Measurement Conversions

Volume Measurements

1 cup	= 8 fluid ounces	= $^1/_2$ pint	= 16 tablespoons
2 cups	= 1 pint	= 16 fluid ounces	
4 cups	= 1 quart	= 32 fluid ounces	
16 cups	= 1 gallon	= 128 fluid ounces	
1 tablespoon	= 3 teaspoons	= $^1/_2$ fluid ounce	

Weight Measurements

1 ounce	= 28.35 grams	
$^1/_2$ pound	= 8 ounces	= 226.8 grams
1 pound	= 16 ounces	= 453.6 grams
1 gram	= .035 ounce	
100 grams	= 3.57 ounces	

Height–Weight Tables

MEN				
HEIGHT		**WEIGHT** (in pounds)		
FEET	**INCHES**	**SMALL FRAME**	**MEDIUM FRAME**	**LARGE FRAME**
5	2	128–134	131–141	138–150
5	3	130–136	133–143	140–153
5	4	132–138	135–145	142–156
5	5	134–140	137–148	144–160
5	6	136–142	139–151	146–164
5	7	138–145	142–154	149–168
5	8	140–148	145–157	152–172
5	9	142–151	148–160	155–176
5	10	144–154	151–163	158–180
5	11	146–157	154–166	161–184
6	0	149–160	157–170	164–188
6	1	152–164	160–174	168–192
6	2	155–168	164–178	172–197
6	3	158–172	167–182	176–202
6	4	162–176	171–187	181–207

WOMEN				
HEIGHT		**WEIGHT** (in pounds)		
FEET	**INCHES**	**SMALL FRAME**	**MEDIUM FRAME**	**LARGE FRAME**
4	10	102–111	109–121	118–131
4	11	103–113	111–123	120–134
5	0	104–115	113–126	122–137
5	1	106–118	115–129	125–140
5	2	108–121	118–132	128–143
5	3	111–124	121–135	131–147
5	4	114–127	124–138	134–151
5	5	117–130	127–141	137–155
5	6	120–133	130–144	140–159
5	7	123–136	133–147	143–163
5	8	126–139	136–150	146–167
5	9	129–142	139–153	149–170
5	10	132–145	142–156	152–173
5	11	135–148	145–159	155–176
6	0	138–151	148–162	158–179

Data assumes 5 lb clothing for men, 3 lb for women. Age range 25–59.
(Courtesy Metropolitan Life Insurance Co., New York)

Tests

Two tests are now available that might help determine what is the best diet for you:

The *Apo E Isoform Test* tests a gene contributing to cholesterol metabolism.
The *LDL Gradient Gel Electrophoresis (LDL-GGE)* tests the nature of your LDL ("bad" cholesterol) particles.

For more information about these tests, how they can help you, and where you can get them, you should contact your personal physician, the laboratory used by your healthcare provider, or you can contact the author at P.O. Box 220, Saratoga, NY 12866-0220.

Index

The Problem of Changing Formulas and Changing Ratings

This book attempts to convey accurate information about food products. Because of the dynamic nature of the food industry, however, any compendium of product-specific nutritional advice represents a snapshot of the rich landscape of food available at the time of data acquisition for *The Food Report Card*. This doesn't present a problem for generic and natural foods; the makeup of a carrot or a slice of beef will always remain largely the same. It does present a problem for certain brand-name foods, however.

As I noted at the beginning of the book, old foods are constantly being reformulated or discontinued while new foods are forever being introduced. Because of this, you will no doubt encounter products not appearing in these listings. You will also be confronted with the problem of seeing an old food with a label stating something like "improved formula" or "reduced fat" and wondering if this has affected the food's rating. Many times a food is reformulated with no indication of the change on the product label. The tip-off in these cases is the calorie value of a serving size will not coincide with what is listed in this book (be careful to compare identical serving sizes). In all of these cases, you should be able to very quickly determine your own ratings for such a food. This allows the principles guiding this book to be carried forth and used indefinitely into the future.

For this purpose, I'll show you a quick and painless way you can derive your own ratings straight off the standard food label.

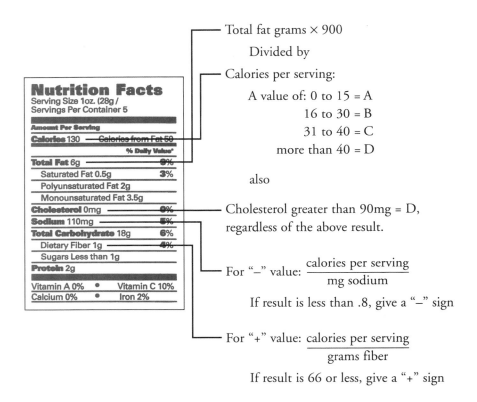

Nutrition Facts

Serving Size 1oz. (28g /
Servings Per Container 5

Amount Per Serving

Calories 130 — Calories from Fat 50

% Daily Value*

Total Fat 6g — 9%

Saturated Fat 0.5g — 3%

Polyunsaturated Fat 2g

Monounsaturated Fat 3.5g

Cholesterol 0mg — 0%

Sodium 110mg — 5%

Total Carbohydrate 18g — 6%

Dietary Fiber 1g — 4%

Sugars Less than 1g

Protein 2g

Vitamin A 0%   •   Vitamin C 10%

Calcium 0%   •   Iron 2%

Total fat grams × 900

Divided by

Calories per serving:

A value of: 0 to 15 = A

16 to 30 = B

31 to 40 = C

more than 40 = D

also

Cholesterol greater than 90mg = D, regardless of the above result.

For "–" value: $\dfrac{\text{calories per serving}}{\text{mg sodium}}$

If result is less than .8, give a "–" sign

For "+" value: $\dfrac{\text{calories per serving}}{\text{grams fiber}}$

If result is 66 or less, give a "+" sign

NOTE: *The calorie value used in the A-B-C-D rating calculation is often rounded by the manufacturer to the nearest 0 or 5, so if a discrepancy between the rating in the book and the one you obtain exists, double check using this more elaborate formula:*

$$\frac{\textit{total fat grams} \times 900}{(\textit{total fat grams} \times 9) + (\textit{protein grams} \times 4) + (\textit{total carbohydrate grams} \times 4)}$$